WORKING WITH THE FAMILY IN PRIMARY CARE

WORKING WITH THE FAMILY IN PRIMARY CARE
A Systems Approach to Health and Illness

Edited by

Janet Christie-Seely, M.D.

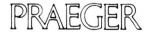

Westport, Connecticut
London

R729.5
.G4
W66
1984

Library of Congress Cataloging-in-Publication Data

Main entry under title:

Working with the family in primary care.

   Bibliography: p.
   Includes index.
   1. Family medicine.   2. Family medicine—
Psychological aspects.   I. Christie-Seely, Janet.
R729.5.G4W66   1984   610   83-17772
ISBN 0-275-91424-0 (alk. paper)

Library of Congress Catalog Card Number: 83-17772

ISBN: 0-275-91424-0

First published in 1984

Praeger Publishers, 88 Post Road West, Westport, CT 06881
An imprint of Greenwood Publishing Group, Inc.

Printed in the United States of America

The paper used in this book complies with the
Permanent Paper Standard issued by the National
Information Standards Organization (Z39.48-1984).

10   9   8

To our families,
who inspired the product
and survived the process

CONTENTS

CONTRIBUTORS

Dorothy Barrier, M.S.W.
Director of Marriage Counselling
Services
CLSC Guy Metro
Montreal, Quebec

Lewis P. Bird, S.T.M., Ph.D.
Eastern Medical Director
Co-Director, Medical and Family
Counselling Services
Christian Medical Society
Medical Center of Havertown
Havertown, Pennsylvania

Maria Bybel, B.S.W., M.S.W.
Social Worker
Family Medicine Unit
Queen Elizabeth Hospital
Montreal, Quebec

Suzanne Charbonneau, M.D.
Fellow, Kellogg Centre for Advanced
Studies in Primary Care
Montreal General Hospital
McGill University
Montreal, Quebec

Janet Christie-Seely, M.D.
Family Physician/Family Therapist
Coordinator, Family Teaching
Kellogg Center for Advanced Studies
in Primary Care
Associate Professor
Department of Family Medicine
McGill University
Montreal, Quebec

Jennifer Craig, R.N.
Fellow, Kellogg Centre for Advanced
Studies in Primary Care
Montreal General Hospital
McGill University
Montreal, Quebec

Roxanna Fernandez, M.D.
Fellow, Kellogg Centre for Advanced
Studies in Primary Care
Montreal General Hospital
McGill University
Montreal, Quebec

Joan Ford, R.N., M.S.W.
Assistant Professor of Nursing
University of Alberta
Edmonton, Alberta

Herta Guttman, M.D.
Psychiatrist
Director, Family Therapy Training
Program
Institute for Community and Family
Psychiatry
Jewish General Hospital
Montreal, Quebec

Monique Jérome-Forget, Ph.D.
Assistant Deputy Minister
Policy Planning and Information
Branch
Health and Welfare Canada
Ottawa, Ontario

Michael R. Liepman, M.D.
Director, Alcohol Dependence
Treatment Program
Veterans Administration Medical
Center
Assistant Professor of Psychiatry
Brown University Medical School
Providence, Rhode Island

Margaret Lock, Ph.D.
Associate Professor
Medical Anthropology
McGill University
Montreal, Quebec

xi

Jacqueline McClaran, M.D.
Assistant Professor
Department of Family Medicine
McGill University
Gerontology Program
Department of Community Health
Montreal General Hospital
Montreal, Quebec

Dawn McDonald, R.N., M.S.W.
Fellow, Kellogg Centre for Advanced
Studies in Primary Care
Montreal General Hospital
McGill University
Montreal, Quebec

Henry C. Mullins, M.D.
Chairman, Department of Family
Medicine
University of Alabama College
of Medicine
Mobile, Alabama

Celia Oseasohn, R.N.
Associate Professor
School of Nursing
McGill University
Montreal, Quebec

Gilles Paradis, M.D.
Fellow, Kellogg Centre for Advanced
Studies in Primary Care
Montreal General Hospital
McGill University
Montreal, Quebec

Yvonne Steinert, Ph.D.
Assistant Professor
Department of Family Medicine
McGill University
Psychologist
Herzl Family Practice Centre
Jewish General Hospital
Montreal, Quebec

Yves Talbot, M.D.
Director, Family Practice Unit
Mount Sinai Hospital
Toronto, Ontario

Renée Turcotte, M.D.
Fellow, Kellogg Centre for Advanced
Studies in Primary Care
Montreal General Hospital
McGill University
Montreal, Quebec

Margaret Warner, M.Sc.A.
Assistant Professor
School of Nursing
McGill University
Montreal, Quebec

Yvonne Whittaker, R.N., M.S.W.
Senior Lecturer
Community Health Nursing
Lincoln Institute of Health Sciences
Melbourne, Australia

Norman J.B. Wiggin, M.D., Ph.D.
Editor
Associate Professor
Department of Medicine
McGill University
Montreal, Quebec

Marie Yaremko-Dolan, M.D.
Family Physician
Assistant Professor
Department of Family Medicine
McGill University
Education Coordinator
Family Medicine Unit
Queen Elizabeth Hospital
Montreal, Quebec

FOREWORD

W.O. Spitzer

In the designation *family medicine,* the word *family* is half the phrase. In other primary care disciplines, there is increasing acknowledgment of the importance of the structure and function of families in determining the health and well-being of each one of its members. But even in teaching centers that exist to develop manpower in family medicine, community nursing, clinical social work, and related primary care disciplines, the concept of family systems in relation to illness is often neglected in the descriptions and characterizations of primary care workers. Curricula frequently ignore the fundamentals of family dynamics that would permit emerging practitioners to prevent deterioration of family function, diagnose dysfunction, and intervene judiciously when warranted in the interest of physical *and* emotional health.

Teaching a family systems orientation is not easy. It is particularly challenging, even to the most dedicated proponents of the family as a determinant of health or disease, because of the dearth of teaching material and the absence of a clear consensus about the content and priority of a family dynamics curriculum within the larger professional syllabus. Another ubiquitous obstacle is the confounding of family health protective strategies with the methods of family therapy as practised by several clinical sub-specialties in the behavioral sciences.

Since 1976 the faculty of the Kellogg Centre for Advanced Studies in Primary Care of McGill University has promoted the notion that scholarly work in family dynamics is an essential activity in the further development of the primary care sciences. Theoretical advances are important; the need for empirical testing of theories and studies of effectiveness of clinical interventions for families requires that research in the field be given a high priority.

We have held the view that the principles and practice of family care must be part of the training of every health worker who encounters distressed families daily. Teaching health workers how to work with families and showing future teachers of family practice how to impart such skills to students and residents have had a high priority at the Kellogg Centre in Montreal. The W.K. Kellogg Foundation has encouraged us, morally and financially, to promote a family-oriented scholarly program in primary care. Several members of our faculty have responded to the challenge with a great deal of energy, enthusiasm, and imagination.

Dr. Janet Christie-Seely, a Fellow of the Kellogg Centre in its inaugural year, has emerged as the leader of a group that over the span of 6 years has given a major impetus to the development and teaching of family dynamics as a basic science for those who work clinically with families. Writing a foreword for such dedicated confreres, from the position of an interested observer of their work, gives me a welcomed opportunity to acknowledge, with gratitude, that they have forged a center of excellence in the field. We, their colleagues at McGill University, are proud of their achievements and delighted to see the appearance of this text. It reflects the concern of Dr. Christie-Seely and her collaborators that innovative theory, sound tactics for clinical practice, and the fruits of recent investigation be diffused from the research center to teachers of clinical care and practitioners in an efficient and pedagogically acceptable way. Professor Medalie of Case Western Reserve University underscores the timeliness and relevance of this text in the introduction that follows. It is my hope that *Working with the Family in Primary Care* will be a useful resource to those who teach and practise family-oriented primary care. I hope, too, that it will not only point out the gaps in our knowledge but also motivate centers throughout the world to undertake the difficult research that is urgently needed by science and society.

Walter O. Spitzer, M.D.
National Health Scientist of Canada
Professor of Family Medicine and of Epidemiology
Director, W.K. Kellogg Centre for Advanced Studies in
Primary Care
McGill University
Montréal

May, 1983

ACKNOWLEDGMENTS

I would like to acknowledge with gratitude the enormous contribution of N.J.B. Wiggin, M.D., Ph.D., Editor of Clinical and Investigative Medicine and Associate Professor in the Department of Medicine at McGill University, in editing large sections of this book. His wit and broad perspective on the whole of medicine kept us on target, and, I hope, clear.

I would also like to thank the Director of the Kellogg Centre for Advanced Studies in Primary Care, Dr. Walter O. Spitzer, for his great personal support and faith in a long project, and for his enthusiastic forward to this book. The Kellogg Foundation itself was responsible for the focus on the Family at the Kellogg Centre and for its funding.

Leaders and teachers in Family Medicine outside Montreal have given much support and encouragement: most notable are Dr. J. Medalie, who wrote the introduction; Dr. H.C. Mullins, who enriched the work with a chapter on the genogram; Dr. G. Smilkstein; Dr. T. Davies; and Dr. M. Glenn and members of the Society of Teachers of Family Medicine Task Force on the Family.

Several Kellogg Fellows have helped in producing this book as well as contributing to its contents. I would like particularly to thank Margaret McGovern, M.S.W. (Sydney, Australia), Marquis Fortin, M.D. (Laval), Mark Yaffee, M.D. (McGill), Wikke Wallop (for unfailing humour and crisis interventions), and the editing group: Judy Mueller, Suzanne Charbonneau, M.D., Roxanna Fernandez, M.D., Gilles Paradis, M.D., and Renée Turcotte, M.D.

Finally, this book owes its total existence to two hard working sisters, Heather Deer and Elna White, whose good humor and fortitude as well as excellent technical and management skills produced the manuscript. Elna White's patience during the final typing was particularly appreciated, as was the support of the rest of the staff.

HIERARCHY OF SYSTEMS

MEANS OF FEEDBACK

SYSTEM LEVEL

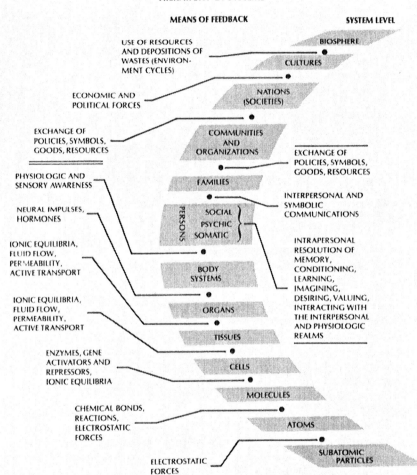

Source: Brody H: The Systems View of Man. *Perspect. Bio. Med.* 17: 71-92, 1975.

PREFACE

Janet Christie-Seely, M.D.

The word *family* has many meanings. Throughout this book a family is defined as a group of people—often but not necessarily related by blood or marriage—with a commitment to live with and care for one another over time. Many types of family structures now exist: blended or stepfamilies, single-parent families, homosexual couples, etc.; the traditional nuclear family is now a small minority. Each family, however, functions as a system, as did the family each one of us comes from and which we carry within us for life.

The natural world consists of hierarchical levels of systems (see facing figure), each governed by similar principles. Each level is a subsystem of a larger system with which it interacts; each contains within it smaller subsystems. The subject of this book is the family level and its relationship with the systems that contain it and are contained within it.

This book is written primarily for family physicians and nurses working in primary care, but is equally appropriate for any professional in the health care team. The family physician or nurse should be able to comprehend complex systems involving more than one individual when the need arises. Other health professionals such as community or social workers, psychologists, or psychiatrists working as members of a primary care team will have more experience in understanding the psychosocial systems; but they must be able to integrate such knowledge with the biomedical aspects of physical and psychological symptoms as inseparable aspects of disease.

Section I provides the conceptual framework for the book, primarily systems theory, on which family assessment and interventions are based. Section II describes the larger systems in which families live and which have an important influence on health and illness. Section III outlines the research linking family and illness. Skeptics about the relevance to the physician of a family orientation should read this section first.

The phrase "Working with the Family," originally coined by Dr. Yves Talbot, denotes working in a collaborative relationship with families over time with a focus on promotion of health and treatment of illness. This contrasts with family therapy, in which there is a contract for change in the family system. The skills required for working with the family are different from those of family therapy and are described in Section IV. Applications of these skills to specific areas of primary care are elaborated in Section V. Finally, the important area of the health professional's own family is the topic of Section VI with a plea for family self-awareness illustrated by genograms.

This book is the product of a multi-disciplinary group, the Kellogg Task Force on the Family, and we hope that the three years of exciting work will stimulate the same excitement in the reader about this topic.

Introduction

Jack H. Medalie, M.D., M.P.H.

The primary care movement took on a new lease of life when general practice became the recognized backbone of National Health Services in the United Kingdom and Canada, and family practice was recognized as a medical specialty in the United States. With this recognition came the development of graduate or residency training programs and the introduction of changes in almost every medical school. Accepting the family as the core of family practice, which has been the norm in some rural settings, has gradually increased in all practice settings over the last decade. Currently most practitioners are receptive to the idea, and increasing the importance of the family in family practice[3] and primary care is both a top priority and a realistic objective.

For decades primary care practitioners, particularly those in cities, dealt with people when they were ill and followed their diseases using the traditional biomedical model. It gradually became evident that the biomedical model was inadequate for chronic illness and disease, as well as for many aspects of acute conditions. The emotional, social, and cultural aspects of the individual, the family, and the community must be taken into account when formulating the appropriate curative as well as preventive measures, and a model even more comprehensive than the biopsychosocial one suggested by Engel is needed.[1] I believe the family epidemiologic model[2] (see Chapter 2), which takes into consideration the interaction between the host (family-individual), environmental variables, and stressors, is suitable for family practice and family-oriented primary care although it implies that the primary care practitioner knows how to assess and manage families. To help carry out these functions, the discipline turned to the various models used by behavioral scientists, including the structural-functional, psychoanalytic, conflict, developmental, symbolic interaction, exchange, holistic, and system approaches. Although many features derived from these different models are used, I agree with the authors of this book in their belief that the systems approach is the most suitable one in helping us understand families and their patients throughout the transitions and crises of the life cycle.

The rapid changes in society are affecting the family structure in major ways and are causing the family to try many new forms in an effort to readjust. During this transitional period, the family, in whatever form, still plays a vital

1

role; consequently, meeting the needs of the changing family becomes an important goal for all primary care practitioners. In developing their theme of "working with families," the authors use the family systems approach and show its relevance whether the primary care practitioner is working with an individual patient and using a family orientation, or with the entire family as the unit of care.

The publication of this book is timely and is helpful to the current developmental stage of family practice and primary care. The authors not only discuss the principles of and evidence for the relation between the family and disease, but also go on to discuss the application of the family systems theory in everyday practice. The discussion of the family in primary care also comes at an opportune time because surveys have shown that in practice residency-trained family physicians spend more time per patient and do more counselling than their nonresidency-trained counterparts.[4] Many professionals feel that family therapy should become an integral part of our practice. The authors face this issue by distinguishing between "working with families," helping families use their own resources to change themselves, and "family therapy," a specialized skill in which the therapist actively changes the family system.

In summary, the publication of this book is an important landmark because it provides necessary guidance in the application of the family systems approach at a critical period in the development of society and of primary care.

REFERENCES

1. Engel GL: The need for a new medical model. *Science* 196:129, 1977.
2. Medalie JH, Kitson GC, Zyanski S: A family epidemiological model. *J Fam Pract* 12:79, 1981.
3. Ransom DC, Vandervoort HE: The development of family medicine: problematic trends. *JAMA* 225:1098, 1973.
4. Rosenblatt RA, Cherkin DCD, Schneeweiss R, et al: The structure and content of family practice. *J Fam Pract* 15:581, 1982.

FAMILY THEORY

Chapter 1

The Family System

Janet Christie-Seely

A little reflection on the nature and function of systems, whether natural or man-made, will make it readily apparent why an understanding of them is highly relevant to good family medicine.

CHARACTERISTICS OF A SYSTEM

Any living cell is a system that is more complex and subtle in its design and workings than the most sophisticated system yet devised by man. Natural and man-made systems share, however, certain basic characteristics that support the validity of their classification as systems, including the following:

1. They are composed of interacting components;
2. The component parts differ from one another;
3. Each of the component parts subserves a specific function that is not fulfilled by any of the other component parts;
4. The component parts interact with one another in an orderly manner;
5. The orderly interaction of the component parts is the result of some form of communication and feedback, whether it be chemical, mechanical, electrical, emotional, or verbal;
6. By virtue of the coordinated interaction of its specialized component parts, a system is able to perform functions or to achieve goals that lie beyond the capability of any of its component parts.

For example, by the interaction of its components the system known as a simple amoeba is able to do the following:

1. maintain a chemically stable environment within its cell wall that is conducive to the functioning of its components despite variations of its external environment, within limits
2. maintain a boundary around itself that permits necessary exchange of food, water, and electrolytes, but prevents the ingress of noxious materials and preserves the cell's integrity

3. take in materials necessary for its continuing functioning and survival
4. eliminate harmful by-products of its internal functioning by excreting these to the environment
5. process "raw" materials taken in to provide energy for the cell's functioning and the synthesis, replacement, and repair of its component parts
6. replicate all its component parts and organize them into another living cell like itself to foster survival of its species

Each and every one of the characteristics and functions listed above is essential. If any one of these is missing or impaired, the healthy functioning and survival of the system as a whole are threatened. Although vastly more complicated, a human family has all of these attributes and more.

Every system (cell, organ system, person, family, community)[5] is more than a collection of parts; it behaves as an organic whole surrounded by boundaries through which defining interactions occur between the system and its environment. Within the system a controller subsystem (the nucleus, the cortex, parents, government) receives information, makes decisions, and then transmits the information that organizes the activities and processes of subsystem units. A closed system is fixed and static with no communication with the environment; an open system is dynamic and fluid, allowing for differentiation (or separateness) and growth of its component parts through adaptive communication with the environment. It is self-regulating, and relationships among the component parts of a system are maintained in equilibrium by feedback mechanisms.

The Endocrine System as Analogy

Another model, the endocrine system (Figure 1-1) can be used to illustrate five concepts of general systems theory.[3] The clinician's knowledge of this system can be transferred to the family system. The concepts are familiar:

1. The whole system must be understood to understand the diseased organ;
2. Homeostasis is essential and is maintained by complex positive and negative feedback mechanisms;
3. Not only the organs themselves must be considered but also the hormones they secrete, because the latter affect endocrine interrelationships and are indices of how the system is functioning and of the effects of therapy;

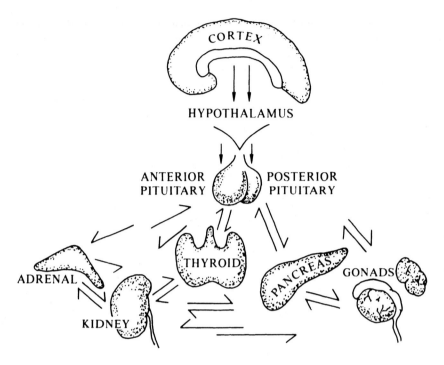

Figure 1-1. The endocrine system characterized by homeostasis and a feedback system of communication through hormones.

4. Changes may occur in areas remote from the primary focus of pathology so that all organs in the system may be affected by a change in one of them;
5. The system is hierarchical and its healthy functioning depends on good communication between its components and effective control through the cortical-hypothalamic-pituitary axis.
6. In a healthy system organs and hormone production change over time to adapt to the needs of the individual life cycle.

A Family Example

These six characteristics of systems are illustrated by an example of an actual family;[6] the analogy with the endocrine system is shown in Figure 1-2. (Any family with problems in which family relationships are known can be used; the visual image facilitates transfer of knowledge from the organic system to the family system.)

The individual family members had a series of physical and psychological problems which in the linear model would have been seen and evaluated separately:

Mr. B. presented to the family physician with a bleeding peptic ulcer and hypertension. His poor compliance with antihypertensive medication was later associated with accelerated hypertension and renal failure. His second wife, the mother of his two youngest sons, Mark and Michael, visited the physician with frequent headaches. Two older sons, Peter and George, in their twenties, had unstable relationships with their girlfriends and intermittently returned home. First Mark and then Michael developed abdominal pains. The one daughter, Ann, had several episodes of delinquency and suicide attempts. Both parents and two sons had thalassemia minor. Two family members had giardiasis.

The family orientation requires that each family member be understood as part of a whole (Concept 1). Further information came from family members once the physician had become a trusted family confidant:

The father's first wife died at the birth of Ann, the third child, and the father clearly had unresolved guilt over her death. That she had hemorrhaged at home after the birth was a family secret, and the father was ostracized by her family, who held him responsible. The father in turn ostracized his son, George, when he eventually married a girlfriend of whom the parents disapproved. The second wife had difficulty relating to the three older children. The family showed a pattern of denial and avoidance of difficult topics, which resulted in physical illness or severed relationships (The father said of George, "He is dead as far as I'm concerned.").

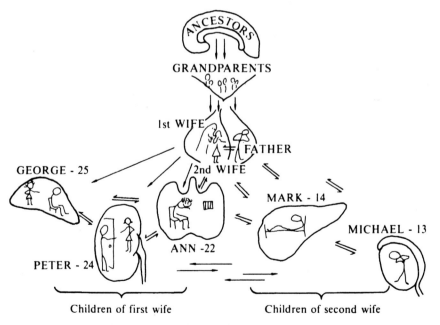

Figure 1-2. A family example illustrating the parallel between a family system and an organ system.

Homeostasis (Concept 2) was disturbed by Ann's developing sexuality and resemblance to her dead mother, which increased her stepmother's insecurity and her father's guilt. The father's renal failure, which was never discussed, and the older boy's leaving home further disturbed the equilibrium. Feedback mechanisms maintained the avoidance of conflict areas. Rather than openly face the father's illness and its implications, the family prompted the sons to come home periodically, ostensibly because of problems with their girlfriends, but in fact to take over the roles of fathering and breadwinning. Ann, the third child, similarly maintained the family pattern of denial by diverting the attention of the family and those providing medical care from the father's illness to herself through delinquent and suicidal behavior. Ann's feelings about her mother's death and her father's illness could not be dealt with directly without altering the family system.

To treat this family it was essential to understand family relationships (Concept 3), which could not be assessed without observing the family members' interaction together, since conflict was denied by individual members. In a family interview the second wife's power became apparent. Normally reticent when seen alone, she was in complete control during the interview. She answered all questions directed to her husband and exacerbated his dependent role by being overprotective. The second wife demonstrated obvious but unspoken jealousy of the dead wife and resentment of her stepdaughter, Ann, in fact, she was unable to tolerate Ann's presence in the same room, although she said she got along very well with her stepdaughter when asked about the relationship.

Diagnosis, treatment, and compliance were all improved by understanding how individual symptoms or illnesses supported the disturbed functioning of the family. The father's initial poor compliance was associated with feelings of guilt about his first wife and with resistance to the increasing power of his second wife. Although one of the younger sons had had guiardiasis a year earlier, their abdominal pains were found to have no organic basis and disappeared when the similarity of these pains to the father's ulcer symptoms was discussed. Diagnosis and appropriate treatment of the daughter's odd behavior, which was first thought to be manic-depressive psychosis or fugue on initial individual evaluation by a psychiatrist, was only possible in the context of the family system. Similarly, helping the older sons in their relationships with their girlfriends entailed helping them and their parents with their difficulty in leaving home. Treatment involved improving communication between the parents and clarifying roles. As can be seen, unresolved conflict over the death of the first wife and the subsequent communication block led to far-reaching effects in every family member (Concept 4).

As in most dysfunctional families the couple's relationship was poor. The husband's hidden anger and abdication of parenting were a reaction to the second wife's control over the family. The older sons attempted to wrest control from the second wife on their father's behalf. Thus, an unclear hierarchy and masked or absent communication result in poor function of this system (Concept 5).

Finally, the orderly progression of the family life cycle in which children grow up and leave was disrupted by the presence of unresolved issues, particularly around the death of the first wife. The family was stuck at an earlier stage of development; compliance with medication and adaptation to illness were poor. Dysfunctional patterns of communication prevented growth and adaptation to the needs of individual members and to life stresses occurring over time (Concept 6).

Premises Associated with a Cybernetic or Systems Orientation

A systems orientation implies interactional or cybernetic thinking about illness and families. Far from negating the medical model, it includes it and expands it. It does not deny the relevance of the individual patient but asserts the importance of systems larger than the individual.[5] Engel has used the term "biopsychosocial model"[6] to emphasize the importance of all systems levels, including the biomedical.

There are three premises or attitudes that tend to distinguish those persons who have learned to think systemically. Two of these premises concern dichotomies familiar to the medical world: health versus pathology, and body versus mind. A third dichotomy, very important to the Western mind, is the individual versus the group. All three tend to be discarded or at least blurred by a systems perspective.

Health versus Pathology

Zola[24] has pointed out that physical symptoms of illness are in fact present in society at all times: only in certain individuals or under certain circumstances are these symptoms labelled as illness, and only a percentage of those individuals with symptoms decide that a visit to the health professional is warranted. It is quite inaccurate to label those who see a physician as sick and those who do not as healthy.[2] To designate states as healthy or unhealthy or as pathological ignores the continuum of well-being and disease. Rather than viewing illness as a discrete "pathological" entity with a specific etiologic agent, the clinician with a systems orientation tends to consider symptoms or illness as an adaptive response to a disruption of equilibrium. Illness or dysfunction becomes part of the equilibrium between organism and environment in which pathogens, physical and chemical noxious agents, and stressors are ubiquitous. As Antonovsky[2] has pointed out, the ability to stay healthy in the face of a very hostile environment is in fact what requires explanation, and the fact that many of us have some symptom or other much of the time is not surprising. Similarly, it is misleading and often unfair to label a family as "pathological." Family dysfunction is a result of multiple crises, poor coping, and poor problem solving.

A useful concept, first elaborated by Selye,[18] is that of illness as an exaggeration of a system's normal adaptive response. Stress disturbs homeostasis and adaptive mechanisms come into play. Symptoms emerge when these mechanisms become overloaded. Kerr[11] has indicated in a description of family systems theory that the symptom that develops is often a complication or exaggeration of the original protective mechanism; the cardiovascular system is used as an analogy to illustrate the dynamic and adaptive aspects of the family system. The initial mechanisms to adjust to a failing heart are the same ones used in daily activities: an increased heart rate and a booster dose of adrenalin. As failure progresses, homeostasis is further disturbed, the failing circulation triggers aldosterone release, fluid retention ensues, and venous return increases and primes the pump. But with increasing fluid the system becomes congested, and ankle edema and orthopnea begin insidiously.

In the past the symptom was directly treated: the ankles were drained of fluid. This procedure might seem logical but actually achieves nothing; in contrast, a diuretic deals directly with the adaptive mechanism that has become the problem. Kerr[11] suggests that alcoholism or schizophrenia should be considered in this frame of reference. Both reactions were originally behavioral defenses to emotional stress, but over time have become exaggerated and fixed:

> To define them [alcoholism and schizophrenia] as pathological states is to fail to recognize the intensity of the problem in the larger system that created the need for these mechanisms in the first place and also the adaptive aspects of the behavior. This is not an argument for calling alcoholism and schizophrenia normal, but to emphasize that they are exaggerations of mechanisms present in all people, designed to adapt to a system problem.

To view illness as part of an interactive field is not to deny genetic, biochemical, immunologic factors that are present. The evidence for a genetic factor in both alcoholism and schizophrenia is clear, but plays only a small role in the illness. Similarly, a fractured hip in an old lady who can no longer cope at home and whose family only visits when she is sick may be only partly due to osteoporosis and poor balance. (Mechanisms of disease and the links between stress, the family system, and illness are discussed at greater length in Section III.)

Mind versus Body

Western philosophy has made a very firm distinction between mind and body (in the past, the soul was a third entity). Dualistic thinking, consolidated by Descartes, is part of our unconscious assumption about the nature of man. In phrases like "control yourself," "pull yourself together," and "get your body in shape," we reflect Freud's thinking that the mind or bodily impulses are precariously controlled by the ego: we believe that the body is the car and we are the driver. If the car goes wrong we send it to the mechanic, the doctor, and hardly consider the possibility that it may be the driver who went wrong. We recognize even less that driver and car are really an inseparable whole. Both modern philosophy and neuroendocrinology have negated this dualism.

Dualism permeates medical thinking—in clinician and patient alike. The patient asks, "You mean it's all in my head, doctor?" Terms such as "functional" versus "organic" and "psychological illness" versus "physical illness" underscore the assumption that brain and body are separate entities. That metabolism and neural hormones vary with some mental illnesses, and that medications alter schizophrenia are seen as evidence for physically or genetically caused illness, rather than as physical reflections of an organism disturbed by its environment. That streptococcal pharyingitis or cancer occurs more frequently with stress (see Section III) is met with incredulity by many persons trained in medical school.

Clearly there is a continuum from functional illness to actual organic change; worry *is* different from an ulcer. But teaching the biopsychosocial model of illness would emphasize the different systems levels that are a part of any disease and would dispense with such a simple philosophical opposition.

Individualism versus the Social System

Western philosophy and psychology have also emphasized individualism and the solidness of the boundary around the individual. In contrast, Eastern thinking and culture place more importance on collective humanity. Alan Watts has described the Buddhist approach: individuals are just loops in the same piece of string—part of the endless knot of nature rather than a lonely island of consciousness, "an ego in a bag of skin."[22] As Watts points out, Western science has become much less dogmatic since the turn of the century; with the cybernetic revolution, Western thinking has grown closer to Eastern philosophy:

> it becomes clearer and clearer that we do not live in a divided world. The harsh divisions of spirit and nature, mind and body, subject and object, controller and controlled are seen more and more to be awkward conventions of language. These are misleading and clumsy terms for describing a world in which all events seem to be mutually interdependent—an immense complexity of subtly balanced relationships which, like an endless knot, has no loose end from which it can be untangled and put in supposed order.[22]

Laszlo[12] emphasizes this radical change in scientific thinking from simple causality to cybernetics in *The Systems View of the World*.

Language with its forced linearity makes a cybernetic model difficult to express and understand. It requires us to look at causality in sequential terms: A leads to B and B leads to C. There is a strong tendency to stress the question, Why?—which assumes unidirectional causation from the past. We neglect asking, How? or What is happening?—questions that focus on patterns of interaction in the present. Moving from linear view to the causal chain, or even multiple causality to the systems view is a quantum leap for the average practitioner (Figure 1-3). Illness B is no longer considered in isolation or thought to be caused by A; A is not the only causal factor, but part of a larger pattern or feedback system.[6]

THE ANATOMY AND PHYSIOLOGY OF THE FAMILY SYSTEM

The family system must be seen as a whole to be understood. Conversely, a single individual, whether sick or well, may be seen as one part of the family or some other social grouping which constitutes the whole. As Whittaker put it, "I don't believe in people any more, only in families—people are just bits

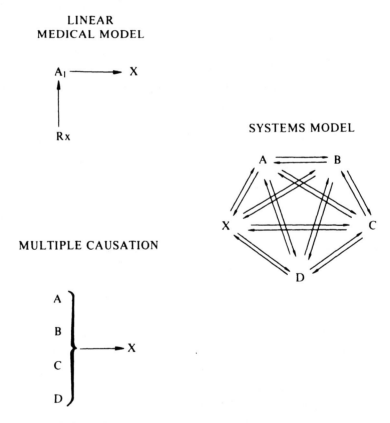

Figure 1-3. Schematic representation of the linear model of thinking (single and multiple causation) compared to the cybernetic system model.

of families."* Minuchin[14] compares the family to a living organism, "a multibodied animal," that is constantly growing and adapting to its environment. Figure 1-4 shows the family "genogram"(more correctly a phenogram) already familiar to doctors and nurses; boundaries define the two families of origin and the family of procreation or nuclear family. (The use of a more extended genogram in family practice is described in Chapter 11.) Within the family there are subsystems, such as the parents and the sibling subsystems, that have their own boundaries. Similarly, the nuclear household represents a subsystem of an extended family, a neighborhood, a village, a city, or a country.

Boundaries can be described as open, closed, or diffuse. Open boundaries around a system or subsystem allow the flow of free communication with minimal distortion. Closed boundaries can be exemplified by the barriers to communication with the environment that exist around a recently immigrated family. To protect its identity such a family may close ranks, refuse to learn the customs or the language of its new environment, and prevent its adolescent members from dating with outsiders. In some cultures, relatively closed boundaries are the norm—little communication takes place between family groups. In contrast, diffuse boundaries may exist around a newly-wed couple or a couple with its first baby: grandparents move too freely in and out of the recently created family system, giving unsolicited or solicited advice, and potentiating in-law conflicts between the couple. Similarly, intergenerational boundaries may be open (when a couple spends appropriate time alone, but has many activities and easy communication with its children), closed (when a couple has *no* communication with the extended family), diffuse, or even nonexistent (when one of the parents is in effect one of the children, or when neither parent is effectively parenting or spending time with the other and the family organization is chaotic).

Homeostasis, in physiologic organ systems is maintained by feedback mechanisms. There is a balance of forces between individuality and togetherness, as well as a balance of roles and status and power. Every family member reacts to a disturbing influence until equilibrium is restored. Negative feedback operates to ensure members respect family rules that are often neither conscious nor explicit. For example, adults as well as children are reproved if they ignore subconscious family beliefs such as conflict is dangerous or leads to divorce; the repression of feeling is masculine; to show love is to give power to the other; or the belief that "Mother is weak and vulnerable and may have a heart attack if you are bad." Negative feedback may be verbal disapproval but is more often nonverbal and outside of the family members' awareness; a statement that contradicts a family myth may not even be heard or may be acknowledged only by a change of subject. Official sanctions

---

*Comment at a workshop by Carl Whittaker in Montreal, 1981.

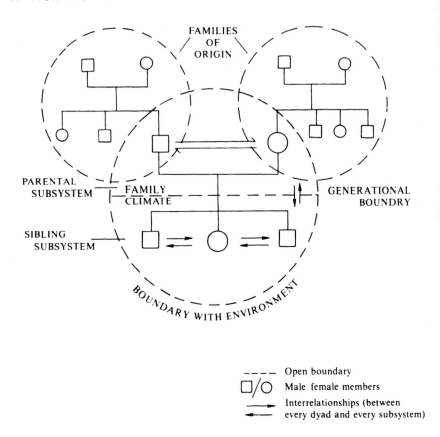

Figure 1–4. Family Tree or Genogram

may be contradicted by more powerful and less conscious sanctions. For example, a policeman father who often beat his delinquent 10-year-old son described the son's behavior with a glint in his eye, thus maintaining the son's role as the family's major problem and avoiding the subject of marital conflict. In this case, the family's belief is that the son is always a bad boy; any examples of good behavior will be ignored and not reinforced.

However, the external environment is constantly changing and family members inevitably change and grow: some disequilibrium and adaptation must occur in the healthy family. A negative feedback system (analagous to a thermostat) maintains the status quo; positive feedback (analagous to a catalyst in a chemical reaction) in contrast amplifies oscillations in a system, encouraging change. Positive feedback from the environment encourages greater flexibility or change in the family rules; positive feedback from within the system at critical times (when children reach adolescence) encourages individual growth and a wider repertoire of family behavior.

There are normal crises with each stage in the family life cycle which if weathered appropriately lead to increased family strength (see Chapters 2 and 3).

A family can be thought of as being composed of *dyads*, or pairs of individuals, each with a particular relationship. The most important dyad is the *couple subsystem*, who set the tone for the whole family. Tension naturally arises in any relationship because of two natural opposing forces: a force toward individuality or autonomy and a force towards togetherness or fusion.[4] The balance between these instinctual forces is never static. As Kerr[11] points out, such forces operate outside of our awareness and should not be considered either positive or negative. They are universal in natural systems. In some individuals one is stronger than the other because of childhood training or experience (for example, early loss of a parent may produce a strong fear of separation). Typically, in many marriages, one person appears to be the pursuer or the dependent, inadequate one (someone who is more afraid of separateness or loss of the other); the other member is the person keeping a greater distance (someone who is more afraid of intimacy or engulfment by the other). Yet if roles are reversed by persuasion or therapy the same degree of intimacy and distance is maintained by the couple; despite surface appearances the optimum level of closeness or distance is the same in both partners. If the dependent member becomes less dependent the independent, cool, detached member will become aware of increased anxiety and his or her own dependence. Many marriages show a pattern of alternating between intimacy, which threatens fusion and triggers a fight, and distance which threatens to separate and triggers reconciliation.

When tension is high, therefore, a fight or reconciliation may result; alternatively one member may submerge his own real feelings, and compromise his functioning for the sake of the relationships, and may become symptomatic (physically or psychologically ill). Another alternative is to bring in a third person to re-establish stability. This third person may be the partner in an affair, with whom husband or wife can play out greater intimacy without the threat of commitment, and almost always with the overt or covert knowledge of the spouse, or it may be an in-law or a child. Such a situation occurs so frequently that it has given rise to an important concept in family systems theory, that of *"triangulation."* Triangulation diffuses tension by making a third person the scapegoat, often a child who adopts a delinquent or sick role when tension arises between the parents. This phenomenon occurs in all human groupings or systems. (It can be seen in a bar where two drunks will insult the barman to avoid a quarrel between themselves.) It may occur in a work system in which tension between the person in charge and a subordinate may make the junior member the company's scapegoat. When tension in a system remains high, a series of fired secretaries or resigned officials may result: one after another person has become the scapegoat in the pattern of triangulation. With greater tension a series of interlocking triangles may form.

(The classic example is the man who comes home after being yelled at by the boss, he shouts at his wife, who shouts at their son, who kicks the dog; each interaction represents triangulation.)

Triangulation occurs in healthy families. The role of scapegoat rotates rather than being permanently assigned to one member of the family. A second form of fixed scapegoating that can be just as destructive is that of the good child. These "white knights" who always had to live up to parental expectations and could never take the role of the bad sibling often have more emotional problems as adults.

No families are without problems. But families vary in problem-solving ability or adaptability. In the systems view no problem is seen as residing in one individual; the entire family system is responsible if there is a problem. Each family member, no matter how bad he or she may seem to the outside world, is doing the best he can with the information and circumstances available. Blaming one member is inappropriate, since the entire family is always involved. Often the problem is that an adaptive response has gone wrong.

Individual characteristics, partly genetic but also to a large extent carried over from behavior in the person's family of origin, play a role in setting up and maintaining problems. But the role of each family member fits with those of the others like the pieces of a jigsaw puzzle. The victim requires a victimizer and vice versa; the alcoholic requires a rescuer; the martyred wife needs the alcoholic or the unfaithful husband; the strong, dependable person or the sane person needs the weak or the insane person to be convinced of his or her strength or sanity.

Mate selection is partly based on unconscious needs and expectations. It has been said that one marries one's childhood's worst nightmare. A woman with an alcoholic father often marries a man who is later revealed to be or becomes an alcoholic. Physically abused wives were often abused as children. That a mate tends to be selected for characteristics, both good and bad, in the parent of the opposite sex, is partly recognized in folklore (as shown in the song "I want a gal just like the gal who married dear old Dad") but often denied by the individuals concerned. Most prefer to see repeat family patterns as "coincidence": for example, one woman whose happy marriage was destroyed in one year by her acutely paranoid behavior after her daughter's second birthday could only later recognize the role of her own father's desertion when she was 3 years old.

We are compelled to repeat history, particularly when we are not aware of it. Repeating childhood experiences at least means we are on familiar territory. There seems to be either a need to repeat early traumatic emotions as an adult or a subconscious optimism that we will solve with a spouse what we were unable to solve with a parent ("You can divorce your wife, but you can't divorce your mother!") Often such emotional patterns involve illness or the sick role. It is sometimes difficult to assess the relative role of genetics and of learned sickness behavior and expectation of developing a family illness. A son who looked after an ailing mother may marry a sickly woman and find himself in the same caretaker role. Huygen, a Dutch family physician, has observed familial patterns of illness.[10] For example, he observed similarity of size of family and life events in a twinned family, two sisters who married two brothers. The fourth child in each of the two families was a daughter and the favorite of the father; these two daughters died at about the same time of different diseases, followed shortly after by the death of both fathers.

The family may also assign differing roles which are then repeated: a second pair of twinned families showed marked differences in their behavior regarding illness; these two sisters had very different roles in the family of origin. The oldest of the two sisters had been responsible for looking after their mother, who was always ill. She became a sickly woman herself, with children who somatized tensions, and stubbornly believed they had all sorts of organic diseases and demanded referral to specialists. Her sister, who had not had the role of caretaker, was much healthier and had a healthy family.

Bowen[4] has described this *multigenerational transmission process.* Marital tension, if it becomes focused on a child rather than expressed as marital conflict, results in that child being emotionally bound up in or fused in the emotional system of the parents. This is true whether the child becomes the scapegoat in a negative relationship or is overinvolved with one parent in a close emotional bond in which the other parent is left out. A physical illness or handicap may be the reason for (or result of) such overinvolvement. Such a child will have greater difficulty developing autonomy as an adolescent and will be an immature dependent adult.

Maturity or *differentiation* is the ability to be a well defined individual in one's own right; it is the ability to separate intellectual from emotional functioning: to be rational and objective in decision making but freely emotional when emotion is indicated. In such an individual the forces for togetherness and individuality are well balanced. As Adler[1] pointed out, true "self interest," as opposed to selfishness, is not opposed to "social interest," or the interests of the group, but complementary to it. A differentiated person can maintain a stand despite pressure from the group to change, but does not, on the other hand, try to dogmatically convince others and is tolerant of opposing views.

The indifferentiated person may borrow parental or societal opinions as his or her own and change them as the group dictates, or may rebel against family beliefs or rules. Whether compliance or rebellion, the behavior is determined by the group, although in the first instance the family of origin may describe that behavior as ideal, in the latter, as unacceptable. Emotional dependency may be denied by an *emotional cut-off*, which reduces the tension level but does nothing for the level of maturity. The same emotional dependency and problems will be reproduced in other relationships. Emotional cut-offs can be accomplished by withdrawing, by avoiding emotionally charged topics, by physical distance, or by totally severing family ties. Extreme cut-offs indicate high tension levels and are associated with the clearest repeating patterns.

Levels of differentiation may differ markedly between siblings. One child may be highly involved in a parental triangle or a parent may project on him bad (or good) parental characteristics. While his autonomy may suffer, other children may be relatively protected from the emotional fusion process. The affected child may remain single as an adult or if he marries will tend to choose someone with the same basic level of differentiation. Many authors[4,11,13,17] have noted that people marry others with the same level of self-esteem or individuation as themselves (self-esteem, basic strength or weakness, individuation or differentiation, and maturity are all closely related concepts). Appearances are often to the contrary. Marriages often appear to have one strong and one weak, or one healthy and one unhealthy member; the usual view is that these are marital mismatches. In fact, the sickness or dependency of the weak member is at the same time his or her strength,[13] while the toughness, apparent conceit, or lack of emotion of the strong one is a cover for felt inadequacies which are expressed by the partner. The strong one feels strong beside the weak partner; the weak (or bad) one protects the other from low self-esteem and borrows from the other's apparent strength to enhance his or her own self-esteem.

Sibling position is another factor determining subsequent relationships. Toman[21] describes ten profiles of different sibling positions and the typical marital result of different combination. Just as oldest children have been shown to predominate in leadership positions and professions, so in marriage do they tend to take leadership roles. The youngest child is more inclined to give responsibility to his or her mate. Two oldest children may produce a highly competitive marriage, while two youngest may have a marriage in which decision making is paralyzed and no one takes the initiative. When these roles are coupled with the still current sex role stereotypes, Toman predicts the happiest marriages occur with oldest sons and youngest daughters, particularly when the husband and wife have had the experience of a younger sister and an older brother, respectively. However, role assignment by parents or triangulation as well as genetic characteristics are major modifying factors.

Differentiation and Stress

Poorly differentiated couples tend to have high levels of stress, less emotional reserve, and more problems. They may be the illness-prone families described by Hinkle[9] (see Section III) who have both psychological and physical illness, early deaths, and high divorce rates. Further stress increases instability. For example, a couple with homeostasis based on one highly functioning, critical, unemotional member, and poorly functioning, dependent, emotional member will respond poorly to stress. He (according to the stereotypes of sexual roles) withdraws further if subjected to stress and she increases her demands for support if subjected to stress; their interaction produces a vicious cycle. In contrast, the differentiated couple is able to withstand external stress because the decreased reactivity of each spouse to the other allows the partner to be a greater support to the stressed spouse. Any family may succumb to repeated stress, as Smilkstein[20] has pointed out, but baseline functioning determines whether a family copes well and treats stress as a challenge or further decompensates.

Education of Families and Prevention

Understanding of family functioning can be conveyed to patients by both a clinician's attitude (for example, not siding with one member, ability to empathize) and by information given over time. Prevention by anticipating problems associated with changes in the life cycle (see Chapter 3) and early treatment of dysfunction is the prerogative of the primary care clinician. It is sometimes useful to give families a description of family function.

These principles of how families operate have been summarized by Peggy Papp.[15] They were written for the benefit of healthy families who wanted to better understand their own functioning.*

How Families Operate

1. Family Systems. The family operates as an emotional unit with no villians, heroes, good people, bad people, healthy or unhealthy members. Family problems result from the way family members relate to one another and not from the behavior of any one person. What each person does affects every other person and a chain reaction is set off. These chain reactions become repetitious and predictable. If one can gain distance, one can study them, observe how they are set off, how they are reinforced, who picks up what cues, and the part each plays in the chain reaction.

2. Labelling. Each family member eventually gets programmed into a specific role in the family and labelled accordingly. Labelling serves a need in the family set-up, and each individual gains some identification from it. Each plays a part in assuming his label and continuing it. Most labels are stultifying, as they prevent growth and have little to do with the true nature of the person. It is possible for families to understand

*Reproduced with permission of Peggy Papp.

their own labelling process and modify it, thus releasing family members to fulfill more of their individual potential.

3. Collaboration. Collaboration is necessary among family members to keep conflicts going. One person cannot carry on an interaction all by himself. By studying how each person is involved in the family merry-go-round, the cycle can be interrupted by any one person changing his behavior. Much frustration can be avoided by concentrating on changing oneself rather than blaming others. The happiest people are those who take major responsibility for their own happiness.

4. Triangles. Triangles tend to form in families because of the close, intense relationships. When one person feels hurt, angry, disappointed, or frustrated with another family member and cannot settle it with him, he tends to bring someone else into the relationship. Parents often use their children to make up for what is lacking between them. Children also involve their parents in triangles by playing one against the other. Sometimes a friend or relative is brought in from the outside to form a triangle. If one person in the triangle changes his position, the whole triangle will shift. It is preferable to have a separate relationship with each person that does not involve any other person and does not form a triangle.

5. Family Ghosts. Family ghosts are passed from one generation to another. Parents tend to assume the same emotional position in their present family as they assumed in their family of origin. They come with prejudices, anxieties, and expectations that are carried over and imposed on the members of their present families. If a parent can understand the way he was programmed into his family of origin and take a step to change it, he will pave the way to do the same thing in his present family.

6. Change. The family system can change by any one person taking a different position and sticking to it.

The Role of the Physician or Nurse

The above principles suggest that the clinician who understands the family as a system will do the following:

1. be nonjudgmental and not side with any one member
2. not compound family labelling by medical labels or diagnoses where these are not necessary
3. not collaborate with a dysfunctional family system to maintain triangulation or blame
4. recognize triangulation and encourage communication of dyads, and avoid becoming involved in triangulation by families or other professionals
5. understand how illness and dysfunction repeat over generations
6. be a therapeutic optimist; emphasize family strengths and ability to change

Whether the clinician likes it or not, what happens in the office with the individual patient will automatically affect the family: an effect on one part of a system necessarily reverberates throughout the whole system.[16] The question, therefore, is not *whether* the clinician will intervene at the family level, but of *how* he or she will intervene. Consequently, it is clearly desirable that the clinician have a sophisticated level of understanding of how families function and know the patient's family well enough to know which interventions will be helpful and which might be damaging. For example, in a family where the grandmother does the cooking and makes all the major medical decisions it might invite family conflict or doctor-shopping to simply tell the daughter-in-law to change her hypertensive husband's diet of spaghetti and pizza. In a patient whose wife's uncle died of juvenile onset diabetes after going blind and having bilateral amputations, a diet to lower his mildly elevated blood sugar may be greeted with skepticism in the office and derision, as well as panic at the diagnosis, by the family at home. Diagnoses like hypertension,[8] arthritis, angina, and even gastroenteritis in a child[19] trigger family overprotectiveness, blaming, labelling, role changes, and suggested treatments. Family relationships or lifestyle may be changed unnecessarily or in a way that is detrimental to the outcome of disease.[23] If the family relationships are understood, the clinician can work with the family in the management and prevention of illness.

Understanding systems theory is basic to both the family-oriented approach and the approach using the family as unit of care. It does not imply family therapy by the physician; such treatment requires further training. The individual will be seen in the office most of the time, but the clinician should be skilled at family assessment and capitalize on opportunities such as home visits to learn more about the family. How to assess and work with the family to promote health is described in Sections IV and V.

REFERENCES

1. Adler A: Superiority and social interest, in Ansbacher HL, Ansbacher RR (eds): Illinois, Northwestern University Press, 1964.

2. Antonovsky A: *Health, Stress and Coping.* San Francisco, Jossey-Bass, 1979.

3. Von Bertalanffy L: *General Systems Theory.* New York, Braziller, 1968.

4. Bowen M: *Family Therapy in Clinical Practice.* New York, Jason Aranson, 1978.

5. Brody H: The systems view of man. *Perspect Biol Med* 71, 1975.

6. Christie-Seely J: Teaching the family system concept in family medicine. *J Fam Pract* 13:391, 1981.

7. Engel GL: The need for a new medical model: A challenge for biomedicine. *Science* 196:129, 1977.

8. Haynes RB, Sackett DL, Taylor DW: Increased absenteeism from work after detection and labelling of hypertensive patients. *N Engl J Med* 299:741, 1978.

9. Hinkle LE Jr, Plummer N: Life stress and industrial absenteeism: The concentration of illness and absenteeism in one segment of a working population. *Ind Med Surg* 21:363, 1952.

10. Huygen FDA: *Family Medicine, The Medical Life History of Families.* The Netherlands, Dekker & Van de Vegt, 1978.

11. Kerr ME: Family systems theory and therapy, in Gurman AS, Kniskern DP (eds): *Handbook of Family Therapy.* New York, Brunner/Mazel, 1981.

12. Laszlo E: *The Systems View of the World.* New York, Braziller, 1972.

13. Madanes C: Marital therapy when a symptom is presented by a spouse. *Int J Fam Ther* 2:120, 1980.

14. Minuchin S, Fishman HC: *Family Therapy Techniques.* Massachusetts, Harvard University Press, 1981.

15. Papp P, Silverstein O, Carter E: Family sculpting in preventive work with well families. *Fam Process* 12:197, 1973.

16. Ransom DC: The rise of family medicine: New roles for behavioral sciences. *Marr Fam Rev* 4(1/2):31, 1981.

17. Satir V: *Conjoint Family Therapy.* California, Science and Behavior Books, Inc., 1967.

18. Selye H: *The Stress of Life.* New York, McGraw-Hill, 1956.

19. Sigal J, Gagnon P: Effects of parents' and paediatricians' worry concerning severe gastroenteritis in early childhood on later disturbances in the child's behaviour. *J Pediatr* 87:809, 1975.

20. Smilkstein G: The cycle of family function: A conceptual model for family medicine. *J Fam Pract* 11:223, 1980.

21. Toman W: *Family Constellation: Its effects on Personality and Social Behaviour,* ed 3. New York, Springer Publishing Co., 1976.

22. Watts A: *Nature, Man and Woman.* New York, Mentor Books, 1958.

23. Watzlawick P, Weakland JH, Fisch R: *Change: Principles of Problem Formulation and Problem Resolution.* New York, Norton, 1974.

24. Zola IK: Culture and symptoms: An analysis of patients' presenting complaints. *Am Soc Rev* 31:615, 1966.

Chapter 2
The "Healthy" Family

Janet Christie-Seely
Joan Ford
Margaret Warner

An open system with flexible boundaries that encourages growth or individuation of its members is considered "healthy"—that is, it is adaptable and can function well in its environment. (If the environment is itself rigid and repressive as in Nazi Germany a closed boundary and a family at odds with the suprasystem may well be considered healthier. One may question whether conformity to modern North American life and standards is healthy.) The term, "healthy," like "pathological," carries certain connotations and should not be used as a fixed label.

In every family a balance is needed between the requirements of closeness and togetherness, and between conformity to family rules and a stable organization and the opposing need for individuality, creativity, and growth. These oppositions reflect the paradox of all systems that a hierarchical order is needed for stability, whereas decentralization, with specialized but flexible individual roles, is needed for growth and adaptability. Either extreme—togetherness (enmeshment) or separateness (disengagement)—can destroy the system. Most families or couples fluctuate between uncomfortable closeness and uncomfortable distance.[2] Fighting and making up occur at the respective limits of tolerance. The more individuated the members of a family are, the less they are threatened by loss of identity through intimacy or by fears of abandonment during separation.

Incidence of Illness

The higher the level of individuation is in a family, the lower the family's level of stress is. Such families also have a greater ability to cope with stress when it does occur. Families that function well have a lower incidence of illness.[6] Dysfunctional families have poorer ability to solve problems, and problems compound one another. Poor communication results from excessive protectiveness of fragile egos, paranoia, and power struggles. This in turn increases stress and decreases mutual support, both of which are factors in the development of illness (see Section III). Illness may become a means of escaping from problems or avoiding conflict; it may also be a metaphor for communicating distress as well as a physiologic response to chronic stress. Pratt[10] showed that healthy or "energized" families had better health care practices and lower rates of illness. The degree of parental conflict and use of punishment and the degree of role rigidity correlated with increased illness, accounting for 30% of the variance.

The task of psychotherapy can be seen as that of converting the closed system characteristics of "sick" individuals and families into more open systems with more open boundaries. The healthy system is preoccupied with increasing its knowledge. This includes knowledge of unknown parts within itself (which may be denied, repressed, or unconscious) as well as unknown or distant parts of the suprasystems.

For all systems a clear hierarchical order and effective communication between subsystems is essential for health or adaptive functioning. For members of the Palo Alto school[5] all behavior is communication. The directness and clarity of communication in what is called the "instrumental" (practical) and emotional areas define a family's health. The clinician working with a family contributes to its health or coping to the degree he or she facilitates communication and strengthens appropriate hierarchical organization.

Health Orientation Versus Disease Orientation

Health can be viewed as a quality that does not simply denote absence of disease. In fact health and physical illness can co-exist. Two notions of health are in vogue, particularly in the field of nursing practice. The one proposed by Ralph Audy[1] states the following:

> Health is a continuing property, potentially measurable by the individual's ability to rally from insults, whether chemical, physical, infectious, psychological, or social. Rallying is measured by completeness and speed. Any insults may have a "training function" and recovery will often be to a slightly higher level of health. The person or body learns something.

The basis of this concept is that individuals deal with disturbing situations in a fashion that is healthful and as a result learn the process of coping—that is, they learn to be healthy. Health is therefore viewed as a developmental phenomenon, and in theory it can expand or be augmented over time. The important idea is that the capacity for coping (rallying) is an attribute of health: an individual can react healthily to physical illness or disability.

The second definition is taken from Bruhn and Cordova: "Wellness behavior is the development of an individual's ability to actively seek and change his life situation so that he can function at his perceived maximum capacity and satisfaction."[3] Appropriate ambition and the harnessing of strengths and resources to the work of achieving life goals are healthy behaviors.

To summarize, health is a behavioral and developmental phenomenon characterized by ways of coping with situations in life, ways of moving toward life goals, and ways of mobilizing strengths and resources. The family currently represents the primary context of learning and developing ways of being healthy. The family responds in the same way as the individual; stress or challenge results in adaptation or growth in a healthy family providing stress is not excessive. These concepts will be developed further in the section on Working with Families.

CHARACTERISTICS OF THE "HEALTHY" FAMILY

Research Findings

Wesley and Epstein pioneered the assessment of the "healthy" family in "The Silent Majority,"[17] a study of McGill University (Montreal) first-year students and their families. Further studies[7,9,10,11] assess the characteristics of the healthy family. No single variable can be used; instead multiple interrelated variables are outlined. Family therapists such as Virginia Satir[12] have compared dysfunctional families and derived characteristics to distinguish the two.

One specific study by Reiss[11] should be mentioned. Reiss' sophisticated research has been useful in clarifying the characteristics which distinguish a healthy family from those with a dysfunctional member (similar studies of families with physical illness would be of great interest). Reiss studied problem solving in three populations of families: those with a schizophrenic child, those with a child who had a character disorder, and those with children who had no known disorders. In the study, parents, the symptomatic child, and one sibling were required to sort 15 cards into a patterned sequence. Cards were fed to each family member in separate rooms. Members were able to communicate with one another by phones and were encouraged to share information about their cards as well as their ideas on the solution to the problem. The correct hypothesis for sorting cards was arrived at most effectively when there was sufficient communication within the family, as well as when full use was made of incoming information (the cards) arriving from the environment to each individual. Families with schizophrenic members were inefficient: although they were in close communication with one another, they were walled off from outside; consensus was of prime importance to these families, who preferred to be wrong rather than fight. The environment was experienced as threatening and dangerous, and the test situation was considered a threat to be warded off as fast as possible.

In contrast, those families with severe solitary delinquencies worked well with cues from the external environment but not with cues from each other. Each family member acted as an independent agent who did not need the help of the rest. As a result, they also did the test poorly. The normal or problem-free families were environment-sensitive and maintained an optimum balance between their internal communication and ability to use cues from the environment.

Although each of the research sources and clinicians like Satir used a different approach, the following five characteristics recur in their findings:

1. *Flexibility of Rules/Role Relationships—Morphogenesis*

Although generational boundaries are clear in "healthy" families, family rules (often implicit or unconscious) concerning behavior are subject to change. Adaptability in times of stress (for example, the hospitalization of the household breadwinner or cook) produces change in the roles of family members. Specialization of function and definition of roles are not so rigid that changes in rules or roles are difficult. The healthy family is capable of morphogenesis,[16] change in its own rules. Such change is characterized as real or "second-order" change, which is distinct from "first-order" change, in which true morphogenesis does not take place.[15] In first-order change the symptom of stress may change, or there may be a change in the identified patient in a family, but the basic problem remains the same. If the problem is poor communication or inability to change the rules of discipline to accommodate adolescent development, the family may need a push from outside the system which will help the family change itself.

Most families seen by the family practitioner are "dynamic": healthy and capable of instituting change or benefitting from minimal help. In contrast, families seen by a family therapist are more "static," requiring massive input or "induced morphogenesis"[16] from outside the family before change occurs (see Chapter 16). Such families rigidly adhere to a familiar way of functioning and resist change; inappropriate solutions to problems are repeated, compounding the original difficulties.

2. *Personal Autonomy or "Individuation"*

Family members recognize, respect, and treat each other as individuals.[9] Children are not seen as extensions of the parents and are allowed age-appropriate behavior. Individuation, the ability to be one's own person, results in a high degree of intimacy. The person with low individuation avoids true intimacy because of the fear of loss of identity or fusion with the other. Self-esteem[12] is a related concept; high self-esteem is associated with the ability to develop secure relationships without loss of the sense of self.

3. *A High Degree of Involvement Within and Without the Family*

A strong parental coalition, resulting from a firm affectional bond and sexual satisfaction, is characteristic of healthy families. There is family unity, loyalty, and intra-family cooperation. The family as a unit demonstrates high levels of initiative and is able to help itself and seek and accept help outside the family when needed.[9] In addition, family members assume responsibility in community relationships, with a link to society that is open and hopeful.[12] The family as a whole is able to realistically appraise its level of functioning; their self-appraisal is congruent with that of a competent observer outside the system.

4. *Open and Honest Communication*

A healthy family is able to communicate in a direct fashion and in depth. There is consensual decision making or clear allocation of responsibility in different areas based on open communication, and an ability to face and resolve conflict. Although parental authority is clear, children feel they have a say in plans affecting them. (It is perhaps surprising to note that several studies have shown that healthy families have rather chaotic communication patterns with frequent interruptions, simultaneous speech, and disagreements, in comparison to the more rigid, controlled, and turn-taking communication in families with delinquents or schizophrenics.) There is more expressiveness and responsiveness in the healthy family, indicating more actual exchange of information and freedom for all members to contribute to problem solving.[13]

5. *A Warm, Caring, and Supportive Environment*

The ability to provide for the family's emotional and spiritual needs as well as physical needs is a prime function of a family. If this is present, members will be able to reach out to others because they expect each encounter to be a caring one.[7] Development of trust is a function of family relationships and trust is an essential part of open expression of affection and well-developed capacity for empathy.[4] A *sense of humor* is also found to characterize the healthy family.

6. *Growth Enhancement*

This characteristic both for individuals and the family unit, has been described only by Otto[9] and Pratt,[10] who looked at families over time rather than by a single assessment. The healthy family is able to use crisis as a means of growth, and fosters growth-producing relationships and experiences within and without the family.[9] Pratt found that the type of family structure that enabled a family unit to serve its members' health needs most effectively was that of the "energized" family model:

The term energized family derives from stimulation and exchange that occur between family members who interact a great deal, both within the family and with outside groups, and who generate ideas and learn to cope with the pressures and demands of contemporary society. The energized concept refers to the unleashing of people's potential so that they may develop themselves to their fullest capacity.[10]

The Family Epidemiological Model

Medalie[8] has developed a conceptual model to depict the interacting factors of family, environment, and specific agents of disease over time (see Figures 2-1 and 2-2). In Figure 2-2 health is essentially represented by the overlapping area of the Venn diagram, which is termed "resultant adjustment."

The family system as host is central to the model seen in Figure 2-3; disturbed homeostasis and dysfunction are reflected by disease in one or more members. Each individual may experience a state of health, or exhibit symptoms belonging to a continuum of malaise, undifferentiated syndrome, enhanced susceptibility to disease, and a defined disease capable of being coded. The environment consists of "all conditions, circumstances, and influences" affecting health, whether they increase and protect health or are deleterious to health. Included within the environment are a person's economic status, social systems, cultural values and beliefs, geophysical factors, and biologic factors. Agents causing stress include biological, chemical, physical, mechanical, nutritional, and psychosocial factors.

The major characteristic of any family, as Medalie points out, is change. Family structure, economic base, educational standards, place of residence, recreational patterns, types of social contact all change as children are born,

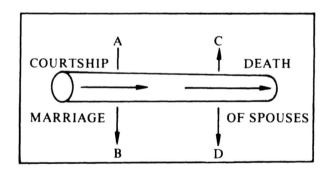

Figure 2-1. Family life capsule

From: Medalie JH: A family epidemiological model: A practice and research concept for family medicine. *J Fam Pract* 12:79, 1981.

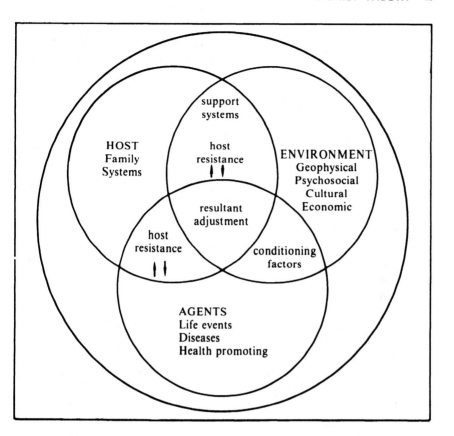

Figure 2-2. Family epidemiological model
From: Medalie JH: A family epidemiological model: A practice and research concept for family medicine. *J Fam Pract* 12:79, 1981.

grow, and leave, and as the couple's relationship develops or deteriorates. The surrounding culture changes rapidly (particularly in our time: the role of women, sexual mores, and technology are the most obvious examples). It is inevitable that the health of every family will fluctuate in its ability to cope. Health, therefore, is not fixed; it must be assessed for a given point in time.

In summary, the healthy family is durable. What Lewis Thomas said about the human organism could be said about the human family:

> We are paying too little attention and respect to the built-in durability and sheer power of the human organism. Its surest tendency is toward stability and balance. It is a distortion, with something profoundly disloyal about it, to picture the human being as a teetering, fallible contraption, always needing, watching, and patching, always on the verge of flapping to pieces; this is the doctrine that

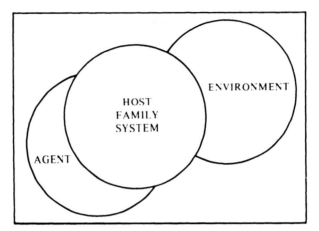

Figure 2-3. The host (family system) as the center of the epidemiological model

From: Medalie JH: A family epidemiological model: A practice and research concept for family medicine. *J Fam Pract* 12:79, 1981.

people hear most often. . . . When we ought to be developing a much better system for general education about human health, with more curricular time for acknowledgement, and even some celebration of the absolute marvel of good health that is the real lot of most of us most of the time.[14]

REFERENCES

1. Audy, RJ: Measurement and Diagnosis of Health. (Unpublished paper, 1967 [copyright 1970]).

2. Bowen M: *Family Therapy in Clinical Practice.* New York, Jason Aronson, 1978.

3. Bruhn JG, Cordova FD, William JA, Fuentes RG: The wellness process. *Community Health* 2:209, 1977.

4. Boszormenyi-Nagy I, Sparks G: *Invisible Loyalties.* New York, Harper & Row, 1973.

5. Jackson D: The study of the family. *Fam Process* 4:1, 1965.

6. Hinkle LE Jr, Plummer N: Life stress and industrial absenteeism: The concentration of illness and absenteeism in one segment of a working population. *Ind Med Surg* 21:363, 1952.

7. Lewis JM, Beavers WR, Gossett JT: *No Single Thread: Psychological Health in Family Systems.* New York, Brunner/Mazel, 1976.

8. Medalie JH: A family epidemiological model: A practice and research concept for family medicine. *J Fam Pract* 12:79, 1981.

9. Otto H: A framework for assessing family strengths, in Quin M, Reinhardt A (eds): *Family-Centered Community Nursing.* Saint Louis, C.V. Mosby Co., 1973.

10. Pratt L: *Family Structure and Effective Health Behaviors: The Energized Family.* Boston, Houghton Mifflin, 1976.

11. Reiss D: Varieties of consensual experience. *Fam Process* 10:1, 1971.

12. Satir V: *Peoplemaking.* California, Science & Behavior Books, 1972.

13. Speer DC: Family systems: Morphostasis and morphogenesis or "Is homeostasis enough?" *Fam Process* 9:259, 1970.

14. Thomas L: *The Lives of a Cell.* New York, Bantam Books, 1974.

15. Watzlawick P, Weakland JJ, Frisch R: *Change: Problem Formation and Problem Resolution.* New York, W.W. Norton, 1974.

16. Wertheim E: Family unit therapy and the science and typology of family systems. *Fam Process* 12:343–376, 1973.

17. Westley WA, Epstein NB: *The Silent Majority.* San Francisco, Jossey-Bass, 1969.

Chapter 3

The Family Life Cycle—Its Importance in Working with Families

Yves Talbot
Janet Christie-Seely
Suzanne Charbonneau

The role of the family life cycle in the context of life and illness seems very familiar and ordinary but is also a process of which we have very limited information. Longitudinal studies based on family observation have not been done. Yet clinicians aware of life cycle stages increasingly believe that most of what is called illness in textbooks and in our diagnostic nomenclature is merely outward evidence of inward struggles to adapt to life.[11,30,31] For the young clinician, whether nurse or physician, awareness of family development is limited to a distant memory of the stages in his or her family of origin, although the difficulties of adolescence may be too fresh to recall with comfort. For the older married clinician, a vivid memory of a baby's impact on a marriage, of a daughter's first date, or of the first time the couple spent a peaceful but hollow week alone together without the children will help the clinician understand families in his or her care.

Clinicians of any age may lack awareness about stages distant from their lives or be intolerant of people who have chosen different routes in life (the migrant artist, the unmarried, the childless). Life cycles of other cultures may not be understood: the Caribbean mother who works in Canada to support children being reared by their grandmother 3,000 miles away may be quite content and productive in her life because she knows that her old age will provide her with a second career of mothering her own grandchildren. The framework which follows is necessarily culture-bound and ignores class differences (see Chapter 5, an attempt to address cultural differences).

STAGES OF THE INDIVIDUAL LIFE CYCLE

Erikson[8] first described the stages of the life cycle of the individual and the concept of stage-specific tasks. Duvall[7] is one of few authors to apply

Erikson's concepts to the family unit. Erikson's stages for the individual and Duvall's stages for the family were juxtaposed by Medalie[23] and are reproduced in Table 3.1; there has been little or no research on the family as a system adapting over time.

The changing culture and development of new family forms, which are very different from the traditional mythology of how a family ought to be, may make current conceptual models inaccurate or obsolete. The popularity of a book like Gail Sheehy's *Passages*[28] suggests increasing hunger for information and the recognition that growth and development do not cease with the end of adolescence. Sheehy's account of the dramatic lives of a nonrandom sample of individuals, over half of whom were divorced, like the author herself, is highly subjective. As she admits, "Gradually I weaned myself away from dependence on the authorities, I came to rely on the richness of life stories I had collected to test and inform the theory and to add original insights. I began to feel comfortable with my own authority."[28]

Levinson and colleagues[18] studied 40 men in mid-life; the group included ten blue-collar workers, ten business executives, ten university biologists, and ten novelists. He noted several transitions, often heralded by "marker events" such as marriage: transition to adulthood (17 to 22 years) in which a person is engaged in separation from parents and forming an initial adult identity; early adulthood (22 to 40 years) in which a life in the adult world is developed, culminating in what is termed "becoming one's own man" (38 to 40 years); mid-life transition (45 to 55 years); and the transition of late adult life (60 to 65 years). As many have noted the turns of each decade seem to have particular significance. For a person 20 years old, individuation and separation from parents and career choice are the prime tasks. Early marriage (particularly if used as a means of such separation) adds another major task to an already difficult period, one in which personal change is still rapid enough that growing in different directions is a real possibility. By age 23, the tasks of individuation are accomplished and mate selection can be pursued with less difficulty resulting from old parent-child bonds and conflicts. The stress of turning 30 years old correlates with the "seven-year itch" of marital relationships when restlessness and re-evaluation set in. The mid-life crisis tends to be combined with the stress of adolescence and the looming "empty nest." Adjustment to loss of the children and recognition that life has a time limit may alter priorities and values.

Vaillant[30] followed 95 men from Harvard University for 40 years in a prospective study that described typical ways in which the men defended themselves against stress. Use of mature coping mechanisms (humor, altruism, sublimation, and suppression) increased fourfold between adolescence and middle life; in the adolescent immature mechanisms (denial of reality, fantasy, paranoid projection, and blaming others) were twice as likely to be used as mature mechanisms. Physical health and happy marriages correlated strongly with the use of mature mechanisms by the age of 47.

Vines[31] summarizes these studies of adult development and uses the term "adult unfolding" to describe what is considered an essential ingredient in marital homeostasis. The couple may not develop at the same time: the 40-year-old woman looking for her first job, gingerly feeling her way into the adult world 20 years later than her husband, is a good example. Vines points out the remarkable difference in the average American woman of 1880 and her counterpart of 1966. Because the average American woman in 1966 had an earlier marriage and had given birth to her children sooner, and had a greater life expectancy as well, she expected to live an average of 32 years after the year of her last child's marriage; in comparison, the average American woman in 1880 expected to live only 13 years after the year of her last child's marriage.

A key role of the family is to provide a nurturing environment which will allow each individual to develop to his or her fullest potential. Adaptation to growth is essential. Distress and physical and psychological symptoms develop when this process is disrupted or when the challenges or tasks of one stage are not met before the family has to deal with the tasks of the next stage. For instance, pregnancy very early in marriage (or even precipitating marriage) may mean that negotiating the couple's relationship is deferred because the role of parenting takes up all time and energy; later, the relationship resurfaces because the children have left home. This concept of stage specific tasks is central to a sophisticated understanding of the context of illness and to clear goals of intervention (see Section IV). If life stress is seen as a backdrop for stress symptoms to which adjustment is the goal, medication or psychotherapy may stabilize symptoms instead of using them as nature's warning that a change is needed in the system or situation. As Haley[12] points out the goal of the health professional should be to help a family or person to increase the variety and richness of life and to broaden options, not to adapt to a confining reality that prevents growth.

In our discussion of the family life cycle, we will consider the life-cycle stages described by Duvall,[7] who describes eight critical periods and the tasks related to each of them.

VALUE OF THE CONCEPTS OF LIFE CYCLE STAGES AND TASKS TO THE CLINICIAN

The family physician or nurse uses developmental tasks and understanding of family development for two main purposes: The first of these is to provide anticipatory guidance about the challenges to be faced in the developmental stage of a given family, based on knowledge of the family's strengths and successes in managing the previous stage of its life cycle. For example, a young couple who have not achieved appropriate autonomy from their families of origin, and are dealing with conflict by denying it will have difficulties with a new baby or with the autonomy and conflict problems of a

2-year-old. Similarly, an older couple who have lived (and argued) through their children, will have great difficulty letting them go in late adolescence; they may never have achieved the couple tasks of the first stage of the life cycle, having submerged those tasks for many years until faced with the empty nest.

The second reason for familiarity with the family life cycle is improved understanding of the context of symptoms or illness. The current demands put on each member and the family system during a given period of their development may produce stress that becomes converted into physical symptoms or illness.[6,22,24] Symptoms of young mothers or frequent illness in their children may be clues to difficulties of the couple in role or parenting issues; delinquency,[9] severe asthma, labile diabetes, anorexia nervosa in a child,[25] and schizophrenia[11,19] may be symptoms of submerged couple conflict and distorted communication, particularly in later adolescence when the illness may serve to keep the child dependent on the parents who can then continue in parenting rather than marital roles. A mother may use illness to escape into the hospital from a brood of small children, or a widow may use illness to keep her adolescent children from leaving home.

The term "normative crisis" implies the degree of stress engendered by normal development during the life cycle. Perhaps the most stressful is the combination of adolescent turmoil, mid-life crisis, or menopause in one or both parents as they adjust to the empty nest.

STAGE 1: A MARRIED COUPLE

Why do people get married? What are the characteristics of a happy marriage? Who marries who? These topics pertinent to the beginning of the married life will be discussed in the chapter dealing with problems of couples. The major developmental tasks for the young married couple are as follows:

1. the establishment of a mutually satisfying relationship;
2. increased autonomy from their family of origin and a new relationship with their kin network; and
3. decisions about parenting and the adjustment to pregnancy and possible parenthood.

An essential aspect of marriage often ignored is the joining of families. The couple must negotiate two different systems in which family traditions (Christmas, Thanksgiving) and ways of doing things (communicating, visiting, present-giving) may be combined.

The Establishment of a Mutually Satisfying Relationship

During the early years of marriage, a period extending well beyond the honeymoon, the couple must learn to accommodate to each other's needs and perceptions. The new partners come from two different family systems where each has learned particular ways of behaving and communicating: when the couple unite to form a new unit, they have to establish the rules and practices that will characterize their own family organization. Consequently, as they form themselves into a new family, some unavoidable developmental tasks may become sources of potential conflict between husbands and wives. For example, the early years of marriage usually coincide not only with the requirement that the husband in a traditional family arrangement devote himself to his work and to the development of his career but also with a natural desire on his wife's part that he be interested and actively involved in the daily affairs and tasks of the new household. If the wife works outside the home, this may also be a cause for conflict. Although some men welcome this arrangement, others perceive it as a threat to their status as the breadwinner.

Role allocations

A number of allocations of responsibility are made during the first 2 years of marriage: some are decided on the basis of interest, others on the basis of competence, but the result should be a division of labor that is satisfactory to both partners. Having a working wife often makes it easier for the man to accept an equitable arrangement regarding who will do the laundry, the cooking, or the buying of the groceries. The fact that both members of the couple are working outside the home increases the requirement to share the responsibilities associated with their living quarters.

Bader[2] has studied the establishment of new roles and the division of labor in a longitudinal study of 57 couples. These couples were interviewed 3 months before the wedding, and 6 months after, 1 year after, and 5 years after the wedding. Household chores were a major focus for discord: 87% of couples marked this area as problematic after 6 months of marriage; after 1 year 91% considered chores to be a source of discord.[2] This high level of irritation is not surprising when both spouses work full-time—neither spouse feels particularly energetic arriving home from work to face cooking supper, washing dishes, doing the laundry, and cleaning the apartment. Often neither member has acceptable role models for the division of labor, all they know is that they don't want to do things the way their parents did.

Women who work outside the home, as opposed to those who make careers of working inside the home, often marry at a later age, when they have more training and more marketable skills. When both members of the couple work outside the home, it is important for them to apportion their financial responsibilities, to make decisions about the kind of lifestyle they will have, and to recognize the financial resources required to support such a lifestyle. These same matters should be discussed, established, and decided mutually when the couple has agreed that one of the partners will work within the home to the exclusion of an external career: responsible, loving care of children and the creation of a warm, nurturing home environment are no less real or valuable contributions to the family than bringing home a regular pay check.

Money and budget

Whether one or both partners have paying jobs, agreeing on adhering to a realistic budget is a very important mutual responsibility; failure in this area is a major source of discontent in a marriage. Other areas that must be worked out include how the couple spends free time: Are hobbies and interests shared as a means of expanding horizons, or do they become a source of conflict? Are vacation preferences similar or in conflict, and is vacation together a source of the relationship's renewal, or is vacation apart a sign of division or of individuation? Are values and the sense of life's meaning and goals similar? Are religious views shared? One couple, incredibly, had dated 5 years without ever asking about each other's religious views. Only on arranging the wedding did the couple discover they were very different; in this case a premarital task (assessing compatibility in major areas) had not been accomplished at the appropriate stage.

Intimacy—psychological and sexual

The couple must also seek to become one, emotionally and sexually, to the extent that they succeed in establishing a mutually supportive relationship that will enable each partner to be truly intimate with the other, to be creative, and to grow as an individual. Sexual adaptation or adjustment is often a source of confusion for couples. Some of the difficulties may stem from inaccurate knowledge or subtleties of individual sexuality or sexual desires that lead to unrealistic expectations and disappointment. Sexual harmony is closely related to the quality of communication and adjustment taking place between the couple as expressed in the presence or absence of shame, indecision, guilt, or hostility, and their consequent impact on the early sexual adjustment of the marital pair. The development of strong bonds between the couple depends on an open system of communication that allows both to reach toward the other for comfort, love, understanding, sympathy, loyalty, and a sense of purpose.

Autonomy and Problems with In-laws

The second task is leaving home.[29] If one or both of the couple have difficulty extricating themselves from emotional entanglement (positive or negative) with a parent jealousy or irritation is aroused in the spouse, and often crises in the family of origin reverberate through the new family. Because families that hang on to their children prevent them from growing up emotionally and psychologically, the newly-wed may be looking for a parent substitute rather than an adult relationship. This will make self-reliance and responsibility hard and parenthood even harder. Triangulation may occur: the husband may use his strong-willed wife to stand up to his parents, or a mother may blame her daughter-in-law for keeping her son from visiting her.

Finally, psychosomatic problems, and in fact any illness, is more likely to occur in people still emotionally entangled with their families. This should be kept in mind when illness presents in early marriage. The converse of enmeshment—cut-off or disengagement of the spouse with his or her parents—often disguises continuing immaturity, and the spouse's sorting out of emotions is simply postponed until later.

Bader's study showed that the wife's relatives are more problematic before the marriage, presumably because of involvement with wedding preparations. When the first Christmas celebration was negotiated between the two families, 67% of the couples in the study claimed disagreement over the husband's relatives, 71% over the wife's relatives. A major area of disagreement, according to Bader, was "time and attention with conflict over the competing demands of work, friends and the families of origin." Again, the new couple's essential task is to create space in which their own relationship can develop.[2]

Interacting successfully with in-laws and relatives is a very important part of the early adjustment of a couple because it involves the establishment of the boundaries between the newly formed couple as a unit and their extended family. Although the extended family can be a significant source of support, it is essential that the new couple clearly delimit the area of decision-making and support that properly belongs to them. Turning to extended families or allowing them to intrude when conflict arises frequently precludes the development of the couple's own problem-solving strategies and skills. Another crucial moment when in-laws seek ways of being intimately involved in the life of the new family occurs when a child is born. If the new parents are to develop their own parenting skills, they must exercise their right to learn them from their own experience, even though the grandparents can be used as a source of support and information without the parents relinquishing their own responsibility for their child.

The Question of Children

Another matter of great import in the early stages of marital adjustment is making decisions about having children. The arrival of a child means that the family must alter its budget and possibly its priorities in order to meet, not only costs immediately associated with a baby (hospital, furniture, clothing, maternity wardrobe, baby food, diapers), but also the long-term costs of raising the child to adulthood. Such costs may mean a change in lifestyle or even in the couple's choice of friends since pregnant couples have a tendency

Table 3.1 Relationship of Individual and Family Life Cycle to Age*

Age†	Individual Life Cycle	Tasks	Family Life Cycle
	Infancy		
0-1	Oral	Basic trust vs mistrust	
	Childhood		
2-3	Early: anal	Autonomy vs doubt and shame	
4-5	Middle: preschool	Initiative vs guilt	
6-11	Late: latency	Industry vs inferiority	
	Adolescence		
12-17	Early	Identity vs role	Courting
	Middle	confusion	Going steady
18-21	Late: pulling up roots		Marriage: associated couple
			Pregnancy
	Adulthood		
22-27	Early: leaving family transition	Intimacy vs isolation	
28-39	:the "30" transition		First child
	:"settling		Multiple children
	down"	Generativity vs stagnation	First child leaves home
			First grandchild
40-59	Middle: midlife	Ego integrity vs	
	:the "50" transition	despair	Last child leaves home
			Multiple grand-children
60-69	Late		Couple again: empty nest
			Widowhood
	Old Age		
70+	Adjustment to death		Termination

*A composite picture based on Freud, Erikson, Levinson, Lidz, Duvall, Gould, Glick, Hill, and others.
†Age groups are approximate as the life cycle stages show a great deal of variation and overlap.

From Medalie JH: The family life cycle and its implications for practice. *J Fam Prac* 9:47, 1979.

to seek other pregnant couples—people who are sharing a similar experience. The most important requirement to be met is that each of the prospective parents have a deep sense of having actively participated in arriving at the decision to have a child; thus, they can be of genuine and continuing support to each other during the course of pregnancy and the inevitable adjustments that ensue. Some joint endeavor during the pregnancy may be desirable; for example, both parents may work together learning what is involved in becoming parents for the first time. One of the adjustments may be to resolve the conflict generated by the husband's being increasingly drawn toward male circles around work because his wife is preoccupied with pregnancy.

Premarital and Prenatal Examination—Key Moments for Prevention

It is worth emphasizing that premarital and prenatal examinations are often the key moments when the family practitioner encounters a new family during its formation. Part of the assessment of the new family is evaluation of adaptation to the current developmental stage and the successful resolution of past stages and tasks. Support and information about sexuality, pregnancy, and common difficulties in marriage and on coping strategies can be provided if the couple requests it. Anticipatory guidance of the family in the prenatal period is often a crucial function of the family physician. Supporting the husband and getting him involved with prenatal classes and with the pregnancy often relieve some of the feelings of estrangement felt by husbands in the early part of the childbearing process. Other anxieties, those concerning conception, fetal abnormalities, and breast feeding, should also be discussed.

> Mr. and Mrs. A. came to the doctor's office for Mrs. A's third prenatal check-up. Mrs. A. talked about her difficulty in carrying on with her daily routine and complained particularly of some back pain; Mr. A was concerned about a gastrointestinal upset. The family doctor, after reviewing the current pregnancy with the couple, elicited from Mrs. A. that she was concerned about the amount of work her husband had to do in the office. Mr. A. had just been given a promotion which was not only very important for him but would also allow them to buy a new house as originally projected. Because the couple had recently moved into a new neighborhood, Mrs. A. felt that she knew very little about the neighbors and that she was relatively alone in her pregnancy.
>
> The family doctor, understanding the current situation, suggested that Mr. and Mrs. A. both join a prenatal class. Mrs. A.'s face brightened immediately because the idea had not occurred to either her or her husband: this would be one way for both of them to be involved in the pregnancy, and she could find out whether she was doing the right things and whether the baby would be normal. Mr. A. also thought it was an excellent idea because it would allow him to learn more about the meaning of pregnancy for his wife and to feel more helpful. In addition to giving Mrs. A. the feeling of being more supported by her husband during her pregnancy, it would give her the opportunity to develop a support group in the new neighborhood with other families taking the course.

Prenatal visits frequently provide an opportunity for the physician to deal with other fears or concerns about such things as sexual intercourse during pregnancy and after delivery, childbirth, and child care.

STAGE 2: CHILDBEARING FAMILIES

Stage 2 spans the interval between the birth of the first child and his or her arrival at preschool age. The main tasks facing a family during this period are adjustment to and encouragement of child development, and establishment of a home that is satisfying for both parents and infant(s). With the birth of the first child, the family has to go through some reorganization as it changes from an intimate unit of two to a unit of three. Time, roles, and possibly space have to be redistributed as the former husband and wife unit transforms itself into the new family group of father, mother, and child.

Modern marriages can be started as a trial relationship with divorce as a possible escape if the going is difficult: a baby may remove this possibility of escape as an easy route. The extended family may also have seen the marriage as temporary until the birth of a child, which clearly unites the two families, occurs. A pregnancy occurring too soon in a marriage may cut short the couple's development and comfortable intimacy in which open negotiation and constructive anger are seen as helping rather than harming the relationship. On the other hand, the long period of contraception now possible allows for a close relationship between the couple that may put off the threat of an interloper until advancing maternal age precipitates the decision to reproduce. Physical symptoms or depression in the mother during or immediately after the pregnancy may reflect concern about parenthood or loss of the couple relationship. Alternatively, the husband or a relative such as a widowed mother affected by the changing roles and the new mother's preoccupation with the baby may become depressed or physically ill.

History Repeats

The couple are now reminded of difficulties with their own childhood; they may wish to be quite different from their parental role models. The first child often gets the brunt of these difficulties for two reasons: we learn from the mistakes with the first and adjust discipline and decrease anxiety over rearing subsequent children. The less obvious reason exists on an emotional or unconscious level: there is a tendency to repeat poor child-rearing practices on the first child. This finding is reminiscent of Harlow's[13] studies of monkeys. Baby monkeys reared by wire dummies with an attached food source proved to be terrible parents as adults. The females (impregnated despite abnormal mating behavior) seemed unable to develop affection for their first born and constantly abused the baby or pushed it away. Like children for whom negative attention is better than none the baby monkey kept coming back for more. However, with subsequent babies these primate mothers became much more capable of caring for their offspring with affection. Similarly, child abuse or neglect in humans repeats in the next generation. Family violence and abuse is dealt with in detail in Chapter 23.

Adjustments to a Threesome

After the baby's arrival, the family's daily routine usually becomes child-centered as a matter of necessity. When the child awakes, the parents awake; when the child goes to sleep, the parents go to sleep as well. The new parents also have to adjust to a new and probably unequal sharing of their time, which may suffer by comparison with the comfortable situation existing before the birth of the baby. The couple's satisfaction with the marriage then decreases. As a result, couples may return to making statements beginning with "I" rather than with "we." Time may also dictate a change in friends; childless couples are often left behind so that the new parents can have more time for the development of relationships with other parents who have young children. The park playground or the nursery school car pool becomes a source of new friends.

The family's adjustment to the presence of a young child encompasses adapting the house to make it safe for the child, meeting present costs, and making plans to meet the future costs of child rearing (education, insurance, clothing, food, medical care). Parents have to assume joint responsibility for household tasks such as shopping and cleaning; both are also involved in facilitating role learning as the child learns the rules of the household and of communication within the family. In addition, the parents must make decisions about having additional children and planning for them. During this period of adjustment they have to strive to keep family life from taking over the marriage entirely.

Return of the In-Laws

When a child arrives, the extended family tends to become more involved with the young couple. Although their input can be an excellent source of support the young couples must set clearly defined boundaries around child-rearing functions. Too much help can be as much a problem as unconstructive criticism. Money loans or gifts are a hazard (as they are in the first stage of marriage) since they often carry an implicit or explicit right to advise or dictate, and also prevent individuation.

Young Mothers, a High-Risk Group

The modern mother may look forward to having babies as a form of self-fulfillment, yet at the same time be unprepared for the personal frustration of being cut off from the adult world, as well as being unable to use her education or pursue her career. The mother's discontent and envy of her husband may add to his burden within the family and hamper his career.[12] Symptoms in this age-group of women, who are a high-risk group for mental and physical breakdown, should alert the clinician to look at the family unit. The author has seen a young mother with 3 months of hysterical blindness, another mother with severe hypertension that resolved only when her husband began sharing care of their 1 and 1/2-year-old child, and the onset of lupus erythematosis in another.

If the morale of the family is to be maintained at a satisfactory level, parents must go over the day-to-day drudgeries associated with rearing a young child to ensure that much more emphasis is put on persons than on things. An environment characterized by reprimands should be avoided. ("Watch out for that vase in the living room!" or "Don't touch the records!") The main function of the family system is to provide for each individual's growth, which may mean that some of an individual's tasks may come into conflict with another's; a compromise has to be found to make life manageable. For example, the father may be at the point of moving up in his career, but unless he is able to find the time to share in handling the concerns associated with a preschool-age child and in meeting some of the child's needs for parenting, his child may be deprived of an important component at this time for her own development.

The "Ticket of Admission," and the Role of the Clinician

The problem of establishing appropriate balances at any point in the family's development is something that families have to resolve; imbalance or stress will produce symptoms. Finding these balances and exploring alternative situations is an aspect of family life in which the family practitioner is involved. The reasons the family presents for consultation may be temper tantrums in the younger child, tiredness of the parents in handling a crying child, or feeding problems. Often the difficulty reflects a preoccupation or concern of one or both parents. For example, a 3-year-old child's temper tantrums in the supermarket may be a reaction to a mother who is overly concerned with her image as a good mother; the child of a working mother may have bedtime problems partly because of a need for her attention, but also because a sense of guilt on the mother's part may make firmness difficult. Feeding problems arise when a parent is overly concerned with what a child eats; such a mother will see the normal decreasing appetite of a 2-year-old as rejection of her mothering, as a sign of ill health, or as obstinacy. A power struggle may ensue in which the child's natural appetite becomes replaced by eating to please the mother. Families in which eating is equated with love, a cure for depression, or a source of control produce obesity or anorexia nervosa, or both in the child.

The normal developmental stages of childhood are handled more easily or less easily, depending on the parents' experiences in their own family of origin and on the adaptability of the family system. The role of the family doctor or nurse is to provide information on normal development (see Chapter 15) and to help the parents explore the various alternatives that allow optimum use of the family's resources. In cases where family resources are inadequate, some community support such as day-care or neighbors may be enlisted to allow people with young children to have some time for themselves. For example, a neighbor with a young child may exchange child care with another mother so that both can have free time. Support groups on parenting often allow discussion of problems and improved problem-solving as well as the recognition that such problems are normal and shared by others.

STAGE 3: FAMILIES WITH PRESCHOOL-AGE CHILDREN

Some of the main tasks facing a family when their eldest child is in the preschool-age range of 2-and-a-half to 5 years include the following:

1. to provide adequate living space and facilities for the enlarging family;
2. to meet the unexpected as well as predictable costs of family life when there are small children;
3. to assume the more mature roles appropriate to the expanding family; and
4. to maintain a mutually satisfying relationship not only between spouses but also with relatives and with members of the community and their activities and resources.

The provision of adequate space is related to the increased motor capacity of the child and his or her need for more activity. Making that space safe for the child is a very important task and may occur too late unless the new parents are warned ahead. As the child grows physically, the cost of food and clothing increases: as he or she develops mentally and becomes more verbal, there is an analogous increase in the amount of time, energy, and attention required from the parents. It often becomes increasingly difficult for the couple to maintain the level of privacy they had with a baby because young children are much more intrusive and demanding. This is the stage at which young children must learn to knock at their parents' bedroom door rather than simply run in. Grandparents or relatives can be very helpful in providing psychological and tangible support for a couple with preschool-age children, especially if another younger infant is also present. They can assist in taking care of the children, and thus act as a buffer when the young parents are endeavoring to cope with the increased demands confronting them. Such assistance may, however, require that a certain number of clearly defined roles be redefined once again because child-rearing styles may conflict. The child often responds to the inconsistencies of the parental role by persisting in normal (but transitory) patterns of behavior such as temper tantrums, refusal to go to bed, etc.

Increased Community Contact

Young children influence their families in the direction of greater contact with the community; parents are almost certain to meet other parents who may become a family friend through the child's interest in zoos and parks. The growing number of children participating in preschool programs has had a similar effect. Such contact with other members of the community may give rise to some new questions and causes for concern, including the following: How does our child compare with others in the neighborhood? How does our style of child rearing (permissive versus authoritative) relate to that of other parents in the community? What kind of aspirations should we have for our child? It is not unusual for families to bring such worries to their family doctor or community nurse.

Grandparents

Another source of concern for families with preschool-age children is the grandparents' imposition on the young parents with regard to the child's development: the grandparents may apply pressure to seek professional services for dealing with such problems. Children are often brought to the doctor at the age of 4 because the parents think their child is enuretic. A little investigation often reveals that a grandparent's imposed definition of enuresis is that the child does not stay dry overnight by the age of 3. Where extended families participate in the definition of a developmental problem in a child, it is useful to make sure that the entire family understands that there is no problem or, if there is one, they can become involved in its resolution or management. To provide only the mother or father with the appropriate information may not be sufficient and may result in the family going to another physician for advice. Unless the grandparents are directly involved in what goes on in the physician's office, some parents will not feel satisfied with the outcome. Other outside influences such as books on child rearing or television programs may be influencing the parent, who should be questioned about sources of information or worry.

STAGE 4: FAMILIES WITH SCHOOL-AGE CHILDREN

School Entry

The first task of this stage is facilitating the child's transition from home to school and community. The family product is now on display, exposed to evaluation by the outside world. The child must begin to fend for itself. Mothers experience a period of great stress with toddlers at home; a second common period of stress occurs during the first child's entry into the school system. For the mother confined to home, preparing the child for this event is perhaps easier than preparing *herself* for her decreasing role; a child's school phobia is known to be associated with emotional difficulties in the mother, and should be treated by getting the child into school as soon as possible and helping the mother with her difficulty in letting go. A mother's unwillingness to let go of her child may also be related to problems with the husband, especially if the husband is often absent at work, overly critical, unsupportive, or against outside interests or work for the wife. His commitment outside the house may be an inevitable part of career development or it may have been a response to the mother's overcommitment to the child. It is essential to see both parents in such a situation.

New Demands on Time and Money

Certain types of activities, such as verbal exchange between the child and the parents, or taking the child to community activities, place greater pressure on parents with school-age children than on parents with preschool-age children. Since children's activities place a definite limitation on parents' privacy and living space, rules must be made to ensure that some reasonable balance is maintained—for example, children should not be allowed to leave their belongings lying all about the house and cause an unnecessary and unproductive diversion of parental time and energy into picking-up after them.

School-age children may make financial demands that are much greater than those made by the preschool-age child; books and supplementary educational requirements such as music or figure skating lessons, more expensive toys, and athletic equipment can be major expenses. Parents have to balance the demands against the budget so that everyone has some of his or her needs met; parents are in effect called on to support childhood socialization. Children at this age often like to work with adults and to devote time to some shared activities and the learning of new skills. Although school becomes a very important socializing element in the lives of children, parental attitudes exert a very powerful influence shaping their likes or dislikes about school, and are also the primary factors in stimulating reading, artistic interest, and working habits within their own household.

A Couple's Time Together

Parents of school-age children usually report a serious decrease in marital satisfaction (see Chapter 25), but it appears that the decline may be more related to the greater emphasis and time spent by the couple on parenting when children reach school age. However, it is just as important for them to keep their close relationship as a couple through these years as it was during the previous stages of child and family development. Increased attention to child rearing or a career orientation by both parents may have the effect of moving them apart. It is not unusual for families or couples at this stage in their development to arrive in their family physician's office with a communication problem. Although the children are now attending school and there has been a consequent increase in the amount of time available for each other, they may have lost the habit of relating to each other or may be building up tension around the unrelenting daily demands of home, school, and work. A decrease in the conflict often occurs when the family leaves the household for a holiday. A study by George Brown[4] showed that mothers with three or more young children were particularly prone to depression, but that work outside the home played a definite protective role.

Community Influences

Another result of the onset of a child's schooling may be the re-establishment of linkages with the community on the part of the parents and other members of the extended family. In the process of establishing ties with the community, parents also monitor the kind of friends their children have. Deciding that some individuals are undesirable as friends because of violent or antisocial behavior may be commendable, but keeping a child from coming into regular contact with other children because of differences in religion or race may seriously curtail a child's chances of healthy social development.

School-age children pass through a spectrum of important changes in their moral development as described by Kohlberg:[16] the child moves from pre-conventional avoidance of punishment through conventional conformity with avoidance of blame to a post-conventional form of behavior in which the child's conscience takes over and good behavior avoids self-condemnation. It is often difficult for parents to adapt to these different stages of moral development in children who may, for example, suddenly begin to test the adult-imposed rules of politeness or cleanliness in annoying ways. Children may also try to change the family's rules about such matters as how much or what kind of television program will be watched; the children's wish to change the rules is often based on the different rules or absence of rules they have observed in the homes of their friends. Parents often find it necessary to make clearly defined distinctions between what happens in the community and what is considered acceptable at home, clarifying the boundary around the family unit.

STAGE 5: FAMILIES WITH ADOLESCENTS

At present the interval between the time when the eldest child enters puberty and the moment when he or she leaves home is unusually prolonged in North America. As a consequence, the young adult stage—the period after age 17 or 18 when many children remain in their parents' home while they attend a university—is important in contemporary society. Families with adolescents have the task of helping their children to grow and mature very rapidly over the relatively short period of 5 to 6 years.

A Normative Crisis: Adolescence, Menopause, and the Mid-Life Crisis

In our own culture and period of incredibly rapid change the generation gap is often enormous. A British general practitioner, Dr. Peter Tomson (personal communication) has aptly described the "4-year age gap" in parental and adolescent perceptions: the parent perceives the child as 2 years younger than his actual age, whereas the child believes he is 2 years older. The clinician can help decrease this age gap by facilitating communication.

Although adolescence is widely recognized as a period of turmoil for the developing youth, it is far from being an easy stage of development for the family. In some cultures, however, adolescence is less stormy, possibly because of clearer roles and responsibilities. In some cultures too the empty nest is not a problem since children stay in the same neighborhood or the grandmother rears the grandchildren. It is interesting to note that in areas where single parenthood and multigenerational families are the norm, symptoms of menopause are unknown.[20]

Certain adaptations must occur if each and everyone's growth is to be fostered. The two principal tasks confronting the family with an adolescent or adolescents are as follows:

1. striking a changing balance between freedom and personal responsibility as teenagers mature and undergo the process of individuation;
2. laying the groundwork for the post-parental interests and careers of the parents as individuals continuing to grow.

In addition to these basic developmental requirements, the parents of adolescents have to grapple with current social challenges posed by drugs and drinking, the sexual activities of teenagers, teenage pregnancy, and contraception. The dilemmas facing families with adolescents therefore include achieving a currently appropriate balance between the following:

1. family control versus the freedom of the adolescent (guidance by the parents who have greater life experience versus allowing the adolescent to learn from his or her own mistakes);
2. personal responsibility versus the freedom given to the adolescent;
3. social versus academic activity;
4. openness of communication versus the personal privacy of the adolescent; and
5. personal dedication versus lack of commitment towards life and society in general.

Parents may have to make major changes within the household to accommodate the more elaborate and differing social needs of their adolescents as they meet with friends or give parties; at the same time, the basic requirements of privacy, reading, and study must be provided. While sharing responsibilities continues to be an important part of family life, the need to disengage from the family often makes the adolescent somewhat rebellious about performing a number of previously acceptable chores. At this point, children often decide that they will stop participating in family outings and would prefer to make their own plans for their holidays or weekends. At the same time the adolescent feels that he or she has a right to the use of the car. It is very important that adolescents in the midst of these changes come to understand and appreciate that they too have responsibilities to the rest of the family in arriving at a reasonable and equitable sharing of the living quarters and facilities.

Although adolescents actively participate in decision-making they must also recognize that the ultimate responsibility for decisions remains in the hands of the parents, particularly for areas that concern the family as a whole. It has been observed[4] that mothers who work at least part-time outside the home seem to have less of a problem with their children's growth than those who do not. The lesser amount of time spent by such mothers in child-watching gives the adolescents a greater sense of freedom, enabling them to develop their own skills. Such an arrangement also affords an excellent opportunity for the parents to prepare themselves for the alternate roles they will assume after their children have left the household.

The Marital Relationship

Despite the clear demands that developing adolescents make on their parents, it is more important than at any other period that the parents, as a couple, keep their primary focus on their marital relationship. No one can or should be taken for granted. The maintenance of communication between the spouses is just as important as it is between parents and adolescents. Their willingness to listen to one another and to continue to give and accept affection from one another are the key ingredients in dealing successfully with adolescents during a period of rapid change.

Just as children of any age need the love, confidence, and respect of their parents, so do parents need the same psychological and emotional response from their children, whether they are adolescents or young adults. Success and accomplishment in this realm gives parents a deep sense of satisfaction in the worthiness of the very considerable personal and monetary investment they will have made in their family.

The Clinician's Role

Family practitioners are frequently consulted when some of the concerns that have been cited are affecting families and their adolescent members. Such clinician-family encounters usually occur at highly dynamic points, when people are in the process of rearranging the pattern of their lives together.

The Potential for Triangulation of the Clinician between two warring parties—the adolescent on the one hand and the parents on the other (or, more often, the adolescent and the parental rescuer on one side and the parental persecutor on the other)—must be recognized and guarded against. If parents enlist the aid of an older physician as an authority figure to regain control of a rebellious adolescent, a nonjudgmental focus on improved communication, and age-appropriate autonomy balanced by age-appropriate responsibility may lead to resolution of the crisis. Taking sides—a younger physician with the dominated adolescent, an older physician with the parents against the adolescent's rude or obnoxious behavior—ruins the opportunity to help. *Every* family member must experience the clinician as empathic and understanding (see Section IV).

The Triangulated Adolescent. When one parent is overtly or covertly supporting the adolescent or when parents are alternatively strict but undermine the other, hidden parental conflict should be suspected. In extreme situations, when the family has problems such as delinquency, alcoholism, or drug abuse, this is usually the case. It then becomes essential to clarify the problem as poor teamwork or disagreement over parenting, and if efforts to help the parents agree on a united front are not successful, referral for family therapy may be indicated.

In caring for a family with one or more adolescents, the family practitioner must be aware of the organizational changes and tasks that the family must accomplish. For example, when assessing an adolescent asthmatic who is not complying with treatment, it is important for the family practitioner to recognize that the adolescent's non-compliance is not only related to the establishment of personal autonomy, but also may reflect the parents' concern about their own future possibilities and needs. The adolescent's behavior may be supported by one of the parents; or it may provide the couple with the means to handle some of their differences or to resolve some of the anxieties they feel in relation to each other. By talking about the child's basic problem rather than by simply dealing with its manifestations, the family physician can help the parents to arrive at some mutually acceptable alternate way of increasing their child's autonomy. This action has the effect both of focussing on the parents as a couple and of allowing the adolescent to have a desirable degree of autonomy and control over the illness. The clinician can be a parental role model and encourage autonomy by suggesting to the parents that teenagers should make their own appointments for health care or for advice, and that their child need not come with the parent to the office.

Tasks of the Adolescent

The essential tasks for the adolescent are the basic tasks for any individual and include individuation, the ability to be independent with a sense of identity and self-esteem. Individuation cannot occur in an enmeshed system in which no member is given permission to be an individual and family self-esteem is low. The ability to love another, usually of the opposite sex, and to be loved in return is another primary task. Adolescents who socialize very late may not catch up with their peers. In the animal kingdom, mating and status are interdependent, and parallels exist in human society: persons who cannot find a mate or close friend become peripheral to the society. Haley[12] describes the health profession as the haven for such individuals; unlike animals we do not expose peripheral members to predators but we may institutionalize them or consider them sick. The clinician can be helpful to the adolescent trying to escape the clutches of the family but must be careful not to involve the young person in long-term therapy, which can prolong financial support from parents and be a way of avoiding relationships in the real world. It is preferable to refer the enmeshed family for therapy as a unit in which parental difficulty in letting go is seen as the main problem. The final task is that of finding satisfying work. Educational success must be seen as benefitting the adolescent and his future, not parental pride. Career choice in our culture must be free of parental pressure.

STAGE 6: FAMILIES LAUNCHING YOUNG ADULTS

This stage of the family life cycle begins when one of the children becomes the first to leave home as a young adult and ends with the departure of the last child. The tasks that face the family during the "pre-launching and launching phase" include the following:

1. Making changes in the sharing arrangements regarding physical facilities and resources which the young adult may require for courting.
2. Meeting the expenses associated with helping a child leave home; family expenses often peak when the oldest child is about 19 years old and there are still one or more other children in the home.
3. Re-allocating responsibilities among parents and grown and growing children; as children assume an increasing level of personal responsibility, the child-centered mother may be problematic to the children's growth so that the children turn to watching father as a role model. When one child has left home, those remaining step into new positions.
4. Rediscovery by the parents of one another as partners. Husbands and wives are, not infrequently, entering the middle stage of their development when some may undergo a period of self-questioning about their lives and their success as people as well as parents.
5. Caring for elderly or sick parents. This is another task imposed on couples at this stage; just when they sense freedom of responsibility from the younger generation, they find themselves faced with a dependent older generation. (As one mother put it, "My adolescents were nothing compared to looking after Aunt Floss." Faced with Parkinson's disease, Aunt Floss had turned to alcohol and was on her third hospitalization for a fracture after an inebriated fall.) The "sandwich generation" may be pressed both financially and emotionally by the needs of the young still dependent on them and the newly dependent elderly.

STAGE 7: THE MIDDLE-AGED COUPLE

The period between the departure of the last child and the retirement of the couple has been described by Duvall[7] as being a particularly important phase of family development for the family practitioner to understand. This period often coincides with the man and woman going through their own developmental mid-life crises, as well as with the appearance of such medical problems as cardiovascular morbidity, adult diabetes, and menopausal changes. The group of people around the age of 50 is continuously increasing in size, resulting in an absolute increase in the number of individuals at risk for adult morbidity. The family practitioner therefore must be familiar with this stage of development, and be aware of which patients in the practice are entering it. The main tasks of the family going through mid-life, as described by Duvall,[7] are as follows:

1. *Providing for Comfort, Health, and Well-Being as a Couple*

After the children have left home it is important for the parents to re-organize the house. In North America, parents may choose to reduce costs and housework by renting part of the house or moving to a smaller house or apartment. Moving can be a difficult adjustment, involving a perceived change in status and the loss of autonomy and familiarity associated with one's home. Couples often become much more health conscious and limit their consumption of alcohol or cigarettes and may take up new forms of physical exercise, sometimes too abruptly. They are often very conscious of the importance of regular medical check-ups, and are increasingly aware of heart disease, cancer, or strokes in their own age group. Observing these diseases first hand in their parents or in their siblings or friends may increase the concern.

2. *Financial Planning*

Current resources must be re-allocated despite the fact that the husband or wife may still be at a peak level income. They have to start planning for retirement, which represents a drastic change in the family finances. Often, planning for this period means the husband must recognize the likelihood of his wife surviving him and the need to provide her with financial security. Because increasing numbers of women are working, financial planning is easier but must also include planning the wife's retirement. Anticipatory guidance by the clinician includes a well-timed and tactful enquiry about such preparation.

3. *Growth and Meaning: The Prime of Life or the Empty Nest*

The third important task for the couple as described by Duvall is to develop new patterns of complimentary interests that will provide enjoyment and meaning for later life, when the children are gone and when careers are over. The middle years alone together before retirement may be as long as their life as parents; most adults describe this period as being a happy one. They enjoy watching the developing independence of their children and rejoice in their new freedom, decreased financial responsibility, and the chance to be themselves. Other parents, on the other hand, who have been very absorbed in their parental role and who are distant from each other, may fear this period, finding it hard to face each other. Such couples may have developed separate interests which they can benefit from by sharing. More leisure time together and more mutual activity before the children leave smooths the transition; the astute clinician can help by some well-timed questions and suggestions.

Anticipation of retirement is an important preventive measure for post-retirement morbidity. Often this period can be one of expansion rather than narrowing of life. Studies of individual development[18] have found that in the middle years, men who used to be very involved in their work and in the community no longer feel the need to achieve and become more involved in their own personal development; on the other hand, the woman who was previously housebound may become more expressive of herself and become active within her community. The development of her career while her husband is becoming aware of the importance of home and family may be complimentary or a source of conflict.

Values and Religion. A renewed interest and involvement in religion and the meaning of life frequently occurs at this age, but may not be shared by both spouses. Values may be reassessed and become a source of differences.

Sexual Relationship. At this age, persons can consider themselves as either uninterested in sex or wanting to maintain sexual relations. Marital interaction and sexual satisfaction depend on a healthy attitude. Both lay and medical literature describe changes in sexual activity associated with middle age; considerable controversy exists concerning the male and female climacteric. There is general agreement that in order to go through the physical and psychological changes of this period, communication and intimacy are necessary to provide each spouse with support, understanding, and respect, and to ensure mutual satisfaction. Couples are often much more satisfied with their relationship after their children have left home; Kinsey[15] has noticed an increased interest on the part of the women in their intimate relationships. Persons in middle age have been noted to have feelings of sexual inadequacy that may be related to boredom, job preoccupation, and mental and physical fatigue. Alcohol is often used as an anodyne and may become a problem. Although some important changes are occurring, it remains true that most couples that have remained married are happy during this period of their life; the increased level of communication and respect for each other fosters this continuation of growth and satisfaction.

Grandparenthood. When the couple has released most of their children, the family circle is enlarged by the marriages of their children and by their involvement with the grandchildren. The development of a mutually satisfying relationship between generations is crucial in facilitating further growth in their children; the parents may be useful as consultants on parenting or marriage. Mutual respect and clarity of boundaries between the new nuclear family and both sets of in-laws are known to be important factors in family development. In-laws are the target for jokes in the popular literature, which emphasizes the rivalry of the mother-in-law, and the competitiveness, jealousy, envy, and comparisons between families; but in-laws can also be a major family resource. Grandparents give to the new family a sense of continuity and history, as well as a sense of belonging, which is so important to human development; the extended family adds richness and diversity to relationships, and family stories and legends add color to the identity of growing children. Families of black North Americans who have lost their "roots" and Jews who have lost their relatives and records in the Holocaust can especially understand the extent of this richness and debt to the past. Largely unconscious, the sense of indebtedness is a powerful determinant of behavior (this indebtedness is the focus of Borszomenyi-Nagy's[3] work, *Invisible Loyalties*).

In this stage of development, the family practitioner is likely to meet each member of the couple more frequently than during the previous periods. Visits are a great opportunity for the introduction of ideas concerning preparation for retirement, development of other skills than those of the current career, the necessity of physical fitness and health maintenance in preparation for the next and last phase of family development, and the importance of communication and mutual support.

STAGE 8: THE AGING OF FAMILY MEMBERS—WIDOWHOOD

This period extends from retirement to the death of one spouse. The aging couple or individual continues to be definitely part of the family of their children. The major task for the aging individual is the preservation of ego integrity; he or she must maintain a satisfying level of activity and productivity to fulfill his or her potential as a person and retain a sense that life is meaningful. There is evidence that a loss of this sense of meaning, which may occur in a man who has stopped his life's work, is associated with illness and death.[10,26] For many aging couples, children and grandchildren are a major source of such meaning; these couples continue to play a significant role in the families of their children. If the children are too busy or the old people too needy and demanding (or overly critical to disguise their uncomfortable dependence), painful conflict may arise. The clinician can sometimes help with a tactful and well-timed comment to the younger families that grandparents are good for children and useful as babysitters or to the older couple that more independence through senior citizens groups would improve the quality of contact with children and grandchildren. It is important for the clinicians who see the aging as a large part of their clientele to understand the developmental tasks that the aging couple must face.

Duvall[7] describes eight developmental tasks of the aging couple after retirement (see Chapter 27). We illustrate here some of the main tasks that are relevant to the family practitioner.

Housing and Finance

Satisfying living arrangements are essential and often hard to find in days of inflation and small pensions. Many aging people are moving into downtown communities and cheaper dwellings, and some join retirement communities or, if they have the resources, move to a warmer climate. The snow and ice of northern regions may make fractured hips a major hazard for those who stay and do not remain housebound in winter. Other people who are debilitated by illness sometimes are faced with no choice but to move to nursing homes. Such a move is usually seen as the last resort, representing a total loss of freedom and personal integrity. In Canada, provinces vary widely in the facilities for housing, homes, and hospital beds for the elderly. Financial distress is a major worry. Many professionals, doctors, lawyers, and the self-employed postpone the moment of retirement for as long as they can to curb the financial deprivation of old age. In countries such as England or Canada, where health care is nationalized, the vast health care requirements of the elderly population can be well taken care of. In the United States, where Medicare is still providing only partial coverage to the elderly, illness can be a source of great financial hardship.

Too Much Togetherness

Most families must change some of their established patterns of living; retirement means a change of routine for both man and wife. For the wife this may mean welcome help as the man starts sharing daily tasks such as laundry, cooking, ironing, vacuuming or paying household bills, or it may mean trouble: "He's under foot all the time." The increased amount of time together may mean increased intimacy or increased time and opportunity for friction. The man who may have been home only for brief periods of time on weekends and holidays is now there for much longer periods of time; often he has little to do and misses the stimulation and sense of purpose of the work environment and his colleagues. If the wife has not worked outside the home, her routine is now disrupted; if she has, she must face the same adjustments as her spouse although her dual role as homemaker and breadwinner is some protection against disruption. The necessary rearrangements of time, activities, and togetherness are best anticipated well before retirement. A single brief question posed by the family physician or nurse years earlier may set in motion the thinking and planning required.

Health

Both members of the couple must protect their physical and mental health. Confronted with a regular decrease in their hearing and sight, and with the aches and pains of aging, old people do their best to avoid illness, which is costly to their financial and overall well-being. Often in the North American family the husband becomes ill first, requiring a shift in roles within the family; the wife becomes the caretaker while the husband is in a position in which he can give little support. When presented with such a couple, the family practitioner must help the couple mobilize community or extended family resources.

A very important part in the health of the elderly person is nutrition; the "Tea and Toast syndrome" is increasing as inflation or solitude affects the diet. (The hazards of too much medication, and diagnostic errors and the importance of the family in health care are discussed at greater length in Chapter 27.) Evidence supports the fact that elderly married couples are happier than those who are single or divorced and are freer of disease.[21] Mutual support gives meaning to people's lives and acts as a protection against illness.[23] There is also evidence that sexual activity in aging people persists at least into the seventies and eighties and that it is highly beneficial to health. People who are physically more disabled are more likely to show marital dissatisfaction. Chronic illness can be very destructive to the partner,[5] but marital support is a key element in adaptation to the physical and psychological changes happening within each member of the couple.

Self-worth and the community

Our culture, with the cult of youth and individualism, and the great mobility of the North American family do little to help the old. People from India and the East are amazed at our callousness and disrespect of the aged. Accummulated wisdom is wasted, as is experience that could be used in teaching and consulting and working with people in community organizations. Physical barriers such as lack of transportation and accessible resources increase the isolation of the elderly. Often lack of family support and isolation are greater handicaps than biological aging; a person's lack of a role in the family or community often makes his or her life meaningless and increases illness. The clinician should recognize that a support network represents a powerful adjunct to the aging family member, and should encourage activity with community groups and resources as preventive maneuvers in the middle-aged or during the first years of old age. It is hoped that as the proportion of elderly in the population increases, communities will respond by increased concern and facilities.

Facing Life Alone

Death of a spouse is listed by all cultures as the most traumatic life event to be faced.[14] If this represents the loss of a life-time, beloved companion all sense of meaning in life may be lost for the survivor. The increased morbidity and mortality of the bereaved has been well documented.[17,26] It is interesting to note that an ambivalent relationship with the spouse may produce greater difficulty in the bereavement period because of excess guilt and anger. This topic and the problems for a family associated with fatal disease are dealt with at length in the chapter, "Terminal Illness and Death" (Chapter 22).

Facing life alone is the lot of many North American women whose husbands die prematurely, often from heart disease. As more women join the ranks of those in the competitive professions and marketplace it seems that their mortality rate is increasing as well. The young widowed are most at risk for illness, and the widower fares worse than the widow[17] (see Table 8-1). However, remarriage is a greater possibility for the young, and they are less dependent on a spouse and find it easier to ward off the isolation that is so common in the elderly. For many couples, friends have moved or died and children are in another province or state. Starting friendships anew at this stage is very difficult. The clinician can be an invaluable resource in stimulating new interests or participation in groups, if that clinician is sufficiently aware of what is available in his or her community. He or she may be an interim substitute for the lost relationship and must encourage working through psychological dependence on the lost spouse to more appropriate relationships with friends and extended family.

Although apparently alone, the widow or widower is as much a part of a family as the young adult looking for a mate. The truly solitary person with no family or substitute family is relatively uncommon. (Such groups as the Legion or clubs or the church often function as a family; these represent a "group of people with a commitment to one another with a past, a present and a future"[27] who will care for each other if illness strikes.) Serious or fatal illness often brings forth relatives that were seldom contacted when the person was healthy. The extended family both affects and is affected by the health of the old person. Death often produces a ripple effect of illness or dysfunction in family members, who are often removed geographically or quite distantly related. The role of the family physician or nurse with a family facing death can be important in facilitating communication and emotional expression and sharing. This topic is covered in detail in Chapter 22.

In summary, the family life cycle forms a context for both the development of illness and for prevention. It is an important aspect of family assessment (see Chapter 14) which often gives the clues to aid diagnosis and understand the individual and family's compliance and response to illness.

REFERENCES

1. Antonovsky A: *Health, Stress and Coping.* San Francisco, Jossey-Bass, 1979.
2. Bader E, Microys G, Sinclair C, et al: Do marriage preparation programs really work? A Canadian experiment. *J Mar Fam Ther* 6:171, 1980.

3. Boszormenyi-Nagy I, Sparks G: *Invisible Loyalties*. New York, Harper & Row, 1973.

4. Brown GW, Bhrolchain MN, Harris I: Social class and psychiatric disturbance among women in an urban population. *Society* 9:225, 1975.

5. Downes J: Chronic disease among spouses. *Milbank Memorial Fund Quar* 25:334, 1947.

6. Duff RS, Hollingshead AB: *Sickness and Society*. New York, Harper & Row, 1968.

7. Duvall EM: *Marriage and Family Development*. Philadelphia, J.B. Lippincott, 1977.

8. Erikson EH:*Childhood and Society*, ed 3. New York, Norton, 1963

9. Ferrerra AJ: The double-bind and delinquent behaviour. Arch Gen Psychiatr 3:359, 1960.

10. Frankl V: *Man's Search for Meaning*. New York, Pocket Books, 1963.

11. Gartner RB, Fulner RH, Weinshall M, Goldklank S: The family life cycle: developmental crises and their structural impact on families in a community health center. *Fam Process* 17:47, 1978.

12. Haley J: *Uncommon Therapy: The Psychiatric Techniques of Milton H. Erickson*. New York, Norton, 1973.

13. Harlow, HF: The nature of love. *Am Psychol* 13:673, 1958.

14. Holmes TH, Rahe RH: The social readjustment rating scale. *J Psychosom Res* 11:213, 1969.

15. Kinsey AC: Sexual Behavior in the Human Female. Philadelphia, W.B. Saunders Co., 1953.

16. Kohlberg L: Moral development, in *International Encyclopedia of Social Science*. New York, Macmillan Free Press, 1968.

17. Kraus AS, Lillienfeld AM: Some epidemiological aspects of the high mortality rate in the young widowed group. *J Chron Dis* 10:207, 1959.

18. Levinson D, et al: *The Seasons of Man's Life*. New York, Alfred Knopf, 1978.

19. Lidz T, Fleck S, Cornelson A: *Schizophrenia and the Family*. New York, International Universities Press, 1965.

20. Lock M: Models and practice in medicine: menopause as syndrome or life transition? *Cul Med Psychiatry* 6:261, 1982.

21. Lynch JL: *The Broken Heart: The Medical Consequences of Loneliness*. New York, Basic Books, 1977.

22. Medalie JH: *Family Medicine: Principles and Applications*. Baltimore, Williams & Wilkins Co., 1978.

23. Medalie JH: The family life cycle and its implications for practice. *J Fam Pract* 9:47, 1979.

24. Meyer RJ, Haggerty RJ: Streptococcal infections in families. *Pediatrics* 29:539, 1962.

25. Minuchin S, Baker L, Rosman BL, et al: A conceptual model of psychosomatic illness in children: family organization and family therapy. *Arch Gen Psychiat* 32:1031, 1975.

26. Parkes CM: *Bereavement: Studies of Grief in Adult Life*. London, Tavistock Publications, 1972.

27. Ransom DC: The rise of family medicine: new roles for behavioral sciences. *Marr Fam Rev* 4(1/2):31, 1981.

28. Sheehy G: *Passages.* New York, Dutton, 1974.

29. Stahmann RF, Hiebert WJ: *Premarital Counselling.* Lexington, Massachusetts, D.C. Heath & Co., 1980.

30. Vaillant G: *Adaptation to Life.* Boston, Little Brown, 1977.

31. Vines NV: Adult unfolding and marital conflict. *J Marr Fam Ther* 5 (2):5, 1979.

Section II
THE FAMILY AS PART OF LARGER SYSTEMS

Chapter 4

The Community

Monique Jérome-Forget
Gilles Paradis

The natural evolutionary tendency for all living organisms is specialization of function and regrouping and consolidation as systems. The common feature of all systems is that they are composed of many different components that are capable of fulfilling specific complementary roles (see Chapter 1). As a whole they are able to carry out functions or to achieve goals which cannot be carried out by any of their components acting alone.

A community is such a system of networks and channels of communication. It is a rich fabric made up of many interwoven threads that do not end within, but project beyond its borders. The community represents the next step in social reorganization after the family.

It is true that an individual family can survive alone in a suitable natural environment and that the basic biological unit of humankind, man and woman, is in a very real sense plenipotentiary in that it can maintain and reproduce itself. It is nevertheless also true that the survival of the individual members of such basic families is much more precarious and the realization of their full human potential is more severely limited when they live in isolation, in comparison to human achievement when the individual becomes a part of the community.

Each community seems to develop a particular character or flavor, making it more than the sum of the various value systems, life styles, and local color of its family groups.[5] The community is determined by its internal factors, such as the background of its individuals, families, and ethnic groups, as well as by the history, membership, and leaders of its agencies.[4] The way the community relates to external factors such as mass media, the national character, provincial or state objectives, and neighboring cultures also influences its identity.

The impact of the community on the lives of families is so pervasive and continuously present that we take it for granted and become almost oblivious to its existence. We may fail to appreciate this fact of life because we often see families living in relatively isolated rural settings; we do not recognize that, despite outward appearances, these families are still very much part of the community which supplies electricity to their homes; teachers for their children; firefighters, policemen, doctors, and nursing care in times of emergency; information about the world; and music, entertainment, and communication with their extended families and friends via radio, television, and telephones.

ROLES AND COMMUNITY NORMS

The community, like the family,[1] is an arena where two fundamental issues must constantly be addressed: how to meet one's need to belong and how to simultaneously individuate. The sense of belonging to a community determines a person's attitudes, beliefs, and values, and is protective of that person's health (see Section III). However, the family must develop its own identity and have a distinct "self."

The manner in which these goals are reached or fail to be reached determines the roles, functions, and contributions a family or an individual makes to the community. The process of individuation is subordinate to feelings of security, of self-worth, and of being cared for. These feelings, in turn, allow the integration and internalization of societal norms.

Families need to feel that they are collectively and individually making a worthy and recognized contribution to the life of the community, whether the contribution be as teachers, electricians, homemakers, members of the hockey team, carpenters, policemen, paperboys, or gardeners. At the same time, families must have a sense of identity and competence that permits them to derive satisfaction from being who they are, from being able to fend for themselves in providing the most basic requirements of family life, and from being able to make up their own minds about appropriate individual behavior and social attitudes in a responsible fashion.

Norms are essential to ensure the progress and the survival of any given community. Norms clarify the relationship between the different elements of a community; they confer security through peer acceptance to those who observe them and they predict what behavior will be rejected as deviant or threatening to its stability.

Social clubs, political parties, baseball leagues, states, and countries all have rules, written or unwritten. In the "healthy community," rules are flexible and promote adaptative responses to stress. A dynamic relationship exists between members of the community permitting reappraisal of its norms in answer to internal or extraneous factors. These factors can be the arrival of a significant new member, technological innovations, pressures from groups, or important events both within and outside the community.

Flexible norms enhance the realization of its members' full human potential, whereas rigidity leads to stagnation and laxity to anarchy. Dysfunctional communities preclude individuation and produce enmeshed families with poor defense mechanisms who are not well adapted to confront new problems. Their response to stress is either authoritarian or chaotic and may well lead to violence or abuse. The mass suicide of 900 of Jim Jones' followers in Georgetown, Guyana in 1978 is an example of a violent reaction in a pathological community.

These societies will often be the center of intense emotional conflicts. Anger, rage, frustration, and aggression are deflected from their original object. The scapegoating of the Jewish people in Germany during World War II is an example of such triangulation.

Deviant Behavior

As much as society needs norms and rules it also needs people to defy them and adopt deviant behaviors. The most common deviant behavior is criminal activity, which represents an outlet for the expression of tensions and conflicts that exist within any community. This inherent potential for destruction and self-destruction poses a serious threat to the system's[1] stability and survival. To reduce its anxiety level and its feelings of helplessness and vulnerability it will find scapegoats, who through so-called "societal factors" (income, socioeconomic class, employment, education, family background) will become its criminals.

The degree to which the community system meets the needs to belong and to individuate determines the extent of violent behavior. This is a reason why the rate of crime is at its highest in large urban areas, where alienation pervades and where individuation is lost within anonymity.

Norms within a society play a fundamental role both because some persons observe them and some do not. For example, great advances have been made in the sciences, arts, and medicine, by non-conformists who are later called "pioneers."

COMMUNICATION

Effective communication pathways and feedback mechanisms coordinate functions within a community and make it possible for people to be teachers, plumbers, musicians, nurses, lawyers, electricians, actors, doctors, etc. In the absence of communication, specialization and assuming specific roles are not feasible; activity is limited to hewing wood, drawing water, gathering or hunting food, and guarding against the hostile elements of the environment.

When studying these mechanisms we must consider not only the content of the messages themselves but also the various ways communication is carried out. "The medium is the message," claimed Marshall McLuhan. Indeed, the modalities and patterns of interaction between individuals, families, and groups reflect the system's prevailing beliefs and attitudes towards all aspects of community life.

In a small community the lines of communication are generally more obvious and simple than in large urban areas. They constitute good indications of the power and influence yielded by the different elements of the system. These lines are not always straightforward; as we have seen, communities can triangulate and scapegoat their members in the same way families do.

By observing the interrelationships of its subsystems (the police system, the court system, the health care system, the church or religious system, the school system), the clinician can often find explanations for tensions and crises that burden the community and increase office visits.

The same interactions occur on a larger scale but they are more difficult to analyze. In a large urban area, for example, communication pathways are much more complex because of the greater number of systems that compose it. Every individual is part of a number of systems, and the degree of emotional attachment and significance each represents in a person's life determines the impact these systems are capable of having. The family, for example, is usually the most important of these systems. Hence the greater consequences of this system's communication lines.

The tremendous technological advances in this field have not been associated with a parallel improvement of the psycho-social and emotional sphere of our society. Television more than any other media has altered our relationship with the world. Marshal McLuhan's concept of a global village illustrates how we gain access, instantly, to the world through this medium. However, one of television's problems is that it takes away the unique perspective for individuals by pre-processing and editing what it shows us. Furthermore, it conveys a limited range of values and norms and establishes models by which people can assess each other. We have yet to discover sensitive and responsible ways of using this refined communication tool.

IMPACT OF COMMUNITY ON HEALTH

The community is a complex human system; each of us is embedded in it, interacting with it every day of our lives. It is therefore inevitable that the nature and quality of such interaction is a significant component of our physical and mental well-being, as well as our capacity as individuals and families to cope with the challenges of life in a healthful way.[2]

The mobilization of community resources to support and provide various kinds of care to a family or its members when faced with an emergency, stress, or a problem that exceeds their coping ability is discussed in a later chapter. Nonetheless, we wish to emphasize the important health implications of a satisfactory relationship between a family and at least some of the more significant elements in the community system.

Pleasant and friendly feelings about the family's neighbors, reasonable satisfaction with what and how the children are being taught at school, a positive attitude toward the constructive role of the various community agencies, and pride in the physical appearance and natural beauty of the community are a few of the community-related dimensions of a healthy family. When discomfort, dissatisfaction, and suspicion characterize or poison these relationships, they constitute a stress that is just as potent a factor in determining a family's state of health as internal forces. A peculiar family dysfunction may lead to difficulty in relating to the community, which in turn will rebound and aggravate the system's internal conflicts. Moreover, the community itself creates comfort or tension within the family, largely influencing the family system's equilibrium and having an unequivocal impact on its health and its ability to cope with health problems.

The clinician must be able to perceive the consequences of the constant interaction of the various components of his or her community. The clinician's own input and that of the health care network in producing and maintaining certain situations are very important within the community; therefore, the clinician's role and responsibilities are extended and the field of health care is broadened to include knowledge about the dynamics and the functioning of systems, and the actions a clinician can take to bring about change (see Chapter 18).

BASIC DESCRIPTION OF A COMMUNITY

Age and Sex

Age and sex are basic demographic factors that strongly influence the types of services a physician or nurse are called on to perform. A young suburban community is bound to request numerous services for children, whereas a center city area is often composed of a large proportion of elderly whose more chronic problems require quite different therapeutic approaches. (For example, in a Montreal city district attached to a university teaching hospital, 13% of the population is over 65 years old, as opposed to 6% in a suburb.)

Communities are becoming older, particularly in the center of cities where poor living conditions often prevail. Women are more often found living in these areas because they outlive their husbands and have little or no source of income. This group, which is increasing, typically lives below the poverty line. Often the elderly have inadequate housing, heating, and nutrition, and few if any relatives or friends. Working with the elderly therefore frequently requires that health care workers use judiciously the resources of their community.

Culture

Ethnicity and culture are important determinants of health care needs and of the expression of these needs. For instance, biological and genetic predisposition are known to be responsible for very serious diseases (thalassemia, sickle cell disease, etc). Furthermore, patterns of illness and requests for services change according to the different cultural approaches to health and disease. For example, whether a person does or does not seek medical attention for a symptom depends on the ethnic background of the individual.

Risk Factors

The health care professional should be able to identify potential risk factors for the population that is being served. The following are a sampling of the questions one should try to answer: What health hazards exist in this community? What is the age and sex distribution? What socioeconomic classes do the people belong to? Is unemployment a problem? Are there industries located in the community? If so, are they potential health hazards for the population? What specific risks do the workers of these industries face? What are the physical characteristics of the community which can predict health problems (housing, recreation areas, highways, etc.)?

Socioeconomic Factors

Establishing an income profile and gathering data on the socioeconomic class and on the lifestyles of clients allow the clinician to measure the impact of life events or disability on families. For example, if a family relies totally on the income of the father, the loss of work for that person will obviously be felt more acutely than if the spouse had a salary.

Case Number 1:
  An urban development project recently shattered a downtown neighborhood where Mrs. X, a 71-year-old woman, lived with her spouse. The husband died shortly after the development project, and now the wife has no friends or relatives near by. Both her children live in another city where they are involved with their own family. Her income is minimal and puts her well below the poverty line. Feeling abandoned she has become increasingly depressed, and now is afflicted by numerous physical ailments.

Traditional medical treatment does not suffice in this case. The appropriate community resources should be approached to help alleviate Mrs. X's isolation and help manage her small income. She may, in fact, need to be moved to less expensive accommodations. The health care worker should give the impetus to this process and should be available for the greater support Mrs. X will need during this period.

Case Number 2:

Mrs. Y is a 38-year-old female who has devoted all of her life to her family. She has three children, aged 13, 14, and 15. She had recently been feeling that the relationship with her husband had deteriorated; he had been increasingly absent from the home. He had admitted that he was having an affair and that he was planning to divorce her.

Mrs. Y left her job when she got married, 18 years ago and she now feels incompetent, insecure, and isolated. She feels incapable of starting over again. Mrs. Y will also have a smaller income because her husband will be supporting two households: hers and his own.

Mrs. Y now feels lethargic, depressed and she does not know how to be functional again. She suffers from insomnia and is very edgy with her children.

The physician will probably be the first person to whom Mrs. Y now turns. He should insist on seeing the children with her since her distress is surely to be experienced by them as well. Furthermore, he should be aware of the existing resources of his community which may help in supporting her to go back to work.

Case Number 3:

Mr. and Mrs. Z and their three children (aged 3, 6 and 9 years old) were war refugees from Cambodia. They had been sponsored by a Canadian organization and were given a free home and food for the first 12 months of their stay. The whole family was attending language classes offered by the government to facilitate their transition. After the first year, the family started experiencing more acutely the stresses of adapting to a new environment. They had not yet mastered the languages spoken in their new community and were isolated and unable to find work or support themselves.

The youngest child became ill and Mrs. Z brought him to the nearest physician and tried to tell him what her child's problem was. She was, of course, unable to tell her physician all the problems the family was experiencing in this new environment.

The necessary first step in this case would be to find ways of improving communication between this family and their milieu. The physician might recommend an interpreter whom the family could call when the need arises or refer the family to a Cambodian physician who could give them help and advice in periods of crisis.

The physician should bear in mind that the investment made in investigating the environmental resources of his or her community is long-term. By knowing what exists in alternative resources and complementary services, he or she builds alliances that will pay off tremendously in his practice (see Chapter 18). While some effort is needed to start and then maintain these contacts, the gains made are well worth the effort.

KNOWING THE COMMUNITY RESOURCES

The back-up support existing in a community can be classified into two large categories: the formal resources are those that belong officially to the existing government agencies. The informal resources, which are less organized, involve the immediate family and the neighborhood.

Formal Resources

Formal resources which exist within most modern countries consist of a large array of services, from pre-natal classes to placement for the elderly. The quantity and variety of resources are such that the clinician can rely on them to help him assume his role completely and fully.

Informal Resources

In addition to the well-established formal resources in the community, the physician has at his disposal an informal network. The foremost resource a clinician can call on is the family. A spouse, a sister, a mother, or a grandparent is often called on to help in critical situations; the clinician should assess the dynamics of the system to determine if help from a relative or involvement by a spouse would adversely affect the illness of the identified patient. When calling on a brother or cousin for help, the physician should remember that there are limits to family resources. The availability, skills, intellectual ability, and emotional stability of the potential helper should be evaluated to avoid jeopardizing the outcome of treatment.

The professional can also use the neighborhood for additional help, especially with regard to isolated families (immigrants, the handicapped, etc.). The nurse or social worker in a community center is often aware of these resources. Also, the local parish is still a source of valuable information on services that are available through local associations.

The schooling system can be of great help to the physician. Usually the principal and the teachers know what is going on in the community. In addition, most schools have a nurse, a social worker, or a psychologist as a part of their services.

Economic constraints imposed on government agencies have resulted in curtailment of services; the client's experience of the agencies' shallowness and impersonalized style has generated new trends in the field. Many communities are filling in where the official channels have left off. The exchange of services in a Canadian city through a link project is such an approach. For example, an elderly woman who finds it difficult at certain periods of the year to go out shopping exchanges baby-sitting services with a younger family who does her shopping. Another example is a university student offering to shovel snow for an elderly person in exchange for food. This trend is bound to increase in popularity: it promotes autonomy, reinforces independent behavior and adds the personal touch associated with self-care services. (In the appendix of this chapter the reader will find a list of services that can be found in most urban areas. Obviously the list is not exhaustive. It can nonetheless provide assistance in deciding what type of support one should seek when faced with certain problems.)

Some family systems, however, are incapable of calling on community resources even in a time of crisis. It is well known that the upper middle-class makes more use of the health care system than the lower class. There is a learning process involved in using health services. Some people do not know how to gain access to these resources; others are suspicious or do not want to get other people involved in their private lives. The family physician must develop a strategy on how to promote the services that are available; at the same time the family's right to privacy must be respected.

In contrast, many dysfunctional or illness-prone families[3] may overuse the health care system. These families use illness and professionals to provide nurturing that is unavailable or not given by their own families. More appropriate community sources of caring and comfort may decrease the need for illness and decrease health care costs. A knowledge of systems functioning permits the family physician to understand and make the best use of the community's network. The physician's management of the individual's or family's problem is aided by such knowledge, and a good doctor-patient relationship is maintained.

APPENDIX: A Sample Listing of a Community's Support and Service Network

ALCOHOLISM AND OTHER
  TOXICOMANIAS
Association for friends and relatives of
  alcoholics
Alcoholics Anonymous
Centers for rehabilitation of drug
  addiction
Detoxification clinics
Rehabilitation centers for alcoholics
Salvation army
Drug information centers

CHILDREN AND YOUTH
Awareness of legislation related to the
  youth
Youth courts
Social services
Reception centers
Group homes for children from broken
  homes
Re-educational treatment centers
Day care centers
Association for day care centers

School boards
Association for autistic children and their
parents
Association for emotionally disturbed
children
Learning disability centers
Rehabilitation centers
Speech and hearing clinics
Big Brother Association
Children's psychiatrist
Young People's Defense
YWCA, YMCA

EDUCATION
School boards
Universities
Center for continuing education
Department of adult education
Nursery schools

ELDERLY
Old Age Security
Day centers
Golden Age associations (in Canada; in
U.S.A. the equivalent organizations
are the Senior Citizens)
Homemakers care services
Nursing homes
Meals-on-Wheels services
Volunteer bureau

EMPLOYMENT
Unemployment agencies
Immigration center
Workmen's Compensation Commission
Vocational training centers
Minimum wage commission
Guidance centers
Placement agencies
Labor unions

HANDICAPPED
Government services
Association of the handicapped
Sports and activities for the handicapped
Citizen Advocacy
Rehabilitation centers
Sheltered workshop
Reception centers

Society for crippled children
Special education division
Wheel-chair dealers (sale, rental, repairs)
Institute for the blind
Cerebral Palsy Association
Association of hearing-impaired adults
and children
Paraplegia Association

HOUSING
Rental commission
Housing offices
Tenants association
Hostels and shelters
Salvation Army
YMCA and YWCA

IMMIGRANTS
Immigration offices
Immigration counselling and placement
Employment offices
Citizenship office and courts
Office of various ethnic communities

LEGAL SERVICES
Legal Aid
Charter of Human Rights (its applica-
tion)
Youth division
Criminal division
Legal clinics
Ombudsman

MENTAL HEALTH
Psychiatric clinics
Psychiatric youth services
Community psychiatric centers
Mental health centers
Out-patient services
Mental Health Association
Rehabilitation centers
Half-way houses
Parents Anonymous (for parents who
abuse children)

MENTAL RETARDATION
Association for the mentally retarded
Center for training retarded children
Homes for the mentally retarded

Day care for the mentally retarded
Sheltered workshops

ONE-PARENT FAMILIES
Association of one parent-families
Therapeutic groups of one-parent
  families

WOMEN'S ASSOCIATIONS
Council for women
Associations of women
Information and referral centers
YWCA
Widow's group
Mastectomy club
Agencies for divorcees

REFERENCES

1. Bowen M: The use of family theory in clinical practice. *Compr Psychiatry,* October:345, 1966.

2. Brownlee AT: Community Culture and Care: A Cross-Cultural Guide for the Health Worker, in *How to Assess the Community.* St. Louis, C.V. Mosby Co., 1978.

3. Hinkle LE Jr, Plummer N: Life stress and industrial absenteeism: The concentration of illness and absenteeism in one segment of a working population. *Ind Med Surg* 21:363, 1952.

4. Leigh H, Reiser MF: *The Patient: Biological and Social Dimensions of Medical Practice.* New York, Plenum, 1980.

5. Paul BD (ed): *Health Culture and Community: Case Studies of Public Reactions to Health Programs.* New York, Russell Sage Foundation, 1955.

Chapter 5
The Relationship Between Culture and Health or Illness

Margaret Lock

Cultural background is a powerful influence in shaping the unique way families handle and understand stress and illness. The physician's understanding of cultural factors can provide a context for medical care that is molded by the values of patients and their families rather than by the physician's own cultural orientation and belief system.

People in all cultures seek explanations for unwanted events such as illness and other misfortunes and devise techniques for averting them. During the early period of socialization, children are taught concepts relating to health and hygiene, such as why illness occurs and how to express and deal with pain and other symptoms. Explanations and methods of coping vary considerably from one society to another, reflecting the environment and culture in which a person is raised. Furthermore, in every culture there are individuals who maintain esoteric medical knowledge. These persons may also hold important political or religious posts in technologically undeveloped societies. With the introduction of technology and the division of the work force into specialized roles and occupations, the profession of medicine usually becomes secularized.

When patients come to a doctor, even in urban industrialized societies, they bring with them a set of preconceived ideas about such things as the information needed to make a diagnosis, the appropriate way to conduct themselves with the doctor, the cause of their problem, the kind of therapy they might need, and the kind of support their family should give them. It is now well documented that these acquired concepts and behavior patterns regarding health and illness not only vary according to ethnic background and social class but also frequently persist for many generations after migration to a different environment. Some examples will help to illustrate these behavioral differences.

Chinese, Japanese, and Koreans are usually taught, as part of their shared Confucian heritage, that cooperation and harmony within the family are of prime importance, and that expression of negative emotional feelings concerning human and especially family relationships is to be regarded unfavorably. Kleinman,[23] Lin,[31] Tseng,[51] and others have shown that although East Asian patients often focus on apparently minor somatic complaints when they arrive in a doctor's office, these complaints may mask feelings of depression and guilt that the patient is unable to express even when encouraged to do so. Tseng has concluded from his experience with East Asian patients that if the physician ignores the somatic complaints and tries to concentrate on the problem of depression, so much guilt may be induced that the problem will merely be aggravated. If, however, the somatic complaints are acknowledged as real and are discussed and treated when appropriate, the patient frequently recovers spontaneously from the depression or becomes more receptive to dealing with the psychological aspect of the problem. The patient and the patient's family want to focus initially on the physical problem because "somatization" is the culturally acceptable way of dealing with unacceptable emotional tension. If the physician attempts to deal with the psychological problems first, patient dissatisfaction is likely.

In a classic study, Zborowski[58] observed the differences in reaction to pain among various ethnic groups in a New York City hospital. He noted that Jewish and Italian patients responded to pain in an emotional fashion, in contrast with "Old Americans," who were more stoical and "objective," and persons of Irish descent, who more frequently denied pain. A difference was also apparent in the attitude underlying Italian and Jewish concern about pain: Italian patients primarily sought relief and were relatively satisfied when such relief was obtained, whereas Jewish patients appeared to worry mainly about the meaning and consequences of pain in relation to their future health and welfare. Accordingly, Italian patients seemed relieved when given analgesics while Jewish patients were reluctant to simply accept medication.

Such differences in attitude frequently go unnoticed by the clinician or, if perceived, are often regarded as being irrelevant to good medical practice. Since the dominant mode of clinical reasoning interprets symptoms as manifestations of underlying biological reality, the primary task of the physician is usually thought to be labelling diseases through the decoding and classification of particular symptoms; the "accurate" labelling of disease is considered a "true" reflection of biological reality, although it is widely recognized that cultural differences can contribute to this distortion. There is a tendency, therefore, to reinterpret or to ignore verbal data that in the physician's opinion do not readily accord with information obtained from the physical examination and laboratory tests.

A different kind of example is furnished by patients from the Caribbean, most of whom believe that a balance should be maintained within the body between substances defined as "hot" and "cold." If medication classified as "hot" (for example, penicillin) is prescribed, the patient is unlikely to take it if his or her illness is also believed to be "hot" because, according to the patient's belief system, "hot" medicine can only help a "cold" illness. Harwood[15] has shown that the rate of noncompliance in taking medication is very high if these beliefs are not acknowledged and accommodated by physicians.

Among black and southern white Americans and Haitians, there is particular concern about the generation, volume, circulation, purity, and viscosity of blood, based on the belief that diet can make blood volume go up or down and lead to conditions known as "high blood" and "low blood." Confusion of "high blood" with high blood pressure[45] can lead to misunderstanding and noncompliance since the patient assumes that the problem can be alleviated by a change of diet and taking folk medicines (for example, drinking brine and eating pickles). The idea that medication should be continued over a long period is rejected since "high blood" is not thought of as a chronic complaint.

Attitudes towards and expectations regarding the behavior of medical practitioners vary enormously: an East Indian patient who is accustomed to traditional medical practice in India expects a diagnosis to be made without his answering many questions or offering much information. A doctor who needs to ask numerous questions to make a diagnosis is regarded as doing a poor job.[17] Class differences have also been shown to play a major role in shaping patients' criteria for consulting a doctor: lower-class patients studied in the United States tend to wait until they regard a medical problem as being serious before they seek professional help, and they rarely acknowledge or present with psychological or social problems since these problems are usually regarded as being inevitable and unchangeable.[38]

Although patients' beliefs and attitudes are involved in every aspect of the medical encounter and can lead to serious difficulties in communication, no practitioner can reasonably be expected to be aware of all the differences among the members of an urban population in North America. Furthermore, there are dangers of stereotyping and even racism inherent in paying overdue attention to cultural values. Individual responses to events are frequently culturally patterned but are *not* culturally determined nor fully comprehensible through an understanding of the culture in question alone. The meaning of the illness experience to the individual patient should be taken into consideration *whatever* the patient's cultural background or class may be, not simply to encourage cooperation but because an understanding of it, by both patient and doctor, is an intrinsic part of the healing process.

The Distinction Between Organic or Physiologic Abnormalities and Clinical Illness: The Health Belief System

Students in contemporary medical education learn how to diagnose and treat abnormalities in the structure and function of body organs and systems. Patients and their families, in contrast, suffer a complex of physical, psychological, and social disorders commonly referred to as illness; the experience of illness is endowed with meaning, and is usually associated with negative affect and with concern about possible disruptions in lifestyle. There is no simple relation between clinical symptoms of illness and organic or physiologic abnormalities. Similar degrees of organ pathology may generate quite different reports of pain and distress in different patients;[59,3] illness may occur in the absence of organic or physiologic abnormalities (it is estimated that half of visits to the doctor are for complaints without a demonstrable biological basis); and patients can have a disease but experience no symptoms (such as hypertension). The course of a disease can be different from the accompanying symptomatology; for example, the physical symptoms are removed but the patient continues to feel depressed.

Drawing on clinical experience, Kleinman[24] concludes that it is essential to elicit the patients' explanation of the illness. Some questions that will help patients express their beliefs and concerns include the following:

1. What do you think caused your problem?
2. Why do you think it started when it did?
3. What do you think your sickness does to you?
   How does it work?
4. What are the most important results you hope to receive from the treatment?
5. What are the chief problems your sickness has caused you?
6. What do you fear most about your sickness?

Wording of the questions will vary depending on the personality of the patient, the nature of the medical problem, and the setting, but the goal in each case is to gauge and record the extent of the patient's understanding of the cause, implications, and meaning of the illness. The physician should always explain to each patient his or her understanding of the illness in simple terms. The two explanations can then be compared and, when required, interpretations and accommodations can be made to create a therapeutic alliance.

Several studies[25,55] have shown that patient satisfaction and compliance are directly correlated to the way in which information is transmitted; noncompliance and dissatisfaction occur when patients believe that the information they have received regarding their illness is insufficient, contradictory, or confusing. There is also a growing body of evidence demonstrating a relationship between effective transmission of information and beneficial physiological and psychological changes in patients during hospitalization, especially for surgical procedures.[7,10,18,44] The healing process is actually enhanced when patients feel that they are well informed regarding their medical problems. Good communication also improves medical history taking and medical records. Good and Good[12] have demonstrated that helping patients and their families to explore the meaning an illness has for them can also foster healing.

Traditional medical practitioners routinely make use of symbolic processes and ritual in their therapeutic sessions.[16,27,49,52] Such rituals, although often dismissed by observers as irrational behavior, are performed with the express purpose of attributing a meaning to the illness which makes sense in relation to the patient's experience and social context. A similar approach is routinely used by psychiatrists and clinical psychologists; comparisons of the techniques of the shaman with those of the psychotherapist have been made several times.[28,29,50]

Exploring the meaning of illness can be particularly important when a problem is chronic and can, as Remen[39] points out, "make the difference between someone who is invalided and someone who is able to live fully within the limitations set by his or her physical condition." There is now scientific evidence to justify such an approach,[1,22,40] which has recently been adopted by some pediatricians, oncologists, and general practitioners, and has been applied to a wide range of medical problems.[39,43]

THE FAMILY AND HEALTH CARE

It has been estimated that 70% to 90% of all sickness episodes in North America are handled without the help of the established health care system.[60] Popular and folk sectors of the society, particularly the family, self-help groups, and heterodox healers, provide a substantial part of all health care. Recent immigrants are especially reluctant to use established care; language barriers and unfamiliarity with the system are deterrents for this group of persons.

Alternative Medical Systems

Biomedicine* is now available to some extent in all societies with the exception of a few isolated tribal groups; nevertheless, it has not replaced the use of traditional medical systems anywhere. (In southeast Asia, for example, only about 15% of the population have access to modern health care facilities.[53])

Medical systems can be divided into three broad groups:

1. biomedicine
2. classical, literate medical traditions such as traditional Chinese medicine, the Ayurvedic systems of India, or the Yunani system used in the Middle East. The explanatory models used in these medical systems are based on ideas very similar to those underlying the

---

*Since medical practice based on a scientific approach to the human body takes a variety of forms around the world, it is referred to as biomedicine rather than as a Western medicine or modern medicine.

concept of homeostasis. The system is always secular and practice is limited to trained professionals.
3. folk medical traditions in which medical practice is frequently, but not exclusively, associated with religious beliefs and rituals.

Every medical system provides explanantions for the cause of disease, a classification system to aid diagnosis, therapeutic techniques, and a set of concepts regarding preventive medicine.

The study of beliefs about the etiology of disease and diagnostic practices brings the relation between medical beliefs and their cultural context to light. Lieban[30] states: "Since etiology is so inextricable from its socio-cultural context, explanations of the occurrence of illness are at the same time representations of the world as it is experienced and comprehended by members of the society." The purpose of the diagnostic procedure in any medical system is to facilitate appropriate therapeutic action, but in many cultures diagnosis does not depend to the extent that it does in biomedicine on observing physical signs and eliciting symptoms. Even when physical symptoms are observed, the most important part of the diagnostic process is frequently the determination of what set of events caused the patient to become ill. The process of identifying these events may take the form of what Young, drawing on the work of Foucault, has described as "externalizing" and "internalizing" discourses.[57] Young visualizes medical discourses as forming a continuum:

> At one end are the discourses that rely on etiological explanations. For convenience's sake, we refer to these as externalizing discourses since they concentrate on events and relations that are external to the sick person's body. Externalizing discourses appear to be limited to some technologically simple societies. At the opposite end of the continuum are discourses relying on functional explanations, i.e., internalizing discourses. While most of the world's medical discourses are located somewhere between the extremes, Western medicine is an extreme example of internalizing discourse.

It is typical of externalizing discourses that agents such as spirits, witches, and insects are used as explanatory devices for the occurrence of illness. These agents may be thought to induce physical changes in the human body, but the particular agent cannot be discerned by a study of physical symptoms. Divination is the usual means of determining the original cause of the illness. In this type of explanatory system the onset of illness is not regarded as an arbitrary event, but as an indication of social or cosmic forces that have been disrupted in some way. Thus, friction in interpersonal relationships or between members of a society and supernatural powers,[2,19] for example, can precipitate illness. Such explanatory systems, therefore, locate most of the important changes and events outside of the sick person's body. Religious beliefs, kinship relationships, and economic and political organization are believed to play a role in illness, and these variables must be manipulated as part of the therapeutic process. Such beliefs are widely disseminated in North America today[11,14,26,45] and have been documented among white groups living in the Bible Belt, rural black groups, native Americans, and groups of Caribbean or Mediterranean origin.

Internalizing discourses focus on objects and events inside the body. The cause of illness may be accounted by a single factor such as a specific bacillus or by a number of factors such as diet and emotional states (as in the literate medical traditions of Asia). The question of why one person and not another becomes ill at any given time is readily explored using a multi-factorial approach.

The purpose of labelling a disease and the choice of therapy vary from culture to culture depending on which types of signs and symptoms are considered significant. Traditional medical systems focus on the *experience* of illness, sometimes at the expense of dealing with the disease. This means that a traditional practitioner is often able to establish good patient communication and rapport rather easily, since he or she can focus on the psychological and social aspects of the problem likely to be uppermost in the patient's mind. Furthermore, a traditional practitioner usually draws on a shared set of culturally derived values to provide an explanation for the patient and the patient's family. Traditional practitioners take for granted that the family should be actively involved at every stage of the therapeutic intervention and that behavioral adjustments will be expected on their part as well as on that of the patient.[8]

Popular Medicine

The explanatory model that patients construct to deal with illness is derived from the ideas of health and illness which people learn everywhere as part of their socialization process. These ideas are known as the "popular health care system," and include all those beliefs and practices that are carried out in a lay context without the participation of health care professionals or institutional advisors. Emphasis in the popular domain is on health maintenance, but also included are ideas about the labelling and evaluation of an illness, selection of the appropriate action to take when ill, and judgments about efficacy of treatment. Knowledge obtained during the early socialization process from the educational system and the religious system are closely related to and form part of the popular medical system. Philosophical ideas, such as beliefs about the nature of reality and the concept of self, are integral to the popular health care system, as are psychological concepts, such as the management of dependency, nurturance, aggression, sexuality, etc. Beliefs about healthy family functioning, personal relationships of all kinds, and the role of society vis-à-vis individuals and families are also important.

Some ideas in the popular system about the structure and mechanism of the human body and some of the lay therapeutic practices are derived in part from the professional and folk medical systems of the society in question. In a pluralistic society like North America, the popular medicine of some families are influenced largely by biomedicine, but in many other families popular medical practice draws on traditional medicine or a mixture of the two.

Family Structure and its Function in Dealing with Illness

There is considerable cross-cultural variation in the structure and function of the family system, and some knowledge of this variation is important in the clinical setting, since there are wide differences in what is considered "normal" and "healthy" behavior. These cultural attitudes can affect the way illnesses and behavioral problems are labelled or even if they are labelled at all. For example, in all Asian families vertical relationships take precedence over horizontal relationships; the closest ties are between parents and children and not husband and wife. Even in contemporary Japan it is considered "normal" for parents to bathe and sleep with their children, often until early adolescence.

Writing of Southern European families living in North America, Sumic[48] states:

> Boundaries against "outsiders" and "foreigners" are continually strengthened through parental authority, appeals to moral absolutes, and negative stereotyping, while at the same time family unity is emphasized as the primary bastion of obligation, fulfillment, and security. One manifestation of this mentality is de-emphasis of the concept of privacy and private property within the home, combined with a prevailing ethic of secrecy and rejection in respect to persons outside this tight-knit group.

In such families, the concept of individual rights is at great variance with what is considered usual for North America. With immigrant families, difficulties can arise in adolescent medicine and in gynecology where confidentiality between patient and doctor to the exclusion of other family members is not considered acceptable.

In North America problems of acculturation and isolation are often very severe in immigrant and refugee families, and the situation is exacerbated for young people who have been raised in extended families and socialized for a life involving close inter-dependency with several family members. In an extended family, male and females roles are usually quite separate, and a very close relationship between husband and wife is not expected or very common. Male members of the household maintain very strong ties with other males both within and outside of the family and actually spend very little time each day with the women of the household. Similarly, women develop strong ties with other women. The husband / wife relationship is thought of as a contract between two families; friendship may arise from it but it is not usually regarded primarily as a romantic or highly intimate relationship. Young couples from families such as these who decide to set up a separate household frequently find it extremely hard to sustain an intimate partnership, and severe psychological and social problems can arise which are often exacerbated by ostracism from the older generation. Establishing some links with similar first-generation nuclear families of the ethnic group in question might be useful in such cases. Much more research is needed on intergenerational conflict in immigrant families and its effect on health.

The role of the family during illness also varies cross-culturally. Responsibility for dealing with an illness is usually regarded as being within the family; the task of handling illness particularly falls on the mother or grandmother. The physician is an expert consultant but not someone to whom one turns over all responsibility.[47] Medical advice and recommendations are discussed within the family; if the family has strong ties to the ethnic community, it is highly likely that alternative types of medical care will be considered or made use of.[16]

Moreover, for first-generation immigrants, being separated from family members during hospitalization can be extremely traumatic for a patient. The family may experience guilt, producing considerable hostility towards hospital-based medicine. Asian patients and many North African and Southern European patients expect family members to come and go in the hospital ward quite freely and perform many of their personal chores for them.

Responsibility for preventive medicine is also a family matter. Beliefs about prevention of illness are often particularly resistant to change, since they are frequently positively associated with family nurturance and care. During acculturation and in times of stress, one way in which a family often adapts positively is to reinforce ritual behavior in the home. Food and the process of eating is one such area and is laden with symbolic associations and meaning.[5] By re-introducing or emphasizing a traditional diet, the strength and continuity of the family can be reaffirmed. If dietary changes are indicated in illness, then they should be designed, if possible, to fit into the traditional dietary patterns of the ethnic group in question.

It has been shown that the use of traditional healers increases in a population which has recently migrated to an urban environment and that the availability of the healers actually facilitates the process of acculturation.[37] Other studies have demonstrated that it is important for people to maintain some traditional values even though they are trying to adapt to a new environment; maintenance of core values appears to provide a resistance against the incidence of diseases associated with stress.[42,34]

Another body of research has been directed towards examining the social support system of individuals. Cobb[4] argues that the presence of social supports facilitates coping with stress; this hypothesis is now supported by several studies.[6,13,35] To facilitate both therapeutic and preventive medicine, therefore, it may be important for a family practitioner to act positively in connection with a patient's ties to his or her ethnic community in addition to the family, and also in the use of traditional medicine if it appears to offer an acceptable support system.

The Meaning of Illness

The meaning attributed to illness depends on an individual's personal experiences and on his or her particular cultural background. A complete symbolic analysis of the experience of an illness entails an intimate knowledge of both the life history and the culturally derived value system of the patient.

An example from Japan illustrates the close relationship between cultural beliefs and the epidemiology of disease. It is well known that Japanese people suffer inordinately from stomach problems and that when they contract cancer it is frequently in the stomach. Diet certainly is a contributing factor to this problem, and so possibly is genetics, but there may be other factors. The abdomen, *hara* in Japanese, occupies the place corresponding to that of the heart in many Western cultures, culturally, linguistically, and as a locus of disease. From early historical times the abdominal region has been viewed as the center of the body, the source of emotions, and, if one is properly trained, the origin of great physical and mental powers. Many everyday terms in Japanese used to express emotional states make use of the word *"hara."* For example, the literal translation of *hara no okii* is "the abdomen is big," meaning "to be big-hearted, generous," and to have a black *hara* means to be "black-hearted," "evil," or "wicked."

Japanese people today still show great concern about their abdominal regions. In modern Japan, the classical concept of *hara* has become blurred with that of the biomedical concept of stomach (*in Japanese.*) The psychological and symbolical significance of *hara* and of the classical East Asian medical terms for the abdominal region have been transferred in the minds of many Japanese to their anatomical stomachs, where their concern is compounded by the high incidence of actual disease. Stomach diseases are greatly feared because it is believed that if the stomach is functioning poorly the whole body will be out of balance. In a sample of 250 informants, 78% said that mild tension first becomes manifest as a stomach problem; more medication is prescribed for stomach complaints than for any other type of problem in Japan.[32] Concern with this part of the anatomy is demonstrated in several ways; one example is that many manual laborers wear a *haramaki*, a 6-inch-wide wool or cotton band, around their upper abdomen to keep that region at a constant, warm temperature. Even in the Tokyo summer the *haramaki* is not uncommon.

Another example is a seizure-like disorder that occurs predominantly among black Americans, who label the problem "falling out"; among Bahamians, who call it "blacking-out"; and among Haitians, whose term for the problem is "indisposition." Fairly extensive studies indicate that the physical manifestations of this problem are very similar in all three cultures, as are the popular explanations for the cause of the disorder. Since the problem is not usually dealt with in medical clinics it is difficult to estimate its prevalence; however, in one study in Haiti, 43% of 69 respondents in a non-random sample reported having had "indisposition," and 72% had seen people with it.[36] The symptoms are described by Weidman:[54]

> In each instance the state described is one in which the individual collapses. For some this occurs without warning; for others it is preceded by feelings of "dizziness," "swinging" or "swimming" in the head. At times there is a degree of salivation but usually not. The episode generally occurs without convulsions without tongue-biting and without bowel or bladder incontinence. These are all points which help to differentiate it from grand mal epilepsy and psychomotor seizures. The eyes are ordinarily open, but darkness is said to come "before" them. Thus, the individual tends not to "see" in the psychological sense, even though he may have no defect of vision in the neurological sense. He usually hears and understands what is going on about him but feels powerless to move.

If patients with such symptoms undergo a neurological examination, the EEG findings are usually within normal limits and the most frequent diagnosis is of "idiopathic epilepsy." Rorschach tests given to ten young Haitian subjects with this condition indicated that they were not hysterics.[36] In Weidman's experience this problem, "whether encountered in neurology, family medicine, or psychiatry, falls into a 'left-over' or 'hard to diagnose' category."[54]

The popular explanation for the origin of this condition is that it is due to either "high" blood or "low" blood. "High" blood is thought to be caused by an emotional shock or heightened emotional state; the blood "rises" in the body. "Low" blood is caused by a poor nutritional state, or it can be linked to menstruation or other forms of blood loss; in this case, insufficient blood is sent to the head. In both instances, the result is an episode of "falling out" or "indisposition." The use of states of dissociation in religious and other ritualized contexts is common in the Caribbean, particularly Haiti, and among people belonging to pentacostal groups in North America. An occasional occurrence of "falling-out" in a suitable social context is regarded as normal but should the problem persist, then home remedies are resorted to. If the episodes become progressively debilitating, then witchcraft will probably be considered as the major cause of the problem and a traditional healer may be consulted. Very few informants believe that a medical practitioner is suitable for this type of illness.[36]

Relatively few people who experience "falling-out" become chronically debilitated, but those who do become socially isolated and withdrawn.

Weidman[54] interprets such behavior as an attempt to handle stress which threatens to be or is already overwhelming, and documents cases involving sexual conflict, extreme fear, or anger. Given a world view in which the environment is perceived as a basically hostile place and in which fear of witchcraft and attendant social ostracism for such belief is dominant, a mechanism for withdrawal can generally be interpreted as an adaptive response. The most suitable therapeutic setting for this kind of problem is in a medical and religious context in which the sufferer is socially and psychologically reintegrated into family and community, often through the positive use of dissociative states. Researchers dealing with this syndrome unanimously recommend closer cooperation between medical personnel and traditional healers; a fully documented account of a case study involving such cooperation is given by Rubin and Jones.[41]

The complexity and ramifications of the experience of illness, therefore, become apparent through a study of popular medical beliefs and practice. Such an analysis clearly cannot be undertaken for every patient, nor is it necessary. But by eliciting the patient's explanatory model of illness, it is possible to gain some insight into the patient's point of view, the meaning of the illness episode, and the expectations brought to the medical encounter.

A brief examination of the meanings attributed to a normal life-cycle transition will provide the final example in this section. Major changes in the life-cycle, particularly birth, death, and the attainment of adulthood, are events that are a source of considerable ambiguity and stress. Usually the result is some form of loss necessitating a reorganization on the part of the group involved; eventually, if the reorganization is successful a new equilibrium is attained.

Menopause is one such transition in which cultural values and the previous life history of the individual shape the meaning and experience of the event. The physiological changes at menopause act as a marker for the sociocultural event, the "change of life." At one level there is a clear, unambiguous message attached to this experience: the end of fertility. But the meaning of the process is profoundly influenced by the status, roles, and values of the woman in question and can be viewed as either a positive or negative event.

Among the Rajput of North India a woman who no longer menstruates can come out of purdah, visit other households more freely, and join the men of her own household without restrictions. Flint's[9] Rajput informants described a symptom-free menopause which she believes can be linked to their increased social status at this time. Among the Gisu, in contrast, La Fontaine[27] discusses the rejection of women by their own husbands and families once they can no longer give birth to children. She does not consider the relationship of this change in social status to the incidence of physiological symptoms during menopause but does link it to the high suicide rate in this age group. Kaufert and Syrotuik[21] point out that the cultural bias toward menopause stereotypes for all members of the society the experience of menopause; even the symptoms that are expected are included in the stereotype. Rajput women expect no symptoms; on the other hand, Manitoban women believe that most women are depressed and irritable at menopause.[20] Kaufert and Syrotuik[21] hypothesize that women whose self-esteem is high will not be as susceptible to a negative stereotype as women whose self-esteem is low. They suggest that women of low self-esteem are more liable to psychological distress and possibly to fluctuating hormone levels during menopause in societies in which there is negative stereotyping.

Previous life experiences also influence the event. Single working mothers of large families who are grandmothers by the age of 50 may hardly notice menopause because they can at this point be supported somewhat by their own children and are no longer extremely vulnerable financially. On the other hand, professional women who believe, rightly or wrongly, that maintaining their place in the competitive work environment means the denial or suppression of events associated with female biology may be vociferous in their demands for estrogen replacement therapy.[33] The practicing clinician, of course, stereotypes menopause according to his or her personal experiences. In an urban North American setting, this experience is unlikely to correspond with more than a minority of the patient population. It is important, therefore, for clinicians to explore not only the meaning of an illness or life-cycle event with a patient but also to examine their own preconceptions and biases that are brought to every medical encounter.

Ethical Dilemmas

Good communication between practitioners, patients, and families, and some insight into the illness of the patient are essential for family practice. Most frequently, such knowledge leads to a direct improvement in medical care,[24,12,39] but sometimes it can raise ethical dilemmas for the medical practitioner. Several brief case studies will illustrate this problem:

Mrs. C. is a first-generation Greek immigrant to Canada and the mother of a 20-month old, obese child. She believes her baby to be healthy and developing well, but each time she sees her pediatrician, he tells her that her child is overweight and should be given a more appropriate diet. Mrs. C., her mother, and her friends have lost confidence in the pediatrician because they believe that this advice is inappropriate since, for them, a fat baby is the epitome of good health, living proof of maternal care, and of the family's adequate financial resources. Because of her dissatisfaction, Mrs. C. plans to try out other pediatricians.

In this case, the value system of the mother is causing her to treat her baby in an unhealthy way according to the pediatrician. There is considerable scientific evidence to back up the pediatrician's point of view. He would be compromising his values not to chastise the mother even if he understood her viewpoint; yet it is probable that if the mother's belief system was elicited and sympathized with, and if the doctor spent some time explaining his reasoning to her, then a compromise might be reached. In the present situation the mother will simply look for another doctor. Another example raises the issue of diagnostic labelling and the implication of certain labels for family support of the patient.

A young Chinese male, 22 years old, was brought by four members of his family, his parents and his older brothers, to the out-patient department of a psychiatric hospital. The family had been referred there from the general out-patient department where they first presented themselves. The family, with great reluctance, said that the young man had been behaving strangely and described symptoms that the psychiatrist called "unusual thought content, hallucinatory experiences, and retarded motor behavior." Throughout the interview the family appeared very warm and supportive towards the patient and described in detail their care of him at home, including special diet, herbal medicines, extra personal attention, and some religious rituals. They went on to state that they wanted the young man to marry as soon as possible and to ask if the illness would interfere with these arrangements.

The psychiatrist, establishing that the patient had been exhibiting the symptoms for at least eighteen months and possibly longer, concluded the interview by telling the family that he thought the problem was a very serious psychiatric problem. He also told the family that the patient needed some tests and that he probably would eventually have to be hospitalized. The family did not keep their next appointment with the psychiatrist nor other subsequent ones that were made. About 6 months later the patient appeared in the evening in the emergency department of the hospital. His mother brought him, but while he was being examined, she disappeared. The patient was hospitalized, but the family never visited him and despite the efforts of a social worker, no contact could be re-established between the patient and his family.

To a Chinese family the diagnostic label of severe mental illness induces great shame and guilt; the illness is most frequently viewed as a punishment for moral misconduct by either the patient or family members and the whole family feels threatened with possible ostracism by their community. A psychiatric department is usually the last resort for family members who have tried all available forms of traditional Chinese medicine and have focused on the somatic rather than the behavioral aspects of the problem. They probably have labelled the illness with one of several Chinese terms that indicate that the problem is physiological in origin. Exploration of psychological factors and family dynamics in connection with such a problem is seen as entirely inappropriate unless pursued indirectly in the context of a Chinese temple. The hope of family members when they finally meet a psychiatrist is that, since all else has failed, he or she may be able to give them some effective medication.

Once the label of severe mental illness was applied, the family's fear of social retribution became so great that all warmth and care lavished on the patient while he was thought of as physically ill ceased quite abruptly: to save the family the individual was abandoned.

In such a case, the psychiatrist probably could not have elicited many details from the family about their expectations and hopes without first establishing good rapport over a period of several weeks or months. One possible way to do this would be to focus on the somatic aspects of the illness, to avoid overt psychiatric labelling of the problem, and also to avoid hospitalization unless absolutely necessary. Under these circumstances the family probably would have continued to be supportive of the patient, especially if the psychiatrist could demonstrate that he was not completely opposed to alternative healing systems. It is possible that the patient and his family could only survive as a unit if there was some sort of cooperation between the psychiatrist and a traditional shamanistic healer.

A 15-year-old girl was brought by her mother, a first-generation immigrant from Greece, and her aunt to the family practice department of a Montreal hospital. The aunt acted as translator. The girl was slightly obese; she complained of an inability to sleep properly and repeated headaches. She appeared withdrawn during the interview and, after a physical examination, was diagnosed as a case of mild depression. The physician asked the mother to allow the girl to come for her next appointment alone, hoping that he could talk more comfortably with her; this strategy proved ineffective. The physician then talked to the aunt on the telephone and, as a result of this conversation, came to the conclusion that intergenerational conflict was a key to the girl's depression; the patient had spent her childhood in North America but, when not in school, was expected to have all her free time monitored closely by family members.

The physician still hopes to win the girl's confidence and to be able to discuss her feelings towards her family with her. He states that his understanding of the situation ensures that the case will not become overly "medical." His therapeutic stance should be that all first-generation families have to deal with acculturation, that the problem is gradually resolved with the passage of time, and that if the symptoms do not get worse he should not run the risk of meddling in a problem relating to important family values which are alien to him.

This third example is more complex. The physician in charge of this case feels incompetent to handle Greek family dynamics, and, in any case, is too young to be an acceptable confidant for the family. Moreover, it is quite possible that the physician's psychosomatic model for the cause of the illness is at variance with that of the patient and her family. If the family members make no connection between family relationships and the incidence of headaches and insomnia, then they will probably be dissatisfied with the medical encounters, since the physician is providing neither medication nor any other kind of relevant treatment, as far as the family is concerned. An exchange of explanatory systems may help the situation. If the family should then become amenable to a discussion of their relationships to one another, then the young physician will have to refer them to an older colleague who, ideally, would have some knowledge of Greek family organization, or the network of support in the Greek community, or both.

> An elderly Italian man had been diagnosed as having lung cancer and expected to live only a few more months. Several members of his immediate family came to the physician in charge of the case and through a translator asked that the man not be told of his impending death. They said that if this knowledge were given to him and to other family members, it would erode his authority and the position of respect that he enjoyed and valued above everything else. The physician agreed to maintain secrecy, and even when the patient himself asked if he was going to die did not give him any information. The physicians and nursing staff involved felt that by respecting culturally patterned family beliefs, they were acting in a sensitive fashion to this patient's needs.

In this instance, patient and family wishes are clearly in conflict. After discussion of the case with some of the staff involved, it appears that being "culturally sensitive" may simply have been the easiest way out of a frequent dilemma for hospital staff. It is a temptation to avoid informing patients of their approaching death; in this case, such a course of action was justified in terms of the family wishes and respect for Italian values. Further discussion with the family about the patient's wishes appears warranted; following cultural norms may not have been the most appropriate course of action. (Further discussion of the "conspiracy of silence" and cultural values can be found in the chapter on death and dying, Chapter 22.)

The meaning and implications of an illness event must therefore be understood independently by both patient and family members. Explanations and behavior, although mediated through socialization into a culture, are ultimately idiosyncratically created. Both levels of interpretation need to be considered, as well as intrafamilial variation.

It is important to understand that popular medical beliefs and practices are part of a complete cultural system and not simply random behavior occuring in isolation. For this reason, it is extremely difficult to produce changes in such behavior because it is always related to other important aspects of the patient's life and existence. Much behavior is learned very early in life and is therefore associated with the development of an awareness of concepts such as nurturance, dependence, and belonging. It is taught in association with feeding, bathing, and other types of close parental contact and is therefore often laden with affect. These beliefs may be reinforced by the religious system and the educational system and become part of a central value system which is essential to the survival of humans in social groups.

Research indicates that it is necessary for patients to try to answer not only "how" they became ill but "why" they became ill; physicians can answer many of the "how" questions but very few of the "why" questions. In order to cope with an illness successfully, a patient must turn to his or her family, support groups of various kinds, and to a cultural heritage to attribute meaning to the event. The medical practitioner's role in this process should be to facilitate the patient's exploration of his or her reactions to the illness while at the same time attending to the process of the disease.

REFERENCES

1.   Amkraut A, Solomon GF: From the symbolic stimulus to the pathophysiologic response: Immune mechanisms. *Int J Psychiatry Med* 5:541, 1974

2.   Beattie J, Middleton J (eds): *Spirit Mediumship and Society in Africa*. London, Routledge & Keagan Paul, 1969.

3.   Beecher HK: Relationship of the significance of wound to the pain experienced. *JAMA* 161:1609, 1956.

4.   Cobb S: Social support as a moderator of life stress. *Psychosom Med* 38:300, 1976.

5.   Douglas M: *Purity and Danger: An Analysis of Concepts of Pollution and Taboo*. London, Routledge & Kegan Paul, 1966.

6.   Dressler W: Coping dispositions, social supports, and health status. *Ethos* 8(2):146, 1980.

7.   Egbert LD, Battit GE, Welch CE, et al: Reduction of postoperative pain by encouragement and instruction of patients. *N Engl J Med* 270:825, 1964.

8.   Fabrega H, Silver DB: *Illness and Shamanistic Curing in Zincantan*. Stanford, Stanford University Press, 1973.

9.   Flint, M: *Menarche and Menopause of Rajput Women*,thesis. New York, City University of New York, 1974.

10. Frank J: Mind-body relationships in illness and healing. *J Int Acad Prev Med* 2(3):46, 1975

11. Garrison V: The "Puerto Rican Syndrome" in psychiatry and *Espiritismo*, in Crapanzano V, Garrison V (eds): *Case Studies in Spirit Possession*. New York, John Wiley and Sons, 1977.

12. Good B, DelVecchio Good MJ: The meaning of symptoms: A cultural hermeneutic model for clinical practice, in Eisenberg L, Kleinman A (eds): *The Relevance of Social Sciences for Medicine*. Boston, D. Reidel Pub Co., 1980.

13. Graves TD, Graves NB: Stress and health: Modernization in a traditional Polynesian society. *Med Anthropol* 3:23, 1979.

14. Hand WD: *American Folk Medicine.* Berkeley, University of California Press, 1976.

15. Harwood A: A hot-cold theory of disease implications for treatment of Puerto Rican patients. *JAMA* 216:1153, 1971.

16. Harwood A: Puerto Rican spiritism. Part 1. Description and therapeutic functions in community psychiatry. *Cult Med Psychiatr* 1:135, 1977.

17. Henley A: *Asian Patients in Hospital and at Home.* Tunbridge, Wells, Pitman Medical Publishing Co., 1979.

18. Janis IL: *Psychological Stress: Psychoanalytic and Behavioral Studies of Surgical Patients.* New York, Wiley, 1958.

19. Janzen J: *The Quest for Therapy in Lower Zaire.* Berkeley, University of California Press, 1978.

20. Kaufert, P: The perimenopausal woman and her use of health services. *Maturitas* 2:191, 1980.

21. Kaufert P, Syrotuik J: Symptom Reporting at the Menopause. *Soc Sci Med* 15:173, 1981.

22. Kiley WF: From the symbolic stimulus to the pathophysiological response: Neurophysiological mechanisms. *Int J Psychiatry Med* 5:517, 1974.

23. Kleinman A: *Patients and Healers in the Context of Culture: An Exploration of the Borderland between Anthropology, Medicine, and Psychiatry.* Berkeley, University of California Press, 1980.

24. Kleinman A, Eisenberg L, Bood B: Culture, illness, and care: Clinical lessons from anthropologic and cross-cultural research. *Ann Intern Med* 88:251, 1978.

25. Korsch BM, Gozzi EK, Francis V: Gaps in doctor-patient communication: Doctor-patient interaction and patient satisfaction. *Pediatrics* 42:855, 1968.

26. La Barre W: *They Shall Take up Serpents: Psychology of the Southern Snake Handling Cult.* New York, Shocken, 1969.

27. LaFontaine J: Homicide and suicide among the Gisu, in Bohannan, P (ed): *African Homicide and Suicide.* Princeton, Princeton University Press, 1960, pp. 94-129.

28. Lederer W: Primitive psychotherapy, in Cos RH (ed): *Religious Systems and Psychotherapy.* Springfield, Thomas, 1973.

29. Lévi-Strauss C: *Structural Anthropology.* Garden City, New York, Anchor Books, 1967.

30. Lieban RW: Medical anthropology, in Honigman J (ed): *Handbook of Social and Cultural Anthropology.* Chicago, Rand McNally, 1973.

31. Lin T, Lin M: Love, denial and rejection: Responses of Chinese families to mental illness, in Kleinman A, Lin T (eds.): *Normal and Abnormal Behavior in Chinese Cultures.* Dordrecht, D Reidel Publishing Co., 1981.

32. Lock M: *East Asian Medicine In Urban Japan: Varieties of Medical Experience.* Berkeley, University of California Press, 1980.

33. Lock M: Models and practice in medicine: Menopause as syndrome or life transition? *Cult Med Psychiatr* 6:261, 1982.

34. Marmot MG, Leonard S: Acculturation and coronary heart disease in Japanese-Americans. *Am J Epidemiol* 104:225, 1976.

35. Nuckolls KB, et al: Psychosocial assets, life crisis, and the prognosis of pregnancy. *Am J Epidemiol* 95:431, 1972.

36. Philippe J, Romain JB: Indisposition in Haiti. *Soc Sci Med* 13B:129, 1978.

37. Press I: Urban folk medicine. *Am Anthropolgist* 80(1):71, 1978.

38. Rainwater L: The lower class: Health, illness, and medical institutions, in Millon T (ed): *Medical Behavioral Science*. Philadelphia, W.B. Saunders, 1975.

39. Remen N: *The Human Patient*. Garden City, New York, Anchor Books, 1980.

40. Rogers MP, Dubey D, Reich P: The influence of the psyche and the brain on immunity and disease susceptibility. *Psychosom Med* 41(2):147, 1979.

41. Rubin JC, Jones J: Falling-out: A clinical study. *Soc Sci Med* 13B:117, 1979

42. Scotch NA: Sociocultural factors in the epidemiology of Zulu hypertension. *Am J Pub Health* 53:1205, 1963.

43. Simonton C, Matthews Simonton S, Creighton JL: *Getting Well Again*. New York, Bantam Books, 1979.

44. Skipper JK, Leonard RC: Children, stress, and hospitalization: A field experiment. *J Health Soc Behav* 9:275, 1968.

45. Snow L: Folk beliefs and their implications for care of patients. *Ann Intern Med* 81:82, 1974.

46. Sontag S: *Illness as Metaphor*. New York, Farrar, Straus and Giroux, 1977.

47. Stimson G: Obeying doctor's orders. *Soc Sci Med* 8:97, 1974.

48. Sumic A: White ethnic and Chicano families: Continuity and adaptation in the new world, in Tufte V, Myerhoff B (eds): *Changing Images of the Family*. New Haven, Yale University Press, 1979.

49. Tambiah SJ: The cosmological and performative significance of a Thai cult of healing through meditation. *Cult, Med Psychiatry* 1:97, 1977.

50. Torrey EF: *The Mind Game: Witchdoctors and Psychiatrists*. New York, Emerson Hall, 1972.

51. Tseng WS: The nature of somatic complaints among psychiatric patients: The Chinese case. *Compar Psychiatry* 16:237, 1975.

52. Turner V: *The Forest of Symbols: Aspects of Ndembu Ritual*. Ithaca, New York, Cornell University Press, 1967.

53. Vogel EF: *Japan's New Middle Class: The Salary Man and His Family in a Tokyo Suburb*. Berkeley, University of California Press, 1968.

54. Weidman H: Falling-out: A diagnostic and treatment problem viewed from a transcultural perspective. *Soc Sci Med* 13B:95, 1979.

55. Williams TF, Martin DA, Hogan MD, et al: The clinical picture of diabetes control, studied in four settings. *Am J Pub Health* 57:441, 1967

56. World Development Report: Washington, The World Bank, 1980.

57. Young AA: Mode of Production of Medical Knowledge. *Med Anthropol* 2:97, 1978.

58. Zborowski M: Cultural components in responses to pain. *J Soc Issues* 8:16, 1952.

59. Zola IK: Culture and symptoms: An analysis of patients' presenting complaints. *Am Soc Rev* 31:615, 1966.

60. Zola IK: Studying the decision to see a doctor. *Adv Psychosom Med* 8:216, 1972.

Chapter 6
Value Systems and the Family

Lewis Bird
Janet Christie-Seely
Marie Yaremko-Dolan

VALUES AND THE FAMILY SYSTEM

The family value system is an important component of the family personality. It is the set of principles, goals, and standards accepted and generally adhered to by the members of the family, both as individuals and as a group. It can consolidate the individual family members and yet possess the property of adaptability. Stress from sources external to the family system, as well as from within the family, affect the value system.

The family value system attempts to incorporate into its evolving matrix internal changes such as the aging process, generational gaps, illness, death, and many other crises. Since the family does not live in a void, external forces such as the blending of past and present cultural environments, changing societal demands, and changing religious beliefs must also be assimilated. The final product is a unique cohesive family value system which determines life-style, response to crisis, compliance with professional health care, and ethical decision-making. For instance, the relative virtues of honesty, hard work, pleasure, education, duty to others, and self-actualization vary from family to family: in one family a pregnant unwed teenager will be forced to leave home, whereas in another family with different cultural and societal standards the pregnancy may be celebrated.

A necessary change in values can be a slow and painful process or a welcome experience, depending on the stress which necessitated the change and on the family's ability to adapt to that stress. The clinician may be called on to assist in the process of adaptation and may even be asked to arbitrate intrafamilial value conflicts. A frequent value system change, which often results in conflict, is that experienced by newly immigrated families. As individual members of the family attempt to integrate into their new environment, conflict among them ensues. Often it is the younger generation or the working members who assimilate first; a common source of conflict is adolescent dating. Feelings of bewilderment, loss, and abandonment in the older generation and impatience and frustration in the younger ones surface and need to be explored.

Behavior and Lifestyle

Value systems are reflected in any individual's behavior and choice of lifestyle. Studies of both Mormon[14] and Seventh-Day Adventist[21] populations correlate values with cancer incidence and clearly demonstrate the relation between belief systems and disease patterns. In both of these groups, conservative smoking habits based on religious belief systems correlated with low rates of lung cancer. A similar study of Canadian Hutterite Brethren[9] supports the same conclusion; uterine cervical cancer was significantly less than the expected rate among the women of this isolated religious group. Where personal beliefs support an increased use of tobacco, alcohol, or drugs, whether due to cultural factors, personality needs, or religious usage, increased health risk can be anticipated. Further, the very low incidence of atherosclerotic heart disease in Mormons has been linked to their very low divorce rate: family support offers major protection against heart disease.[13]

Behavior reflects value systems in many ways. Examples include the choice of alcohol as a way of handling the trials of living, the denial of symptoms because illness is considered weakness, or the repression of emotions as "unmanly." Selecting a physician who understands the whole family (or, on the contrary, who "doesn't insist on seeing my wife too and getting into all that psychology stuff") also indicates different values. Family resources, which are so important to coping with crisis, reflect values; religious groups, community organizations, the importance of the extended family, and the attitude to helping agencies are all determined by the family's world view and attitude to asking for help.

In conclusion, the family value system manifests itself in the daily activities of the family members. The values can be a source of strength or conflict within the family, and can determine the health of individuals and their response to illness. Although espousing family independence and self-help in regard to health care is good, second thoughts concerning patient responsibility in the face of family and culturally conditioned health habits merit review:

> Our culture trains us, through its legal, community and family value systems, to seek a leisurely lifestyle of inadequate physical movement, a diet rich in fats and carbohydrates and lacking in essential nutrients, and a reduction of tension through the use of tobacco, alcohol and other drugs. How can you bring up a whole generation on eggs and bacon, only to adjure them to pay attention to their cholesterol levels? How can you bombard the adolescent mind with infinite inducements to pick up a cigarette and then expect the adult mind to protect his or

her heart and lungs? A great deal of energy, brain power and, above all, money has gone into marketing bad health in this country. It is naive and indeed irresponsible to hope that a few single-spaced articles in *Consumers Reports* will turn the situation around. The most likely outcome of this strategy will not be self-responsibility but only self-incrimination. Having been given none of the skills of taking responsibility, having had all too few experiences in their prepackaged lives for actually assuming responsibility, most people will cling to their candy bars and their cigarettes.[23]

UNDERSTANDING VALUE SYSTEMS

Figure 6-1 outlines some of the components of value systems that can apply to some or all system levels. Any natural system can be seen as having goal-directed behavior or values. This is true of nonhuman biological systems, but only at the human level can consciousness of values exist. Unconscious values can also exist at the level of individual, family, community, or culture; it is often conflict between conscious and unconscious or overt and covert values that causes problems.

The health of any system depends on clear communication between its parts, a hierarchical organization, and deference to the goals of the suprasystem when conflicts occur. This centralization and order must be balanced by sufficient decentralization and autonomy to allow individuation and growth of subsystems. Thus flexibility of a system allowing a wide range of possible solutions to a conflict of values is an indication of its health. For example, when various community methods of financing care are available a family financially burdened by raising a child with Down's syndrome need not be limited in the range of ethical solutions available (as seen in the case described in the next section). The community must decide on the extent of the burden on the taxpayer or on appropriate insurance rates. Such practical decisions and ethical guidelines are best made by the larger system. Doctors have been requesting for some time that they not be left alone in the difficult decisions involved in many health care issues.

Ethics and the Health Care System

"Medicine needs urgently to be sensitized to the intersections of values inherent in every medical act"—Edmund Pellegrino's[20] apt observation underscores the current sensitivity to problems in biomedical ethics. The issues which have attracted considerable attention both in the media and in government include abortion, infanticide, euthanasia, fetal experimentation, organ transplantation, surrogate motherhood, etc. These issues are only the more visible concerns of the health care community. In contrast to the public debate, little attention is paid to ethical problems in medical school; even less attention is given to such problems at the postgraduate level.

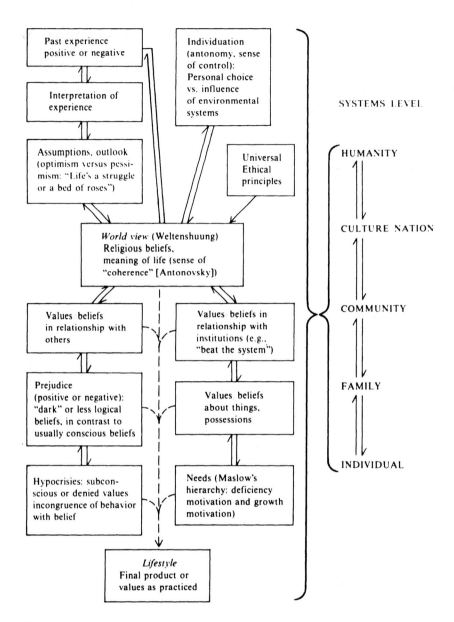

Figure 6-1. Value Systems. Congruence between different areas and between systems results in tranquility. Major discrepancies result in guilt, anger, embarrassment, or conflict between systems (for example, individual and family conflict over religion or lifestyle, especially if individuation is low). Illness may result (an escape into sick role or result of stress). Integration of all areas is complex and rarely fully achieved. Crisis or illness may represent disturbed homeostasis because of change in one area.

Patient care may inadvertently involve a number of ethical issues, including values related to diet, the management of health crises, family planning, sexual orientation and behavior, marital fidelity, terminal illness, surgical procedures, medication compliance, etc. While patients in the past may have offered little resistance to prescribed regimens, at present victims of either trauma or pathology may bring a range of assertive behaviors and assorted beliefs in regard to their clinical situations. Some responses may clarify the patient's expectations concerning treatment; others may only confuse or anger the health management team. Responsibility for decision making is a major contemporary ethical issue, as is excess control by the medical profession. Issues regarding resuscitation and termination of life support efforts are of particular concern. Physicians have been left alone for so long in these ethical dilemmas that they are unused to public debate; many, however, welcome the discussion, considering it long overdue.

The dehumanizing aspects of hospital care have been well documented and described.[8] Responding to this tendency to depersonalize patient care, Balfour M. Mount pioneered a hospice within a hospital, the palliative care unit at the Royal Victoria Hospital in Montreal, with specific regard for personal value systems. In his essay, "Caring in Today's Health Care System,"[18] the recommendation is made for hospital staff members to "increase the emphasis on psychosocial and spiritual issues related to the patient and key family members by assessing these areas, in addition to medical concerns, at the time of admission, establishing distinct goals and drawing up intervention plans."

The following case illustrates a typical sequence in the medical decision-making process in a large hospital where concern for the family's rights and values are peripheral to technical medical issues. Communication between professionals (surgeon, local doctor, clergyman) was almost nonexistent preventing a broader view and more careful assessment with support for a family at a time of crisis.

A six-day-old baby with Down's syndrome, a bowel obstruction, and jaundice was admitted to a children's hospital. The baby underwent tests which confirmed the mongolism, identified the obstruction as duodenal stenosis with possible atresia lower in the tract, and indicated a bilirubin level of 17 mg.

The parents of the child were young (the father was 21 years old, the mother 18 years old), and the father's position as an hourly worker suggested modest means. This had been the woman's first pregnancy. Operative permission was sought from the parents both for an exchange transfusion in the event that the baby's hematologic status did not stabilize and for surgery to correct the bowel obstruction. The parents had discussed the prognosis for the child with both their local physician and their clergyman. At their request, the baby had been baptized. When asked for permission to operate, they refused to grant it.

It was the opinion of the attending physician that the future for this child as pictured by the local doctor had been unduly pessimistic. The tenor of the conversation with the clergyman was not known. The hematologic condition did in fact stabilize overnight, forestalling the need for a transfusion. At a meeting of a wider consulting group the next morning, sentiments of varying degrees were expressed both for and against the decision of the parents. Parents in that state were financially responsible, according to their means, up to an amount of $3000 or more per year, for the upkeep of a child in the state hospital. The responsibility lasted until the child was 15 years of age.

This example and others in this chapter are used to illustrate the dilemmas of practice. There are no right solutions, although some solutions are better than others. Principles given later in the chapter may clarify issues in ethical decision-making.

Every system level has a set of values or goals: universal ethical principles theoretically provide normative values for mankind at large; each culture has a value system; social classes and communities have differing values; and each family and each individual within it has a unique set of values. The medical and nursing professions each have their own set of cherished values and goals, which sometimes differ considerably from those of the public. Since many medical decisions have an ethical component the problem lies in which of these levels should be consulted and what weight should be given to a particular opinion when opinions differ. Most clinicians feel it is a right of the patient to decide his or her own fate. The family may have to act as the patient's advocate when the age of the patient, or coma, confusion, or depression interfere with the ability of the patient to judge.

Ethical problems arise when there is conflict between universal principles or between value systems. This may be conflict within a system or between systems. There are many examples of such conflict: a surgeon may wish to perform a disfiguring operation to save life while a family physician is arguing for quality of life and an end to the family's suffering (conflict within the health care system); a patient's lifestyle may be at odds with the value he places on a long life (conflict or poor integration of values within the individual); a patient's lifestyle may be at odds with his family's lifestyle (conflict between systems); and finally, the clinician's and the patient's value system may conflict:

A young female patient presents with a 10-week pregnancy. She is an ambitious unmarried law student who lives alone. The pregnancy is unwanted at this time in her life and she requests an abortion. The physician, on the other hand, is married, has a wife devoted to rearing their five children and belongs to the pro-life movement. If the physician recognizes the patient's right to her own personal value system he may decide to avoid engendering guilt feelings in the patient or in himself by referring her to another doctor.

Management of conflict of values can be very difficult but is aided by understanding the components of value systems and the implications of decisions at each system level.

Universal Ethical Principles

While opinion is divided among professional ethicists about the existence of universal principles, a review of several specific universal principles in biomedical ethics may be useful.[4] These ethics usually govern the therapeutic relationship between practitioner and patient.

1. *Primum, non nocere* (First of all, do no harm)
2. The Sanctity of Human Life
3. The Alleviation of Suffering
4. The Confidentiality of the Physician-Patient Relationship
5. The Right to Truth
6. The Right to Informed Consent
7. The Right to Die with Dignity

Most difficult ethical decisions, however, occur when two or more universal principles conflict. The best decision in most instances is the one that weighs all known factors and judges which of two conflicting principles (such as the sanctity of human life versus the relief of suffering) should be upheld in this particular case. A case in the practice of one of the authors illustrates the limits of medical knowledge, the complexity of ethical decision-making, and the problems of medical responsibility.

Debbie is a 27-year-old woman with a rare congenital disease, Werdnig-Hoffmann's anterior horn cell degeneration. Normally fatal in patients by age three it is one of the causes of the "floppy baby syndrome." Debbie defied medical prognosis: when she lived past 3 years old; doctors said she'd die before she turned 9 years old—"After that they gave up predicting; I guess I've lived on borrowed time ever since." Highly intelligent, she has a warm, cheerful disposition but a distorted and paralyzed body. Her personality clearly was a means of survival in a woman who could eventually move only two fingers. She was totally dependent on a family that also had to cope with tuberculosis in the mother, and with a pituitary adenoma in the son, who grew to a height of six foot ten; alcoholism, obesity, and depression were the understandable sequellae in several family members.

At age 20, after a childhood lived in bed and wheelchair, Debbie developed a severe respiratory infection. She weighed 37 pounds. Debbie was essentially a very functional head on a useless, contorted but pain-free body. Five days after hospital admission she was severely dyspneic and cyanosed; she had been clearly asking for help, "do something or I'll die." The family physician, who had known her family for 2 years, and an intern, who also knew her, could get no opinion from the rest of the medical team as to whether a tracheostomy was justified. Given that the patient's wishes were clear, that the family also requested treatment, and that a few days or weeks of respirator care was predicted, these two physicians made the decision to do a tracheostomy.

For months after the operation the patient stayed on the respirator, unable to communicate unless laboriously writing with her two still functioning fingers. Incredibly she remained cheerful. Once she was depressed for 2 days and the family physician considered pulling the plug of the respirator; she decided that she would consider it seriously if the patient remained seriously depressed for more than 10 days. Five years later, 6 months after the patient was weaned from the respirator, the physician admitted her dilemma to the patient who responded with a laugh, "Thank God I didn't get depressed." To the patient life was more than worth it. On one occasion, chasing a friend with her new electric wheelchair in a park, she was confronted by a stranger who asked why she was smiling. Embarrassed, she said she was happy, then listened to him tell a tale of drug addiction, restless travelling, and failure. More and more angry at her contentment, he suddenly left. Her comment afterwards implied sympathy: "people . . . have so many problems." Her total lack of self-pity or martyrdom tends to arouse guilt in others.

Is her life worth the cost to society? Debbie lives in a hospital, making forays with friends to shops, movies or pubs; her family cannot cope with suctioning and nursing care. In Canada the cost to the taxpayer in a system of universal medicare and free hospitalization is enormous. Yet she educates all who meet her and enriches the lives of any who know her. She was a better teacher to a class of 160 medical students than any professor: she told them of the problems of the handicapped, of how different doctors helped or hindered, of how important is a doctor's humanity and kindness to patients who have no inner resources left. This patient's humanity, despite her appearance, and her knowledge of her own disease and physiology leave an imprint on students that probably affects their future contacts with the handicapped and helpless. Her spirit is infectious. She can say of the decision to do the tracheostomy: "It's a difficult decision for doctors. I don't know if it's right to keep me alive." She is the counsellor for the hospital's nurses, has been interviewed by newspapers, radio and television, and would like to write a book.

Does this productivity give her the right to live? Was the decision to put her on the respirator an ethical one? Would it have been right if she were depressed, unintelligent, not so helpful to others? If she were to live at home and cost less to the state but the family broke up under the stress, would the decision have been ethical? Who should make the final decision? If there is time for consultation, who should be consulted? How many Debbies can the state afford? The latter is the question currently raised about dialysis—if not everyone can afford dialysis, how can someone be ethically chosen for treatment? How important is the family in such a decision?

In many ways the family's view must be considered along with the impact of the decision on family function. If the family is a unit, to some extent what is good for one member will be good for the whole. A systems orientation clarifies conflict of values within the family. Usually facilitation of communication improves the situation for every family member and may resolve the conflict. In the rare situation in which differences are irreconcilable medical ethics demand that the doctor be the patient's advocate if a choice must be made. For the truly family-oriented clinician this situation should occur rarely; neutrality can help the family understand one another. Similarly, a systems view of the family addresses the problem of a family's privacy, which is often given by the physician as a reason not to see the family. Family secrets are often destructive to the individual as well as the family; they often are in fact already known but are hidden issues. In most, but certainly not all, instances the family benefits from their open discussion.

Values Clarification

Values clarification is a technique that can be taught.[22] Questions can be asked: To what extent are values cherished or publicly affirmed? Are the values freely chosen from alternatives after the consequences have been considered? Are values acted on consistently? (This technique may have particular merit with classes in comprehensive prenatal health care for pregnant adolescents, drug addicts, alcohol abusers, child abusers, etc.) A range of specific patient problems may warrant exploration of a patient's values; discrepancies between belief and behavior may be intruding on disease processes.

A patient making lifestyle decisions or health choices against his or her own interest or against the interest of others can be helped by a discussion of the patient's own values. Sometimes fear or lack of knowledge, rather than values, interferes with a decision, as when a patient procrastinates over a breast lump or a parent seemingly ignores a serious symptom in a child.

Morals and Maturity

Probably the most seminal recent work on the development of value systems in the past decade has been done by Lawrence Kohlberg. His research[12] suggests that children progress—or become fixated—along six different levels in their moral growth towards adult ethical maturity. The six levels are outlined and described in Table 6.1. Kohlberg uses the stages of moral reasoning described by John Dewey and Jean Piaget as a developmental framework.

Values may be composed of freely chosen ideals, traditional thinking, and conditioned personality dynamics. The clinician, when confronted by less than mature coping mechanisms or questionable moral development, can explore the level of ethical development in a nonjudgmental fashion. He may then discover the basis for the patient's behavior and with this information he

Table 6.1: Stages of Moral Reasoning

Levels and Stages	Definitions	Application-Patient Behavior
I. Pre-Conventional Levels		
1. Stage One—Rewards and Punishments	Unquestioning deference to authority figures. "Good" behavior contingent on reinforcement.	pediatric patients minority patients who docilely follow instructions retarded patients who docilely follow instructions
2. Stage Two—Need Satisfaction	An instrumental relativism prevails here wherein though a sense of fairness, reciprocity and sharing are recognized values, nonetheless moral behavior is viewed largely in terms of satisfying one's own needs.	tranquilized relief from life's discomforts contraceptive relief from promiscuous risks
II. Conventional Levels		
3. Stage Three—Conformity to Social Mores	"Good boy-nice girl" orientations, moral behavior is highly conformist, peer oriented, usually designed to please meaningful other persons, and often judged by good intentions.	adolescent patients immunization campaigns periodic health examinations

4. Stage Four— Law and Order	A relatively informed obedience to authority and the maintenance of one's basic social order are paramount. In contrast with stage one, obedience to authority figures is perceived as supportive more of community than of personal concerns.	most adult patients (prevailing North American morality?) patient compliance with drug and diet regimens
III. Post-Conventional Levels		
5. Stage Five—Social Contracts	Assuming equality of human rights and a respect for personal values, this stage seeks negotiated contracts wherein mutual rights are affirmed and a consensus achieved. As justice is sought, laws may be changed and new social contracts designed.	well-educated patients patients seeking a second opinion patients struggling with issues such as abortion, amniocentesis, terminal illness, etc. . . . .
6. Stage Six— Universal Ethical Principles	The highest integration of personal integrity, intellectual comprehensiveness, and logical consistency would combine with community awareness to achieve a universally admired moral behavior. Emphasis here is upon a highly developed social conscience and intellectual rigor.	(Does this stage exist?)

From: Kohlberg, 1968[12]

may be better able to understand the patient's behavior and assist in resolving the problem.

Environmental Influences and Moral Maturity. The level of moral maturity correlates with the systems with which the individual interacts. The small child focuses on himself and on rewards and punishments: good behavior is contingent on reinforcement by parents and later by teachers. Later the peer group and conformity become important. At this level moral behavior is consistent with loyalty to the group, which determines the level of honesty and consideration of others and the need for self-preservation. Phrases like "beat the system," "he's an outsider," "foreigner," and "not one of the family" imply different treatment of people or institutions perceived as alien. Prejudice, whether positive or negative, does the same. As individuation proceeds so does the ability to look beyond self, family, and social group to what is best for the greatest number and the question of absolute truth or value.

Life Experience, Personal and Ancestral. This is a major determinant of beliefs and attitudes; life may be perceived positively or as a struggle. This perception in turn contributes to future life experience since expectations of life usually become self-fulfilling prophecies. The ability to cope and see crisis as opportunity or catastrophe depends on past experience. Also, as Maslow[15] points out, human beings cannot pay attention to the higher values of life when basic needs for survival, food, shelter, physical safety, and psychological security are unmet.

Health Beliefs, and the Meaning of Illness

If a clinician is unaware of the significance of a symptom or an illness to a patient, inappropriate decisions may be made. The patient's health belief model may be very different from the clinician's.[7] A clinician who has worked with Navajo patients defines the problem well:

> . . . patients have concerns about the origin and meaning of their symptoms that may be more important to them, and ultimately to healing, than the purely descriptive aspects of pain or vomiting. Illness is not value-free or meaning-free, although medical education has not placed much emphasis on this fact. The physical world, as studied in natural science, is , for us, an abstraction. Where we really live is in what Eric Cassell calls 'semantic space'. We live in a world of symbols and interpretations, and the physician must collect data about patient beliefs just as he or she collects other relevant data.

Unscientific or anti-scientific folklore or mythology need not be incorporated into patient regimens, although it is wise to recognize that the patient may do so. However, cultural and religious beliefs provide a supportive and interpretative framework for trauma or pathology; if they do not violate rational norms, they may serve well the clinician who values the patient as a whole person.[6]

In the cross-cultural studies analyzed by Kleinman, Eisenberg, and Good[11] a larger awareness of a patient's value systems was reflected than is sometimes the case with traditional studies. In seeking to apply their social science concepts to clinical strategies, Kleinman and colleagues[11] observe that the patient's and family's explanatory models of illness may differ markedly from clinical models: "Such models reflect social class, cultural beliefs, education, occupation, religious affiliation, and past experience with illness and health care." This belief system should be elicited by the clinician since it determines the patient's concepts of etiology; onset of symptoms; pathophysiology; course of illness; and treatment. It may markedly affect the patient's history of the illness and his compliance with treatment. As discussed in the previous chapter on culture, open comparison and negotiation of belief models may lead to better understanding, cooperation, and teamwork between clinician and family.

Religion and World View

Holistic approaches to patient care cannot ignore the spirit of the patient, although the physician may need time to feel comfortable with this aspect of treatment. Simply noting the patient's religious preference can provide a basis for future exploration when indicated. Comprehensive care has physical, psychological, social, and spiritual dimensions that are best described by workers in the hospice movement.[16,18] Such care would incorporate the chaplain's services. The adoption of mature coping mechanisms[27] that are enhanced with responsible belief systems[3] can offer the patient significant support and make the tasks of the health care team easier. Antonovsky[1] has postulated that a sense of coherence, of a place in the world, is a major factor promoting health (see Section III).

VALUES AND THE HEALTH PROFESSIONAL

The health professional is an individual, with a personal value system and a family from which values are in part derived. Most health professionals bring a middle- or upper-class value system to their medical practice. Their belief system may be colored by specific religious or nonreligious factors, by special cultural or ethnic folkways, and by enhanced educational and travel opportunities. Consequently, the clinician's value system will greatly influence the choice of lifestyle, type of medical practice, attitude towards patients, and response to their personal belief systems.

Awareness of one's own value system is particularly helpful to the health professional. Knowledge and personal comfort with one's beliefs is crucial when initiating dialogue with patients. At times, such an awareness may be an asset in establishing special rapport with patients having similar beliefs, or with patients having opposing beliefs if openness and honesty is valued by such patients. Self-awareness also precludes the communication of either verbal or nonverbal judgmental attitudes when a meaningful and fruitful clinician-patient relationship is being attempted. Recognition that the values of one's own family have influenced one's own views makes for tolerance of another person's values; one may hold beliefs while recognizing they may not be the only truth.

The Clinician's Lifestyle

Health professionals often do not practice what they preach. A physician may strongly advocate nonsmoking and smoke two packs of cigarettes a day. That the health professional be the paradigm of all that is healthy and virtuous and be competent, caring, and effective is not implied. But the discrepancy between belief and practice underscores the clinician's humanity, as well as the need to temper expectations of patients with compassion and realism. Hence, the health professional's advice and subsequent patient compliance is facilitated if both value systems are explicit and conscious.

The health professional may neglect his or her own health and family in favor of caring for patients. Physicians as a group are highly prone to problems of drug and alcohol abuse, marital dysfunction, and a tendency to early death and suicide (see Section VI).

Conflict within the Health Profession

The health profession itself has a value system, one that is at times different from that of the public it serves. Family medicine and nursing have their own value systems, which may conflict with other areas of the health care system:

A family physician had left his practice to become a surgeon. He retained his attitudes and skills with families that he had learned in practice. On rotation in an intensive care unit he found himself allied with the nurses who were very aware of the pain and misery inflicted on patients who were clearly dying. He was disturbed that the attending surgeons had to continue in their attempts to save a person's life when all reasonable hope of survival or of any quality of life had gone. In one case, a patient with terminal hepatic and renal failure was given repeated blood transfusions for bleeding esophageal varices which had been repeatedly sclerosed. On one occasion, blood was consequently unavailable for another patient with an aneurysm.

The patient's family was too disturbed by the sight of the respirator, central venous lines, and monitors to visit. Family members were told only that "His condition is stable" when they enquired. The resident, used to helping families with the grieving process, arranged a family conference with the surgeon and himself. Once the patient's condition was understood the family insisted that no more active measures be taken. The surgeon was doubtful that the condition was completely irreversible.

For the attending surgeon the possibility of saving one patient outweighed the misery inflicted on those who did not survive, many of whom he felt were comatose and unaware. He also felt that letting his patient go seemed akin to a punitive response because he was alcoholic. He had never had an operation himself and separated himself from the pain so many patients in the unit experienced. Some did recover and returned later to thank him. However, he was aware that teamwork suffered when nurses and residents undermined decisions to actively treat the patient. He therefore agreed to monthly ethics rounds with a consultant medical ethicist. An outsider helped facilitate team communication and to clarify the many opposing ethical views.

Ethical decisions are increasingly problematic in emergency rooms and intensive and coronary care units. Discussions of ethics are essential if an atmosphere of conflict is to be avoided. In such a situation the primary care clinician may be caught between patient and family and intensive care unit staff and may not be aware of conflicts already present. He or she may be powerless to intervene and may be discouraged from visiting. An understanding of the various systems, of their organizational hierarchy and their values, and communication with those in power will help avoid conflict and prevent unnecessary suffering.

Family medicine and surgery have different value systems that need to be understood. Skillman's text on intensive care[25] has an excellent chapter on ethics and recognizes the underlying problem that "We cannot accept death for our patients, because we cannot easily accept our own ultimate mortality." Skillman writes the following:

> The fear that the removal of machines that prolong life in apparently irretrievable patients will lead to a permissive situation in which physicians will arbitrarily decide to "pull the plug" in patients who may be salvageable with superhuman effort should not detract us from responsible decision-making. Evasion of this responsibility produces a serious deterioration in the morale of personnel in the intensive care unit. Nurses in particular put their sweat and tears into the care of the critically ill. When it is clear that a patient has no chances of recovery, the continuation of intensive care becomes a mockery of their physical and emotional efforts. Nor is it fair to remove an irretrievable patient to another floor of the hospital to die.[25]

The family is briefly mentioned by Skillman, who feels "decisions for continuation or discontinuation of therapy must not be placed on the family's already heavily burdened shoulders, for they are frequently racked with grief and guilt and look to the physician for guidance and counsel." Such decisions may avoid subsequent guilt but may also remove a family's right to choose, particularly when they know the expressed wishes of the patient and are pleading for an end to suffering. The family physician or nurse would be much more likely to grant the family a part in the decision-making process if it so wishes.

For McWhinney[17] the "justification" of family medicine is expressed in the following quote:

> To restore the primacy of the person, one needs a medicine that puts the person in all his wholeness in the center of the stage and does not separate the disease from the man, and the man from his environment — a medicine that makes technology firmly subservient to *human values*, and maintains a creative balance between generalist and specialist. These I believe to be the aims of family medicine. Awareness of value systems as part of family assessment and care is apparent from the family assessment schemata of Arbogast and Smilkstein,[2,26] but evidence that this is demonstrated in practice is lacking. Often rhetoric is forgotten in the day to day time pressures of practice.

Conflict Between Family, Patient, and Health Professional Value Systems

In treating a wide range of ethnic groups with diverse belief systems in a pluralistic culture, the health practitioner cannot help being in conflict with various values held by some of the patients. Responsible clinicians do not permit conflicts to intrude on good health care. However, this does not imply that the practitioner must provide all of the requested services an afternoon's slate of patients may expect. Society's policeman protecting the privileges of the sick role from abuse, the practitioner must use clinical judgment and honesty.

Another area of ethical debate concerns the provision of contraceptive advice to minors. Differences between members of the health profession reflect differences in the public as cultural values change. A study of Canadian nurses[10] showed that although the Canadian Nurses' Association affirms that sick leave, insurance payments, and contraceptive information and devices should be available to all persons needing them, 57% of the students and 39% of the graduates did not know this. Only 31% thought that most adults were in favor of making contraceptive services available to sexually active high school students. Forty percent agreed that many physicians are not willing to prescribe the birth control pill to these adolescents. While an earlier study[24] had found that only about one half of nursing students and nursing faculty surveyed agreed that married women under 18 years old should be provided with contraceptive services, this more recent investigation disclosed that 89% of the respondents supported the provision of contraceptive information and devices to high school students. In the face of changing social mores, this socio-medical problem is only one of many that could be cited to illustrate the changing perceptions of health care practitioners regarding their responsibility to contemporary patient populations. In the following case physician, nurse, patient, and family all have different points of view:

> A 12-year-old girl came with her parents on a return visit to the County Hospital pediatric emergency clinic for a follow-up report on a pregnancy test, VDRL, and gonorrhea culture smear taken earlier. Her initial complaint had been irregular menses and amenorrhea for 2 months, and during the original interview with her alone she had indicated a very active sexual history for her age. All test results were negative, however, showing that she was neither pregnant nor infected. The irregularity of her menses was considered normal for her age. Because of the onset of another menses since her previous visit, the resident physician who talked to her felt the problem was resolved and was ready for the next case. However, the medical student who had been observing the interview stopped him in the hallway outside the patient's room. She asked: "What if she does get pregnant? She's not married, quite naive, but certainly sexually active. Should we instruct her now on birth control methods, and, in fact, initiate oral contraceptives?" The resident seemed surprised because he had not thought of the possibility. He said: "She's so young . . . You're right, though, she's sexually active . . . Birth control at her age? Her parents don't even know why she is here. I don't see how I could recommend the pill to her."[28]

In addition to his own attitudes, the resident should be aware of the law in his region: for example, parental consent may be required for dispensing contraceptives to children under 14 years old. If he is aware of the family as a system he may recognize the girl's complaints as an indication of a disturbed family system; such a family needs help in the area of communication even if he chooses to give the girl the choice of raising the issue of sexuality.

Although the health practitioner's role a decade ago in the care of sexually active, non-married adolescents may have been controversial, changing morals have stimulated changing procedures. Whether the issue be non-marital sexual activity, abortion, blood transfusions for Jehovah's Witnesses, or many other problems of moral consequence, thoughtful clinicians seek to establish a relationship with the patient in such a way that the values of both may retain their integrity. Another common situation in the area of sexual morality is represented by the following case:

> A 47-year-old white Protestant male presents with venereal warts. He has been a patient known to the practice for over a decade with a history of minor illnesses only. His wife is also seen in the practice. Her only major medical problem is control of her diabetes. The marriage has appeared to be stable. Upon explanation to the patient that his warts were infectious, he insisted that his wife be treated under subterfuge, without any awareness of his other sexual outlets. Should the physician maintain patient confidentiality and treat the wife with circuitous explanations or arrange to explore the marital dynamics?[28]

Although both the clinician and the patient may strive for a good working relationship, there are instances when irreconcilable differences may exist. The clinician, aware of gaps between his beliefs and those of the patient, may need to exhibit particular sensitivity such that he can establish meaningful rapport. A therapeutic alliance must be often forged in the face of value conflicts. Alternatively, the clinician and the patient may choose to acknowledge their differences and agree to referral of the patient to another colleague.

The following example illustrates the compatible resolution of differing values between physician and patient by referral:

> Dr. Z and the Birk family had a good working relationship over a 2-year period. Jennifer, the 3-year-old daughter, was then discovered to have a congenital renal malformation necessitating surgical repair. Dr. Z was well aware that the family members were Jehovah's Witnesses and that their belief prohibited blood transfusions. Their religious differences had not interfered with their relationship in the past, but came to the forefront with Jennifer's need for surgery. The parents, aware of the potential loss of blood, refused consent for blood transfusion and accepted the possibility that Jennifer could die from the surgery. Dr. Z could not morally permit himself to allow the child to have, while under his care, surgery within these restrictions. Hence, both he and the family agreed that the family be referred to another physician.[28]

Self-awareness, coupled with patient sensitivity, can bridge both cultural and moral barriers to clear communication and a viable treatment plan.

ETHICAL ISSUES IN WORKING WITH THE FAMILY

A systems-oriented clinician is by definition nonjudgmental. Siding with or having greater empathy for a particular family member implies that the clinician has been drawn into the family system because of the power of that system and its need to blame or victimize one member; that objectivity has been lost because of similar problems or similar personalities in the clinician's own family system, or that the clinician lacks true understanding of systems and is judging members on appearances. A systems perspective encourages an ethical egalitarian approach by tempering the human response to those who whine or dominate, to the bully, the martyr, the victim, the persecutor, and even the abuser. It puts each person in context and endeavors to understand the behavior even when it is irritating or horrifying. Each person is seen as doing the best he or she can with the abilities and circumstances fate has given. Each person's behavior is determined by the other members of the system.

Many of the ethical problems cited by those who do not understand the family as a system—confidentiality, privacy of the individual, conflict of interests, independence—fall away when individuals and their illnesses are seen as inextricably interwoven with family function. In general, facilitation of communication within the family improves the health and well-being of family members; family secrets and hidden agendas are often in fact known but not discussed. Ventilation may produce enormous relief, providing the choice to do so is the family's and is not imposed by the clinician. Clearly, an assessment of the family and expertise in handling the family, as well as knowledge of one's limits and the indications for referral, are essential. As in profession of surgery, harm can ensue if skill is deficient or diagnosis is incorrect. (The ethics of intervention depend on many aspects covered in detail in Section IV.)

The goal of the systems-oriented clinician is to improve the health of the individual and the family. True independence or individuation is optimum for both; excess dependence on either family or clinician is detrimental. Thus, independence in a teenager for example is encouraged, not by denying the ties with parents but by working through the relationship to encourage separation. Those who espouse only individual therapy for the disturbed adolescent do not recognize the power of parents to keep children immature and at home. Family therapy can often be more powerful in facilitating independence and maturation.

Finally, the most important ethical consideration is that the clinician is going to influence the family whether he or she wishes to or not. When the clinician knows the family, the influence is hopefully a contribution to family health; when the family is not known the influence is haphazard—it may be beneficial or it may be highly destructive to family or individual. (For example, a woman was hospitalized and permanently labelled with a psychiatric diagnosis after a marital fight that took her to the emergency room.)

ETHICAL GUIDELINES

To summarize, the following guidelines for managing ethical decisions have been found helpful:[5]

Because of the privileged nature of the confidential physician-patient or physician-family relationship and because health practitioners are usually sought for medical rather than ethical or pastoral care, our culture assumes that physicians and nurses will not impose their values on patients; it has not been as clear whether patients' values are to control medical intervention. Extreme positions are problematic: the physician who asserts his or her values too much is in danger of being assailed as a moralizer, but if the patient's values are given too much weight, the health practitioner is in jeopardy of becoming society's clinical technician and no more.

Whatever the issue—abortion, premarital contraception, deviant sexual behavior, adolescent pregnancy, venereal disease, marital problems, divorce, insurance forms, drug addiction, lifestyle, child abuse, blood transfusions, retardation syndromes, chronic care, terminal illness—if integrity is to be preserved for the health practitioner, for the patient, and in the therapeutic contract, these specific guidelines are recommended:

1. If the *integrity* of practitioner and family and patient is to be protected, then it should be assumed that the family brings moral values into their relationship; that these values may be implicit or explicit in their relationship; that not every treatment necessitates an evaluation of ethical principles; and that some clinical procedures are so ethically demanding that a clarification of the principles involved is incumbent on both practitioner and patient or family if personal integrity is to be preserved.

2. If the *vulnerability* of the patient is to be protected, then it must be remembered that any ethical discussion is not necessarily a moral debate among equals, but rather a consideration of alternatives and consequences in which the focus is on the patient's total health. The patient's distress, weakness, candor, insecurity, apprehension, and human uniqueness must be recognized.

3. If the *identity of specific moral principles* is to be recognized, then the clinical situation needs to be recognized not so much as a forum for debate, but rather as a place where diagnosis and therapy for people with problems is primary, where the ethical implications may merit discussion, and where concern for the person must find obvious supportive expression. In the clarification of moral principles, the health practitioner's role includes the following: aiding the patient in discovering the direction, the alternatives, and the consequences of their intended action; sharing values with the patient; challenging patient assumptions which may not be valid; and bringing empathy, understanding, rapport, and supportive care to the patient's dilemma.

4. If the *dignity* of the patient is to be enhanced, then recognition of the human rights and responsibilities inherent in being fully human should be incorporated in the dialogue between health practitioner and patient.

5. If the *family* is valued as a unit, the clinician must work to facilitate communication between family members and help the family communicate with outside systems, particularly the health care system. The values of the family must be recognized and respected.

6. A *nonjudgmental* understanding of every family's part in contributing to the family's structure and values[19] enables the clinician to facilitate problem solving and family and individual independence.

REFERENCES

1. Antonovsky A: *Health, Stress and Coping.* San Francisco, Jossey-Bass, 1979.

2. Arbogast RC, Scratton JM, Krick JP: The family as patient: Preliminary experience with a recorded assessment schema. *J Fam Pract* 7:1151, 1978.

3. Belgum D (ed): *Religion and Medicine: Essays on Meaning, Values, and Health.* Ames, Iowa, Iowa State University Press, 1967.

4. Bird LP: Universal principles of medical ethics, in Frazier CA (ed): *Is It Moral to Modify Man?* Springfield, Ill., Charles C Thomas, 1973.

5. Bird LP: Statement on moral values between physician and patient. *Christian Med Soc News Rep* Feb/Mar, 1980.

6. Clyne MB: Racial and cultural factors of relevance for the general practitioner. *Proc Roy Soc Med* 69:635, 1976.

7. Coulehan JL: Navajo Indian medicine: Implications for healing. *J Fam Pract* 10:55, 1980.

8. Duff RS, Hollingshead AB: *Sickness and Society.* New York, Harper & Row, 1968.

9. Gaudette LA, Holmes TM, Laing LM, et al: Cancer incidence in a religious isolate of Alberta, Canada, 1953-74. *J Natl Cancer Inst* 60:1233, 1978.

10. Herold ES, Thomas RE: Attitudes of nurses to providing contraceptive services for youth. *Can J Pub Health* 68:307, 1977.

11. Kleinman A, Eisenberg L, Good B: Culture, illness and care: Clinical lessons from anthropologic and cross-cultural research. *Ann Intern Med* 88:251, 1978.

12. Kohlberg L. Moral Development, in *International Encyclopedia of Social Science.* New York, Macmillan Free Press, 1968.

13. Lynch JL: The Broken Heart: The Medical Consequences of Loneliness. New York, Basic Books, 1977.

14. Lyon JL, Klauber MR, Gardner JW, et al: Cancer incidence in Mormons and non-Mormons in Utah, 1966-1970. *N Engl J Med* 294:129, 1976.

15. Maslow AH: *Toward a Psychology of Being.* New York, D. Van Nostrand Co., 1968.

16. Markel WM, Sinnon VB: The hospice concept. *Can J Clin* 28:225, 1978.

17. McWhinney IR: Family medicine in perspective. *N Engl J Med* 293:176, 1975.

18. Mount BM: Caring in today's health care system. *Can Med Assoc J* 119:303, 1978.

19. Papp P, Silverstein O, Carter E: Family sculpting in preventive work with well families. *Fam Process* 12(2):197, 1973.

20. Pellegrino ED: Medicine and philosophy: Some notes on the flirtations of minerva and aesculapius (monograph). *Soc Health Hum Val* 1974.

21. Phillips RL: Role of life-style and dietary habits in risk of cancer among Seventh-Day Adventists. *Cancer Res* 35:3513, 1975.

22. Raths L, Harmin M, Simon S: *Values and Teaching.* Columbus, Ohio, Charles E. Merrill, 1966.

23. Shapiro J, Shapiro DH: Some second thoughts on holistic medicine. *N Engl J Med* 301:211, 1979.

24. Shea F, Werley H, Rossen RA: Survey of health professionals regarding family planning. *Nurs Res* 22:17, 1973.

25. Skillman JJ: *Intensive Care*. New York, Little, Brown, 1975.

26. Smilkstein G: The family APGAR: A proposal for a family function test and its use by physicians. *J Fam Pract* 6:1231, 1978.

27. Vaillant GE: Theoretical hierarchy of adaptive ego mechanisms. *Arch Gen Psychiatry* 24:107, 1971.

28. Veatch RM: *Case Studies in Medical Ethics*. Cambridge, Mass., Harvard University Press, 1977.

Chapter 7
The Meaning of Illness, Crisis, and Growth

Janet Christie-Seely

The human family, like the human individual, is constantly adapting to the stresses and crises of life and to the progression of changes inherent in the family life history. The opportunity for growth of personal and family understanding and strength provided by the misfortunes that bring the patient or the family to the physician or nurse's office is often overlooked or rejected. Naomi Remen, in her book *The Human Patient,*[9] has given detailed attention to the individual's response to illness and the potential for growth the individual may derive from the experience of illness. The helpful principles set forth in her book can be expanded to include the family system:

> The ability to learn something of value from experience seems to be a natural and innate human capacity. Crisis events such as illness seem especially rich in this potential and the subjective gain in understanding, wisdom, insight, and compassion that may result from such experience can ultimately become integrated into our daily lives and enrich us.
>
> Yet people commonly look to their health care system only to eliminate crises, irradicate problems, and anesthetize pain, not realizing that challenges, problems, and crises are the norm; they are life. To retreat from them is to retreat from life. To see them only negatively is to see life itself as negative. The skill of being fully alive does not lie in expertly avoiding crisis; crisis is not usually avoidable. Rather, healthy living seems to involve meeting problems in such a way that something of value is learned.[9]

The nursing profession has focused its attention on health as opposed to disease. Like Dr. Remen, nurses have described the healthy way to have a disease (see Chapter 2). The clinician, like the patient and the family, may choose to see the positive or the negative aspects of the situation. He or she may focus on pathology, or look for the strengths and potential in each patient. His or her attitude will either help or hinder the family's efforts to adapt to illness or other crises in a healthy way.

What can be learned from an illness will depend on the type of illness, the limitation it is felt to impose on the patient, and the significance of the illness for the family and for continuation of the accepted role of the patient as an individual within the family as well as within the larger context of the meaning

115

of life. Viktor Frankl[6] believes that a sense of meaninglessness is a core problem in the person who responds poorly to life stress or disease and is a possible cause of illness. The significance of meaninglessness, hopelessness, or loss of a goal to the function of a system will be elaborated in Chapter 8.

THE STAGES OF ILLNESS

Remen has described three stages of illness in the *individual* (See Figure 7-1). The level of functioning represented by the box, "daily life," drops abruptly as the consequence of a health crisis but gradually returns to normal as recovery occurs.) To many, the concept of serious illness embraces permanent disability or at least diminished function and a greater awareness of advancing age. Nevertheless, as Remen points out, function may not only return to normal but may reach a higher level as a result of enhanced insight, a change in behavior, or a new perception of the value and meaning of things previously taken for granted. If such is the outcome, daily life will have been enriched by illness. Some cultures are more aware of this potential than others: the Japanese use the same character to represent both misfortune and opportunity.

Patients are particularly prone to becoming withdrawn, preoccupied with self, and dependent during the first stage of an acute serious illness such as a myocardial infarction. They are in a state of psychological as well as physical shock during which they not only allow but welcome decisions being made for them by others, and may well be compliant and unquestioning in their acceptance of all therapy. Family members often show parallel states of shock, acquiescence, and dependence on the medical team. The family or patient, or both, may also be angry and may use denial in a manner that parallels recognized stages of mourning over the death of a relative.

Passing from the passivity of stage one to the struggle of stage two when patients are trying to regain control, both of themselves and of their illness, is often heralded by refusal to take pills or efforts to sign themselves out of the hospital. Such manifestations, when misinterpreted by the staff as indicating poor compliance, often lead physicians and nurses to make a special effort to push the patient back into stage one. This type of patient behavior should, however, be seen as a valiant attempt to re-establish control and to adapt to the illness. The patient's attention is turned outward by a desire not only to understand the cause of the illness but also to prevent its recurrence. The following questions may surface: Why did this happen to me? What did I do to get myself into this, and why now?

Most of us live by habit, unaware of the reasons for our choices and of our values; illness not only gives us time out from busy lives to meditate (an activity notably lacking in most Western lives) but also forces us to re-examine our values and our own inner selves. An executive whose sense of identity

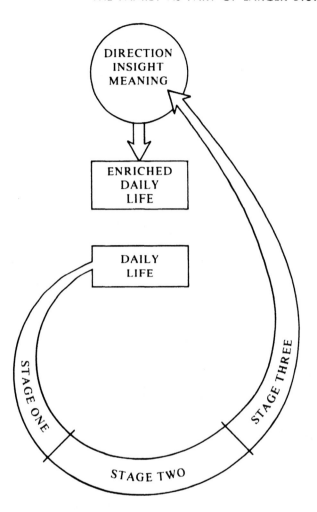

Figure 7-1. The Spiral Trajectory.

Reprinted, by permission, from Remen N. *The Human Patient.* New York, Anchor Press, 1980.

depends on his competence and indispensable leadership at work and who prizes only his breadwinning role at home, may, after having had a heart attack, decide that his relationship with his teenage children is of higher priority than his executive image. Remen describes a physician whose gastric ulcer enabled him to obtain a more balanced perspective and to recognize that his self-esteem and his value to his patients should not be dependent on self-denial to the point of self-destructiveness. Such reassessment of lifestyle, of personal relationships, and of possible causes of the illness, as well as achievement of an understanding and control of the illness, are characteristic of stage two. One prominent physician-teacher summarized his experience with a chronic health problem by saying, "I have learnt to make friends with my psoriasis; in the morning I look at my elbows to see how I feel inside, particularly when I have to give a lecture-tour. I have my own built-in feedback system!"

The influence of this stage on family members is often a similar reassessment of behavior and relationships. A nagging wife of a man stricken with an infarct may feel acute guilt and resolve to change; this decision may be part of a bargaining process with God or fate for the life of the patient. Even more distant relatives may be affected. (For example, in one woman the news of her 46-year-old brother-in-law's hospitalization for an infarct led to changes in the destructive behavioral patterns that were clearly causing stress to her husband, who was only a year younger than his brother.)

Enough change may occur during stage two of a serious illness to improve the patient's original level of functioning and family relationships; and the patient may become more efficient at work through better use of relaxation and recreation. The experience of stage three does not always occur and may depend on the person's age and on the seriousness of the illness: stage three involves a farther reaching assessment of the meaning of the illness and of life in the wider context of what Remen describes as the level of universal meaning. Although it is not usually acceptable to talk of spiritual values or universal consciousness in medical circles, Viktor Frankl and Naomi Remen believe that exclusion of the higher levels of consciousness restricts our understanding of human nature as much as would exclusion of the subconscious level.

Response to illness, particularly serious illness such as cancer, correlates highly with the individual's sense of the meaning of life and of spiritual values. One study of people who attempted suicide, as reported by Frankl,[6] showed that 85% felt that life was meaningless; another study of suicide produced a figure of 100% who felt the same way. Frankl has also observed that survival in a concentration camp correlated with the sense of purpose of the individual (whether the person had someone or something to live for). The meaning ascribed to life is unique to each individual; it may spring from an important purpose or life work, from a love relationship, from a belief in a supreme being or, as Frankl has pointed out, from transcendence of personal suffering. A new sense of meaning has often been described following serious illness of either oneself or a loved one: life afterwards may be approached with renewed vigor or a new sense of peace.

THE NATURE OF SUFFERING

Eric Cassell[4] has distinguished between suffering and physical distress. Suffering is experienced by persons and their families, not merely by bodies. A person may be in pain but not suffer (for example, labor pains or pain diagnosed as caused by a renal stone and not from cancer) because the pain does not imply loss or destruction. Pain causes suffering when the person feels out of control, when pain is overwhelming, or when the source is unknown or the meaning is dire. When pain is chronic the person may adjust or suffer silently because others are bored with complaints and can no longer sympathize or adjust their roles.

Suffering usually means loss in many ways: there may be loss of a role that is so ingrained it is hard to change (role of mother or of doctor); loss of a relationship; loss of a perceived future; loss of daily routine; loss of hopes or fantasies; and even loss of a political role. The handicapped feel politically powerless: one of my patients, in a wheelchair and permanently confined to the hospital, arranged for a televised ambulance trip to a voting booth to encourage others. This particular patient apparently suffered little despite 5 years on a respirator and almost total disability (see Chapter 6). She was a major support to others, recognizing that the health professional is a major resource for patients who have no more strength left. As Cassell put it, physicians must lend strength to such a patient, "As though people who have lost parts of themselves can be sustained by the personhood of others until their own recovers."[4]

Such strength may be needed by the family. Only by open discussion can such needs be known, particularly in families who find communication difficult. When the needs of a family are not known, the results can be tragic: a diabetic husband had a leg amputation and was believed to be coping well because he said he had no problems with the loss. Signs of family dysfunction suggested a family interview but the patient asked to go home. On arrival he said he had come home to die and that day developed a mesenteric thrombosis; he died a week later. It then became apparent that his wife had been unable to look at his amputated limb and unable to express her feelings of revulsion to anyone, and that the patient's apparent peace of mind masked a hopelessness he could not share.

FAMILY RESPONSE TO CRISIS

Smilkstein[11] has described a "crisis trajectory" for the family as a unit in terms very similar to those of Remen (Figure 7-2). The level of functioning of the family drops in the face of crisis in the same way it does in the individual. Relationships are strained, conflict increases, role allocations may be disrupted, and performance at work or school may decline. The first phase is one of disorganization, denial, or crisis. Gradually, adjustment takes place, problem solving occurs, and the family returns to a new level of functioning. In the dysfunctional family, or the family that has encountered a series of closely spaced crises, the level of performance after recovery may be lower than it was originally. Tension level may be higher, adaptability and flexibility

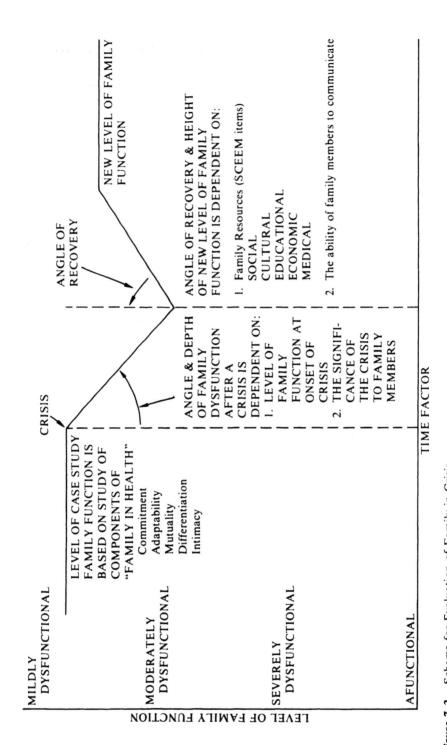

Figure 7-2. Schema for Evaluation of Family in Crisis

From: Smilkstein G. The family in trouble – how to tell. *J Fam Pract* 2:19, 1975.

decreased, conflict avoidance more evident, and rules more rigid. In contrast, the healthy family may return to a normal level of functioning or, as Smilkstein points out, may even reach a higher level. During crises a family's flexibility may attain its maximum and facilitate changes that were previously impossible.

Crisis intervention has long been recognized as having special attributes and effects. A clinician who sees a family when one of its members has been diagnosed as having cancer or is on the verge of death has a rare opportunity to help that family to reorganize and to change its communication patterns in a way that could never come to pass while its life was flowing uneventfully. This fact underlies the observation that no marriage is truly solid unless it has gone through the threat of divorce. Crises frequently force the recognition of problems; without such recognition problem solving is exceedingly difficult.

> A man of 66, dying of lung cancer, had not seen his three children for 20 years. Surrounded by his siblings and his second wife, he was stoical about his disease. When asked if he wished to see his children he said "No, they'd just think I was wanting sympathy." Nevertheless, when it was suggested that the doctor could phone them as a matter of hospital policy and not as a request from the patient, he agreed readily. The eldest son, aged 29 and long taught by his divorced mother to see his father as the villain in the marital break-up, eventually agreed to visit. He discovered a man with great courage, able to joke despite pain not fully controlled by large doses of morphine; in two visits he became reacquainted with his father. The son was glad he had come and probably communicated some of what he had seen and learned to his brother and sister who had not had the same courage. For the father the visit was of great significance; indeed, it seemed that he had waited for the second visit because he died very soon after, apparently at peace. After the father's death, his extended family remained in communication with his son.

Those who work in hospices are familiar with the correlation between the timing of death and the conclusion of unfinished business. An extremely emaciated woman, dying of advanced cancer of the cervix, lived on with virtually no nourishment for 6 weeks beyond the time when her death had been considered to be imminent. When I asked her what was keeping her alive, she replied, "My time has not yet come, I still have to look after my son Mark." True to her word, she waited for Mark to get his own apartment and a girlfriend; then she quietly died. It is not unusual to see patients, who have accepted their own death, wait for acceptance of it by the family; sometimes, they even verbalize this need for the family's permission to die. If the family is helped to share its grief and to break what has been termed the "conspiracy of silence," there is some evidence that it will experience less difficulty and less morbidity during the bereavement process (see Chapter 22). The crisis of death is the most dramatic of family crises but the principles of helping the family interact apply to most, if not all, crises. When the family is able, with the aid of a health care professional, to discuss the anxieties, fears, and myths associated with a traumatic event, the potential for growth through the experience and the attainment of an improved level of functioning is greatly enhanced.

DISEASE AS LABEL

Labelling by the Health Professional

Classification and diagnosis are characteristic components of science in general and of medicine in particular. However, affixing labels is stultifying.[8] A diagnosis may mean ending prematurely any further thought about the nature or cause of a problem. At best, a diagnostic label refers to present reality and possibly to only part of that reality; it seldom includes what new realities may ensue. The limitations and stigmata imposed by a diagnosis are particularly obvious in the field of psychiatry. William Glaser, in *Reality Therapy*, states, "If there is a medical analogy which applies to psychiatric problems, it is not illness but weakness. While illness can be cured by removing the causative agent, weakness can be cured only by strengthening the existing body to copy with the stress of the world, large or small as the stress may be."[7] He describes the meeting of two psychiatrists who discovered they had had a patient in common. One commented on the very positive outcome reached at the end of therapy; the other, in surprise, exclaimed, "But didn't you know he is a schizophrenic?" Remen describes a similar sad case of an excellent mother who was psychotic and was accused of child abuse when an intern discovered a "bruise" on the child's shoulder. The "bruise" was later diagnosed correctly as a birthmark but the mother expressed her continuing despair to the family physician, who knew her well:

> You are a nice person, doctor, but you don't understand. They don't care. They don't see me and they don't hear me. I'm a 'crazy,' doctor. . . . Sometimes when we talk I forget that I'm a 'crazy'. *I* am a good mother. How could a crazy woman be a good mother? I love my baby. But you won't be here forever. Some day you'll leave. Then they'll hassle me, and I'll get scared and say something or do something they think is wrong, and the first chance they get, they'll send the police again and take my baby away.[9]

Disease labels can be physically restricting. Remen describes a grandmother disabled for many years by an incorrect diagnosis of angina that was never questioned because every member of her extended family was in the medical or nursing profession. Then a consultant became involved, who indicated that the squeezing pain she experienced, particularly when conflict occurred in the family, was related to her rather oppressive and overbearing husband. The pain was vague and accompanied by nervous breathing, and disappeared once she learned to express her own feelings openly. The original diagnosis may have been accepted by her physician simply because the patient herself was a nurse.

The terms "organic" and "functional" are similar labels with which patients get transfixed. A resident once expressed concern when I suggested that the division between organic and functional was not that clear; he said, "Then even more patients will be discounted and not taken seriously by their doctors." This may indeed be a hazard of pointing out the psychological components of physical illness.

Labels like "crock" or "turkey" reveal the hostility that physicians feel toward those they believe they are unable to help. (Strategies for management of such patients that have proved helpful are described in Chapters 15 and 19). A systems orientation helps understanding of the chronically sick or pseudo-sick and avoids the blame that is often attached to labels. Empathy then becomes possible. Families may be similarly labelled. An understanding of the background of families on welfare, of multi-problem or illness-prone families, of "difficult" or "demanding" families helps the clinician to empathize and to see family strengths.

The need to classify and diagnose serves an obviously essential function in clarifying therapy. It is also protective to maintain distance in difficult situations. Although distance from psychological distress or dysfunction, from fatal illness or from deformity and disability may be unfortunate and destructive, it may be necessary for the physician or nurse to maintain equilibrium. Staff stress is highest in emergency rooms, intensive care units, and in the hospice setting, and mechanisms to diffuse this stress are necessary if distancing is not used (see Chapter 22, "Terminal Illness and Death").

Labelling by the Individual

The patient is likely to label himself *as* his disease, particularly when he or she first learns the diagnosis. Statements such as "I am an epileptic, a cripple, a diabetic" can make the disease loom larger than the person and obscure the facts. This problem is most obvious in the chronically obese, who need to be helped to lose weight by obtaining some distance from their fat self and finding the slim person inside. The strategy of visualizing the fat on a chair in front of the patient and dealing with it as if it were a separate entity will help separate the inner identity from the overload of adipose tissue. Remen and many others, including Berne,[1] have seen the individual as a system made up of many different identities. The identity as a sick individual may take over at the expense of other identities; or, because of the perceived threat to his identity the individual may deny illness in a self-destructive way. The clinician can help put such identities or labels into perspective.

Disease as limitation is also a part of the labelling process. The words "I can't" are often a substitute for "I won't." As Remen points out, if the patient can learn to accept the latter words as part of what he or she is feeling, new insight and some potential may be regained. Limitation obviously depends on the person's previous skills and career. Blindness is an obvious catastrophe for an artist, although creativity may perhaps be able to be channelled through touch or other senses, or some other unused potential in the person may be tapped. A surgeon who shattered his right shoulder may be spurred on to a full recovery because of his need to maintain his career. There are many examples of people who have overcome handicaps and travelled far beyond them. Remen discusses the impact of illness on individuals in whom the intellectual, physical, or emotional aspects predominate, depending on whether they have emphasized development of mind, body, or feelings. To a person with intellectual pursuits, hip disease may seem small limitation, whereas to the skier or golf enthusiast this will be a major problem. The physician or nurse can help the person live within their limitation and maximize possibilities in other areas of ability. The person who persists in living beyond his limitations will be in a state of constant frustration.

Labelling by the Family

Genetics is usually assumed to be the explanation of the familial incidence of hypertension, heart disease, cancer, and diabetes. A genetic origin was recently found in patients with premature onset of coronary artery disease: one half to two thirds of these patients had normal cholesterol values but high titers of lipid-binding protein.[12] However, in many genetic studies the information from which the phenograms are made is usually obtained from the individual whose family is being studied, or by observation of facts well known to the family's members. It is therefore sometimes unclear to what extent the person's conscious knowledge of family incidence makes him prone to the disease, as opposed to influence at the genetic level. Little research has been done on people's expected year of death as a self-fulfilling prophecy but there is much anecdotal evidence that anxiety levels become very much higher on reaching the expected year (as predicted, for example, by a physician, an individual, a fortune-teller, or by an assumption that death will occur at the same age as it did in the parent of the same sex). People certainly do die with uncanny frequency at the time predicted. Voodoo death has been well documented in certain cultures,[3] but the concept of control of time of death is not well accepted in our culture.

The family labelling process may, therefore, include the illnesses to which it knows it is predisposed. The family genogram can be used to identify patterns of illness in past generations and questions about expected longevity can elicit useful data. The information gleaned can outline genetic risk and form a basis for a plan of action for remedial changes in lifestyle that will give the person a sense of control over his or her destiny. If risk factors can be altered, he or she need not expect to die at the same age a parent did.

The family labelling process covers many possibilities. The name given to a child at birth may not be without impact. A baby boy may be named after his Uncle John and may, thereafter, be expected to develop Uncle John's personality traits and even to follow Uncle John's career. In a family known to the author, every male by the name of William became alcoholic. The predominance of one name in a family is sometimes striking. In one family the mother, the daughter, and the son's girlfriend were all called Suzanne; in another family the father was named Bob, his son was named Bob, and two daughters married men named Bob. That personality traits may be prophecied for a baby and be reinforced during childhood—"You're just like your grandmother"—need not be elaborated here.

Disease labels can also be assigned by the family. Research on the vulnerable child syndrome has revealed that even minor illness early in life can result in a predisposition to illness later or to behavioral problems resulting from the increased protectiveness or expectation of illness by the family. For example, one study showed that gastroenteritis necessitating hospital admission early in life was followed by behavioral problems 6 years later.[10] These children were labelled as weak and vulnerable by their families and were treated differently from the other children in the family. Such children may become targets for scapegoating if family stress levels rise to uncomfortable proportions as the children grow older. It may be these children who develop anorexia in adolescence or who are "chosen" to be the delinquent family members. A family seen by Minuchin because of an anorectic adolescent who had been born with a club foot is a good example of children developing illness to fulfill expectation.

Peggy Papp has pointed out that all permanently affixed labels are stultifying.[8] The "good" child (white knight) in a family has been shown to have more problems in adulthood than the "bad" child (black sheep). The "weak" child is liable to develop a personality that depends on illness as a means of obtaining caring, an example of maximum secondary gain. The ability of such children to see themselves as competent functioning individuals may be permanently stunted by their families; as shown in the study of patients with gastroenteritis, this stunting process may be actively aided and abetted by the pediatrician or family physician.[10] To remove a label once it has been solidly affixed may be extremely difficult because the family system will have reorganized around the concept of that person as being ill; the illness may have been a solution, at its onset, for a family problem. For example, in his studies of asthma and diabetes in childhood, Minuchin described how psychosomatic families see themselves as loving families, deny any conflict, and consider their only problem to be the child's disease (see Chapter 8).

Alcoholism is the most obvious example of a destructive label. Although application of the label may be a highly useful step in breaking through the denial system of the alcoholic, it also carries the risk of producing pessimism regarding therapeutic outcome in family, friends, and the health profession as well.

GROWTH AND MEANING

In many people, cessation of growth of personality and character may be felt as meaningless.[9] The adult whose life and personality remain fixed at a level of development appropriate to adolescence avoids the satisfaction as well as the pain of growth. Such an adult is prone to difficulties in relationships as the family's life history unfolds; he or she adapts poorly to stress and is at greater risk of illness. Growth, change, and adaptation are also vital characteristics of families. If a family encounters stress at one time and becomes more rigid and less well adapted as a consequence, it may not accomplish the tasks that must be fulfilled during that stage of its development. As a result, the family is increasingly in trouble during later stages of its development (see Chapter 3).

Murray Bowen has looked at the growth of families over many generations[2] (see Section I, Chapter 1). He has observed that some lines of a family displayed increasing individual differentiation. The families produced by persons in these lines were flexible, healthy, and productive, and tended to have less physical illness. Other lines of the same family tree exhibited decreasing individual differentiation accompanied by increasing incidences of psychosis, severe physical illness, and family disruption:

A 56-year-old divorcee presented with a long history of arthritis since her early twenties, Sjogren's syndrome, and depression of 3 years' duration. She looked about 70. Her demeanor, clothing, and behavior radiated a poor self-image and severe depression. However, her primary complaint concerned her 13-year-old son, who was severely overweight and had shown signs of behavioral problems for several years. He had stolen money from her purse and had been found putting the cat in the refrigerator.

The patient was requesting help with disciplining her son, but her profound depression elicited questions about her life history. Her mother had died 3 years previously. The patient was the seventh child in a family of seven daughters and three sons. The patient had been her mother's favorite, but had been severely beaten by her father, possibly for that very reason. The last daughter, who was 1 year younger than the patient, had died at age 5 of rheumatic fever. As the survivor next in line and as the child affected by triangulation, the patient was clearly the vulnerable member of the family.

Attempts to learn more about the family were curtailed by the fact that the patient's mother had come to Canada from England, alone, at age 13. Of her grandparents, the patient knew nothing. Her mother had been raised in an institution and had one brother and one sister, who also eventually came to Canada. The mother never spoke of her family, and no questions were asked. The patient's father came from Ontario, but the patient never met his family, although her paternal grandparents were alive through her childhood.

The patient also had three other children who had left home. The obese child with whom she had so close a relationship was her fourth child; born a year after the mother's divorce from her husband, he was the son of another man. Because this boy was born at a time when his mother felt particularly vulnerable, he became the vulnerable child as his mother had been. Like the other males in the family, he was labelled as aggressive and unreliable. Nevertheless, he was the only person with whom the patient had a close relationship; she indicated this, saying "It's funny that we fight like man and wife."

The treatment plan included socialization for both mother and son. The few friends already attached to the family were asked to help. An attempt was also made to help the mother understand how she maintained the boy's obesity to keep him close to her. She accepted the suggestion that her son was close to her in the same way that she had been close to her mother, and that she had stocked the refrigerator with fattening foods so that her son would not lose weight. Open discussion of her mother's death, of which she had not spoken to anybody, also helped the delayed mourning process. However, limited goals were suggested by this lady's very low degree of personal differentiation.

This example illustrates the sad results of an extremely deprived childhood resulting in a marital relationship that was distant and conflicted. Affected by an overly close involvement between parent and child in two successive generations, the 13-year-old boy was aggressive, delinquent, and given to overeating. The families of the mother's brother and sister did not seem to have fared so poorly and displayed better individual differentiation than the patient's family. Enabling mother and son to separate before worse pathology developed required a knowledge of community resources, the use of a health care team, and behavioral approaches to reduce the involvement. Also, techniques were used to help the patient mourn for her mother with whom she had been so closely involved. Helping the patient to see herself as a strong woman who had coped with a great deal, despite a family background that had given her little, was central to therapy.

THE ROLE OF THE HEALTH PROFESSIONAL

When illness disrupts the functioning of an individual or a family, and when conflict or behavioral problems indicate family dysfunction, an outsider may provide the understanding needed for change. The primary role of the clinician is to help the individual or the family to step back into the role of "observer," as Remen puts it, in order to gain a proper perspective. A family that sees itself as the "perfectly happy family" can be helped to see its affection and closeness as a strength that will not be weakened by fighting or expressing different opinions. The couple who are so close they never part can be told that holidays spent away from each other can only be safely considered by couples like themselves. In contrast, the family with a negative label, whether covert or overt—the "inferior family," the "ne'er do well," the "failures"—need help to see their strengths. Cohen and colleagues[5] have described depression as arising in families (often from minority groups) who felt inferior and put pressure on one child to prove the family could amount to something, only to see this child respond later on with depression.

As individuals, we are all caught up in our identity of the moment, whether that identity be the Dedicated Doctor, Noble Nurse, Harried Housewife (or Harried Executive), Creative Person, He-Man, Athlete-of-the-Day, Worthless One, Unappreciated Martyr, Best Hop-Scotch Player, etc. We all have many identities, but at any one time we tend to be one of them and to forget the others. The role of observer enables us to step back and assess where we are at a point in time. Some people, probably those who have made the least progress in developing their own individuality, are rarely given to observing themselves. They can be helped by a professional to view themselves with at least a little distance.

Achieving some degrees of objectivity is particularly necessary for the patient whose identity and illness have become interrelated, when, for example, the patient's predominant identity is that of the "victim" or the "bereaved one." The therapist can help the patient to recall older forgotten identities. The football player who has lost his leg can be reminded that he used to write poetry, or that the teamwork of football was the essential part of the activity for him. In one case, a patient was able to use his enthusiasm for teams in an entirely new way in his career and to accept his inability to play a sport with equanimity. It took time to help this man understand what football truly meant to him, but arrival at this understanding made a major contribution to his adaptation to his handicap and constituted a turning point in his life.[9]

Illness may be an ally in any endeavor to clarify a person's identity. It forces a personal change in role, provides a period for reflection, and induces modification in the role structure of the family. Even a child's role in the family may be clarified; hospitalization of the "bad" child may result in misbehavior by the previously "good" child. Conversely, hospitalization of the good, affectionate child may enable the parents to become closer to the one previously labelled as bad or distant, or increase their expectations of the one labelled unhelpful. Even a single symptom may enable change to occur.

Many techniques may be employed to facilitate change; each requires a different amount of time, some requiring one to several sessions, others only a few minutes. A single well-timed question or statement may induce change. In dealing with the individual, positive imagery may be used as described by Remen. With the family, the clinician may change the system by simply raising topics that the family has avoided, by using words such as cancer, death, anger, conflict that have evoked fear in the family, and by demonstrating his or her own comfort with these subjects. Tact and care in choosing the right time and approach for such interventions are essential. One's diagnostic impression of the role of illness in the family can be enough in itself to stimulate change: for example, the mother of the obese son was surprised and intrigued by the suggestion that she was helping him to stay fat to keep him close to her. In some situations, relabelling a problem is the essential first step to its removal. Re-awakening optimism and belief in the possibility of new options often help a family to set a different course.

If the clinician is generally pessimistic about the possibility of change, perhaps because he feels unable to change the circumstances of his own life, he will have difficulty in seeing the potential for change in other people. Remen uses the analogy of the acorn—a small object whose potential one could never guess. To see people as acorns is to maximize the possibility of their growing into oak trees.

REFERENCES

1. Berne E: *Transactional Analysis in Psychotherapy*. New York, Grove Press, 1961.
2. Bowen M: *Family Therapy in Clinical Practice*. New York, Hason Aronson, 1978.
3. Cannon WB: Voodoo death. *Am Anthropol* 44:169, 1942.
4. Cassell EJ: The nature of suffering. *N Engl J Med* 306:639, 1982.
5. Cohen MB, Baker G, Cohen RA, et al: An intensive study of twelve cases of manic-depressive psychosis. *Psychiatry* 17:103, 1954.
6. Frankl V: *Man's Search for Meaning*. New York, Pocket Books, 1963.
7. Glaser W: *Reality Therapy. A New Approach to Psychiatry*. New York, Harper & Row, 1965.
8. Papp P, Silverstein O, Carter E: Family sculpting in preventive work with well families. *Fam Process* 12:197, 1973.
9. Remen N: *The Human Patient*. New York, Anchor Press, 1980.
10. Sigal J, Gagnon P: Effects of parents' and paediatricians' worry concerning severe gastroenteritis in early childhood on later disturbances in the child's behavior. *J Pediatr* 87:809, 1975.
11. Smilkstein G: The family in trouble—how to tell. *J Fam Pract* 2:19, 1975.
12. Sniderman A: Hyperapobetalipoproteinemia, a syndrome of atherosclerosis. *Proc Nat Acad Sci USA* 77:604, 1980.

Section III
RESEARCH ON ILLNESS AND THE FAMILY

Chapter 8

Research Linking Stress, Illness, and the Family

Janet Christie-Seely
Herta Guttman

Stress is a popular lay concept today. What is the evidence that stress plays a role in illness, and what is the link between illness and the family? Two major breakthroughs have paved the way to a new perspective on disease and medical practice:

1. A simple questionnaire, easy to use and quick to apply, was developed by Holmes and Rahe[36]: "The Social Readjustment Rating Scale" (Table 8.1). This scale was a subjective rating of stressful life events and led to numerous retrospective and prospective studies of almost every common disease, adding up to impressive evidence that the incidence of both serious and minor illness of all sorts increases following stress.

2. A new way of thinking about illness in its family and social context has developed from the interaction of family systems theory with the practice of medicine, reaffirming what all doctors know but often deny in their practice and medical terminology: that mind and body are one and that illness is defined in a psychosocial environment. Interactional, systems, or "organismic" thinking (the "biopsychosocial model"[21]) are various names for looking at illness as but part of a complex matrix in which culture, the community, the family, the individual, and his organ systems and genes play a role in the definition, development, and cure of disease. The impact of stress, the protective value of family support and the impact of family on illness have been looked at separately, but are in fact inseparable aspects of an interacting system.[72,78]

Medicine has been slow to leave the simple, linear model of specific disease causation (for example, genes and diet contribute to increased cholesterol level, causing coronary atheroma, which in turn produces an infarct). However, as Engel comments, "Most lay people have taken for granted that a person's frame of mind has something to do with his pro-

132

Table 8.1 Social Readjustment Rating Scale

Rank	Life Event	Mean Value*
1	Death of spouse	100
2	Divorce	73
3	Marital separation	65
4	Jail term	63
5	Death of close family member	63
6	Personal injury or illness	53
7	Marriage	50
8	Fired at work	47
9	Marital reconciliation	45
10	Retirement	45
11	Change in health of family member	44
12	Pregnancy	40
13	Sex difficulties	39
14	Gain of new family member	39
15	Business readjustment	39
16	Change in financial state	38
17	Death of close friend	37
18	Change to different line of work	36
19	Change in number of arguments with spouse	35
20	Mortgage over $10,000	31
21	Foreclosure of mortgage or loan	30
22	Change in responsibilities at work	29
23	Son or daughter leaving home	29
24	Trouble with in-laws	29
25	Outstanding personal achievement	28
26	Wife begins or stops work	26
27	Begin or end school	25
28	Change in living conditions	24
29	Revision of personal habits	23
30	Trouble with boss	20
31	Change in work hours or conditions	20
32	Change in residence	20
33	Change in schools	19
34	Change in recreation	19
35	Change in church activities	18
36	Change in social activities	17
37	Mortgage or loan less than $10,000	16
38	Change in sleeping habits	15
39	Change in number of family get-togethers	15
40	Change in eating habits	15
41	Vacation	13
42	Christmas	12
43	Minor violations of the law	11

*The mean value assigned to each item on the scale is based on the weighted value attached by the research population to each life event in terms of its tendency to induce stress.

From: Holmes TH, Rahe RH: The social readjustment rating scale. *J Psychosom Med* 11:213, 1967.

pensity to fall ill and even to die. . . . This is a theme that has been common-place in popular thinking in folklore and literature throughout the ages."[22] That critical family life events and stress are somehow related to illness and death is enshrined in folk wisdom and sayings such as "He died of a broken heart" or "It made me sick to my stomach." Galen observed the increased mortality among the bereaved and the depressed; Napoleon's soldiers suffered severe diarrhea before battle. Reports of "voodoo death" from other cultures have been well documented[14] and have forced a recognition that the mind alone can bring about death in a few days. In medical teaching, it has been traditional to note that thyrotoxic disease is often preceded by an emotional crisis of some kind, that rheumatoid arthritis is aggravated by psychological factors, and that infectious mononucleosis and furuncles are associated with stress, particularly that of medical school. Nevertheless, the major emphasis in medicine is on the physical, chemical, and biologic agents of disease.

Engel ascribes the loss of past insight to the tremendous breakthroughs in the biological sciences, which resulted from the powerful tools which could only study the biochemical and physical alterations of the body and were poorly adapted to study the connections between mind and body. Even the brain was studied without reference to its psychological functions! But the emphasis has changed: "The development of an organismic point of view is finally making it possible to understand how the individual functions within an environment and how mind and brain act as mediators and regulators of the body economy."[22]

Several authors[4,25,53] in family medicine have reviewed the reserach demonstrating the following:

1. that stress is frequently followed by illness;
2. that family support protects from stress;
3. that illness has an impact on the family; and
4. that the family has an impact on illness.

Although the scientific method necessitates isolation of variables, studies conceived to assess the "impact of X on Y"[75] lead to arguments that do not effectively address the complex interaction between family and illness, particularly chronic illness. Illness and family function are often co-evolving, inextricably interwoven phenomena.

Early Studies of the Relationship Between Life Crisis and Illness

The first studies to look beyond specific causes of disease were triggered by Selye's pioneer work on stress.[80] Previously, the individual had been the focus, and stress was seen as a nonspecific entity. After World War II, American prisoners of war in the Pacific (one third died before liberation) had twice the mortality rate normal for their age during the 6 years after liberation. Nine times the expected number died of tuberculosis, twice the expected number of heart disease, and more than twice the expected number of cancer. Mortality from gastrointestinal disease was four times greater than the normal rate; the suicide rate was doubled, and the accident mortality tripled. In survivors the subsequent hospital admission rate closely paralleled the degree of stress and suffering during imprisonment; those with the worst histories had ten times as many health impairments as control groups. It was also noted that after the wars in Korea and Vietnam suffering was proportional to isolation. The use of a buddy system or larger cohesive groups helped protect veterans against morbidity and mortality; death of a buddy increased vulnerability. The Turks were particularly adept at creating such supportive substitute families and had a much lower rate of illness than the Americans.

In 1952, Hinkle and Plummer[31] and later Hinkle and Wolff[32] began a series of studies that systematically studied the relationship between onset of illness and life circumstances in a large population of people. They studied the work records of American working men and women in relation to illness. They studied Chinese and American graduate students and Hungarian refugees. The conclusions they came to were the following:

1. 50% of illnesses were found in 25% of the population.
2. 10% of illnesses were found in 50% of the population.
3. Illnesses occurred in clusters that consisted of months or years during which a number of more or less serious illnesses occurred. Concurrently, a number of significant life events were occuring in the lives of these individuals (see Figure 8-1).
4. In the families of these illness-prone people marked psychosocial disruption occurred, with a high incidence of divorce and poor interpersonal relationships. The families were also illness-prone, both psychologically and physically. The index patients also displayed interpersonal difficulties in their work environments as well as physical illness.[31]

HEALTH, STRESS, AND COPING

Antonovsky[4] has broadened the discussion of disease causality to include the "causes" of health as well as disease. In a stressful environment, what is surprising is not that people get sick but that most of us remain relatively healthy. He argues against the dichotomy between health and disease in favor of a continuum. Medical care studies in the United States and Great Britain suggest that in an average month, 750 of 1,000 adults will experience an episode of illness, of whom 250 will consult a physician. These data led Zola to conclude that "The empirical reality may be that illness, defined as the presence of clinically serious symptoms, is the statistical norm."[87]

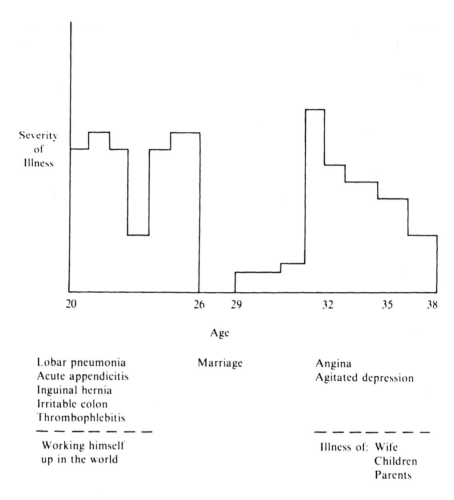

Figure 8-1. American Working Man: Illness Clusters (Hinkle & Wolff)—History of a Young Man's Illnesses in Relation to Life Crises

From: Hinkle LE, Wolff HG: Ecologic investigation of the relationship between illness, life experience, and the social environment. *Ann Intern Med* 49:1373, 1958.

Forty-four percent of the population of Baltimore were afflicted with a chronic condition causing present or future limitation (19% with one condition, 13% with two, and 12% with three or more). Many of these persons are not patients, and many persons who visit doctors do not have disease; therefore, equating the sick with those who visit the health care professional is inaccurate. A more useful concept is that of a breakdown in functioning, as indicated by pain and limitation, which is likely to increase and to require therapeutic intervention. What factors lead to this breakdown? As Antonovsky put it: "Given the 'right' constellation of factors, one will 'look around' for a way to break down. There are, as it were, always additional factors in one's internal or external environment which one 'chooses' and which facilitate the expression of the breakdown in one specific disease or another."[43]

Stressors are ubiquitous. We are constantly bombarded by stressors, whether daily strife, omnipresent endogenous organisms, or abnormal mutant cells threatening our immunologic surveillance system. When internal mental stress (conflict, guilt) and family stress are added life becomes a walk on a tightrope. Antonovsky noted that human experience in exposure to stressors ranges from "fairly serious and lifelong—in, shall we say, the typical experience of many, though far from all, comfortable middle class readers of this book—to the unbelievable hell on earth of so large a part of the world's population."[4] Yet, as Antonovsky pointed out, "Conflict is endemic; breakdown is still happily, relatively exceptional."

Lack of stress, however, means monotony and boredom. Selye[80] coined the term "eustress" to remind us that optimal levels of stress are associated with health; illness may result from too low levels of stress, as in a veteran administration study of 88 chronically ill, marginally employed men, all of whom had very low levels of recent life events (19% had had no life event, except Christmas, in the past year[86]). Like the normal arousal curve for optimum performance level, both low and high levels of stress can be destructive and impair performance.

Stressful Life Events

There has been much discussion as to whether change is the essential component of the stressor in comparison with undesirability.[84] Life events such as marriage or promotion may be desirable but require a considerable degree of adaptation of the individual and can often be associated with the onset of illness if these demands for adaptation are excessive.

The Holmes and Rahe scale (Table 8.1) was developed by asking 394 randomly selected people to rate the amount of social readjustment required for a series of 43 events common to most individuals.[36,51] An arbitrary numerical value of 500 (later changed to 50) was assigned to marriage. If a given event represented more intense and longer readjustment than marriage, a larger number was chosen. These values are called "life change units." Universally, death of a spouse was rated as the most stressful event. This scale has been rated by many different cultures and age groups; a remarkable amount of consistency was found within subgroups of the American population. High correlations were found between the estimates made by Black, Mexican, and Anglo-Saxon Americans.[45] Other studies demonstrated correlations between Americans and two populations of Japanese people.[52] Most recently, groups of Swedish and Finnish people have rank ordered these events in a parallel fashion.[73,85]

Stress as measured by life change units was found in many independent studies to be followed by illness. The amount of life change units is usually highest within the 6 months immediately associated with a major health change, a finding similar to Hinkle's finding that illness has a tendency to cluster.[32] This has been corroborated by Rahe's study of Navy personnel just after the stress of enlistment[69] and by a study of survivors and nonsurvivors of myocardial infarction in Scandinavia. Following an illness, the number of life change units gradually diminishes.[70,71,83,85]

Accumulated stress was even more likely to be followed by illness; for example, in persons with a score of 200 to 299 over a 2-year period 51% reported significant health changes; in those with a score over 300, 79% had such changes.[71]

The scale has been criticized as being overly simple and having poor content validity. For example, according to the scale, 20- to 30-year old persons have twice the number of stressful life events than those over 60 years old, whereas most persons think stress increases with age; illness certainly increases. However, the scale's simplicity has lead to its extensive use in other studies. Rahe's group and other have studied the onset of tuberculosis,[30] pneumonias and other infections,[39] cardiac disease (particularly myocardial infarction),[85] diabetes,[27] inguinal hernias,[70] schizophrenia[47] and accidents[15] in populations in Scandinavia and North America; a consistent correlation was shown between the total amount of stressful recent life events and the occurrence of the particular illness under study.

However, in those studies that looked at stressful life events alone the correlation coefficients are only approximately 0.3; only 9% of the variance of illness is explained.[68] Many people experience terrible stress with no signs of illness; illness often occurs in the absence of apparent stress. It is becoming apparent that the effects of stress are much greater when other mediating (and confounding) variables are added.

CYBERNETIC OR SYSTEMS THINKING AND STRESS

Stress is one variable in a complex matrix (a feedback system of interrelating variables), and can be caused by illness as well as cause illness. It can result from family interaction as well as being relieved by family support. Medical research has been confused by the linear approach in which variables are taken out of context for measurement and not seen in the light of reality. For example, it has been shown that congestive failure and admission to the hospital follow a stressful life event in 75% of cases.[16] This may represent organic changes as a result of stress (the "ripple effect" of disease following the death of a spouse or parent) or an escape from stress into the sickness role: for example, hospitalization may represent a positive adaptation to a partner's alcoholic binge, or a means of avoiding a lonely Christmas after the last child has left home.

Holmes'[36] and Rahe's "Social Readjustment Rating Scale" includes not only external and uncontrollable events such as injury from an accident but also events that are within the control of the individual, such as marriage, imprisonment, and divorce. Many items on the list (29 of the 43)[37] can be symptoms or consequences of illness in themselves.[43] Illness itself can be a major stressor, and part of a vicious circle that produces more and more dysfunction in an individual or family.

The source of stress, as well as mediation of stress, can be from any of the systems levels shown in Figure 8-2. Brody[12] has illustrated a situation in which a national decision has stressful repercussions throughout the community, resulting in organic illness at the cellular level. Conversely, a genetic defect can cause repercussions in the individual, the family, and sometimes the community:

> In one family, the diagnosis of Werdnig Hoffman's Disease in a 1- and 1/2-year-old girl resulted in severe family dysfunction. The family was vulnerable at the outset because the mother had tuberculosis (which has been called "a disease of isolation"[17]), perhaps the result of the woman's isolation in a foreign country with no one but her husband with whom to communicate. The family also had another sick child. Alcoholism in both parents resulted from stress, the lack of support by physicians and community, and the couple's coping styles of denial and avoidance. Obesity and depression in a sister was an outcome of multiple stresses, yet another sister was not affected.

Thus, biomedical factors, the sickness role, coping styles of individuals and of families, the degree of support from family and community, and the characteristics of the stress all must be considered in the evaluation of the stress-illness relationship. Each factor is interrelated with the others.

MEDIATING FACTORS

Mirsky[59] did a pioneering study of young army recruits showing that peptic ulcer developed under the stress of being away from home for the first time, but only in those recruits who were genetically predisposed by high levels of blood pepsinogen, and who had particular personality variables. Spilken and Jacobs[83] found that upper respiratory infections in college students increased after events that provoked a sense of personal failure or social isolation coupled with helplessness.

The concept of the "giving up-given up complex,"[22] the feeling of hopelessness and helplessness following a loss or stressful life event, has been a fruitful concept developed by a group at the University of Rochester (including George Engel, William Greene, and Arthur Schmale.)

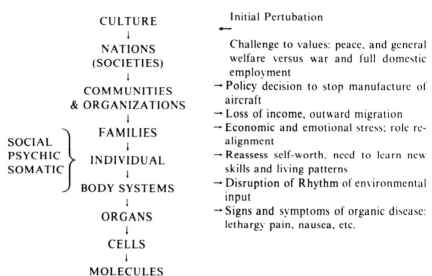

Downward Spread of Pertubations →
Stress Related Illness of Aerospace Engineer

CULTURE
↓
NATIONS
(SOCIETIES)
↓
COMMUNITIES
& ORGANIZATIONS
↓
FAMILIES
↓
INDIVIDUAL
↓
BODY SYSTEMS
↓
ORGANS
↓
CELLS
↓
MOLECULES

SOCIAL
PSYCHIC
SOMATIC

Initial Pertubation
←

Challenge to values: peace, and general welfare versus war and full domestic employment
→ Policy decision to stop manufacture of aircraft
→ Loss of income, outward migration
→ Economic and emotional stress: role realignment
→ Reassess self-worth, need to learn new skills and living patterns
→ Disruption of Rhythm of environmental input
→ Signs and symptoms of organic disease: lethargy pain, nausea, etc.

Figure 8-2

From: Brody H: The systems view of man: Implications for medicine, science, and ethics. *Perspect Biol Med* Autumn, 1973, pp. 71-91.

In four studies that included 190 patients hospitalized with medical illness and in one study of 50 patients hospitalized for psychological illness, Schmale[77] found that 80% had experienced a recent actual, threatened, or symbolic loss that leads to feelings of helplessness and hopelessness. The giving-up process comprised feelings of being deprived, let down, and powerless, despair, futility, and failure resulted. Loss was the antecedent of disease in all categories (infectious, metabolic, degenerative, and neoplastic).

Schmale comments that giving up objects is a repeated part of growth, relating, and aging in every person's life. Early life experiences of deprivation or familial vulnerability might lead to a chronic defensive state in which feelings of helplessness or hopelessness were avoided by dependency on a few key figures and selfless devotion. The psychiatric patients particularly felt that they had had difficult, unrewarding lives with strained interpersonal relationships. The medical patients reported more temporary early losses that were only briefly disruptive because of their activities and supportive environment.

Grant[28] in a longitudinal study of eight adult celiac patients who improved on a gliadin-free diet, correctly predicted relapse in 28 of 30 episodes of celiac syndrome when the episode was preceded by gliadin and the patient's feeling of giving up, or by the patient's feeling of giving up alone, but never by gliadin alone. Parens[65] predicted which student nurses would have a higher frequency of illness in the first 8 months of training by correlating illness rates with a tendency toward depression in the first 6 weeks.

Greene[29] studied the lymphomas and leukemias and found a high incidence of recent loss or separation. Le Shan[48] and Schmale[78] each independently observed the response of hopelessness in patients who developed cancer following loss. A study of cervical cancer by Schmale[78] accurately anticipated the result of biopsies in 76% of patients based on rating their feelings of helplessness and hopelessness. The increased mortality rate from cancer, as well as from other diseases,[40] after the loss of a spouse has been documented now many times. Table 8.2 shows one of the earliest studies done by Kraus and Lillienfeld[46] that demonstrates the increase in the mortality rate of those persons widowed between the ages of 25 and 35 years, in comparison to the married of the same age. The 12-fold increase of tuberculosis in the men is striking. Hawkins,[30] studying the prognosis of tuberculosis, found that all treatment failures were in the lowest third of the social support scale; it has been suggested that alcoholism in young widowers might be one factor in this high incidence of tuberculosis. (It is of note that alcoholics who stop drinking in the absence of social support have a 20-fold increase in the incidence of tuberculosis, compared to those who stop drinking with full social support, whose incidence of tuberculosis is lower than that of the general population[41]).

Characteristics of Stressors

The more intense the life event, the more prolonged the exposure to it, the higher the incidence, and severity of illness that may result. Severe stress such as war or disaster will cause a breakdown in all people exposed to it. For example, there is evidence that individuals who survived the Holocaust all show irreversible psychological effects.[68]

What constitutes a stressor in everyday life? Many people experience extreme changes or difficulties in life and seem to thrive on them. A stressor must be perceived as a threat of harm to the physical self, the psychological self, or to interpersonal relations. McGrath[50] reviewed the psychosocial factors in the perception of stress; five categories were discerned from the examination of 200 studies of stress:

1. *Cognitive appraisal.* The meaning of an event determines its stressful content. The perception of stress depends on the individual's identity, ego strength, circumstances, and belief system. There is some evidence, for instance, that subjects of sensory deprivation studies hallucinate to the degree that they have heard that these hallucinations are to be expected.

Table 8.2 **Average Annual Death Rates for Selected Cases in the Married and The Widowed, for the 25-to-35 Age Group, by Sex, United States 1949–1951 (Deaths rates per 100,000 population in each specified group)**

Cause	Sex	Married	Widowed	Widowed/ Married
Tuberculosis	M	11.2	141.8	12.7
	F	15.4	76.1	4.9
Vascular lesions of the central nervous system	M	3.6	29.3	8.1
	F	4.1	17.4	4.2
Hypertension with heart disease	M	1.7	18.3	10.8
	F	2.3	10.9	4.7
Influenza and pneumonia	M	2.6	20.1	7.7
	F	2.7	13.4	5.0
Arteriosclerotic heart disease	M	8.6	42.1	4.9
	F	2.8	16.5	5.9
Malignant neoplasms	M	16.2	37.5	2.3
	F	20.9	52.4	2.5
Diabetes	M	1.4	4.6	3.3
	F	1.7	4.2	2.5
Motor vehicle accidents	M	32.3	88.2	4.5
	F	7.8	19.8	3.3

Adapted with permission from Kraus A, Lilienfeld A: Some epidemiologic aspects of the high mortality rate in the young widowed group. *J Chron Dis* 10:207, 1959.

2. *Past experience.* Prior experience attenuates the effect of a stressor or situation, particularly if the stressor has evoked an adaptive or "successful" response by the individual.
3. *Negative experience.* "Failure breeds failure." This is a variation of category 1 and a qualification of category 2. Task failure has been shown to increase the level of 17-hydroxy-ketosteroids.[9] Rigid problem-solving behavior and premature closure contribute to repeat failures.
4. *Optimum level of stimulation.* Both too much stress and too little can be stressful. Boredom and sensory deprivation can be damaging physically and psychologically in animals as well as humans: the non-stimulating environment of the old age home leads to deterioration in mental capacity and often to death within months of admission. The optimal stimulus intensity and complexity and the optimal degree of *uncertainty* of a situation depends on its novelty and duration and on the individual.
5. *Social interaction.* As McGrath[50] comments, "We can't live with people and we can't live without them." Social support systems are

important to our health but crowding is hazardous. People generate stress through threats to the ego, conflict, and other interpersonal threats. Again there is an optimal level of social contact, and this level varies with the individual and over time.

Characteristics of the Individual

The individual's response to stress depends on his or her genetic make-up, culture, family belief system, and use of the sickness role, upbringing, and past experiences. A person's own behavior may contribute to stress, both in himself or herself and in others.

Monat and Lazarus[60] describe three ways that stress can lead to illness: disruption of tissue function through neurohumoral influences under stress; coping activities that are damaging to health (smoking, type A life style); and minimization of symptoms and neglect of care, particularly when stress derives from a feared diagnosis. Thus coping style may result in decreased or increased harm to the organism. Lazarus classifies coping processes into two kinds of responses: direct (fight or flight); and palliative (reduction of the emotional impact of stress). The latter includes defense mechanisms such as denial (often highly useful but potentially destructive) and somatic responses such as use of tranquilizers, exercise, relaxation, or bio-feedback. Whether these are effective depends on the physical, psychological, or social level involved, the point in time (short- or long-term), and the particular situation as well as on the value system of the observer.

Antonovsky[4] has described a "sense of coherence" in a person's view of the world as a major determinant of resistance to stress. This is not a sense of control by the individual but a sense that the world at large is under control and that he or she has a legitimate place in it. This concept is reminiscent of Viktor Frankl's views in *Man's Search for Meaning.*[23] Frankl observed that survivors of Hitler's concentration camps had a sense of meaning to their lives derived from work, love, or through suffering.

Life experience, family, and cultural attitudes contribute to a sense of coherence. Culture also may help define the type of response to stress. For example, stomach ulcer and cancer are very prevalent in Japan (see Chapter 6), whereas heart disease is commoner in North America. Factors such as diet are thought to explain these differences but it is of interest that the Japanese consider the stomach the soul or locus of emotion; phrases like "broken-hearted" or at the "heart of things" reflect our own culture's emphasis on the heart and its vulnerability.

Early trauma, particularly death of a parent, seems to predispose to the helplessness/hopelessness response.[21] Uncertainty, lack of knowledge or understanding of the situation, lack of resources, and poor coping mechanisms in the past all diminish coping ability in the present.

Past efforts to isolate *personality* types with specific illnesses [19] or specific conflicts with specific organ responses[1] or organ inferiority[2] are in disrepute. This tradition is maintained, however, in the popular concept linking a type A personality with cardiac disease.[24] Friedman and Rosenman's interest in persons with the type A personality (who are hard driving, competitive with an underlying hostility, and, above all, driven by time) originated in an observation in the waiting room of a cardiologist. The chairs in this waiting room, in contrast to that of other specialists, were worn down at the front edge; the cardiac patients, unable to relax, tended to sit on the edge of their seats. This inability to relax represents a level of chronic stress on which life change events are superimposed.

THE FAMILY AND ILLNESS

Family Characteristics and Support Systems

Individual personalities are developed and maintained in families. The family types associated with cardiac disease have not been studied. However, the type A personality is often supported by a spouse who encourages workaholism (sometimes by complaining about it!) and whose own family pattern was often type A. In a study by Hoebel,[33] a series of such men with cardiac problems were treated with up to five interviews with their wives alone. When the wives' usual approach to their husbands' behavior was altered, the family system that was maintaining the high-risk behavior changed. The so-called "lifestyle diseases" are independently linked with family functioning, regardless of the influence of cigarette smoking, diet, and exercise.

The Framingham study,[42] in which these risk factors were evaluated, did not examine family function. Medalie,[53] however, in a prospective study of 10,000 men in 1973, showed that family dysfunction was a greater risk factor in cardiovascular disease than cigarette smoking, and as important as hypertension and cholesterol. There was a threefold increase in the incidence of angina in families with severe dysfunction compared to those with no dysfunction (16/219 at risk and 50/1636 at risk, respectively) (Table 8.3). Family support decreased the incidence of angina (52/637 with strong support compared to 93/183 with no support).

Nesser[61] found a high correlation between stroke morbidity and the degree of family fragmentation in the black community in counties of North Carolina. Counties with least disruption (divorce, single parent families, illegitimacy, and imprisonment) had an annual mortality rate of 84/100,000 from stroke, compared to a mortality rate of 290/100,000 for those with most disruption.

Table 8.3 Angina Pectoris Incidence (1963-1968) as Related to Psychosocial Factors in 1963

Psychosocial Area	Severity Score*	Number of Subjects	Number of Cases	Age Area— Adjusted Rate/1,000
Family problems	0(least)	1,636	50	31
	1	3,972	125	33
	2	1,836	68	38
	3	865	41	49
	4(most)	219	16	88

*Severity Score: A score indicating the number of times a subject reported serious or very serious problems in respect to questions within the psychosocial area (eg, 0 = no serious problem 3 = a serious problem in each of the three questions related to the relevant problem area).

Adapted with permission from Medalie JH, Snyder M, Groen JJ, et al: Angina pectoris among 10,000 men: 5-year incidence and univariate analysis. *Am J Med* 55:583, 1973

Medalie has found that husbands tend to develop hypertension during pregnancy.[54] Rahe's scale ignores the chronic stress baseline caused by family or work pressures or day-to-day argument with a spouse, which may be more stressful than some life events on the scale.

Meyer and Haggerty[55] assessed the impact of both acute and chronic family stress on streptococcal infection. Throat swabs and blood cultures were taken every 3 weeks from 100 people in 16 families over a 1-year period; infection was found to be four times more likely to occur in the 2 weeks following an acute family stress, such as divorce or death of a relative, than in the 2 weeks preceding it. In families under chronic stress (rated independently by two observers using Bell and Vogel's 16-point rating scale),[8] infection and carrier rates were higher, as was the incidence of elevated antistreptolysin 0 titers per infection (49% of patients compared to 21% in low stress families, $p < 0.05$) (Table 8.4).

Social Support Studies

One of the chief mitigating variables for life stress is that of social support. For example, a study of Nucholls[62] showed that stressful life events alone did not predict the development of complications of pregnancy. However, when the pregnant women were divided into groups with high, medium, and low social support, the occurrence of complications after stressful events during the pregnancy was 33% in women with high social support and 91% in those with low social support ($p > 0.001$). Conversely, in Lynch's *The Broken Heart, the Medical Consequence of Loneliness*,[49] numerous studies demonstrating the effect of isolation on the occurrence of illness are outlined.

Table 8.4 **Beta-Streptococcal Infections in Families***

Level of Chronic Family Stress	Antistreptolysin 0 Response† Episodes, Group A Streptococcal 0 Acquisition			No Evidence of Streptococcal Acquisitions
	ASO Rise	No Rise	Total	
Low	3	11	14	19
Moderate to high	34	36	70	9

*100 persons, 16 families, 12 months
†Two or more tubes ($p < 0.05$)
‡Antistreptolysin 0 titre.

Reproduced with permission from: Meyer RJ, Haggerty RJ: Streptococcal Infections in Families, *Pediatrics* 29:539, 1962.

Cobb[17] divides social support into three components:

1. emotional support, the sense of being cared for and loved;
2. esteem support, the sense of esteem and value and satisfaction given by the recognition of others; and
3. network support, the sense of belonging to one or preferably several networks of mutual obligation and a feeling of having one's place in society.

There is an extensive literature demonstrating the positive effects of social support[5,77] on patient compliance and improved recovery from illness,[35] as well as the protection from illness associated with severe stressful life events.

Berkman and Syme,[10] in a major prospective study of 6,928 adults in Alameda County, California with a 9-year mortality follow-up, showed that lack of social and community ties more than doubled the death rate. Age-adjusted relative risks were 2.3 for men and 2.8 for women. These figures were independent of socioeconomic status, health practices (smoking, alcohol consumption, obesity, physical activity), and utilization of preventive health services. Pre-existent disease as a cause of social isolation was not a factor. Causes of death significantly related to lack of social support included ischemic heart disease, cancer, cerebrovascular and circulatory disease, disease of the digestive system, accidents, and suicide. Four sources of social relationship were examined: marriage; contacts with close friends and relatives; church memberships; and informal and formal group association. Each influenced mortality independently, but the first two were the stronger influences.

Several studies demonstrated that one important component of support is the physician. In a study done by Chambers and Reisers[16] emotional support from the physician had an extraordinary beneficial effect on the course of congestive heart failure. Egbert and colleagues[20] showed that special supportive care by the anesthetist to one group of surgical patients (the surgeons were unaware which patients had the support and which were controls), who, in comparison to controls, needed less pain medication and were discharged 2.7 days earlier.

Studies of the Family System

Family dysfunction can promote illness. Minuchin's studies of children with severe asthma, superlabile diabetes, or anorexia nervosa[57] have shown how interactions within the family can cause or aggravate an illness in a family member with a genetic predisposition to such diseases. These children with severe psychosomatic illness were thought to both manifest physiologic vulnerability and to maintain family homeostasis in a family where conflict was present but denied. Through a psychosomatic crisis, the child protected the parents from open conflict. For example, an asthmatic child anxious about signs of masked parental disagreement might develop bronchospasm that would take him and at least one parent to the emergency room, with the result that parental conflict would be forgotten.

Family therapy (lasting an average of 6 months) improved the organic condition of children in all three disease groups. These children were followed for a minimum of 2 years. Eight of ten steroid-dependent children with intractable asthma, who had lost an average of 3 weeks of school each year, had discontinued steroids by the end of family therapy. One child was free of asthma; seven only occasionally needed bronchodilators and lost no days of school; and two had mild to moderate attacks. Of 25 severe anorectics with a mean weight loss of 30 lbs and amenorrhea, three dropped out of the program at the outset; the remaining 22 patients regained their original weight. None died; usually the mortality rate for anorexia nervosa is 5% to 15%.

Minuchin's studies of diabetic children[58,59] have demonstrated both the relation between home environment and ketoacidosis and the effects of family therapy (lasting an average of 5 months) on acidosis. Of 13 diabetic children who were hospitalized an average of 12 times per year for severe ketoacidosis, three averaged only one admission in 2 years, while ten children had no admissions during that period. Before family therapy the children's diabetes had been easy to control while in hospital but was extremely resistant to insulin when the children were at home (in one girl 500 U were required in 18 hours at home, compared to a daily hospital requirement of 30 U).

Minuchin is one of the few researchers with a family systems orientation. He describes the contrasting models: the familiar linear medical model "links the individual's life situations to his emotions to bodily illness, in a causal chain. But the illness is seen as contained within the individual. Consequently, research and treatment approaches are focused on the individual and this is far too limited a target." In contrast, in the systems model, "Since family interactions affect the psychophysiology of the child in the psychosomatic crisis, disorder is seen as situated in the feedback process of child and family. The artificial boundary between individuals and context no longer handicaps therapeutic efforts."[58] The family then becomes the patient and is the more appropriate target for treatment.

There are two other much less known examples of a systems orientation to health, both of which were influenced by one of the fathers of systems thinking, Gregory Bateson, through his wife, Margaret Mead. In 1926 the "Peckham Experiment"[67] involved an entire community in Cambridge, South London, which was set up for healthy living and for experimental observation along anthropological lines. The concepts on which the study was based were those of a systems orientation; the "family as organism model." The purpose was to document North American family behavior as one would in a biologist's laboratory and to assess the effects on subsequent health of children in a happy environment. Annually there was a "family health overhaul" with physical exam and discussions with the family as a group. The war intervened and the community faded, although some community programs such as Maria Montessori's educational nurseries remained. This little known study has been used by Donald Ransom,[73] one of the pioneers on the family system in family medicine.

The second example is the "Macy Family Study," documented in the book *Patients Have Families* by H.B. Richardson.[74] Richardson's previous training in hospital wards and clinics, animal experiments, electrocardiograms, pathology, and metabolism did nothing to prepare him for the insight, that the family is the unit of illness. His book is a study of family care and teamwork and of disease as a manifestation of disturbed family equilibrium.

In 1943 Huygen, a Dutch family physician, began to record all contacts with patients in a family record.[38] He, like Hinkle, observed clustering of visits and noted that some families were much sicker than others, some were accident-prone, and organic physical illness occurred much more often in families with a high incidence of relationship problems. Housing, hygiene, and finance did not explain the consistently different illness patterns between family units. In a detailed study of 200 families, a striking correlation between children's illness and parental problems was noted. Children needed the doctor more often when their parents tended to avoid conflicts ($p < 0.001$); their mother was little involved in social networks outside the family ($p < 0.001$); and their parents, especially mother ($p < 0.01$), were prone to somatic complaints, and there was a discrepancy in their parents' knowledge of complaints of the partner ($p < 0.01$). These data support the work on psychosomatic families by Minuchin[58,59] and Bowen's[11] theory that the family projection process passes illness down through generations.

A third study describing family patterns of illness was reported by Peachey,[64] who randomly selected 25 families from a rural general practice in the United States. In 21 families, she noted one of four repetitive patterns: constant illness in the family as a unit (there was always at least one member of the family who was sick); regular periodicity of illness; clustering; and simultaneity of visits by two or more family members on the same day. The author, however, did not investigate the reasons for such patterns.

The Impact of Illness on the Family System

That illness in an individual affects the family in many ways may be more apparent to physicians and nurses than the fact that the family can affect the illness. Illness may alter the family member's role and his or her performance of necessary tasks. There are financial implications: both the illness (medications, medical and hospital bills in some settings, appliances, etc.) and the loss of wages in a working adult affect the family adversely. Fear of terminal illness, dismemberment, disfigurement, or simply decreased ability to function and increased dependence may all affect family members as much or more than the afflicted individual. The effects of chronic illness on the family are well described by Bruhn.[13]

Less obvious is the impact of illness on the health of family members. The incidence of illness in a second family member is higher than would be expected by chance.[13] Another family member may develop symptoms similar to those of the afflicted member, and children often develop a parent's complaints. Klein[44] demonstrated that an increase in the level of interpersonal tension and symptoms in a spouse correlated with tension levels and symptoms of the chronically ill patient. Thus families may have periods of frequent illness, and members may respond both to stress in the system and to already developed symptoms in others, in addition to physical factors such as the presence of infectious agents.

Hospitalization may induce a family crisis. The rate at which the family recovers and the level of functioning after the crisis are indicators of family health.[81] Family equilibrium may be so disturbed by illness, particularly that of the mother, that it may not recover. If a second crisis occurs before the family has had time to rally, progressive disintegration may occur. Chapter 20 discusses the impact of illness on the family at greater length.

BIOLOGICAL MECHANISMS

Minuchin[58] studied the association between home environment and acidosis in diabetic children, finding biochemical evidence of transfer of stress from one part of the family system to another. These diabetic children with frequent acidosis and their families were tested in a standardized stress situation against control diabetic children and their families. Free fatty acid values were determined by continuous intravenous measurement in all family members during a family diagnostic interview. (Fatty acids are indicators of emotional arousal and increase with stress in all of us, and are also precursors of ketones in a diabetic). The parents were instructed to discuss a family problem in period 1 (Figures 8-3 and 8-4); in period 2 a therapist went into the room and focused the problems so that the conflict escalated. During this time, the child watched the parents through a one-way mirror. In period 3 the child was asked to enter the room; during period 4 the family relaxed.

Figure 8-3 shows the free fatty acid level of the diabetic children. The lowest curve is that of normal diabetics with no behavior problems or difficulty with diabetic control. The middle curve shows the free fatty acid level of diabetic children with behavioral problems or poor compliance; it rises above the baseline after the child enters the room (period 3) but otherwise is essentially no different from the first group. However, the labile diabetics or "psychosomatic" children, as Minuchin calls them, continue to show a marked rise in anxiety and may be heading towards ketosis.

Figure 8-4 is a comparison of the parent with the higher free fatty acid level and their child. The control group is at the top: the fatty acid levels of the normal parent rise a little above the baseline but indicate little anxiety when the parent is asked to discuss a family conflict. In comparison, the parents of the children with behavioral problems have higher levels of free fatty acids, indicating greater family conflict, as might be expected of parents with a child who has behavioral problems. The lower graph shows the "psychosomatic" families; there is a marked increase in stress in the parent's free fatty acid levels when the therapist comes in to encourage discussion of a conflict (period 2). However, when the child enters the room, the parent's level of free fatty acid abruptly drops. This drop is in contrast to that of the parents of the child with behavior problems, who continue to argue and remain tense as indicated by their levels of free fatty acid in period 3. Thus, the psychosomatic families are showing a transfer of stress from the parents to the child: the parents focus on the child when he or she enters the room to avoid stress and conflict. Diabetes in the context of the family is a very different phenomenon in these three groups and depends on the characteristics of the family.

In one family with two diabetic children[57] there was no biochemical difference between the older child, Dede, who was caught between her parents and felt much more involved in their conflict than her younger sister, Violet. Dede's free fatty acid levels rose higher and stayed high during and after the observed interview. Violet's returned to their usual level once the stress was over. Dede volunteered and played the role of family scapegoat.

Several studies are beginning to elucidate the pathways through which stress influences the body and support exerts its protective effect. Selye was one of the earliest investigators to note the commonalities of disease.[80] His work on stress showed that stressors of all sorts produced a general adaptation

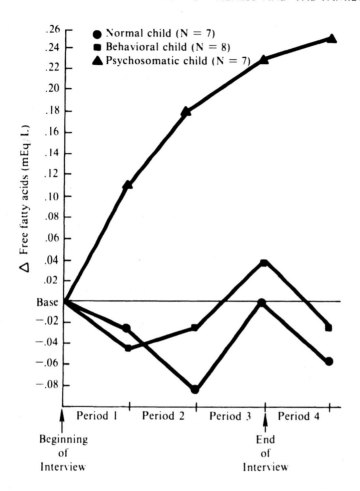

Figure 8-3. Changes in FFA levels of diabetic children during family interview.

From: Minuchin S: *Psychosomatic Families.* Cambridge, Harvard University Press, 1978.

syndrome of three stages. The first stage, alarm reaction, was characterized by enlargement of the adrenal cortex, shrinkage of the thymus, spleen, lymph nodes, and all lymphatic structures, leukopenia with almost complete absence of eosinophils, and deep ulcers in stomach and duodenum. Unless the dose was sufficient to kill the organism during the alarm reaction, more prolonged exposure to any agent causing tissue damage produced a stage of resistance or adaptation with reversal of many of the original changes. If exposure was still more prolonged, a stage of exhaustion ensued, reminiscent of premature aging from wear and tear, with eventual death. The syndrome was also produced by heat, exposure, or by threat of danger and fear. Selye noted that

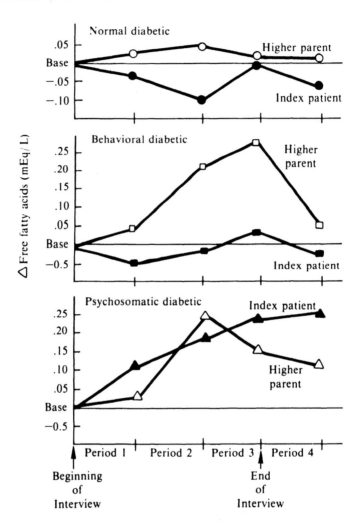

Figure 8–4. Medians of parent with higher FFA response and index patient.
From: Minuchin S: *Psychosomatic Families.* Cambridge, Harvard University Press, 1978.

the disease processes (for example, ulcer formation) resulted from the organism's defense system and not from the noxious agent itself. This concept parallels Freud's contention that the person's psychological defenses against unpleasant stimuli, if extreme or prolonged, produce illness.

An interesting study of parents with children dying of leukemia[85] showed a drop in the parents' 17-hydroxy-ketosteroids before the death of the child; this drop seems to represent a normal period of anticipatory grief. Parents who did not show this drop developed a more precipitous hormonal drop after the death, which seemed to correlate with greater difficulty in adjustment. Bartrop and associates[7] studied the T-lymphocyte function during bereavement and found that the decrease in function was significant, and that it was greatest 6 weeks after death. Gore[26] studied 100 men whose jobs were abolished and showed changes in cholesterol, uric acid levels, norepinephrine in the urine, and serum creatinine. The same study also produced a surprising finding: 41% of men with low social support developed pain and swelling in two or more joints, compared with 4% of men with high social support, and 12% of men with medium social support.

A HEALTHY SYSTEM

In a healthy family, the forces of cohesiveness and individuation are balanced, flexibility is maintained by the ability of the parts to function separately and as a team, and the ability to change the rules of the system to accomodate growth and input from other systems is evident.

Rigidity produces maladaptation. Just as the body's defenses against stress may produce illness by an exaggerated response, so may the family's defenses against a threat produce dysfunction or disease. Symptoms can be seen as failures of adaptation[43] or as exaggerations of adaptive responses to stress. Old solutions that once helped reestablish homeostasis are now inappropriate and contribute to further dysfunction. Anxiety, disorganization, and lack of communication all increase the use of maladaptive defenses and decrease the possibility of second-order change or change in the system rules.

Bakan in *Disease, Pain and Sacrifice* views disease as a breakdown in central organization at a given systems level, whether this is at the cellular, organic, individual, family, or community level.[6] Well-functioning systems show behavior that is goal-directed or purposeful. The term "teleologic" implies that this goal-directed behavior can exist without conscious awareness on the person's part. Studying the hierarchical nature of systems and such behavior at all systems levels, Bakan coined the term "telic (or teleologic) centralization" as the healthy functional state of any system. In such a system, the interests of the parts are subservient to the good of the whole. Decentralization and autonomy of parts are needed for individuation, but needs must be subordinate for the whole to function. The system must in its turn be subordinate to the suprasystem.

For such organization to be maintained communication is essential. Communication may be chemical or physical interaction between cells, genetic hormonal or neural information transfer, verbal and nonverbal communications, or even behavioral communication between nations (the movement of armies). A breakdown in hierarchical organization or communication heralds disease. Cancer cells on a glass slide do not, like normal cells, stop growing when they touch each other. Electrical measurements show that normal ionic transfer does not occur in these cells. Failure of central immune surveillance mechanisms allows these cells to grow and set up a center whose interests are largely opposed to those of its host. Similarly, bacterial antigens or toxic agents may set up defense mechanisms that eventually overwhelm the host. Degenerative diseases and death are all signs of an inevitable process towards telic decentralization. Every system eventually dies, to be replaced by a new, more vital system. Death too becomes part of an overall teleologic system.

In the social system, organizations rise and fall. Their hierarchy and functions depend on effective communication and good government. Times of social disruption have been periods of poor health. Dubos[18] describes examples in the animal world: an accepted pecking order for chickens is beneficial to their health; overcrowding leads to death in lemmings and increased susceptibility to drugs and infections in mice.

At the individual level, it has been proposed that psychosomatic illness is associated with lack of emotional awareness. Nemiah and Sifneos[89] have described "alexithymia," the inability to find words for feelings as a characteristic of the psychosomatic patient. A similar concept, *pensée operatoire* (operational thought), has been suggested by French psychiatrists Pierre Marty and Michael De M'Uzau[88] to imply a person's ability to think only in instrumental rather than emotional terms. It may be that the avenue of verbal catharsis is not available to these people, and psychological tension and organ damage results.

The concept of failed awareness of distress with poor corticothalamic communication supports breakdown of communication within the individual as productive of disease. Freud argued that mental health depends on a strong ego, conscious awareness, and integration, and that denial and repression of emotion causes disease. Loss of meaning or a sense of purpose decreases resistance to a hostile environment such as a concentration camp,[23] and a sense of hopelessness and helplessness seems to be the eiptome of loss of "telos" or hope or goal in the individual organism.

In families disruption of communication and of system organization can also produce ill health and dysfunction of its members. If one member's good ceases to be subservient to the good of the whole, or if the parental subsystem is in conflict or communicates poorly, family dysfunction or symptoms of one or more members will result. If the process continues unchecked, serious illness, antisocial behavior, or family dissolution may occur. Similarly, if the family system communicates poorly or is in conflict with suprasystems, health problems may result.

To summarize, disease often results from a breakdown of adaptation to a stressful environment or from an exaggerated or distorted adaptation. Defenses such as Selye's general adaptation syndrome, denial in individuals, triangulation in families). This maladaptation is both caused by and results in failure of communication, both within and outside the system; failure of goal directedness also occurs. Each system has an optimal stress level ("eustress") and if this is altered by decreasing stimulation or increasing stress, breakdown will eventually result.

Disease may be the stressor or the result of stress; genetic diseases or predisposition to disease, infectious disease when the dose of pathogen is overwhelming, accidents, or injury when clearly not provoked by the system, and iatrogenic disease are all easily seen as stressors rather than as the result of stress. Most other illnesses are a combination of environmental challenge, genetic endowment, and attempts at adaptation. The degree of support and level of stress of the surrounding system (family, community) will be an important factor in promoting both health and recovery for illness. Working with the family means working with and enhancing the hierarchial organization of a family, focusing on family strengths and goals, and facilitating communication. The next section describes, in detail, how this can be done.

REFERENCES

1. Alexander F, French T, Pollack G: *Psychosomatic Specificity*. Chicago, University of Chicago Press, 1968.

2. Ansbacher H, Ansbacher R (eds): *The Individual Psychology of Alfred Adler*. New York, Basic Books, 1956.

3. Antonovsky A: Breakdown: A needed fourth step in the conceptual armamentarium of modern medicine. *Soc Sci Med* 6:537, 1972.

4. Antonovsky A: *Health, Stress and Coping*. San Francisco, Jossey-Bass, 1979.

5. Baekeland F, Lundwall L: Dropping out of treatment: A critical review. *Psychol Bull* 82:738, 1982.

6. Bakan D: *Disease, Pain and Sacrifice*. Beacon Press, 1968.

7. Bartrop RW, Lazarus L, Luckhurst E, et al: Depressed lymphocyte function after bereavement. *Lancet* 1:834, 1977.

8. Bell NW, Vogel EF: Introductory essays, in *A Modern Introduction to the Family*. Glencoe, Ill, Free Press, 1960.

9. Berkeley AW: Level of aspiration in relation to adrenal cortical activity and the concept of stress. *J Comp Physiol Psychol* 45:443, 1952.

10. Berkman LF, Syme SL: Social networks, host resistance and mortality: A nine-year follow-up study of Alameda County residents. *Am J Epidemiol* 109:186, 1979.

11. Bowen M: *Family Therapy in Clinical Practice*. New York, Jason Aranson, 1978.

12. Brody H: The systems view of man: Implications for medicine, science and ethics. *Perspect Biol Med* 17:71, 1973.

13. Bruhn JG: Effects of chronic illness on the family. *J Fam Pract* 4:1057, 1977.

14. Cannon WB: Voodoo death. *Am Anthropol* 44:169, 1942.

15. Cassel J: Physical illness in response to stress, in Levine S, Scotch NA (eds): *Social Stress*. Chicago, Aldine, 1978.
16. Chambers WN, Reiser MF: Emotional stress in the precipitation of congestive heart failure. *Psychosom Med* 15:38, 1953.
17. Cobb, S: Social support as moderator of life stress. *Psychosom Med* 38:300, 1976.
18. Dubos R: *Man Adapting*. New Haven, Yale University Press, 1965.
19. Dunbar F: *Psychosomatic Diagnosis*. New York, Hoeber, 1943.
20. Egbert LD, Battit GE, Welch CE, et al: Reduction of post-operative pain by encouragement and instruction of patients. *N Engl J Med* 270:852, 1964.
21. Engel G: The clinical application of the biopsychosocial model. *Am J Psychiatry* 137:535, 1980.
22. Engel G: A life setting conducive to illness: The giving-up-given-up complex. *Ann Intern Med* 69:293, 1968.
23. Frankl V: *Man's Search for Meaning*. New York, Pocket Books, 1963.
24. Friedman M, Rosenman R: *Type A Behavior and Your Heart*. New York, Knoff, 1974.
25. Geyman JP: The family as the object of care in family practice. *J Fam Pract* 5:571, 1977.
26. Gore S: The effect of social support in moderating the health consequences of unemployment. *J Health Soc Behav* 19:157, 1978.
27. Grant I, Kyle GS, Teichman A, et al: Recent life events and diabetes in adults. *Psychosom Med* 36:121, 1974.
28. Grant JM: Studies in celiac disease. I. The interrelationship between gliadin, psychological factors and symption formation. *Psychosom Med* 21:431, 1959.
29. Greene WH: The psychosocial setting of the development of leukemia and lymphoma. *Ann NY Acad Sci* 125:794, 1966.
30. Hawkins NG, Davies R, Holmes TH: Evidence of psychosocial factors in the development of pulmonary tuberculosis. *Am Rev Tuberc Pulm Dis* 75:5, 1957.
31. Hinkle LE Jr, Plummer N: Life stress and industrial absenteeism: The concentration of illness and absenteeism in one segment of a working population. *Ind Med Surg* 21:363, 1952.
32. Hinkle LE, Wolff HG: Ecological investigation of the relationship between illness, life experience, and the social environment. *Ann Intern Med* 49:1373, 1958.
33. Hoebel FC: Brief family-interactional therapy in the management of cardiac-related high-risk behaviors. *J Fam Pract* 3:613, 1976.
34. Hofer MA, Wolff CT, Friedman SB, Mason JW: A psychoendocrine study of bereavement. *Psychosom Med* 34:481, 492, 1972.
35. Holmes TH, Joffe JR, Ketcham JW, et al: Experimental study of prognosis. *J Psychosom Res* 5:235, 1961.
36. Holmes TH, Rahe RH: The social readjustment rating scale. *J Psychosom Med* 11:213, 1967.
37. Hudgens RW: Personal catastrophe and depression: A consideration of the subject with respect to medically ill adolescents and a requiem for retrospective life event studies. In Dohrenwend BP, Dohrenwend BS (eds): *Stressful Life Events: Their Nature and Effects*. New York, Wiley, 1974.

38. Huygen FJA: *Family Medicine. The Medical Life History of Families.* Netherlands, Dekker and Van de Vegt, 1978.

39. Jacobs MA, Spilken AZ, Nomen MM, et al: Life stress and respiratory illness. *Psychosom Med* 32:223, 1970.

40. Jacobs S, Ostfeld A: An epidemiological review of the mortality of bereavement. *Psychosom Med* 39:344, 1977.

41. Jackson JK: The problem of alcoholic tuberculosis patients, in Sparer PF: *Personality, Stress and Tuberculosis.* New York, International Universities Press, 1954.

42. Kannel WB, McGee D, Gordon T: A general cardiovascular risk profile: The Framingham Study. *Am J Cardiol* 38:46, 1976.

43. Kerr ME: *Family Systems Theory and Therapy. Handbook of Family Therapy.* New York, Brunner/Mazel, 1981.

44. Klein RF, Dean A, Bogdonoff MD: The impact of illness upon the spouse. *J Chron Dis* 20:241, 1976.

45. Komaroff AL, Masuda M, Holmes TH: SRRS: A comparative study of Negro, Mexican and white Americans. *J Psychosom Res* 12:121, 1968.

46. Kraus AS, Lillienfeld AM: Some epidemiological aspects of the high mortality rate in the young widowed group. *J Chron Dis* 3:207, 1959.

47. Langsley DG, Pittman FS, Swank GE. Family crisis in schizophrenics and other mental patients. *J Nerv Ment Dis* 149:270, 1969.

48. Le Shan L: An emotional life-history pattern associated with neoplastic disease. 125:780, 1966.

49. Lynch JL: *The Broken Heart: The Medical Consequences of Loneliness.* New York, Basic Books, 1977.

50. McGrath JE: *Social and Psychological Factors in Stress.* New York, Holt, Rinehart and Winston, 1970.

51. Masuda M, Holmes TH: Magnitude estimations of social readjustment. *J Psychosom Res* 11:219, 1967.

52. Masuda M, Holmes TH: The SRRS: A cross-cultural study of Japanese and Americans. *J Psychosom Res* 11:227, 1967.

53. Medalie JH, Snyder M, Groen JJ, et al: Angina pectoris among 10,000 men: 5-year incidence and univariate analysis. *Am J Med* 55:583, 1973.

54. Medalie JH: The family life cycle and its implications for family practice. *J Fam Pract* 9:47–56, 1977.

55. Meyer RJ, Haggerty RJ: Streptococcal infections in families. *Pediatrics* 29:539, 1962.

56. Minuchin S: *Families and Family Therapy.* Cambridge, Harvard University Press, 1974.

57. Minuchin S, Baker L, Rosman BL, et al: A conceptual model of psychosomatic illness in children: Family organization and family therapy. *Arch Gen Psychiatry* 32:1031, 1975.

58. Minuchin S: *Psychosomatic Families.* Cambridge, Harvard University Press, 1978.

59. Mirsky AL: Physiologic, psychologic and social determinants of psychosomatic disorders. *Dis Nerv Syst* 21:50, 1960.

60. Monat A, Lazarus RS: *Stress and Coping—Anthology.* New York, Columbia University Press, 1977.

61. Nesser WB: Fragmentation of black families and stroke, in Kaplan BH, Cassel JC (eds): *Family and Health.* Chapel Hill, North Carolina, Institute for Research in Social Science, University of North Carolina, 1975.

62. Nucholls K: Life crises and psychosocial assets: some clinical implications, in Kaplan BH, Cassell JC (eds): *Family and Health.* Chapel Hill, North Carolina, Institute for Research in Social Science, University of North Carolina, 1975.

63. Parens H, McConville BJ, Kaplan SM: The prediction of frequency of illness from the response to separation. *Psychosom Med* 28:162, 1966.

64. Peachy R: Family patterns of illness. *GP* 27:82, 1963.

65. Pearse I, Crocker L: *The Peckham Experiment: A Study in the Living Structure of Society.* London, Allen and Unwin Press, 1943.

66. Rabkin JG, Struening EL: Life events, stress and illness. *Science* 194:1013, 1976.

67. Rahe RH, Ransom JA: Life-change patterns surrounding illness experience. *J Psychosom Res* 11:341, 1967.

68. Rahe RH, Holmes TH: Social psychological and psycho-physiological aspects of inguinal hernia. *J Psychosom Res* 8:487, 1965.

69. Rahe RH, Mahan J, Arthur R: Prediction of near-future health change from subjects preceding life changes. *J Psychosom Res* 14:401, 1970.

70. Rahe RH, Paasikivi J: Psychosocial factors and myocardial infarctions. II. An outpatient study in Sweden. *J Psychosom Res* 15:33, 1971.

71. Rahe RH, Romo H, Bennett L, Siltanen P: Recent life changes, myocardial infarction and abrupt coronary death. *Arch Intern Med 133:221, 1974.*

72. Rakel RE: *Principles of Family Medicine.* Philadelphia, W. B. Saunders, 1977.

73. Ransom DC: The rise of family medicine: new roles for behavioral science. *Marr Fam Rev* 4(1/2), 1981.

74. Richardson HB: *Patients Have Families.* New York, The Commonwealth Fund, 1945.

75. Schmale AH Jr: Relationship of separation and depression to disease. *Psychosom Med* 20:259, 1958.

76. Schmale AH, Ker H: Hopelessness as a predictor of cervical cancer. *Soc Sci Med* 95, 1971.

77. Schmidt DD: Patient compliance: the effect of the doctor as a therapeutic agent. *J Fam Pract* 4:853, 1977.

78. Schmidt DD: The family as the unit of medical care. *J Fam Pract* 7:303, 1978.

79. Smilkstein G: The family in trouble—how to tell. *J Fam Pract* 2:19, 1975.

80. Selye, H: *The Stress of Life.* New York, McGraw Hill, 1956.

81. Spilken AZ, Jacobs MA: Prediction of illness behaviors from measures of life crisis, manifest distress and maladaptive coping. *Psychosom Med* 33:251, 1971.

82. Steinert Y: Helping patients cope with stressful life events. *Can Fam Phys* 24:859, 1978.

83. Theorell T, Rahe RH: Psychosocial factors and myocardial infarction. I: An inpatient study in Sweden. *J Psychosom Res* 15:25, 1971.

84. Wershow HJ, Reinhart G: Life change and hospitalization: A heretical view. *J Psychosom Res* 18:393, 1974.

85. Wolff CT, Friedman SB, Hofer MA, et al: Relationship between psychological defenses and mean urinary 17-hydroxy corticosteroid excretion rates. I. A predictive study of parents of fatally ill children. *Psychosom Med* 26:576, 1961.

86. Wolff HG: A concept of disease in man. *Psychosom Med* 24:25, 1962.

87. Zola IK: Culture and symptoms: An analysis of patients' presenting complaints. *Am Sociol Rev* 31:615, 1966.

88. Marty P, De M'Uzau M, David D: L'investigation psychosomatique. Paris, Presses Universitaires, 1963.

89. Nemiah JC, Sifneos PE: Affect and fantasy in patients with psychosomatic disorders. Modern Trends of Psychosomatic Medicine. London, Butterworth, 1970.

Chapter 9

The Relevance of the Family to Medical Outcomes

Janet Christie-Seely
Herta Guttman

Awareness of the family produces better medical outcomes. Thus, the family orientation of the physician or nurse concerned primarily with improving patient's health has proven benefit. It is important to emphasize the benefits of family awareness in teaching and to present the research for critical evaluation by residents early in the teaching process. Nursing students are more likely to recognize the relevance of the family to health since they are less preoccupied with the biomedical aspects of disease.

If clinical research is to fully account for the phenomena of health and illness it must broaden its area of interest to incorporate the systems approach. Ultimately, improved research will improve medical outcomes. At present, much research is hampered by a myopic view of the cell, organ, or individual patient; it rarely conceives of that patient as part of a highly influential system whose impact on health is major. A recent article in the *New England Journal of Medicine*,[12] "Later Development of Inflammatory Bowel Disease in the Healthy Spouse of a Patient," is a striking example. The author cites five references describing the occurrence of Crohn's disease in a spouse and then concludes that this is evidence of an external agent, a "slow virus," which precipitates a genetic susceptibility to disease. No mention is made of the possibility of psychosocial factors. Thus, a biomedical focus allows consideration of genes and microbes but no recognition of the larger levels of organization. From a systems view, a better understanding of etiology would include the influence of stress on changes in blood flow, muscle spasm, the role of mimicry of symptoms, and a specific type of sickness role, as well as genetic vulnerability.

EFFECT OF KNOWLEDGE OF THE FAMILY SYSTEM ON DIAGNOSIS AND TREATMENT

Diagnoses may be missed, incorrect, or incomplete if the family is ignored. Duff and Hollingshead[4] found a misdiagnosis rate of 26% in a New

160

England teaching hospital. Ninety-eight percent of the physicians in this study stated they did not need to know more about their patients. The study revealed, however, that they were unaware of family issues, such as a death in the recent past causing identification with the illness of the dead relative ("anniversary reaction"), which would have clarified the diagnosis. Treating the presenting physical illness may be equivalent to treating a symptom and ignores the underlying problem. Apart from being "tickets of admission," the minor illnesses often seen in the family physician's office may point to family dysfunction as sources of lowered resistance.

Most family practitioners are well aware that physical symptoms often mask problems of living since our culture feels physical complaints to be more acceptable than psychological complaints. The limitations of our traditional diagnostic labels have been recognized by Engel[6] and McWhinney,[14] who developed diagnostic schemata to allow for multiple causality but did not look beyond the individual patient to the family system. The systems perspective takes diagnosis one step further. Dealing with the psychological problem behind the symptom or illness may constitute symptomatic treatment if the individual is considered alone; only treatment of the underlying disturbance in the family effectively eliminates the cause of distress. Clearly Minuchin's studies outlined in the previous chapter indicate that the standard individual treatment for a child with steroid-dependent asthma, labile diabetes, or anorexia nervosa is frequently ineffective, whereas family therapy improved the lung function and removed the need for steroids of the asthmatic children (Table 9.2), reduced the hospitalization rate of labile diabetes (Table 9.1), and restored normal weight and menses in the anorectics (Table 9.3). (The unfortunate absence of controls in this study relates to the ethical problem of a referral center where only severely ill children with life-threatening diseases are seen.)

Other studies supporting the efficacy of family therapy for physical problems include those of Comley[2] and Huygen.[11] Comley showed that simple family therapy done by family physicians resulted in a decrease in visits for physical illness and increased patient satisfaction, as well as improvement of relationship problems in two-thirds of the families. Huygen[11] showed a decrease in medical demands in 45% of families referred for family therapy (50% did not change their demands; 5% increased their demands) and a decrease in number of prescriptions in 42% (57% did not change their demands; 1% increased their demands) (see Figure 9-1).

Outcome studies of family therapy for emotional and behavioral problems have been recently reviewed.[7] Each of the 200 studies reviewed showed that family therapy was equal or superior to individual therapy; therapy for the family or marital system was the treatment of choice for marital problems, sexual dysfunction, and psychosomatic and behavioral problems of childhood, including juvenile delinquency. Improvement occurred in two out of three families. Only well-designed studies were included

Table 9.1 Summary of 13 Cases of Superlabile Diabetes

Case No.	Presenting Problems	Family Treatment, mo	Follow-up
1*	30 hospital admissions in 3 yr	9	4 admissions in 3 yr 8 mo, 3 associated with infection
2*	14 hospital admissions in 2½ yr	5	No admissions in 2 yr 4 mo
3*	35 hospital admissions in 20 mo	9	1 admission in 3 yr 1 mo
4*	18 hospital admissions in 4 yr	12	No admissions in 5 yr 11 mo
5*	24 hospital admissions in 20 mo	9	No admissions in 6 yr 7 mo
6*	6 hospital admissions in 6 mo	9	No admissions in 2 yr 6 mo
7*	20 hospital admissions in 2 yr	7	No admissions in first 4 yr 7 mo, 2 admissions in past 21 mo
8†	Recurrent ketosis, nausea, & frequent school absence	3	Free of recurrent ketosis, no associated school absence 2 yr 8 mo
9†	Chronic acetonuria, 6 hospital admissions in 2 yr to evaluate poor diabetic control, & frequent school absence	9	2 hospital admissions in 2 yr 3 mo; free of chronic acetonuria, school attendance excellent (2 days' absence per year)
10†	Poor diabetic control, & 1 hospital admission for vomiting and 3 for diabetic regulation in 1 yr	3	Good control, no vomiting for 2 yr, lost contact 1 yr 9 mo, no problems reported
11†	Chronic acetonuria, headaches, nausea, & vomiting for 12 mo	5	Acetonuria well controlled, 1-day absence for vomiting, no problems for 4 yr 6 mo
12*	15 hospital admissions in 4 yr	15	No admissions in 15 mo
13†	Lethargy, nausea, vomiting, frequent school absence, & 3 hospital admissions in 3 yr to evaluate poor diabetic control	2	For first 6 mo, less frequent nausea & school absence, 1 incident poor control associated with cold; for past 20 mo, no problems, good control

*One of eight cases of severe relapsing diabetic acidosis.
†One of five cases of chronic acetonuria.

Source: Minuchin S; et al: A conceptual model of psychosomatic illness in children: Family organization and family therapy. *Arch Gen Psychiatry* 32:1031, 1975.

Table 9.2 Summary of Ten Cases on Intractable Asthma

Patient No.	Referral Time: Sex-Age, yr	Age at Onset	Steroid Dependent	Clinical Severity, Grade*	Duration Family Therapy	Current Status, Grade*	Follow-Up Posttherapy
1	F-8	3 yr	Yes	3	7 mo	1	2 yr 8 mo
2	F-12	3 yr	Yes	3	6 mo	1	2 yr 2 mo
3	F-12	15 mo	Yes	3	9 mo	1	1 yr 8 mo
4	M-16	11 yr	No	3	5 mo	1	3 yr 2 mo
5	M-14	18 mo	Yes	4	22 mo	2	2 yr 2 mo
6	M-8	6 yr	Yes	3	8 mo	1	1 yr 2 mo
7	M-11	3½ yr	Yes	3	6 mo	1	2 yr
8†	F-11	1 yr	Yes	3	11 mo	1	1 yr 11 mo
9	M-12	18 mo	Yes	4	Ongoing	2‡	10 mo
10	F-6	6 yr	No	2	Ongoing	1‡	9 mo

*Pinkerton (1970) Scale for Evaluation of Clinical Severity of Asthma: Grade 1, no school loss, mild attacks, occasional need for use of bronchodilator; grade 2, days off school, mild to moderate attacks, need for regular use of bronchodilator; grade 3, weeks off school, more prolonged and severe attacks, steroid plus bronchodilator therapy; grade 4, more than 50% school loss, persistent symptoms, need for special schooling, regular steroid therapy.

†Asthma-free for past 17 months.

‡Treatment continuing for other problems.

Source: Minuchin S: et al: A conceptual model of psychosomatic illness in children: Family organization and family therapy. *Arch Gen Psychiatry* 32:1031, 1975.

Table 9.3 Summary of Treatment and Follow-up of 25 Anorectic Patients

Patient No.	Treatment Duration			Current Statistics			
	Inpatient, Days	Family Therapy	Weight, kg	Weight Gain	Duration Follow-up	Anorexia	Clinical Assessment*
1	11	1 yr	31.8	14.1	2 yr 9 mo	Recovered	Recovered
2	21	1 yr	50.5	17.3	2 yr 5 mo	Recovered	Recovered
3	8	4 mo	25.5	5.0	1 yr 9 mo	Recovered	Recovered
4	13	6 mo	40.9	24.1	2 yr 5 mo	Recovered	Recovered
5	16	4 mo	33.6	10.9	2 yr 5 mo	Fair	Recovered
6	15	6 mo	50.0	11.4	1 yr 2 mo	Recovered	Recovered
7	14	9 mo	35.9	14.1	1 yr 2 mo	Recovered	Recovered
8	7	10 mo	—	—	—	Dropped program	Dropped program
9	13	3 mo	43.2	14.1	1 yr	Recovered	Recovered
10	13	7 mo	51.1	14.8	11 mo	Recovered	Recovered
11	15	—	—	—	—	Dropped program	Dropped program
12	20	7 mo	28.6	10.9	1 yr	Recovered	Recovered
13	22	7 mo	39.5	9.5	1 yr	Recovered	Recovered
14	24	7 mo	51.8	18.6	2 yr 5 mo	Recovered	Recovered
15	25	6 mo	37.3	6.4	5 mo	Recovered	Recovered
16	14	9 mo to date	49.1	10.9	Continuing	Recovered	In treatment
17	14	6 mo	46.8	15.9	11 mo	Recovered	Recovered
Outpatients:							
18		1 yr	52.3	11.4	4 yr	Recovered	Recovered
19		6 mo	61.4	18.2	3 yr 9 mo	Recovered	Recovered
20		1 yr	63.6	27.7	3 yr 9 mo	Recovered	Recovered
21		2 mo	53.6	31.4	2 yr 9 mo	Recovered	Recovered
22		4 mo	46.4	10.9	2 yr 9 mo	Recovered	Recovered
23		14 weeks	46.8	19.5	1 yr 9 mo	Recovered	Recovered
24		—	35.9	9.5	—	Dropped program	
25		1 yr	52.3	15.4	Lost contact	Recovered	Recovered

*Social, school, and family adjustment.

From: Minuchin S: et al: A conceptual model of psychosomatic illness in children: Family organization and family therapy. *Arch Gen Psychiatry* 32:1031, 1975.

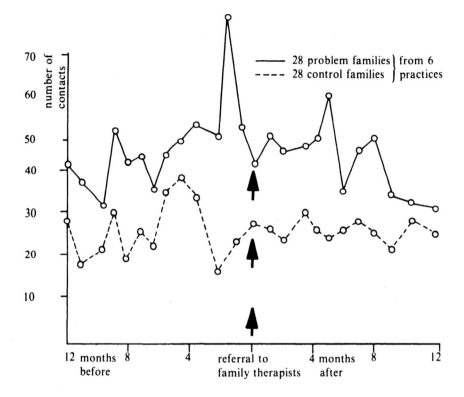

Figure 9-1. Number of Contacts with General Practitioner before and after Referral for Family Therapy

From: Huygen FJA: *Family Medicine: The Medical Life History of Families.* The Netherlands, Dekker and Van de Vegt, 1978.

in this estimate; criteria included random assignment of families to control or treatment groups, follow-up of at least 1 year, inclusion of measures of outcome before and after treatment, predictions of research stated in advance, appropriate statistical analysis, and objectivity of authors (if therapists in the study were also the authors, the study was not included).

One specific study of short-term family therapy should be mentioned. Watzlawick[20] found positive outcomes after an average of 7 hours of family therapy in 71 of 97 families (73%). Success was defined as achievement of the goal agreed on by the family and therapist at the onset of therapy, and, in addition, maintenance of that goal, an absence of new problems, and no other need for therapy at a 1-year follow-up session. The primary care clinician caring for such a child may limit his or her activities to treating the asthma and minor illnesses and refer the underlying emotional or family problem to

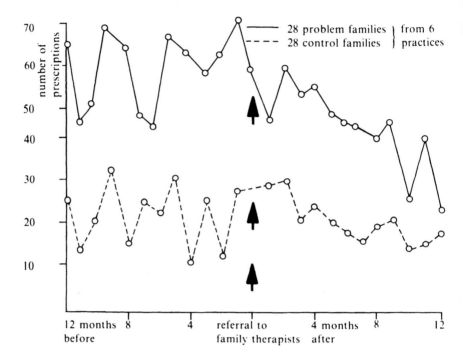

Figure 9-2. Number of Prescriptions before and after Referral for Family Therapy

From: Huygen FJA: Family Medicine: The Medical Life History of Families. The Netherlands, Dekker and Van de Vegt, 1978.

another professional (see Chapter 15), but he or she should be aware of the larger picture.

If the underlying family problem is not treated the symptom of distress may change just as the presenting symptom of an individual patient may change if the underlying depression is not treated. For example, in one family an asthmatic child improved but a sibling developed recurrent boils. Then a second sibling developed eczema. Once the fighting between the children's divorced parents was resolved through therapy, the frequent visits for physical illness stopped dramatically. Many cases in this book demonstrate the importance of diagnosing and treating problems at the level of the family system.

Therapy for part of a family system can be hazardous. For example, individual psychotherapy of one spouse has been shown to lead frequently to partner breakdown or marital breakup.[7] Obese patients undergoing intestinal bypass operations manifested marital problems in the postoperative period when the family dysfunction that had maintained the obesity was ignored.[13] These facts emphasize the role of the family system. At the same time, however, they do not negate the need to treat the individual's medical problem. Assessing the family may increase accuracy of diagnosis and therefore treatment will be more appropriate.

COMPLIANCE AND THE FAMILY

Schmidt[17] has described the main factors influencing patient compliance. These factors include health beliefs, particularly with regard to the perceived threat of the disease and the likelihood of the medical regime to correct this threat; the doctor-patient relationship, including continuity of care; the complexity of the medical regime; the family attitude to the regime; and family stability. A patient's health belief model (see Chapter 5) is strongly influenced by the family; if a family's health belief model is significantly different from the medical model compliance is low. The patient's contribution to the doctor-patient relationship is related to the family's view of doctors and their role and to how the patient has learned to behave with parental or authority figures.

Several studies have demonstrated the powerful influence of family attitudes on compliance. Oakes[16] studied the use of splints by 66 patients with rheumatoid arthritis. Compliance with the splint regime was high when the patient perceived his family as expecting him to use a splint. Elling[5] studied 80 families of children with a history of rheumatic fever. Compliance with penicillin prophylaxis and regularity of visits to the clinic (which correlated also with polio immunization) was greatest in families who identified with the medical model, and where mothers felt the doctors thought well of them. Families with relationship problems—divorce, separation, police involvement in family conflict, hospitalization for mental illness, officially recorded delinquency—showed low compliance. Family disorganization, indifference to the child, and lowered self-esteem in the mother all appeared to be factors. Other investigators have found low compliance associated with family breakdown.[1,3,19] Schwartz[18] showed a greater number of medication errors in elderly when they are widowed, divorced, separated, or living alone.

CHANGES IN LIFESTYLE

The links between the family and habits such as cigarette smoking, drug and alcohol abuse, and exercise and obesity are well known. However, physicians and nurses may be less aware of the data showing that involving the family in prescribed changes in life-style results in much better compliance. Heinzelman and Bagley[8] studied 239 sedentary men with hyperlipidemia or hypertension who were advised to participate in supervised physical activity 3 hours per week. If the wife's attitude towards the exercise was positive there was an 80% chance of good compliance; if it were negative there was only a 40% chance.

Hoebel[9] took family involvement one step further. He showed that persistent high-risk behavior in men with heart disease could be altered by short-term therapy with their wives; there was no attempt to deal directly with the patients themselves. These families had been referred because the men were resistant to change and several months of intensive efforts by the medical team had failed to alter their behavior. At this point most health professionals give up, but that is because they ignore the potential of the family to become a therapeutic ally and the fact that many families unwittingly maintain behavior in the patient. It is, in fact, rather presumptuous of the clinician to expect 15 minutes or even 1 hour per week to effectively counteract the potent verbal and nonverbal influence of the family.

Hoebel's group spent five sessions with the wives of these men who persisted with smoking and poor exercise and overeating. By changing the wives' typical response to the men, a vicious cycle of the spouse's overconcern and taking too much responsibility for recovery was altered. In each case the typical response of the wife was ineffectual and played a part in the negative feedback system. One woman whose role in the family was that of the cheerful optimist had had no success through encouragement. The surgeon's pessimism—"You'll be dead in a few months if you keep that up"—produced some reduction of weight. When the wife with the health care team's encouragement switched to a more pessimistic stance, her husband became less depressed and actively sought to prove her wrong. Such an approach is based on the Palo Alto group's four steps of family therapy[21]: 1) careful description of the problem; 2) description of the family's solution, which is often the behavior maintaining the problem; 3) setting of minimal treatment goals—an objective testable criterion for real change is decided on by the family; and 4) selecting and making behavioral interventions. These steps often represent a major change from the family's original solution, but take into account the functioning of the entire system.

STRESS MANAGEMENT

What are the practical implications of the research on stress and illness? The family physician is often in a unique position to monitor the effects of life stress, particularly in bereaved persons or in persons undergoing a number of stresses at once, such as sickness in the family, job loss, friction with teenaged children, etc.; many patients appear with vague "functional" symptoms which require reinterpretation as stress related. Estimating Rahe's[10] life change units (see Chapter 8) may be helpful in assessing and conceptualizing the patient's complaints.

It is striking that in all cultures and subcultures of the six life events scored highest, four (death of a spouse, divorce, marital separation, death of a close family member) directly involve the person's family life. Many of the other events clearly have a direct relation to family life, whereas others (for example, imprisonment) must affect family supports. For this reason, an inquiry into the family's recent life stresses is essential.

In the popular press, much has been made of a maximal permissible level of life change units per year. The implication is that anything over and above these can spell trouble. Presumably it is fairly easy to monitor and alter actions which are within one's control—moving, going on vacation, changing one's job. However, most of the major unpleasant life stresses, which rate highest on the scale of life change units, such as illness and death, are not within our control. Perhaps these findings can be applied: a person can be advised against making many other concommitant changes in his life if he or she is recently bereaved or has just had a serious illness.

If life stresses in fact affect physical and mental health through their impact on endocrinological and immunological systems via affective states, it is probably worth considering more organized methods of prevention. Stress reduction methods and therapies of various kinds can be offered to patients who are the direct sufferers and to various family members who may be next in line. These therapies include individual, couple, and family therapy; multiple family or group therapy; various self-help groups; relaxation; and biofeedback training. Most important is the mobilization of the patient's and the family's natural support system: extended family, friends, employers. Because the family practitioner is often in contact with some of these people, he or she may be ideally placed to mobilize their aid. Natural networks are probably often more helpful than artificial ones (this is probably the reason for the success of self-help).

Crisis intervention often has significant and long-lasting effects on the level of functioning in the individual and family. During crises, defenses decrease and flexibility and potential for change markedly increase. The principles of crisis intervention are described in Chapter 15.

REFERENCES

1. Alpert JJ: Broken appointments. *Pediatrics* 34:127, 1964.

2. Comley A: Family therapy and the family physician. *Can Fam Phys*, 19:81 1973.

3. Diamond MD, Weiss AJ, Grynbaum B: The unmotivated patient. *Arch Phys Med* 49:281, 1968.

4. Duff RS, Hollingshead AB: *Sickness and Society*. New York, Harper & Row, 1968.

5. Elling R, Wittemore R, Green M: Patient participation in a pediatric program. *J Health Hum Behav* 1:183, 1960.

6. Engel GL: The need for a new medical model: A challenge for biomedicine. *Science* 196:129, 1977.

7. Gurman AS, Kniskern DP: Research on marital and family therapy: Perspec-

tive and prospect, in Garfield SL, Bergin AE (eds): *Handbook of Psychotherapy and Behavior Change: An Empirical Analysis.* New York, Wiley, 1978.

8. Heinzelmann F, Bagley R: Response to physical activity programs and their effects on health behavior. *Public Health Rep* 85:905, 1970.

9. Hoebel FC: Brief family-interactional therapy in the management of cardiac-related high-risk behaviors. *J Fam Pract* 3:613, 1976.

10. Holmes TH, Rahe RH: The social readjustment rating scale. *Psychosom Med* 11: 213, 1967.

11. Huygen FJA: *Family Medicine: The Medical Life History of Families.* The Netherlands, Dekker and Van de Vegt, 1978.

12. Kirsner JB: Later development of inflammatory bowel disease in the healthy spouse of a patient. *N Engl J Med* 306:1148, 1982.

13. Marshall JR, Neill J: The removal of psychosomatic symptom: Effects on the marriage. *Fam Process* 16:273, 1977.

14. McWhinney IR: Beyond diagnosis: An approach to the integration of behavioral science and clinical medicine. *N Engl J Med* 287:384, 1972.

15. Minuchin S, Baker L, Rosman BL, et al: A conceptual model of psychosomatic illness in children: Family organization and family therapy. *Arch Gen Psychiatry* 32:1031, 1975.

16. Oakes TW, Ward JR, Gray RM, et al. Family expectations and arthritis patient compliance to a hand resting splint regimen. *J Chron Dis* 22:757, 1970.

17. Schmidt DD: Patient compliance: The effect of the doctor as a therapeutic agent. *J Fam Pract* 4:853, 1977.

18. Schwartz D, Wang M, Zeity L, et al: Medication errors made by elderly, chronically ill patients. *Am J Public Health* 52:2018, 1962.

19. White MK, Alpert JJ, Kosa J: Hard to reach families in a comprehensive care program. *JAMA* 201:801, 1967.

20. Watzlawick P, Weakland JJ, Frisch R: *Change: Problem Formation and Problem Resolution.* New York, W.W. Norton, 1974.

21. Weakland J, Fisch R, Watzlawick P, et al: Brief therapy: Focused problem resolution. *Fam Process* 12:141, 1974.

Section IV

WORKING WITH FAMILIES IN PRIMARY CARE

Chapter 10

Establishing a Family Orientation

Janet Christie-Seely

A systems orientation implies a way of thinking about people, whether they are patients, colleagues, or one's own family. It does not dramatically alter a clinician's mode of practice; individuals get sick, not families. It will be the individuals who appear in the office most of the time. However, the systemic clinician sees a person surrounded by the invisible family members with whom the patient's history, character, behavior, and illness are inextricably interwoven. Even single people living alone are influenced by their families of origin—the "family in the patient." They are also influenced by social systems of friends, neighbors, extended families, or in some cases by the welfare or health care system only. For the elderly, the Golden Age Club (or senior citizen clubs in the U.S.) may be their family; for many the church or synagogue is family.

There are several practical implications of a family orientation. The setting, arrangement of rooms, and practice hours all give messages that underline or negate a stated orientation to families. If no attempt is made to see whole families, if different family members see different teams or clinicians, if members' charts are all filed separately (with no family coding system) it will be difficult, if not impossible, to develop a family orientation. Registration in the practice by household should be encouraged whether or not the family is seen as "the patient."

The attitude of the clerical staff to family care can set the tone: is a relative's phone call considered a nuisance or a welcome introduction to another family member? Obviously, the attitude of doctors and nurses is important. Attitudes in the community and culture determine those of staff and patients; family care may be seen as a natural and logical part of practice or as an unwelcome invasion of patient privacy, a time consuming and unnecessary complication of true medical practice, or a frightening intrusion into an area of little knowledge where therapy has little effect.

Community Acceptance. In some communities, family registration and family interviews will be treated with suspicion; in others, such an approach is expected. Evening hours may be the only way to attract men reluctant to come to the office in middle- or lower-class communities. Home visits are an

172

essential part of care in some rural areas, while they are greeted with surprise by city-dwellers. In some urban areas specialty care may be the norm; the family physician may need to discourage a patient's decision to go to a specialist for clinical problems, or at least insist on being informed of visits to gynecologist, pediatrician, orthopedist, etc.

The acceptance of a link between family stress and illness varies with community and culture, as does the acceptance of talking with a doctor about topics other than physical symptoms. Community education can achieve remarkable results. In one midwestern small town in the United States a single physician with an engaging manner became involved with the community and educated members of the community to a family systems approach. Over a couple of beers or during a casual lunch the doctor talked to local policemen or firemen about family problems. He often learned about a problem before it became a crisis; then the community network would take care of many of these problems.* In another rural community, on a small island off the coast of British Columbia, the affection and respect given the physician who knew every ferryman by name and could enquire about every family member is another example of the community's respect for family-oriented physicians.

Acceptance of a physician or a visiting nurse is made evident by a crowded or empty waiting room; the community is efficient in passing the word concerning a physician's interviewing skills, perceived competence, office premises, and staff, as well as his or her orientation to family medical care. The importance of proper conduct, language, religion, and even political affiliation can affect a community's response to a new physician or nurse, particularly in a rural area, but also in the city. The concept of working with the community is further developed at the end of this section (see Chapter 18).

The culture of the community must be understood and valued by the clinician. The clinician who is from a different culture must be careful neither to misinterpret nor to give diagnoses or instructions at odds with the culture's beliefs (see Chapter 9).

Premises.   The site, layout, and characteristics of the family practice unit or of the practitioner's office have implications for the practice.[1] It becomes apparent to patients whether the practice is oriented toward the family: a community with families needs easy access to medical care; a large hospital in the business center of the city with poor parking facilities will not serve this patient population as efficiently.

Toys and appropriate reading materials for younger children in the waiting room convey the fact that a practitioner sees whole families.[1] Similarly,

---

*This physician has now written of these experiences in *Family Therapy and Family Medicine* by Macaran A. Baird and William Doherty (New York: Guilford Press, 1983). This book was published after this book was written and is heartily recommended.

if it is evident that the waiting room has been made accessible to the elderly, consideration for the older generation is conveyed. Rooms must be large enough for more than a single patient to be interviewed, or there should be at least one family interviewing room. If this is not available, the waiting room may be used for family sessions after office hours (however, this does not contribute to an atmosphere of family-focused care). In one setting, each room was dominated by a large examining table toward which the nurse propelled the patient, already in an examining gown, clearly giving the message that the physician has little time and is concerned with physical complaints only. The attitude of health care personnel should convey acceptance of families and small children as well as the elderly. Babysitting for small children while the mother is having a gynecological exam might be an additional service.

Practice Hours. Despite the doctor's need to spend time with his or her own family, it is nevertheless important to be able to see patients occasionally in the evening. This is often necessary for treating working fathers unable to visit in the daytime or for sessions with families of school children. Evening hours for a family medicine unit or practice convey the impression of accommodation to the family unit in a way that the nine-to-five routine cannot. Similarly, housecalls when the entire family is at home can be highly productive and can help gain essential information about the family in its own environment.

In many practices time pressures are acute, so that the average session with a patient is 10 to 15 minutes. A half-hour session for a family may disrupt the usual routine. Most practitioners have found that setting aside one-half day a week for half-hour sessions is usually feasible and in the long run pays off in terms of decreased utilization of office time because of underlying family problems. Once a family has been seen as a whole, then sessions with individual family members will be much more productive and based on a clear overall perspective.

Charting. Smilkstein[7] has described a family-problem-oriented medical record, and Green[4] has suggested a uniform recording system to facilitate family research. Family charts have been used in many family medicine units and practices, but in others the argument that they are cumbersome has resulted in the use of individual charts that can be filed in the same location. Physicians who use family charts are usually convinced of their value. Usually, these physicians see individuals as a part of families.[6] A compromise is the use of a family folder with updated information on each family member. A card can be used indicating the visits of each member and the data of these visits.[3] This practice can detail useful information showing responses to family crises, and indicate the possible need for family assessment (see Chapter 9).

More detailed card systems with diagnostic information can be invaluable for research, as well as for understanding illness behavior in a specific family. (Huygen's[5] outstanding work on family patterns of illness is based on a simple recording system.) A family orientation is apparent from the amount of information about the family that is charted and how easily that information can be retrieved. The next chapter outlines the use of the family tree to record information. Chapter 14 describes the acronym "PRACTICE" and a form for recording information derived from a family interview. We have found the combination of a genogram and "PRACTICE" to be a flexible, concise and adequate means of recording family data.

Continuous, Comprehensive Care of the Family

Family medicine is committed to comprehensive and continuous care for the patient in the context of the family,[6] but often falls short in all of these aspects and becomes episodic care. This results in patient dissatisfaction and clinician boredom. Knowing the family and observing its links with illness is to many family physicians an interesting part of primary care, and provides the justification for the specialty of family medicine in that such knowledge improves the quality of care for the patient.

Continuity of care and care of all family members by the same clinician may in fact not occur in many primary care settings.[2] This is particularly true in some teaching environments, where interns and residents have long periods out of the practice and may change practices every two or three years (Canada has a two-year program). In one setting, a husband and wife came in with the common complaint of diarrhea. They were seen by two different physicians — a foolish duplication of work as well as a clear message that the family is irrelevant to the practice of medicine.

In primary care nursing in North America, a family orientation is the rule (although not always from a family systems model) but continuity is often difficult, primarily because the nurse has less opportunity than the family physician to follow families over time or patients during and after hospital admission. The district nurse in Britain, particularly when also the midwife, provides continuity of family care. The general practitioner or district nurse team gives comprehensive care but usually must hand over to specialists their hospitalized patients.

Family Registration. If the practice or family medicine unit insists that only whole families register, a family orientation is emphasized; however, those concerned about individual privacy or family members with an allegiance to another doctor will not be accommodated. The individual living alone may misinterpret the rule and go elsewhere. A policy of encouraging household registration without insisting that all members join the practice allows more flexibility and later registration of other family members once trust is established. Similarly, the suggestion can be made that a family visit will allow the clinician to get to know the whole family at the time of registration. Thus, if a patient becomes ill, he or she already feels comfortable, knowing the clinician and the premises. This approach facilitates later family encounters and gives the clinician essential baseline data on family relationships and structure (see section on Family Assessment). Evening hours make such a family visit acceptable to most, especially if the family members see the visit as a routine and logical way of meeting the clinician and obtaining the family's medical history, rather than an intrusion into their private affairs. A half-hour visit with the whole household quickly establishes who is currently in need of care or preventive measures, and a more accurate health history is obtained in less time than separate visits for every member. However, if a family is resistant to the idea, nothing is gained by insisting on the interview.

Is the Family the Patient?

Whether the family is the patient is a controversial issue. Some clinicians insist that this is so; others feel that the concept confuses the reality of practice (the predominance of the individual visit), professional loyalty (when family and patient disagree), and the public ("I can't go to a family physician as I have no family") as well. From a systems orientation the question seems largely a matter of semantics. In most practices, particularly those built up over time, the clinician will in time meet all family members: when the individual is treated the family is treated too. The physician who diagnoses or treats a family member cannot avoid influencing the family. If the family's character and homeostasis is well understood by the clinician, treatment will be appropriate and the change will benefit both patient and family; if not, it may benefit neither, at best maintaining the status quo. If family and patient disagree in diagnosis or health care management compliance will be poor. The public has been strongly influenced by modern medicine and the relevance of technology and a disease orientation. The mind/body split of our culture is underlined by the dichotomy of psychological versus physical illness in medicine. The public differentiates what is "all in your head" from "real illness". Hence it is not surprising that studies show that a large proportion of people believe a visit to the physician to be appropriate only for physical illness.[7] The public as well as the medical profession must become more sophisticated about mind and body and the role of families and family dysfunction in illness and its management; a systems-oriented clinician has a major task in educating both colleagues and patients.

The clinician as teacher of a systems orientation can help communication on many levels. With peers or colleagues he or she can help prevent labelling that is destructive, promote understanding of the "difficult" patient or family, and avoid aiding family dysfunction. In the work situation or professional health care systems, recognition of triangulation and scapegoating, rigid boundaries, and poor communication between professionals can improve conflict management and avoid blaming.

The clinician's role in teaching systems principles to families is of prime importance. The clinician's questions and empathy and understanding for each family member communicate understanding and tolerance, with the clinician acting as a role model. The paradox of family systems is that while no one is to blame everyone is responsible for change and is capable of changing his or her own behavior and response to illness.

The family systems viewpoint can be conveyed subtly in the individual interview as well as the family interview. Certain questions or comments may broaden a person's perspective of a complaint: "Do you find you handle your husband's drinking the same way your mother handled your father's? Did that seem to stop him or egg him on?"; "You complain your mother treats you badly when you're well, perhaps that makes it easier for you to be sick."; or "Your son isn't taking his medication but he's at a rebellious age; perhaps reminding him to clean his room every day will make him rebel in a less dangerous area."

One of the most effective ways of demonstrating systems principles to individuals is to ask them to draw a family tree. It should be remembered that, unlike a question or comment that reorients the patient's thinking, the genogram takes time. However, many centers feel that the one-half to one hour needed is well worth the increased knowledge for both patient and clinician. The genogram then becomes a part of routine care. Centers more pressed for time can limit the use of the genogram to any patient whose recurrent physical complaints or behavior needs greater understanding. (For example, parents complaining of a drug problem in an adolescent were helped when they drew their family tree, which showed many family members on both sides of the family had alcohol or drug problems.) Repetitive patterns through the generations are noted by the patient without the clinician's comments.

REFERENCES

1. Allmond BW, Buchman W, Gofman HF: The Family Is the Patient: An Approach to Behavioral Pediatrics for the Clinician. St. Louis, C.V. Mosby Co., 1979.

2. Fujikawa LS, Bass RA, Schneiderman LJ: Family care in a family practice group. *J Fam Pract* 8:1189, 1979.

3. Goodman M: The diagnostic index and the family record card. *J R Coll Gen Pract* 19:192, 1970.

4. Green LA, Simmons RL, Frank M, et al: A family medicine information system: the beginning of a network for practicing and resident family physicians. *J Fam Pract* 7:567, 1978.

5. Huygen FJA: Family Medicine: The Medical Life History of Families. The Netherlands, Dekker & Van De Vegt, 1978.

6. Medalie, JH: Family Medicine: Principles and Applications. Baltimore, Williams & Wilkins, 1978.

7. Smilkstein G: The family in trouble—how to tell. *J Fam Pract* 2:19, 1975.

Chapter 11
Collecting and Recording Family Data—The Genogram

Henry C. Mullins
Janet Christie-Seely

Once an orientation to the family has been adopted, and it has been decided to use the family unit in health care, it is necessary to employ a clinical method to collect, store, and retrieve information; and a theoretical framework to process, understand, and give meaning to the information that is collected. The focus of this chapter will be on a method of *collecting, storing,* and *processing* information. The theoretical orientation on which this clinical method is based is the family systems theory described in Section I.

As developed by Murray Bowen, the theory of transmission of behavioral patterns from generation to generation is best illustrated on a family tree—that is, a phenogram or genogram (although phenogram is the correct term, the term genogram is in current usage; we have chosen to use the latter). Patterns of illness are repeated, and are clearly dependent on genetics as well as on environmental factors such as the cultural and family health belief system; role models of sickness; "secondary gain," the increased power a spouse appropriates to balance the power of a partner; and a patient's expectations of developing the family illness. Sickness can also reflect family-transmitted stress and lifestyle, and is part of a feedback system of the family's impact on illness and of the illness' impact on the family.

A family study is the study of the recurrent, predictable, biomedical, behavioral and cultural phenomena that have significant impact on the health and disease of individual patients.

The family genogram (familiar to most physicians or nurses from genetic studies) is a method of collecting and storing family data that provides immediate graphic feedback, allowing rapid interpretation. It serves as a

Much of the information presented in this chapter was provided by the Centre for Family Learning, New Rochelle, New York. The author especially thanks Phil Guerine, M.D., Eileen Pendagast, M.A., M.Ed., Tom Fogarty, M.D., and Charles O. Sherman, B.S., M.A., A.B.D.

skeletal framework on which biomedical, genetic, behavioral and social facts, and relationships may be explored, displayed, and processed. It also enables the physician to diagram, in simple terms, family data including basic information (names, dates of birth, death, marriage) and complex information (repetitive family themes, triangulation, genetics), depending on the appropriateness to the problem under consideration and the interest of the physician.

A genogram or "family study" of some sort (whether simple or complex) is a desirable part of the medical record of all patients cared for by any physician, but especially the family physician. In many practices a family tree is located in the family folder, which is pulled out with the individual chart on each visit. Additional information can be added when it becomes available from different family members, or a single interview may be used to develop a family tree in greater depth and detail. In the Department of Family Practice in southern Alabama the clinician records information from the individual on a large sheet (24 inches × 32 inches) on a flip chart. This method is considered very practical because patient and clinician both are able to see the diagram, and the treatment process becomes an open sharing of information. (Since many people take in visual information more easily than verbal statements, the use of a large diagram is more effective than mere description; later, the sheet is reduced to fit into the chart.) This retrievable record prevents duplication of questions about family history to different family members and to the same member on different occasions, saving time.

Since these data can be derived from an individual patient, a family study of several generations must be distinguished from a family assessment interview in which relationships are observed in the current family or household. Family assessment interviews and a means of recording them, "PRACTICE," are described in Chapters 13 and 14.

The time taken for an in-depth family study is approximately 1 hour. Such a study has provided so much information relevant to patient care that it is now routine in south Alabama to do a study of every family in the practice. Centers beginning to use genograms may feel it necessary to begin with a brief (5-minute) version on all charts, reserving detailed studies for certain situations, including the following:

1. Dealing with the "ripple effect" of serious illness or death.
2. Using the family to manage health problems.
3. Evaluating and managing frequently seen symptoms: headache, backache, abdominal pain, chest pain.
4. Identifying the cause of symptoms rather than focusing on the presenting complaint.
5. Considering and managing acute and chronic biomedical problems influenced by stress such as elevated blood pressure, ulcers, asthma, colitis, and myocardial infarction.

6. Anticipating and preventing biomedical problems precipitated by normative life crises.
7. Recognizing, diagnosing, counselling, or referring genetic problems.
8. Diagnosing and managing emotional and behavioral problems influenced by family structure and function.
9. In marital and sexual dysfunction.
10. In alcohol and other drug abuse.

This list is very similar to the list of indications for family assessment derived by the Montreal group (see Chapter 13). The choice between doing an in-depth family history in an individual interview (or with two or more family members) or a family conference dealing primarily with the present situation depends on the particular situation and the medical or nursing setting. In a setting where many patients live alone or register as individuals and not as households, or where there is little awareness or skill in family-centered care, many clinicians use the family genogram to increase the understanding of both patients and staff that the family is a system influencing current illness. Skills in interviewing the family can then be developed once the importance of the family is recognized. In contrast, if only family interviews are used the awareness of the power of the past may be missing.

Often an hour spent with an individual doing a family study may result in spontaneous changes in the patient and be very cost effective. In one example, a young unmarried girl, who visited the health center frequently for a variety of vague physical complaints and admitted to difficulties in her social life, was able to link dating problems and her complaints with issues in her family of origin. This initiated a process of self-understanding and change that markedly reduced subsequent clinic visits.

For nurses or physicians who do not use such a detailed enquiry and method of mapping that is visible to patient and clinician, the potential power of such family awareness will not be recognized. For medical and nursing students or residents the task of doing their own genogram, including toxic issues (family secrets), triangles, and repeat patterns of illness and behavior, often is effective in helping them to understand the family system in patients (see Section VI). Once the effectiveness of doing a genogram has been demonstrated in one patient, the tendency to consider doing a family study for the next patient increases.

Eliciting Information

The family physician or other health professional elicits information in an orderly and prescribed manner by directing an interview with one or more people knowledgeable about the family being studied. Techniques of interviewing are difficult to learn from a book and are best learned by observing trained interviewers and videotapes of family study interviews, and by participating in family sessions with trained observers and family study conferences where the information from interviews and presentations is processed with an experienced family physician. In initial family training, the student of family interview techniques may record a family study of himself or herself or of a fellow student.

The interview should begin with standard information such as names, dates, illnesses, and moves. An atmosphere of trust and acceptance is essential before eliciting more personal material with such questions as who were you closest to in your family? or what was their marriage like? Sensitive issues might be queried in the following manner: was there any subject people couldn't talk about in your family? or all families have someone who is alcoholic; who was your family's alcoholic? and family members cut-off from the rest of the family could be inquired about with the following question: many families have a person or group of relatives they never see or rarely mention; is that true of your family?

Genuine interest and a nonjudgmental approach often produces a degree of openness that is surprising even when the interviewer is not previously known to the patient. The issue of confidentiality should be raised if family secrets are written onto the genogram and later put in the family chart. An agreed-upon set of codes or initials for problems may protect privacy if this is a concern. A spirit of scientific inquiry avoids the impression that therapy is the goal. Indicating that problems for a family are normal, by statements implying that all families have problems, difficult relationships, secrets (see Chapter 15), reassures patients and often enables them to examine issues previously repressed or ignored and to gain a new understanding of their family and themselves and their illness or symptoms. (Confronting one's family history for the first time is a little like seeing oneself on videotape for the first time, it is a highly educational but sometimes unnerving experience.)

Understanding and Utilizing Data

A completed genogram produces a great amount of information concerning a family. This information can be used to clarify diagnoses to improve management and for patient education. For appropriate and meaningful use of the collected information a theoretical basis must be used. A systems orientation and the ability to see illness and family patterns as part of a non-linear feedback system provides clear understanding of the complex array of family facts.

A genogram can also be used by clinicians with different orientations:

1. For the individually oriented clinician it provides a framework by which diagnosis and management of patient problems can be facili-

tated; *biomedical, behavioral,* and *social* influences are taken into account. McWhinney (see Chapter 9) earlier addressed this issue, suggesting a classification of patient's problems that was helpful to the practitioner. Family studies go a step further and provide a clinical method of integrating and synthesizing information, diagnoses, and management of the patient's problems.

2. For the physician who as a contextual orientation (in which the family is seen as an important context of illness, but thinking remains linear rather than circular, with an emphasis on cause and effect as a unidirectional phenomenon), a family study provides a voluminous amount of information about the environment in which a problem or symptom occurs. There is a cultural shift toward concern with environment in general that is properly reflected in the consideration and management of problems of health and disease. Knowledge and information have greater meaning as the context increases.

Data Collection and Recording

At least three generations of the family should be studied and diagrammed. The latest offspring is the first generation; parents the second generation; and grandparents the third generation. If more than three generations can be studied, family patterns will become more visible.

Symbols

To record information on the genogram, symbols are used: circles indicate women; squares indicate men (the father is on the left side, the mother is on the right). These symbols are joined as in the diagram by the marriage or generational line (Fig. 11-1).

All pregnancies are indicated by vertical lines below the sibship line. The line indicating the first pregnancy should begin at the far left; later births are indicated, according to pregnancy order, by lines moving toward the right. The outcome of each pregnancy is shown using the appropriate symbol. Abortions or stillbirths are represented by small symbols indicating the sex if

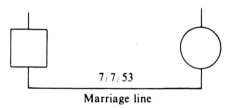

Marriage line

Figure 11-1.

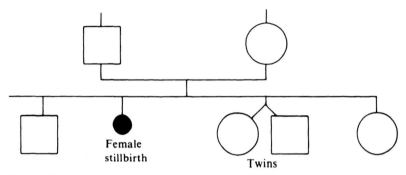

Figure 11-2.

known. All deaths are shown as solid symbols or with a cross through the symbol (see Figure 11-2).

Place the name, date of birth, and place of birth (or other outcome of pregnancy) for each person within or adjoining the appropriate symbol.

Figure 11-3 gives important information about names and dates, which, even if left in this simple form, provide clues that will broaden the perspective of, for example, recurrent illness in either Henry (a "vulnerable child" conceived before the marriage) or Ann (who may be a "replacement child" following the stillbirth of the first girl after whom she was named).

If either spouse had a previous marriage, place the symbols for their marriage partner on the side of the appropriate spouse and connect them by another marriage line. If children were born or pregnancies resulted from the

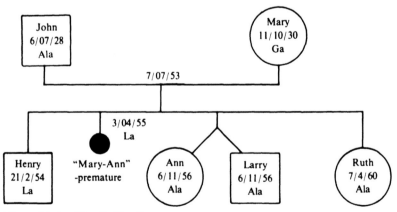

Figure 11-3. The H. Family

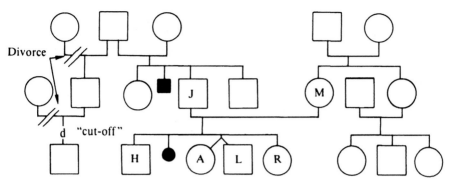

Figure 11–4.   The H. Family (continued)

previous marriages, indicate them by symbols as previously described for children of a marriage.

A genogram includes all people joined together by blood, marriage, adoption, or marriage alternatives over at least three generations. The diagram should include all pregnancies and their outcome (Fig. 11-4). Note the two divorces and the member cut-off from the rest of the family. If the genogram is continued, family secrets, triangles, drug problems, or occupations can be added (Fig. 11-5).

The genogram in Figure 11-5 might alert the clinician to the possibility of an escalating problem with Henry and to his being cut-off in the future. The possibility that John and Ann's overachievement is related to an earlier stillbirth in each family, and the family pattern of drug and alcohol abuse might be made clear to the family if the family were asked to chart the family tree.

BASELINE DATA

For each person represented on the diagram, the following can be recorded on the genogram:

1. Date of birth, miscarriage or abortion (recording dates is better than recording ages, which must be updated and do not show correlations with family events as dates do). Date of adoption if relevant.
2. Name
3. Place of birth
4. Date and cause of death
5. Major illnesses with dates

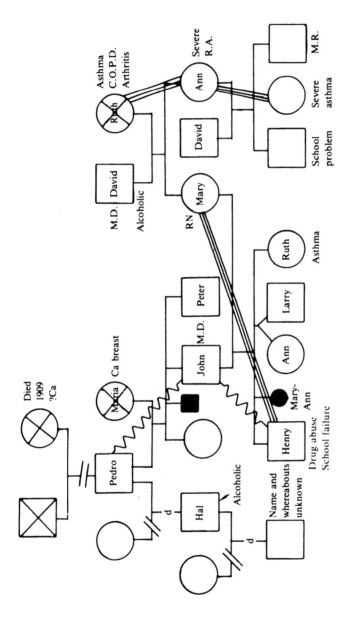

Figure 11-5. The H. Family (continued)

Mary—an R.N., not working. Allergies. On diazepam.

John—hard-working physician. Conflict with father and son Henry (triangulation—masked conflict with wife similar to that between parents).

Henry—left home, rarely writes. Believed by family to take after Uncle Hal.

Ann—an overachiever. Frequent physical symptoms. On diazepam.

Larry—shy, underachiever.

Grandfather (paternal) Pedro—Moved to US in 1920 from Italy. Never visited Italy since emigration.

6. Date of marriage or marriage alternative, separation, divorce. Birth, death, illness, and rites of passage (marriage, promotion) all have emotional impact and create some social reorganization and stress. Dates help clarify coincidence of such events with illness ("clustering" or "ripple effect").

Sibling position is an important factor in relationships in the family of origin and in subsequent relationships and abilities. The oldest learn managerial skills, while the younger are often better able to submit to authority. (Toman's research on sibling position is discussed in Chapter 2.)

After the genogram (pedigree or family tree) has been drawn, ask about anyone on the family tree having the following, and record on the genogram:

1. Cancer or leukemia
2. Other diseases that cluster in families: allergy, skin problems, diabetes, arthritis, rheumatic fever, glomerulonephritis, hypertension, heart disease, eye problems, respiratory problems
3. Problems of reproduction: a history of sterility, spontaneous abortion, induced abortion, stillbirth, congenital anomalies, multiple births, mental retardation, and learning disabilities
4. Problems similar to the present problem
5. Drugs taken (including alcohol)
6. The usual cause of death in the family

These can be recorded on the genogram beside the affected member. An asterisk can be used to indicate a repetitive problem, such as extramarital pregnancies.

Family Information

The more information gathered the more time is required, but the better the system will be understood. Some of the questions listed will be highly relevant in a given family, others less so; greater detail in a given area may be very helpful on occasion (for example, the dating pattern of young adult).

For each member of the core family* and certain other members (those of special significance or with similar problems), the following may be recorded on the genogram or family studies report:

1. Birth weight and gestational age if this is relevant and known
2. Nickname or title. Names and nicknames are often clues to family labels, identities, or expectations. In one example, all members of a

---

*Usually parents and siblings and relatives who live or lived in the same household. Since non-relatives within the family such as a housekeeper or nanny may have been key persons, they can be indicated by symbols placed on the genogram that are unconnected by blood lines.

family named William were alcoholic. First or second names may indicate alliances; a child named after a grandmother is in a sense a gift to her. Family scripts or roles may be indicated by titles "genius," "princess," "blacksheep," "lazy bones," "little mother").

3. Character. It is often useful to ask for two or three adjectives to describe key figures. These can be written beside their symbol and can clarify relationships and identities: William, the patient, describes Uncle Bill as a "hard-driving, intolerant loner." Uncle Bill's death from a massive infarction may help William improve his similar lifestyle since he clearly identifies with his namesake.

4. Problems (social, family, emotional)

5. Geographic changes. Elicit and record the time and place of all geographic locations and changes. Certain questions can be asked: Is it the family tradition to settle close to home or move away? Who in the family has differed from the family tradition by staying closer or moving further away?

6. Occupation. Determine the occupation of each family member: What do people in this family usually do for a living? Who has a job or occupation outside the usual family tradition or standard? Who in the family stresses occupation? Is work important to the family?

7. Education. Determine and record the educational level of each: What is the usual educational level throughout the family? Is education valued? Is there great emphasis on school grades?

Family Contact, Cohesion, and Boundaries

1. How do members of the extended family communicate and how often? Is it only at times of crisis or at specific holidays? Is it by visit, letter, telephone, audiotapes, newsletters? Is there a person central to contact between members of the extended family—the family "telephone operator"? What happens if that person gets sick? Who is the person responsible for health care or for medical information?

2. What are the rules for privacy? Are surprise or extended visits welcome or unwelcome?

3. With which person in the same generation does the patient have the closest relationship? Which person in the parents' generation? Which person in the grandparents'?

4. With which person in each generation does the patient have the least contact? Are these relationships similar? What would happen if the patient initiated or increased contact? What would be the family repercussion?

5. Are there family members cut off from the rest of the family? In most

families there is someone who no one talks about or who has decided to solve problems by leaving. What crisis initiated the family member's being cut off? What crisis might occur if contact is made with the cut-off member(s)?

Toxic Issues and Nodal Events

1. "Toxic issues" or family secrets (issues with intense emotional charge)
   a. Are there things or people never talked about in this family? What are/were the things that, when talked about, made people uncomfortable or argumentative? What topics and issues were talked about freely and with comfort?
   b. What topics were the patient's parents unable to discuss in their families? Did they take the same or opposite position to their parents? What topics does the patient find difficult to be open about with his or her children?
2. Nodal events: some family secrets are linked with nodal events (births, deaths, marriages, separations, divorces, geographic changes, promotions, graduations, serious illnesses, diagnosis of diabetes, economic changes, or job loss). Nodal events often lead to a series of other events and to illness. What major events or changes in status have occurred in this family? What were the repercussions?

Environmental Influence and Relationships

1. Ethnicity
   a. What is the family's ethnic heritage? (If the patient does not understand, an example should be given.) Most families in North America have immigrants in their lineage. What were the circumstances prompting immigration? Is there still a link with the country of origin?
   b. What are the traditions and values of the family heritage? How important are they to key family members? How easy is it to move away from family values and traditions?
2. Religion
   a. Values, health beliefs and attitudes, beliefs in causality and illness as retribution, and the religious family's view of the world are closely linked and should be questioned.
   b. What is this family's religious tradition? Are they church members, regular church-goers? Are rituals important?
   c. Who in the family is more religious or less religious than usual? Is this an issue for the family?

3. Income and Social Status
    a. If it is acceptable to the patient, determine and record the patient's income level. (Determine the income available to the patient at the time of the occurrence of the problem.)
    b. Which family members are better off or worse off economically? Was there a discrepancy in social status between families joined by marriage? Is money a major problem? A source of conflict?
    c. Generally is the family doing better or worse than their parents or grandparents? Is there social mobility?
4. Social Network
    a. How does the patient spend his or her free time? How much time is spent alone? within the family? outside the family? What kind of activities does the patient engage in?
    b. With whom does the patient and family spend time? (Individuals, groups, organized groups, age, sex)
    c. Determine and record the number of relationships outside the family. What are the characteristics of those relationships?
    d. What is the frequency or amount of time spent in social activities? Recreational activities? Dating? (If appropriate, in-depth questioning about dating habits would include the usual dating pattern in this family and of this patient: age at first date, frequency, number of partners, characteristics of partners (age, education, etc.), sexual activity. Also, the time and circumstances of first sexual activity, number of sexual partners, frequency. How are dating partners valued by the family and others?)

Family Relationship Patterns To Be Recorded in the Report (Conclusions Derived from the Preceeding Data)

1. Nuclear Family
    a. Level of differentiation, the degree to which a person can separate intellect and emotions, make decisions, and openly express feelings (see Chapter 1)
    b. Operating principles of spouses, including the degree of intimacy possible, behavior of the "distancer" and the "pursuer," communication
    c. The predominant family process for handling stress (distancing, illness, transmission to a child)
    d. Members involved in triangulation? (see Chapter 1)
    e. Quality of relationships
    f. Child-centered or spouse-centered

2. Extended Family
    a. Repeating patterns over the generations, including repeated triangulation, illness patterns, and behavioral problems such as substance abuse, physical abuse or cut-off of a family member
    b. Unfinished family business (unresolved family conflict)

Chapter 12

Establishing a Working Relationship with the Family

Janet Christie-Seely

Yves Talbot

Trust is the foundation of any effective family-physician relationship. Unless a family places its trust in a physician or nurse, it will not cooperate fully even in the clinician's most sincere efforts to guide its members in the maintenance of health or the management of illness. Nor will the family be able to receive or accept the moral and psychological support it may need to carry it safely through periods of severe physical or emotional stress. That a trusting relationship should exist between family and practitioner is well established, and is frequently mentioned in the medical literature; nevertheless, very little has been written about how it can be accomplished. If the clinician is worthy of being trusted personally and professionally, most families are prepared to entrust to him or her problems or sensitive issues; but the practitioner must have the sensitivity and communication skills to encourage such trust.

WHEN TO ESTABLISH THE RELATIONSHIP

Some situations or moments are more favorable than others for initiating the establishment of a fruitful family-physician or family-nurse relationship, including the following:

1. when an individual or a family joins a practice (This saves time in obtaining health histories and conveys a family orientation.);
2. when a family seeks information (in premarital and prenatal examinations)—husbands are much more likely to respond to a doctor's request for their presence during their wives' third trimester of pregnancy);
3. when a medical crisis such as an acute or terminal illness occurs (these crises are often emotionally charged for the family; anxiety and uncertainty usually prompt the request for assistance and facilitate stronger clinician-family bonding); and

4. during a home visit, which provides an opportunity to see the family in its environment and to perceive the best approach to winning the confidence and approval of the family.

Trust is also built up over time during office visits by individual family members. An interest in family members' overall well-being beyond the presenting symptoms and an understanding of the family context will build up this trust.

STRATEGIES TO FACILITATE A FAMILY INTERVIEW

Specific indications for a family interview are listed in Chapter 13. The entire family may be very willing to come for an interview in certain situations: when the health of children is in question (sometimes the father may be less willing to participate than the mother); or when a family member is hospitalized (it may be easy to have a family interview during visiting hours). If a family physician is known to insist on seeing all members of each family in his practice, new families entering the practice will expect family-oriented treatment. Members of families who do not wish to be seen by one physician may choose to go to specialists or physicians known to have an orientation toward the individual patient. Although the patient's right to privacy and right to choose must always be respected, there are times when family involvement is more or less mandatory for the sake of the patient's health or recovery, just as there are times when unpleasant interventions such as emergency surgery are essential. In such circumstances it may be necessary to use whatever ethical tactics may be required to bring in reluctant members of the family or to persuade the patient that the understanding and cooperation of the family are essential to the recovery process.

In most cases it seems reasonably clear that attendance at family interviews is a direct function of interviewer expectation.[1] Like the patient in a teaching unit who refuses to be videotaped largely because the resident is anxious about it, other family members often do not cooperate with the clinician who hesitates because he is unsure of the value or afraid of the results of the family interview. Satir's statement for family therapists is to the point: "Once the therapist convinces the husband that he is essential to the therapy process, and that no one else can speak for him or take his place in therapy or in family life, he readily enters in."[8]

DEALING WITH FAMILY RESISTANCE

Resistance to participation in a family interview is usually engendered by the fear that members of the family will be blamed for the illness or that family conflict will surface, if the illness is merely its symptom. A wife may agree, for instance, that her husband is part of the problem but state that he will never come in to see the physician or nurse. If it is true, the clinician can only endeavor to understand the family without meeting the husband; if the clinician is sufficiently astute at discerning the nature of the family tension underlying the wife's symptom, he or she may be able to help her change her behavior or role in a way that will decrease family dysfunction and her consequent need to be ill. The wife's statement may, however, be her way of saying "I don't want my husband to come in." The truth may be that she is afraid of losing the clinician as her ally if the husband's point of view is revealed, or is afraid of her husband's reaction to her disclosure of family problems, or is unwilling to relinquish her privileged position as the sick or weak member of the family.

The basis for the patient's statement can often be determined in this situation by suggesting to the wife that she rephrase the request in such a way that the husband might comply. Examples might include the following: "Do you think he would come if we said we needed some help in understanding your behavior or your illness?" (it is important to keep the focus on her as the patient at least until the first interview to avoid his fear of blame); and "Would he come if you said that I always like to meet the family of my patients as a matter of routine?" Requesting the spouse's help in dealing with the patient's problem without intimating that the family milieu is connected with the problem is usually the best first step; it takes some time for most families to accept a family systems approach to their problem. Sometimes challenging the patient can produce results: "I'm sure you know him well enough that you can think of some way of putting it that will make him realize it's important enough (or so he feels sufficiently less scared/nervous/blamed) for him to make the effort to come in." Suggesting an immediate telephone call by the clinician to the spouse to ascertain his willingness to come in for an interview is also helpful. Even if the husband is reluctant to come in, all that may be needed is a "joining" maneuver over the phone that will convince the husband that the clinician will consider his point of view and is not already taking his wife's side.

A separate appointment for the husband before a joint interview may be needed to establish an amicable relationship if the husband is not already known to the clinician; without this relationship, there is a danger that the clinician will be seen by the husband to favor the wife. A separate interview might be achieved casually during a routine visit for a health examination. The spouse of a patient may genuinely claim that it is impossible to come during work hours, and older children may have the same problem during school hours, particularly if more than one visit is required. Such real time constraints must be recognized and accommodated (see Chapter 10).

SKILLS IN ESTABLISHING THE RELATIONSHIP

How the clinician relates to a family is clearly important but rarely described. Like any organization, the family possesses a hierarchy that comprises formal and informal lines of power, cultural values, and rules that regulate its function. All these factors must be considered when a physician or nurse wants to establish a relationship with a family. The astute practitioner adjusts to the given family system and will work with the prevailing lines of authority; when, for example, a mother's strong leadership is perceived during an interview, the physician will go through her to talk to the children, ensuring that she remains head of the household. Working with the person in charge is characteristic of effective contact with *any* system.)

Joining

Joining with each Family Member

Preferably at the beginning and certainly during the family interview, the physician or nurse will make contact or *join* with each family member in such a way that each feels that he or she is being or will be understood, accepted, and liked.[7] Although it is not always possible to like everyone in one's practice, it should be kept in mind that there is evidence that success with patients (psychotherapeutic outcomes)[9] and compliance with medication[4] correlate with unconditional regard for the patient by the clinician.

It bears repetition that just as good clinicians will spend a few minutes getting to know patients on the first visit, they will spend a few minutes talking with every member in a family interview to assure each one, though not necessarily overtly, that the clinician is understanding and on everyone's side. The art of empathizing with and understanding every family member is the secret of the successful family interview and of working efficiently with families.

Much can be learned by watching the verbal and nonverbal behavior of a successful professional: Minuchin, for example, though usually a nonsmoker, smokes with smokers, his position mimicking that of the person to whom he is speaking. He may launch into a discussion of the virtue of different rail routes with railway men, within minutes of their being introduced; or he may speak about football scores with an adolescent. A firm bond with each is established in a short time. The broader a clinician's life experience the easier it will be for him or her to join with people of all ages and walks of life; the younger clinician may have to substitute real life experience with a knowledge of literature.

The younger children must also be included in this process, or they will understandably feel unwanted and disrupt the session, or become bored and silent; the importance of their contribution should be emphasized during the interview. The clinician's behavior while listening even to young children may provide a model of better listening skills for the parents, and essential information that may not have been evident or obtainable from the parent may become available. For example, in one family the father stated that the only problem was his adolescent son's behavior, at that point the 7-year-old daughter asked her father why he had recently left the family for a month. On another occasion, two children playing with puppets resembling their parents contradicted their parents' statement that they had had a peaceful week together by staging a very vigorous fight between the puppets. One father with heart disease and type A behavior said he had slowed down considerably since the operation; his wife agreed, but both son and daughter shook their heads in vigorous disagreement. The truth is frequently told by children who are less practiced in masking true feelings.

Joining with the Family System

The clinician should recognize and support the family's values and should show an interest in the family's traditions. Points held in common with the family are shared by saying, for example, "I have two adolescents like you." On the other hand, if a conflict arises between family members during an interview, the clinician avoids taking sides or being judgmental. Understanding the interactional basis for behavior helps avoid labelling a patient "difficult," or calling the wife the "victim" or "strong one" if the husband is an alcoholic. The clinician must avoid the role of rescuer or judge.

Wise interviewers adapt to the personalities of families; they are quiet with families that are restrained but jovial with those that are more expansive. Bonding behavior between family and clinician is not limited to the initial phase of the first interview; it continues throughout the relationship. Being available when needed and helping family members solve health-related problems enhance the practitioner's credibility. Although all the components of the clinician-family relationship can be established in the nurse's or physician's office, a home visit often expedites the process and gives the clinician important information about the physical and emotional environment in which the family lives. A home visit is one of the most powerful joining maneuvers.

Comfort Level in a Family Interview

Being comfortable during the family interview is the result of experience, a sense of direction, and knowledge concerning family assessment and management. Since most medical and nursing students rarely, if ever, interview more than one person at a time, they must face the anxiety associated with group interviews.

The physician or nurse who is not comfortable with nor skilled in conducting family interviews may not develop a family orientation either. Lip service to the importance of family may be given, but families may be avoided. In one practice that advertised its concern for the family as patient, only three out of 30 nurses and physicians had conducted more than three family interviews, not through any lack of interest or caring but because of anxiety at being confronted with several people at once, and a fear of saying the wrong thing.

Fear of Conflict

Even the clinician who has become confident in handling the one-to-one interview may feel less certain about maintaining control during the group interview, and may fear that the loss of control will permit open conflict or risk the possibility of opening the proverbial can of worms.

Role playing in simulated group interviews is one way of developing self-assurance before engaging in actual family sessions. Such role playing is usually an essential ingredient of residency and nurse-training programs. Assuming different roles in simulated conflict situations teaches empathy through taking the roles of family members and teaches the skill of setting limits when the interviewer role is taken. Students may also be reassured by being reminded that nothing will happen in the office that does not happen at home and that the real problem in most families is avoidance of conflict.

Clinicians often have the same problem; they are healers and helpers and often fear conflict. The need of many physicians and nurses to be actively helpful can be a serious barrier in allowing families to learn to help themselves. Physicians particularly, must be persuaded that more can be accomplished in certain situations by their being willing to become a supportive presence and not actively involved, enabling the family to work through a problem despite its fear of conflict.

The Presence of Children

It is usually easiest to start with interviewing couples and to progress later to the distractions and liveliness inherent to interviews involving young children. Interviews in which children are participating can usually be conducted more easily in the home, where the environment is familiar and more conducive to the children's being at ease. Observing the children and their parents at home also gives more reliable and complete information than it is possible to perceive through their behavior in the office. The general comfort level may also be enhanced for both clinician and family because house calls are still valued as a special service provided by a family doctor or nurse, more so because of their current rareness.

Observational Skills

Most clinicians have mastered the observational skills required in the area of physical diagnosis. They quickly notice any abnormality in color, respiration, gait, or other physical signs as the patient walks into the office. These same physicians or nurses may be oblivious to the patient's facial expression and other forms of nonverbal communication if their attention is focused primarily on signs of physical illness. It is relatively easy, however, for such clinicians to learn how to transfer their observational skills to this additional area. Observation of nonverbal interaction between people can be learned by viewing videotapes of family interviews. These videotapes can be replayed without sound until the clinician's attention is automatically given to the nonverbal as well as the verbal content of the interview. Nurses and social workers are frequently better trained in this skill, although some who have had experience only with the one-to-one interview may feel as uncomfortable and ill-equipped as most physicians to function in the group setting.

Ways to Facilitate Learning

Feedback from colleagues who role-play a family and especially from actors, who create a *"simulated family"* and may be more candid than colleagues, accelerates the acquisition of observational and interviewing skills. "Simulated patients" as developed by Barrows[2] are impersonations of real cases by "actors" who, if properly trained, can not only fool a physician but can also give him or her discerning feedback information after the interview in a constructive and nonthreatening way. Similarly, a real family can also be portrayed by "actors" of appropriate ages who take care to avoid scripts and accurately reflect the dynamics of the real system. Such a family or patient can state specifically which words or manner of the interviewer made them feel more able to talk or display emotion. For example, a patient simulating the difficult role of a patient to be informed of a diagnosis of ovarian cancer was able to cry openly when the interviewer projected real empathy. Another patient said they felt comfortable until the interviewer asked a rather forced question about sexual relations and then rapidly changed the subject. Similarly, a resident in a family role-play can rapidly identify times when the interviewer is favoring one member or is angry with another. In one family, the seeming villain explained how defensive he felt when challenged about his unemployment; the challenger increased his obnoxious behavior.

Observing one's self on videotape is a rapid method of obtaining distance from an interview; it is important to see ourselves as others see us. (In fact, most clinicians thus exposed are overly self-critical and need help to see their strengths.) The skills needed to interact effectively with the individual patient are now taught in most North American medical and nursing schools, and courses in interviewing skills are basic components of training in social work. Older physicians and nurses or graduates from very traditional schools may not have been given training in interviewing or have good role models. The student who was never observed while interviewing and who never observed another professional conducting an interview may never discover that certain habits seriously impede communication and understanding (standing when the patient is sitting, leaning away from the patient with a protective desk interposed between physician and patient, asking three questions in one sentence, or using excessive medical terminology).[5,6] Without the encouragement of a group or the example of a good role model, it may be hard to adopt the practice of leaning forward, making eye contact, and demonstrating interest nonverbally so that the patient understands that the expression of emotions and attitudes is both acceptable and encouraged.

THE CLINICIAN AS OBSERVER OUTSIDE THE SYSTEM

Frequently, the main obstacle to successful interaction in both individual and family interviews is the professional who talks too much. An interesting study of physician-patient interaction in England showed a high number of dysfunctional interviews when both clinician and patient talked at once, neither listening to the other.[3] The compulsion to talk may be a sign of anxiety, or of overvaluing the helping role, or of undervaluing the self-knowledge possessed by the individual or family.

It is particularly difficult for physicians who are accustomed to taking helpful action, to sit quietly, observe, and do nothing other than allow the family to observe and communicate with itself. Instead of being the focus of attention during an interview in which all questions or comments are directed to the physician or nurse, who acts as the hub of the family wheel with spokes radiating outward, the clinician must deliberately stay outside the wheel except to give it the occasional gentle push to keep it turning. A similar analogy applies to working with families as well as to interviewing them: the professional may occasionally be needed to get the family moving in a healthier direction but should never become enmeshed in the family's internal mechanism or, worse still, become an indispensable part of it. This is particularly true when the family is trying to involve the physician in order to transfer responsibility for the illness to him or her by the process of triangulation.

REFERENCES

1. Allmond BW, Buchman W, Gofman HF: *The Family Is the Patient: An Approach to Behavioral Pediatrics for the Clinician.* St. Louis, C.V. Mosby Co., 1979.

2. Barrows HS: *Simulated Patients.* Springfield, Illinois, Charles C Thomas, 1971.

3. Byrne PS, Long BEL: *Doctors Talking to Patients.* Department of Health and Social Security. London, Her Majesty's Stationary Office, 1976.

4. Elling R, Whitemore R, Green M: Patient participation in a pediatric program. *J Health Hum Behav* 1:183, 1960.

5. Kent Smith C, Polis E, Madac RR: Characteristics of the initial medical interview associated with patient satisfaction and understanding. *J Fam Pract* 12:283, 1981.

6. Larsen KM, Kent Smith C: Assessment of nonverbal communication in the patient physician interview. *J Fam Pract* 12:481, 1981.

7. Minuchin S, Fishman HC: *Family Therapy Techniques.* Cambridge, Harvard University Press, 1981.

8. Satir V: *Conjoint Family Therapy: A guide to Theory and Technique.* Palo Alto, California, Science and Behavior Books, 1964.

9. Truax CB, Carkkuff RR: *Towards Effective Counselling and Psychotherapy.* Aldine, Chicago, 1967.

Chapter 13

The Presenting Problems of Families and Family Assessment

Dorothy Barrier
Janet Christie-Seely

Families usually present to the primary care professional through members who are sick or believe they are sick. Individuals also come because of anxiety, worries, personal problems, behavioral problems in children, or direct complaints about family tensions. The extent of these "non-medical" visits varies with the tendency to somatize tensions, the acceptability of psychological complaints by the family and community, and the availability of other resources. Such visits vary greatly from practice to practice and probably depend most on the patient's perception of the clinician's interest and ability to help, and on the doctor-patient relationship that has been established. Behind the presenting patient is often a family asking for help. It is important for the clinician to be responsive to these cues, and to develop a cost-effective strategy of management.

Earlier in this book (in Chapter 2), health was described as a behavioral and developmental phenomenon characterized by successful ways of coping with situations in life, determining and moving toward life goals, and mobilizing strengths and resources. In contrast, patterns of behavior and relationships that inhibit coping, achievement of goals, and the use of resources can be called dysfunctional. To label a family "unhealthy" is to suggest that it has certain fixed characteristics that cannot be changed.

Dysfunctional families are characterized either by rigidly closed borders or by nonexistent boundaries. Individuals who are poorly individuated and cannot develop truly intimate relations fear the loss of identity or the risk of separation and loss; they lack trust. Such persons may be isolated from one another or, overly close. Isolated individuals from disengaged families are less often seen by the clinician as they preserve their independence and seek help later in the course of their illness; they may die at home or on the street with few friends or family to help. The too close or "enmeshed" families lack privacy, which restricts individual autonomy and the possibility of change. Communication may, in fact, be excessive; mind-reading and intrusiveness can prevail.

Jealousy and intrusiveness prevent real communication between two persons because a third person always jumps in to clarify or protect. An "infinite dance of shifting coalitions"[10] occurs along with an unspoken demand to conceal the coalitions. Family members rarely show congruence between internal emotional states and their verbal expressions; therefore, the confusion of messages and of relations makes problem solving extremely difficult. The equilibrium of such a system is precarious and can be easily upset by illness. Because of high levels of chronic stress these families are illness-prone.[7]

An outside professional can easily get caught up in the confusion. A problem first labelled as the illness of one family member may become an argument over financial support, then switch to a complaint of favoritism of one child, which in turn evokes an argument between the children about allocation of household chores. To understand what is happening the clinician requires skill in observing interaction, in assessing roles and structure, and in observing the family process. He or she must not be caught up in the content of discussion, but must observe the process.

Barnhill,[2] in a review and integration of the theoretical literature on family assessment, has isolated eight basic indicators that can assess the functional health of a family. All families have certain strengths, and a family with few healthy characteristics may remain functional if not exposed to stress. Conversely, any healthy family that experiences repeated or extreme stress may develop dysfunction. Unhealthy families display a number of characteristics which can be grouped into four categories: identity processes, coping with change, information processing, and role structuring: The eight characteristics are as follows:

IDENTITY PROCESSES

Enmeshment versus Individuation

Enmeshment refers to poorly delineated boundaries of self, to an identity dependent on others, to symbiosis, and what Boszormenyi-Nagy described as "shared ego fusion."[4] Psychosomatic families tend to show enmeshment.[10] They present themselves as loving, happy families with one or more sick members but exhibit a total avoidance of conflict, constant intrusiveness, overprotectiveness of one another, and excessive awareness of each other's thoughts and feelings.

Disengagement versus Mutuality (Isolation versus Partnership)

Dysfunctional families often display a sense of isolation within the family and a feeling of alienation from others. They may be geographically separate from each other, with no communication by phone or mail. Boundaries around self may be closed; family members may show no warmth or sharing. Cooperation in caring for a sick or elderly family member may be nonexistent. This pattern represents the extreme opposite of enmeshment. The healthy family, whose behavior is found between these extremes, is composed of individuated members who can develop maximum intimacy and mutuality without fear of loss of identity.

COPING WITH CHANGE

Rigidity versus Flexibility

A dysfunctional family shows inadequate resilience when under stress; its attempts at problem solving are inappropriate and unsuccessful. Rigid rules, family secrets, and traditions that are in conflict with the current environment lead to closure of the family boundary and entrenchment of existing roles and rules. Such a family is unable to change its own rules to accommodate growth within the system or new information from outside systems. A common example is the immigrant family, isolated from the community by language and culture, which is confronted by the different sexual mores and greater personal freedom of the new culture through an adolescent daughter. Any attempt to close the family boundary around her is bound to fail because she still must go to school and relate to her peers. The boundary may also be closed to health professionals who are treated with distrust.

Disorganization versus Stability

A lack of stability and consistency of family relationships characterizes some families. In contrast to the rigid family, discipline and rules are inconsistent or chaotic. Parents may ignore a child's behavior one week, and cross-examine him on homework, friends, and activities the next. Joking at a father's expense may be encouraged one day but produce a rage the next. Alcohol may add to the chaos. Clearly, in such a family adding a strict diet or medication regime will be much more difficult than in the highly structured family.

INFORMATION PROCESSING

Unclear (or Distorted) versus Clear Perception

How a person perceives the behavior and communication signals of others depends on self-image and that person's view of the world as being hostile, friendly, or neutral. Confusion of feelings with thought, and distortion of reality are characteristic of persons at the lower end of Bowen's "differentiation of self scale" (see Chapter 1), these persons are less individuated, mature, and autonomous. (An extreme example is the schizophrenic who perceives comments on the radio as referring to him.) Whole families may accept a myth that is out of touch with reality: a mother labelled as "weak and vulnerable" may in fact, control every member of the family through threats of an impending heart attack creating feelings of guilt.

Unclear (or Distorted) versus Clear Communication

Communication will be distorted if perception of its meaning is distorted, or if the communication itself is unclear. In some families verbal statements may be in conflict with nonverbal messages, producing a confusing situation.[3] Communication may be indirect; anger may be directed at a child rather than the spouse. Communication may also be masked; arguments over money can mask sexual conflict or symbolize the stinginess or misspent affection of the partner. Poor communication is often based on mutual protection. Communication about a serious illness, for example, often is avoided or is unclear to protect family members from the pain of clarity.

ROLE STRUCTURING

Role Conflict (Unclear roles) versus Role Reciprocity

The changing role of women often results in role conflicts becoming the basis of tension between spouses, and between parents and children, particularly adolescents. Family roles become important only if there is disagreement or discontent over role assignments, or if no one is assigned to a necessary family task. Flexibility of roles becomes particularly important when there is illness or hospitalization. Maximum family stress occurs during hospitalization of the mother whose nurturing and homemaking role must then be filled by a substitute. Chronic illness of the breadwinner produces similar stress, particularly if no one else can do work to provide money.

Diffuse (Breached) versus Clear Generational Boundaries

The most important area of family assessment for any presenting problem is the strength of the parental coalition. If the parents have a strong affectional bond, the boundary around them as a couple will usually be clear and an alliance between a parent and a child against the other parent will not occur. It is when the generational boundary is consistently vague that problems occur. The clinician may help to strengthen this boundary by suggesting activities for the couple, such as weekends without the children, as well as activities for the children as a group without the parents. This is often helpful for families with adolescents as a way of anticipating the problems encountered when the children have left home. Boundaries with the older generation may be diffuse and produce problems with in-laws; newlyweds who are trying to develop appropriate boundaries are at particular risk. With the arrival of a new baby the grandparents may try to move back in; boundaries must be redefined.

PRESENTING PROBLEMS OF DYSFUNCTION

Dysfunctional families are also illness-prone families.[7] That family stress plays a role in the etiology of disease has been well documented (see Section III). Bowen[5] identifies three possible indicators of family stress:

1. overt marital conflict and sexual problems
2. behavioral or psychosomatic problems in a child: scapegoating, delinquency, and psychosomatic crises (protecting the myth of parental cohesion)
3. illness in one or more family members

These three manifestations of stress are not specific to unhealthy families but tend to persist as fixed patterns in such families due to their lack of resiliency in finding other methods of coping.

The treatment plan of a family presenting with a marital problem is more straightforward and acceptable to the family when requested by the couple. When a couple avoids marital difficulties by involving the children or by reverting to an illness role there may be difficulties in diagnosis and management. Treatment may not be as successful if the family is unable to recognize that a child's or adult's illness may be the result of an unresolved family problem, preferring to regard the ill or misbehaving member as the only problem. Such a situation may well raise an important ethical question: *When should a clinician interfere with the displacement or denial process?* If a child's life is at stake (when the child has diseases such as anorexia nervosa, diabetic acidosis, asthmatic crisis[9]) most agree that the clinician should intervene. If the child has become the scapegoat or is misbehaving, and it is clear the parents are avoiding conflict between themselves, the question that arises is, "Do I have the right to suggest that the couple may have a marital problem?" In this case, the distinction between diagnosis and treatment can be made. The clinician has the responsibility, if consulted, to diagnose illness, but before the patient can be involved in treatment, his or her acceptance of the treatment plan is needed. The same principle applies to family assessment.

FAMILY ASSESSMENT

Family assessment is based on a family interview. One family member cannot provide an assessment of the interrelationships and functioning of the system. When we assess a family, labels such as "unhealthy" or "dysfunctional" are better avoided in favor of focusing on positive attributes like family strengths or ability to cope. The importance of observing the interaction between members during a family assessment interview cannot be overstated. Although it is not practical to assess every family encounted in practice, a brief family interview at the time of registration to discuss the general health status of its members and to obtain a preliminary idea of family functioning makes the clinician's family perspective evident (see Chapter 12).

Signs Indicating the Need for Family Assessment

Certain symptoms, behavior patterns, or situations indicate the need for family assessment. The following list has been found to be useful:

1. Nonspecific symptoms in a patient who visits frequently: headache, backache, and abdominal pains, particularly in the absence of organic disease
2. Overutilization of medical care services or frequent visits by *different* family members
3. Difficulty in the management of chronic illness. (Involvement of the family is always a useful part of chronic disease management, but problems in management make family assessment mandatory.) Examples include difficulties in obtaining drug and diet compliance in such diseases as epilepsy and hypertension; and recurring problems such as diabetic coma or insulin reactions and severe asthmatic attacks.
4. The "Ripple Effect"—that is, when one member of the family presents with the same symptoms of a serious illness or crisis as another member, or a series of illness occur in close sequence within the family.
5. Emotional and behavioral problems, such as "acting out" in the adolescent, depression, or anxiety in the adult
6. Two-person problems (marital and sexual problems), including impotence, infertility, and excessive dependency with or without illness
7. Scapegoating or triangulation: transference of unresolved family stress onto one member, usually a child
8. Diseases causally related to lifestyles and environmental factors (liver disease and alcoholism, lung disease and smoking, peptic ulcer and emotional stress)
9. Activities promoting health and preventing disease in the family, including immunization, genetic counselling, and nutritional guidance

10. Anxiety caused by anticipation of common problems associated with each of the developmental stages of the family, including the arrival and care of a baby, adolescence, mid-life crisis, "empty nest" syndrome, etc

11. Loss of a family member, loss of home or employment, disfigurement or amputation by accident, death, war, separation, plant shutdown, etc

12. Whenever the strictly biomedical model is inadequate—look at the family! (This one is for the clinician unable to "think systems" in every encounter!)

METHODS OF FAMILY ASSESSMENT

Ransom* has described four levels of measurement in family research to date:

1. *Self-report data about the family* from interviews or questionnaires of *individuals*. This level gives information only about individual perception about the family, and usually only what is admitted and conscious.

2. *Data derived from combining or comparing individual responses.* This technique begins to give actual data about family interaction. For example, if the statement, "I am satisfied with the amount of time my family and I spend together,"[15] elicits strong agreement in one member and strong disagreement in another, questions are raised about conflict avoidance and communication.

3. *Data about family structure.* Such data give information about the family as a unit: its size and composition, its stage in the family life cycle, etc. This level is the predominant level discussed in the sociology literature.

4. *Data derived from family interaction.* This level is more difficult to obtain but gives direct information about family interaction. Data include the following:

Observational Description of Family Behavior. A videotaped interview of a family performing a standardized task such as menu selection may be analyzed in segments to assess communication, roles, conflict, and decision making. Measurements can include actual frequency of interrupted versus completed statements by each member; patterns of sequence of response by members; number of support statements (by whom, for whom); decision

---

*Ransom DC, Dallman J: Presented March 9, 1983, Workshop on Family Measurement in Third Annual Meeting on Working with Family, Kansas City.

statements ("Who suggested jello for the final course?" "Who agreed or disagreed?"); or nonverbal items (the number of times members touch one another, direction of gaze when talking, physical positions). Since family processes are said to repeat patterns every 5 to 10 minutes a short section of a videotape provides a rich and often complete source for assessment, particularly if the family is challenged by a task that brings out maladaptive responses.

Observational studies have also been made in the home.[17] However, there the lower stress levels may mean longer time intervals before dysfunction is observed.

Joint Product Data. Instead of investigating the process of family interaction, the study may be designed so that family function is assessed by the product of the family task. For example, a family having difficulty in making decisions will not be able to complete menu selection in the requisite 20 minutes (see Reiss's[13] study Chapter 2).

Individual Responses Measured During Ongoing Interaction. In one study[10] free fatty acid levels were monitored in every family member during a stressful interview (see Chapter 8). This measurement enabled clinicians to correlate a family's behavior with its biochemical response.

Data Derived by Combining or Comparing Individual Responses during Ongoing Interaction. Again Minuchin's study[10] is illustrative; he compared free fatty acid levels of the parents which fell as the diabetic child entered the room, relieving their tension. The child's level continued to rise indicating transfer of stress from one part of the system to another.

CURRENT CLINICAL ASSESSMENT TOOLS

The Family APGAR

Smilkstein has devised the "Family APGAR"[15] as a means of assessing the individual's view of family functioning (level 1 measurement). It is a useful screening tool, particularly if results from different family members are compared (level 2—never actually studied by Smilkstein). The individual is questioned about the family's degree of adaptation, partnership, growth, affection, and resolve (commitment). Each variable has a maximum score of two; a total possible score of ten represents maximum satisfaction with the family (see Table 13.1). This questionnaire, for which construct validity but not predictive validity has been assessed,[16] measures only conscious and admitted satisfaction with family life. It is very similar to scales of social acceptability. Smilkstein recognizes that the response given by members of an

Table 13.1 Family APGAR Questionnaire*

	Almost always	Some of the time	Hardly ever
I am satisfied with the help that I receive from my family* when something is troubling me.	_____	_____	_____
I am satisfied with the way my family* discusses items of common interest and shares problem solving with me.	_____	_____	_____
I find that my family* accepts my wishes to take on new activities or make changes in my life style.	_____	_____	_____
I am satisfied with the way my family* expresses affection and responds to my feelings such as anger, sorrow, and love.	_____	_____	_____
I am satisfied with the amount of time my family* and I spend together.	_____	_____	_____

Scoring: The patient checks one of three choices which are scored as follows: 'Almost always' (2 points), 'Some of the time' (1 point), or 'Hardly ever' (0). The scores for each of the five questions are then totaled. A score of 7 to 10 suggests a highly functional family. A score of 4 to 6 suggests a moderately dysfunctional family. A score of 0 to 3 suggests a severely dysfunctional family.
*According to which member of the family is being interviewed the physician may substitute for the word 'family' either spouse, significant other, parents, or children.

Source: Smilkstein, G: The Family APGAR: A proposal for a family function test and its use by physicians. *J Fam Pract* 15:303, 1982.

enmeshed, conflict-denying family may well be higher than is actually the case; such a family may be so dysfunctional that a member's illness becomes aggravated and even fatal while the family still considers itself close and loving and whose only problem is the sick child.[9]

The Family Circle

A second, more useful screening tool for clinical practice is the "Family Circle."[18] This is a simple projective test in which a patient is given a piece of paper with a circle drawn on it and is asked to represent his or her family in the circle (see Figs. 13-1, 13-2). It is an effective way of obtaining a rapid view of relationships in the household and is an avenue to discussion that conveys to the patient the clinician's interest in the family. (The reader interested in other schemata of family assessment used in family medicine is referred to Arbogast and colleagues[1] and Pless and Satterwhite,[12] who offer tools of assessment that are primarily focused on the individual rather than on the family.)

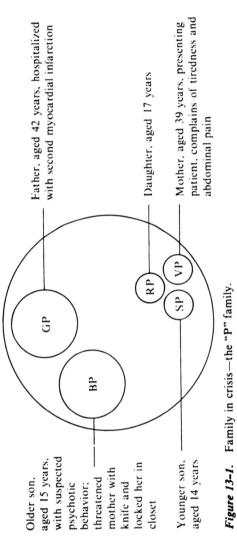

Older son,
aged 15 years,
with suspected
psychotic
behavior;
threatened
mother with
knife and
locked her in
closet

Younger son,
aged 14 years

Father, aged 42 years, hospitalized
with second myocardial infarction

Daughter, aged 17 years

Mother, aged 39 years, presenting
patient, complains of tiredness and
abdominal pain

Figure 13-1. Family in crisis—the "P" family.

From: Thrower SM, Bruce WE, Welton RF: The family circle method for integrating family systems concepts in family medicine. *J Fam Pract* 15:451. 1982.

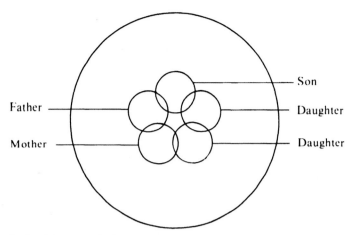

Figure 13-2. The enmeshed psychosomatic family.

From: Thrower S M, Bruce W E, Welton R F: The family circle method for integrating family systems concepts in family medicine. *J Fam Pract* 15:451, 1982.

The Family Interview

Once the need for family assessment has been identified a family interview is essential. Assessment of family functioning through each individual is not adequate because it does not permit accurate perception of the true relationship between members. Nonverbal communication, unconscious interactions, and problems denied by family members that are the true cause of dysfunction cannot be assessed. Once an interview with the entire family has taken place, much can be inferred from subsequent encounters with individual members.

Framework for Interview and Record

A theoretical framework is necessary to make sense of the voluminous data that flows from a family during an interview. Some means of recording the data for future reference and communication with other professionals is necessary. Smilkstein[14] has devised the "Problem-Oriented Record" (POR) to direct attention to three areas of particular importance paralleling the history of present illness, past history, and functional enquiry familiar in medicine:

1. the crisis episode (the present illness or problem);
2. the resources of the family (past history); and
3. the functional status of the family (systems review).

Smilkstein also devised the acronym SCREEM[14] (social, cultural, religious, economic, educational, and medical resources) as an aid in reviewing the strengths and deficiencies in various categories of resources (deficiencies might include social isolation, over-commitment to community activities, educational handicap, inappropriate training, medical underutilization, or major frequent medical-surgical problems). However, this structure is inadequate for a family assessment interview.

The McMaster model of family functioning[6] has been used in the examination of families whose patterns of functioning range across a spectrum from healthy to severely pathologic. This model utilizes general systems theory to describe the structure, organization, and transactional patterns of the family unit and is useful in studying the presenting problems of families. It considers family functioning in the following categories:

1. Problem solving (problems may be poorly defined; family "solutions" often aggravate the problem).
2. Communication (clear, direct or masked, indirect, mixed messages).
3. Roles (clear and flexible, satisfying or rigid, or ill-defined with poor accountability).
4. Affective responsiveness (expression of warmth, affection).
5. Affective involvement (symbiosis/enmeshment or disengagement).
6. Control of behavior (rigid, appropriate and flexible, chaotic).

Another more complex schema using similar variables to those of Epstein[6] and Barnhill,[2] but designed and validated as a research tool is the Beavers-Timberlawn Family Evaluation Scale,[8] which is based on the concept that pathology and health in family organization are on a continuum from chaos through rigidity to flexibility with a clear family structure. Fourteen scales are each rated on this continuum: the power structure, strength of parental coalition, closeness, family mythology (and its fit with reality), negotiated problem solving, autonomy, responsibility, invasiveness, permeability (openness to other's statements), open expression of feelings, mood and tone, unresolvable conflict, empathy, and a global health-pathology scale. A simpler and well validated tool, the circumplex model of marital and family systems underlines two of the most basic variables: cohesion and adaptability.[11]

These models were designed by family therapists primarily for use with families requesting family therapy. In such families, illness is not a primary presenting problem or they would have appeared in the family physicians' offices. It was felt by the multi-disciplinary Task Force on the Family at the Kellogg Centre in Montreal that there was a need for a family assessment tool for physicians and primary care nurses dealing with families that typically present in the offices of family physicians. "PRACTICE" presented in the next chapter was the tool developed. Factors added include: illness (chronic or acute), illness role, health belief system, coping by the family in the past and present with illness and other crises. Roles and structure, communication and affect are similar to the factors described by Barnhill and the McMaster model. The focus is the problem presented to the family physician or nurse, the P of Practice. There is also more emphasis on the time in the family life cycle, a large part of which the family physician is often privileged to view. The acronym "PRACTICE" denotes its use in family practice and emphasizes the fact that repeated practice of family assessment will improve this skill.

REFERENCES

1. Arbogast RC, Scratton JM, Krick JP: The family as patient: Preliminary experience with a recorded assessment schema. *J Fam Pract* 7:1151, 1978.

2. Barnhill L: Healthy family systems. *Fam Coordinator* 28:94, 1979.

3. Bateson G: *Steps to an Ecology of Mind.* New York, Ballantine Books, 1972.

4. Boszormenyi-Nagy I: A theory of relationships: experience and transaction, in Boszormenyi-Nagy I, Framo J (eds): *Intensive Family Therapy.* New York, Harper & Row, 1965.

5. Bowen M: *Family Therapy in Clinical Practice.* New York, Hason Aronson, 1978.

6. Epstein NB, Bishop DS, Levin S: The McMaster model of family functioning. *J Marr Fam Counselling* 4:19, 1978.

7. Hinkle LE Jr, Plummer N: Life stress and industrial absenteeism: The concentration of illness and absenteeism in one segment of a working population. *Ind Med Surg* 21:363, 1952.

8. Lewis JN, Beavers WR, Gossett JT, et al: No single thread: Psychological health in family systems.

9. Minuchin S, Baker L, Rosman BL, et al: A conceptual model of psychosomatic illness in children: Family organization and family therapy. *Arch Gen Psychiatry* 32:1031, 1975.

10. Minuchin S: *Families and Family Therapy.* New York: Brunner/Mazel Inc., 1976.

11. Olson DH, Spenkle DH, Russell C: Circumplex model of marital and family systems: I. Cohesion and adaptability dimensions, family types, and clinical applications. *Fam Process* 18:3, 1979.

12. Pless IB, Satterwhite B: A measure of family functioning and its application. *Soc Sci Med* 7:613, 1973.

13. Reiss D: *The Family's Construction of Reality.* Cambridge, Harvard University Press, 1981.

14. Smilkstein G: The family in trouble—How to tell. *J Fam Pract* 2:19, 1975.

15. Smilkstein G: The family APGAR: A proposal for a family function test and its use by physicians. *J Fam Pract* 6:1234, 1978.

16. Smilkstein G, Ashworth C, Montano D: Validity and reliability of the family APGAR as a test of family function. *J Fam Pract* 15:303, 1982.

17. Steinglass P: The home observation assessment method (HOAM): Real-time naturalistic observation of families in their homes. *Fam Process* 18:337, 1979.

18. Thrower SM, Bruce WE, Welton RF: The family circle method for integrating family systems concepts in family medicine. *J Fam Pract* 15:451, 1982.

Chapter 14

PRACTICE—A Family Assessment Tool for Family Medicine

Dorothy Barrier
Maria Bybel
Janet Christie-Seely
Yvonne Whittaker

A family assessment form has been designed for use in assessing the function of the family as a unit. It is based on a systems approach and acts as a guide and a record for a family interview. The acronym PRACTICE denotes its use by family physicians and nurses, and is a reminder that repeated practice will develop and improve skill in family assessment.

The components of the PRACTICE schema are as follows:

Presenting problem or reason for interview (illness, hospitalization, behavioral or relationship problems).

Roles and structure. Included are hierarchical organization, boundaries and individuation, cohesion (from disengagement to enmeshment), and control (from chaos to rigidity).

Affect (emotional expression) family emotional tone (warmth, sadness, anger, humor).

Communication (verbal and nonverbal).

Time in the family life cycle. The dynamics of developmental stages are experienced differently by each family and may influence the occurrence and response to illness.

Illness in the family past and present. Usually the focus in family practice is on the illness, which may be the presenting problem masking dysfunction in the family unit. Past experience of illness, especially if frequent or serious, will modify response to illness in the present. The meaning of illness, health belief system, health practices, and lifestyle are also determined by the family.

Coping with stress (adaptability, family strengths and resources, coping in past and present).

Ecology and culture (interaction of the family with the environment). Social, cultural, religious, economic, educational and medical resources (SCREEM).[26]

An Educational Tool

The variables chosen have been derived from research on the healthy family[2,22] and from literature on family therapy based on systems theory.[10,20] It has been found useful to associate these assessment variables in an acronym to aid health professionals, particularly residents in family medicine and nurses in training, and to remind them of the various aspects of family function. Once skills in family assessment are fully developed, these forms like other such learning tools may be discarded. The insertion of forms in a patient's file does not necessarily imply good patient care; an informal approach may well be the best. However, it has been our experience that these forms provide a needed transition and structure for the learner and are a convenient means of recording and communicating family data.

The form should not be taken into the interview and filled out sequentially as a check list. The interviewer may or may not want to take notes during the family meeting, but the sections of the form should contain a one- or two-sentence impression of each aspect of family function. (For example, under the heading, Affect, the clinician might write the following: "Family very depressed, unable to respond to jokes or attempt to lighten atmosphere. Denied anger at anyone."; or under the heading, Roles: "Father very rigid, apparently makes all decisions. Mother lenient, undermining. Chaotic interview. Masked conflict between parents."

A list of family members present and absent from the interview should also be included. It should be remembered that it is often difficult for beginners to obtain a family's agreement for and cooperation during an interview. Some members may fail to show up; others may persistently give work or school as excuses for not coming, even when appointment times are flexible enough to accommodate late afternoon or evening hours. The more experienced professional has less difficulty with compliance, partly because his or her conviction that a family interview will be helpful may be greater than the beginner's, partly because he or she will not convey the discomfort of the beginner with such an interview to the family.

A family interview may be seen as very threatening or unusual; that it is a nonthreatening and routine part of care can be conveyed by phrases such as "I usually like to see the whole family if anyone is seriously ill or hospitalized to clear up any questions or worries anyone might have," or "I would like to see your husband too next visit as he may be able to give his perspective and help with your depression." If one or two family members are missing from the interview, despite originally agreeing that they would come, proceeding with the family assessment risks inaccurate data. A member who has not participated in the interview may cause difficulties later. Permitting members to miss the interview may allow the family to leave the problem at home. The missing member is often the most outspoken. In family therapy, the missing member often represents the family's resistance to a family approach and may undermine the process if allowed to remain absent.

Much of the information needed to complete the form may be derived from the discussion of the presenting problem. For this discussion, if the interviewer is skillfull in having the family discuss the issue among themselves rather than answer his or her questions, communication patterns, the roles and structure of the family, and general emotional tone will become apparent. Some idea of the family's strengths and coping and its use of resources will also be conveyed.

Depending on the complexity of the presenting problem, and on the goals of the meeting, the interview and completion of the form can take anywhere from 15 minutes to an hour and a half; experience produces efficiency. An expert can recognize, in the first 5 minutes of the interview, behavior patterns indicative of family structure and themes that will be subsequently repeated. The way the family handles a current problem will tend to be typical of its ability to handle other problems. It has been shown that almost 75% of the information in an individual interview for a medical problem is obtained in the first 10 minutes;[3] similarly, most information about the family is available early on in a family interview if the interviewer is trained to perceive it.

Assessment, A Prerequisite for Action

Family intervention without assessment is like treatment without diagnosis. Assessment, diagnosis, and management are inextricably interwoven; to manage illness or maintain health in the family context means to understand the structure, function, development, and approach to health and illness of that particular family.

For a given problem, assessment of one or more of the items covered in the acronym PRACTICE is important for successful intervention. Rarely do all aspects need assessment. For example, in improving dietary compliance in diabetes the family's roles and structure ("R" in PRACTICE) and their experience with illness and their health belief system ("I" in PRACTICE) determine who does the shopping and cooking, who has the power to influence compliance (positively, or negatively if it produces rebellion), and whether the family believes diet will alter the course of the disease. Affect, communication, time in life cycle, coping, and the environment may be of little relevance to this particular problem.

P—PROBLEM

In identifying the problem of a family, an important step is the art of joining with the family system (see Chapter 12, Joining). The interviewer encourages family interaction, by asking about the presenting problem and testing the family's communication and affect (emotional expression). Particular attention is paid to the mood of the family—whether the family is cheerful, angry, or unhappy. The family's mood is important when the clinician attempts to enlist its cooperation in solving the problem. Family organization and hierarchical structure as well as repetitive sequences of behavior will be noted. Previous attempts at problem resolution should be explored.[31] Thus, information on roles, affect, and communication and coping are often derived from discussion of the problem.

At the beginning of a family assessment the clinician elicits the family's description of the problem(s). The problem may be a physical illness that is causing family difficulties or is suggestive of a broader family problem contributing to the illness. Since the couple is the source of the family system's rules and functioning, they are assumed to be central; conflicts in other parts of the system are often displaced from an unrecognized or hidden problem in the couple. Conflict may be over *practical problems* ("instrumental"), such as money, roles, school and work difficulties, problems of *physiological control* (enuresis, encopresis); or problems of an admitted *emotional nature* ("affective"), such as marital conflict, sexual dysfunction, behavioral problems, and difficulty with the expression of negative or positive emotions. Instrumental and affective problems often co-exist; however, when only one area is a problem, its correction is less difficult.[10] During the stage of problem identification, attention is paid to the question of who identifies an issue as a problem. Is there consensus on the part of the other members or disagreement? Is there evidence of displacement? Is it an individual or a family problem? Has the time of onset been recent or has the problem been present for a long period? Is this the only problem? Often a child is labelled as *the* problem, but questioning about the existence of difficulties in other members may elicit a long list.

Similar to questions concerning physical symptoms, such as pain, the following questions may help make the diagnosis: Who is the identified patient in the family? (analogous to: Where is the pain?); Does the problem affect anyone else in the family directly or indirectly?; Are there any other problems? (Does the pain occur anywhere else in the body or radiate elsewhere?); When did the problem start *exactly*? (When and how did the pain start?); Under what circumstances? Has there been a new arrival in the family, death or illness elsewhere in the family?; What made the problem better or worse? For example, a son's conflict with a mother always became better when the father was away. What solutions have the family tried? (What medications have been tried with what results?) Family solutions (such as skin creams, or laxatives for appendicitis), often make the problem worse. Is the problem simply a normal aspect of living with others? Can the family understand it and solve it alone without exaggerating it into a real problem? (If the symptom is not serious, (eg., hyperventilation), does the patient understand it well enough to prevent recurrence?). Will the family agree to look more closely at the problem through family therapy if the problem is serious and this is required, or is it asking only for symptomatic treatment? (If drastic measures like surgery or long-term medication are needed to stop the pain, will the patient comply?) Does the family understand the treatment and its side effects? Family therapy is successful in two out of three cases[11,31] but may be painful (like surgery) as well as productive of growth for individuals *and* family; Is the therapy available locally, or must the family go elsewhere? A family with an anorectic child may request and be able to afford a visit to Minuchin or a local expert on "psychosomatic families." A rural family may have no one but the district nurse or family physician to turn to. Such a clinician may have to attempt therapy despite inadequate training, or become better trained. Death from anorexia or alcoholism may occur where there are no facilities.

The patient's refusing treatment allows the disease to take its natural course: the patient may recover, become chronically ill, or die; families are often able to recover from even serious dysfunction, they may choose to live unhappily or with continuing secondary physical illness, or they may dissolve through divorce, estrangement of children, or death of a family member. Patients may effectively refuse treatment by doctor shopping. Similarly, for some families therapy is a way of life: each member may have his or her own therapist or several therapists. Like the dissatisfied individual patient who shops around, such families may be turning away from professionals who have failed to reach a correct diagnosis and are treating a symptom rather than the family distress that gives rise to it. Professionals may be failing to communicate or hold opposing opinions on treatment. The family physician may recommend family therapy while the school doctor or nurse has referred the child to psychiatry.

Sometimes more than one interview is required to clarify the issues. However, in using PRACTICE with the average family the clinician should be able to obtain a maximum of information in the first interview. After the interview, the clinician should be able to grasp the problem and decide with the family on the type of intervention (education, anticipatory guidance, support, facilitation, or referral). An important dimension of assessment is knowing when and where to refer a family for therapy; however, families who are in serious need of change and need family therapy by experts for the survival and sanity of their members are a relatively small percentage of the average practice.

If a family is able to use the information obtained from the family assessment to change itself, it is not in need of therapy. The benefit of the diagnostic impression given to the family by the health professional is that the family is given a broader perspective from outside the system and is able to relabel problems in a constructive way. For example, a twenty-year-old woman's noncompliance with asthma medication might be restated as a mistaken way of telling her mother she needed more age-appropriate autonomy. The mother's overcontrol of her dating and higher education may be described as the natural maternal response to that last child leaving home, particularly when father is away all the time and yet does not want her to work. In the presence of the father, the suggestion that his workaholism might be related to the wife's refusal to do things alone with him, will make this restatement of the situation more effective. If the health professional correctly understands the role of the presenting problem in family dysfunction and is able to communicate his or her understanding to the family, the family may be able to initiate changes in the behavior leading to the symptom. The clinician must speak tactfully, indicating ideas as impressions rather than facts; diagnostic error is always possible. Error is less likely if the professional has successfully empathized and joined with all family members and is not covertly or unconsciously protecting a "victim." Such a stance would betray nonsystemic thinking and hence an incomplete family diagnosis.

R—ROLES

Accurate perception of the de facto roles, structure, and organization of a family is a difficult and challenging part of assessment, but the effort expended frequently provides a clue to the role of illness. If, for example, the husband is controlling and dominant and forbids the wife to work outside the home, the wife may express loneliness, boredom, and tension by developing an illness. This unconscious solution on the wife's part effectively corrects the lack of companionship and the balance of power since the sick, "weak" family member can control the attention and activities of family members through illness. The "sick role" is of obvious importance to the clinician (see Chapter 20).

Clear hierarchical organization is necessary for the healthy functioning of any system (see Chapters 1 and 2). The locus of power in a family is determined by who makes the important decisions, which is often a function of who controls the family's income. Power may be indicated by the greater talkativeness of one spouse, or by a spouse's ability to have the last word or to undermine the other spouse's decisions by nonverbal means. Democratic, flexible decision-making by both spouses who have an approximately equal say in major decisions, and who have clearly allocated responsibility for the minor ones, appears to work best in North American culture.

If the most powerful member of the family is not present during the interview, the assessment of the power structure will not only be incorrect, but management decisions made with the clinician may not be carried out or may be undermined: if the grandmother has the final say in family matters but was left out of the interview because she lives next door or in the apartment upstairs, a sick member's compliance with prescribed medication or diet may be very poor. The grandmother may even persuade the family to use the herbalist across the street instead. It should, therefore, be ensured that all effective members of the family system are present if a family interview is indicated, even if this results in a rather crowded office.

Roles cause no problem if they are clear and accepted by all members of a family. If the family defines roles in such a way that conflicts exist with the surrounding social structure, as is the case in many immigrant families, problems result. Roles can be divided into two categories: instrumental and affective. Who does the breadwinning or the dishwashing are instrumental role assignments; whom the child runs to when hurt and whom the mother turns to for comfort when depressed indicate affective roles.

Role allocation and role accountability may be decided implicitly or explicitly by dictum or open discussion. Role satisfaction results when male and female role expectations match the actual roles, and correlates highly with marital outcome.[5] When role expectations change too quickly for adaptation to occur, as is happening in Western culture as a result of the women's liberation movement, or when an individual family moves from one culture to another with very different expectations, role strain and role conflict may result.

Effective behavioral control can only be expected when rules are clear, rewards and punishments are consistent, and parents are in basic agreement. Parents whose own parents were poor role models or who are in covert conflict with one another may exert no effective control; the result is chaos. Poor discipline that allows children to play with equipment in the doctor's office, to interrupt, or to leave the room are obvious clues. At the other extreme, one or both parents may be intolerant of normal childhood exuberance, and their rigid control will be revealed by the timidity or immobility of the family's children or by their covert or overt rebellion. Anorexia nervosa, enuresis, misbehavior or failure in school, or poor compliance with prescribed medication regimens may all be responses to such tight control. Such families may exhibit little tolerance when efforts towards individuation become manifest as the children reach adolescence.

The healthiest pattern, at least for North American families, is clear parental authority that allows increasing flexibility and age-appropriate autonomy as the children mature. Gordon[10] has labelled the three styles of parenting as authoritarian (parent wins), permissive (child wins), and negotiatory ("no win, no loss"). During a child's adolescence, the authoritarian style promotes rebellion, or timidity and repressed anger (the child may hate the parent), the permissive style produces obnoxious, "spoiled" children (the parent may end up hating the child), and the negotiatory style allows a slow, progressive increase in freedom *and* responsibility.

The degree of individual autonomy allowed in a family is a useful measure of health. Families at the two extremes of cohesion (enmeshment and disengagement) are those most subject to pathology. A balance of autonomy and mutuality, deficient in enmeshed and disengaged families, respectively, is essential for individuation, the development of identity, self-esteem, maturity and health. Enmeshed families have blurred boundaries and are overinvolved with and overprotective of one another. Stress to one member reverberates through the system because every member is excessively responsive to every other. Roles tend to be confused; there is a lack of autonomy and independence:

> In one family with five children, the mother had bulimia, anorexia, and colitis. All family members took turns accompanying her to the bathroom because of diarrhea and vomiting. The 9-year-old girl with enuresis was advised and taunted by the other members of the family, who knew all the details of her doctor's visits and looked in her dresser to see her chart of dry and wet nights. The mother accompanied even older adolescents on their visits to the doctor, and all family members read each other's diaries and listened to telephone conversations.

In such an enmeshed family, triangulation is a common occurrence and conflict is never resolved between two individuals without a third becoming involved. There is an emphasis on love and affection but true intimacy and honesty are absent since conflict tends to be avoided or detoured through another member. In contrast, disengaged families lack a sense of belonging and a capacity for interdependence. Boundaries are rigid and individual members have maximum autonomy but provide little support for each other when in difficulty. There is tolerance for a wide variation in behavior and stress has little effect on the family as a whole. There may be no response even when one is needed (as in the case of a delinquent child whose behavior was largely ignored by the parents until the police intervened). The children become adults with little ability to form satisfactory relationships.

Family structure can be illustrated graphically in one of two ways: by the family tree (genogram) particularly as developed by Bowen (see Chapter 11); or by family mapping.[20] Elaborate symbols can be used in the genogram to indicate triangulation, and close and conflictual relationships; or marginal notations regarding the character of individuals and the nature of their relationships can be made on the regular genogram. Boundary lines (around members of a household) and double or dotted lines (for close and conflictual or distant relationships respectively) can be added where important. The advantage of obtaining a detailed family tree has already been described (see Chapter 11).

Family roles can be diagrammed using Minuchin's method of "mapping" the family. This technique gives added information about the family hierarchy in the current family, but says nothing about the family of origin. It has the advantage of indicating the power structure and relationships by a special arrangement of symbols. In a map of the family,[20] the letters M, F, G, C, and PC represent Mother, Father, Grandparent, Child, and Parentified Child, respectively. The symbol for the strongest member of the family is put at the top of the diagram.

For example, a family with a frequently absent father, a mother, and "parentified" child and two other children would be diagrammed as follows:

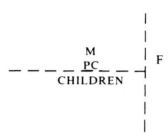

The same family, if reorganized into more satisfying relationships would be represented by:

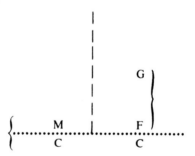

A family with a dominant grandmother, a weak parental subsystem, a coalition between the father and his mother, and between the mother and her child would be represented by:

Symbols used include the following:

Boundaries: _ _ _ _ _ _   ....   ————————————
                clear   diffuse   rigid, closed

Affiliation: ————————   Overinvolvement: ════════════

Conflict: —||—   Coalition: }   Detouring: ⇊

The "scapegoated" or "triangled" child with conflict avoidance in parents can be diagrammed as:

M —||— F
  \ /
   C

Diagrams can indicate change following illness, as in:

```
    F                                              M
 _ _M_ _ _      ———— Father's ————▶      _ _ _F_ _ _
    C            myocardial infarction            C
```

```
                     _ _ _G_ _ _
          or              F
                     _ _ _M_ _ _
                          C
```

A—AFFECT (EMOTIONAL EXPRESSION)

Healthy families are capable of expressing a wide range of emotions, both positive and negative. If one emotion not only predominates but is used even when another would be more appropriate, the family may be in considerable difficulty. Individual members of a family may differ in their individual abilities to express both positive and negative emotions as appropriate. The presence of emotion in a family member, whether overt or covert, and also to whom it is directed should be noted. One member may be assigned the role of expressing anger or sadness for everyone, relieving the others of the need to express this emotion by giving a clue to how they may feel underneath. If one person is crying or very angry it is useful to enquire if others are feeling the same way. Children, particularly, frequently express the feelings of a parent, often the one of the same sex. An argument or fight between children often parallels a parental conflict.

Awareness of the characteristic emotional tone and observation of the family's ability to change this tone when challenged is important in family assessment. The family that can show a wide range of affect in one interview usually has a good prognosis for coping with stress.

Culture has a vast influence over the acceptability of different emotions or of their open expression; the tone of the interviewer, as well as his or her cultural or social class and language origin, influences the family. If the interviewer has difficulty recognizing or accepting emotions like anger, depression, or physical demonstrations of affection, the family will behave in a restrained manner for the sake of the professional.

Assessment should not imply value judgment. Family atmospheres vary widely in families who function well. Openness of expression may be overvalued by family professionals in North America. To impose the values of the family therapy movement or to be judgmental can be presumptuous, invasive of other persons' values, and unethical; however, to assess a family and predict coping ability is not to judge them. Empathy with the family precludes judgmental approaches; unconditioned regard for the family safeguards the principle that the clinician must not do any harm. A clinician's persistent dislike of one or more family members should suggest to him or her that transferring the family to another professional would be best. The systems approach facilitates empathy for all members of a family and decreases the likelihood of such dislike.

Empathy with the family can itself facilitate expression of emotion. Even a single interview can be helpful, especially at a time of crisis such as the terminal illness of a family member. Expression of repressed emotions, with the encouragement of a trusted professional, can result in a permanent change in the closeness and communication of that family. So often a clinician, afraid of releasing anger or sadness, ignores clues (tears in the eyes or a break in the voice) indicating stress that can be transformed by a brief comment into much needed emotional release.

C—COMMUNICATION

Communication is so important an aspect of functioning that many therapists[24] base assessment and treatment on this area almost exclusively. As in any system, health depends on both effective communication and effective hierarchical control (see Chapter 2).

Communication is the process by which people convey messages to each other. Expression of emotion and effective social communication are linked, but clarity of communication implies the transfer of information in a form that results in the correct message being received. Messages may be verbal or nonverbal and are usually a mixture of both in direct face to face contact. All families have their own patterns or methods of communicating. In family therapy, communication is described as being "direct" or "displaced" and "clear" or "masked." Four different ways in which a husband may communicate anger to his wife can be seen in the following examples:[12]

Clear and Direct:	"I am angry at you!" (said to the wife)
Masked and Direct:	"I don't like the way you comb your hair!" (said to the wife)
Clear and Displaced:	"I am angry at you!" (said to the daughter, when the husband is feeling angry at his wife)
Masked and Displaced:	"Women are so lazy!" (said to the daughter, when the husband is feeling angry at his wife)

A clinician can encourage direct communication *to* other members rather than *about* other members: ("Your father's here, why not say it to him, not me.") Mind-reading or speaking for another person can be discouraged. Family members can be encouraged to use "I-messages" instead of "you-messages";[11] for example, a woman might say to her husband, "when you come home late I feel lonely and depressed" instead of "you always come home late; you're so inconsiderate." The former states feelings and conveys an important message; the latter is accusatory and elicits similarly accusatory responses.

Families communicate in a variety of ways, and each family does so in a way that is very particular and identifiable as part of its personality. Knowing how a family communicates is an essential part of understanding how a family is organized. Even though words are the most obvious means of making a statement or expressing oneself, nonverbal messages (a sigh, a shrug, a side-ways glance) can be just as effective and perhaps more convincing. Bateson[4] has written about "meta-messages," messages about the message and about the state of the relationship. In the healthy family these meta-communications, which are usually unconscious and nonverbal, do not contradict the verbal messages. Satir[25] has described nonverbal communication as a right brain function reflective of current emotional content and the actual status of the relationship; verbal communication, a left brain function, is considered to be a factual reference to the past or future.

Family communication is complex. "What did you do today?" can be an interested enquiry, a statement of affection, a routine meaningless greeting, or an accusation depending on which word is emphasized. The message will be altered by various nonverbal communications such as facial expression, tone of voice, distance of the questionner, and physical stance. Satir[25] has described the four most common positions in dysfunctional relationships (blaming, placating, super-reasonable, and irrelevant), which can be represented by physical positions such as the accusatory stance with a pointing finger.

Family rules control communication and meaning, particularly as to what constitutes "value messages" and "devalue messages." Strayhorn[29] describes how newlyweds must discover the meaning of each others' value messages. For example, help offered by a husband in cooking meals is, for him, a sign of caring and wanting to share in the household; the wife from a very traditional family perceives the offer as the implication she is a poor cook. A wife interprets her husband's long work hours as a sign of lack of love and her own complaining as a sign of her love and need for him; the husband sees his hard work as a major sign of his commitment to his family's support and her nagging as lack of caring and appreciation. In one family, everyone is always late and no one worries about it; in contrast, the in-laws are always on time unless angry with one another. Such "non-correspondent rules" must be clarified.

Channels for value messages can be positive (helpfulness, physical contact, tidyness, time spent together, sexuality) or negative and painful. Negative channels include jealousy and possessive love, overfeeding and overeating to please each other, fighting for the sake of eventually making up, or the use of alcohol, which may increase closeness and physical contact.[28] Very destructive or "toxic" channels such as suicide threats to elicit messages of caring may be used if no other channels are open. Sickness may be a very often used channel in families who find it easy to care for the sick but otherwise cannot show affection. Getting fat may mean keeping oneself unattractive to others of the opposite sex (one study showed that marital problems followed intestinal bypass operations for obesity[18]). Cigarette smoking may be so tied up with an exchange of value messages that it is difficult to stop without helping patients become aware of the unconscious messages and linking them to a different behavior.[8,19,30] Development of positive channels must occur before one attempts to eliminate negative ones.[29]

The communication process is, without question, complex. One cannot hope to modify a family's response without first understanding its pattern of communication. Since physical symptoms have often been considered a mode of communication both to other family members and to the clinician,[1] their part in communication must be understood.

T—TIME IN LIFE CYCLE OF FAMILY

The particular time of the family life cycle may determine both occurrence of illness and the response to it. (Details of the stages of the life cycle and the family developmental tasks associated with each stage are discussed in Chapter 6.) Satisfactory completion of these tasks meets the needs of the family members and promotes the continued growth and development of the family unit.[8] No two families are alike, and "each experiences its own dynamics of formation, growth and dissolution."[7] At each developmental stage families go through normal transitions such as marriage, birth, adolescence, menopause, and retirement, but may also experience unexpected or tragic family life events.

Difficulty in coping with family transitions may lead to a visit to the family physician. For example, the birth of the first child in a family will require, at the very least, adjustment of roles and autonomy of the parents, learning child-care skills, and change from dyadic to tryadic interaction. Some families adapt with ease; others may lack the skills to cope with the change. A young mother under the stress of change may present with headache and fatigue or may focus on her child's symptoms of colic, constipation, or cold. Awareness of developmental stress in the family life cycle alerts the clinician to probe beyond this presenting symptom.

There are periods in the life cycle when visits to the doctor's office are frequent, partly because these are prescribed (immunization in infancy, premarital check-ups), partly because stress is generated by a family transition. Illness-prone families have a higher incidence of conflict and stress[15]; there are also illness-prone periods during the family life cycle. At the end of life we all become illness-prone, but the time at which this occurs is partly dependent on the stage in family life (widows and widowers are more illness-prone than married people of the same age) and on successful handling of previous challenges such as retirement and departure of children. The active octogenarian who leads a full life may do so despite arthritis or heart disease, or may remain free of illness because of an active, full life. The lonely pensioner with no interest in life is more likely to succumb to disease and disability.

Some authors[14] believe that the way families cope with each stage of the life cycle is the major factor in the development of illness. Illness reflects failure at a given developmental stage. It can also reflect stress or represent a solution to or an avoidance of a task: a mother overwhelmed with child-care responsibilities may lift her child in such a way as to slip a disc and force her reluctant husband into helping out with domestic tasks. Negotiation of tasks can be replaced by using sickness to change roles. A widow may threaten to have a heart attack if an adult daughter leaves home to get married, thus using illness to avoid the task of facing life alone and developing resources outside the family. Assessment of life cycle stage and apparent success with completion of previous stages is a key part of family assessment.

I—ILLNESS

To the health care provider the role that illness plays in the family is a crucial part of the family evaluation. The meaning of illness to a family will depend on many factors:

Family History of Illness.   The history of illness in the family of origin and in the present nuclear family is a major determinant of family reactions. Frequent acute illness or chronic illness in the past will have an impact on the interpretation of new symptoms. It is possible that the expectation that illness will occur at a given time of life, in certain individuals in the family or in a given organ system, will sometimes lead to such an illness. Such expectations and concern (for a particular part of the body) may play a role in the apparent genetic transmission of some diseases, or in a family organ vulnerability such as peptic ulcers or atherosclerotic heart disease. However, as Huygen[16] has pointed out, family patterns of disease often follow genetic tissue type (for example, families whose various secretory organs of dermal origin are predominantly affected). Interpretation of symptoms will be highly dependent on family experience. To a family with a strong family history of arthritis, an aching leg may be cause for great concern. Experience with health care providers in the past will color a family's expectations in the present. When suspicion or pessimism about the efficacy of drugs or doctors are passed through several generations, almost no effort on the part of the health care providers can reverse the belief. Indeed, such families' expectations and behavior usually lead to self-fulfilling prophecies by antagonizing medical staff. Discussion of the past and expression of empathy may help; hostility reinforces the family's beliefs.

Culture. The family diagnosis and the acceptance of illness or ill health are in part culturally determined: a patient from northern Europe, seeing illness as weakness may be highly stoical when compared to a patient from Greece. Denial may result and serious symptoms may be ignored. The Japanese individual is taught greater body awareness from early childhood and to the Western doctor may appear hypochondriacal.

Tertiary Gain (family need for a sick member).[6] The concept of secondary gain in the context of the family changes to a concept of maintenance of family homeostasis in which all family members are involved; this is called "tertiary gain." The mother who uses illness to induce guilt in children and to manipulate her husband is matched by a husband who accepts her dominance to excuse his alcoholism or absences from work. The child who focuses attention on himself or herself through frequent asthmatic attacks may also be protecting the parents from conflict. Madanes[17] has explored the role of illness in marriage when the sick role may maintain the balance of power. The question must be asked, Is it an advantage in this family to be sick? A question that is of enormous value in eliciting the role of recurrent sickness in a relationship or in a family is as follows: "If by some miracle you were to become completely better now, what would you do, or what would happen differently in the family that is not possible with your sickness?"

> In the M. family in which the wife had incapacitating back pain for 2 years, both spouses were asked this question in separate interviews. Mrs. M.'s answer was: "Oh, I guess I'd leave my husband." She had tried to leave him twice before but on each occasion he had threatened a heart attack. This helped Mrs. M. avoid facing her need for him and maintained the couple's belief that she was independent and could manage emotionally without him. The relationship was charac-

terized by conflict; Mrs. M. was clearly boss of her ineffectual husband. When Mr. M. was asked the same question he said, "If she weren't sick she'd be back in control. This way I can keep the students out of the house, at least to some extent." The students of his wife, an artist, had clearly been having affairs with her in the past. The role of sickness in this family is dealt with in more detail in Chapter 20.

Sick-role assignment may occur in families with a vulnerable member: in one family, a child with a clubfoot became the family member who developed anorexia nervosa.[21] Family resemblances or even names may become the basis for expected behavior or illness, for example, a family in whom every member called Charles eventually became alcoholic. A family member may be inappropriately labelled as sick: Remen[23] gives an example of a woman in whom the whole family insisted on a diagnosis of angina. If the patient is cured another may take his place, indicating the need for sickness in such a family.

The Role of the Sick Member.   Serious illness obviously has an impact on every family member. This may be because of the threatened loss of the sick member, or of his or her roles in the family; the loss of the important nurturing role of the mother has serious consequences. In most families more family disruption and subsequent illness or stress in other members occurs when the mother is seriously ill than when the father is ill. If there is complete financial dependence on the father, the only possible breadwinner, the converse may be true. An only child may produce overprotective concern for minor symptoms. A child born after the death of a sibling may have a special replacement role for his parents, and may be a "vulnerable child" as a result.

Recurrent Crises.   Recent or remote family deaths, particularly if inadequately mourned, are a very major cause of subsequent pathology (see Chapter 21). Particularly if other crises occurred in the same period, a family may never regain its original functional level,[26] and the "ripple effect" of serious illness, mental breakdown, or other deaths in family members may follow.

C—COPING WITH STRESS

Adaptability is perhaps the most important characteristic of a family; with cohesion, it forms Olson's circumplex model of family function.[22] A focus on family strength and coping is both therapeutic and necessary to mobilize family resources to deal with a given problem. The family's history of coping with past stresses is a useful predictor of future coping. The history of illness, of stresses such as accidents, deaths, change of job or environment, and cultural change in both the nuclear family and families of origin should be elicited. General questions ("Has your family had a lot of stresses in the recent past?" "Have you had to deal with this sort of thing before?" "How did you cope when that happened?") quickly give a picture of past stress and the response to it. If the family has been previously well and cannot recall a serious problem, then past coping cannot be assessed. However, such a family is likely to adapt well if it has maintained such a problem-free life style in the past. The occasional rigid or brittle, but previously lucky, family may succumb to the current stress as a result of the family system's poor adaptability. In contrast, illness-prone families may go from crisis to crisis and still hold together despite or because of the crises.

Information about past examples of a family's ability to cope may serve as a warning signal to the professional; as in the following examples: the son of a woman with cancer had developed ulcerative colitis after his father's death; although the son was less close to his mother, he was at risk for serious illness since her death would remind him of the earlier death of his father. In another family, injury to a daughter resulted in mutual recrimination between the parents. This couple reacted with anger at each other whenever a health crisis occurred, making the marriage vulnerable in case of serious illness, particularly of a child.

E—ECOLOGY OR ENVIRONMENT

Ecology, for the purpose of family assessment, is the study of the interaction of families with their environment and of the available environmental resources. The environment includes all the other systems that influence, or are influenced by the family system: the extended family, friends, school, employment, government agencies, religious and other community organizations, and the subculture and culture to which the family belongs.

The interaction of spouses with their families of origin has been observed to affect the incidence of problems and symptoms in the family. Emotional distance or closeness is deemed to be the important variable and is unrelated to a family's living in close proximity or far away.

Relationships outside the immediate family may compensate for inadequate family relationships and thus help the family to adapt in times of transition: if a pregnant woman is not having her increased psychological needs met by family members, it is important to find out if these needs are being met by the family of origin or by friends. A family with loose ties in which members tend to ignore family relationships may use community resources to carry out functions that could be done by the family system. This may be of immediate benefit but may also lead to overdependence on community resources.[13]

A closely knit family system may not allow members enough freedom to develop relationships in the community; in such a family, if the breadwinner is also the dominant member and becomes incapacitated, the other members of the family might be unable to reshuffle roles or obtain help from the environment. This can lead to breakdown of the system.

Smilkstein's acronym SCREEM[26] (see Chapter 13) is useful as a reminder of the important environmental resources of a family: Social, Cultural, Religious, Educational, Economic, and Medical.

PRACTICE

McGill Family Assessment Form

Family (or household) members present in interview. Names and ages.

Missing members. Names and ages.

Presenting problem(s) or reason for family interview. (Description, identified by whom? Onset, attempted solutions by family.)

Roles—structure, organization. (Who is dominant, nature of parental coalition, characteristics of boundaries, role flexibility. If possible, draw family map.)

Affect. (Predominant emotional tone, range of affect in this interview, difficulty in expressing emotion.)

Communication. (Clear, direct, masked, displaced, congruent. Who talks? Who listens to whom? Nonverbal communication.)

Time in life cycle of family. (Courtship, family in formation, child bearing, child rearing, child launching, contracting family, retirement, widow(er)-hood.)

Illness. (History or presence of serious illness, chronic or frequent acute illness. Sickness role—who tends to be sick in this family. Recent deaths.)

Coping. (Adaptability. Family strengths and resources. Coping in *past* and *present*.)

Ecology. (Relationship with families of origin. Financial status. Use of community, school, professional resources. Recreation.)

Overall rating
Does this family express the need for help?
            □ YES   □ NO   □ DON'T KNOW
Do you believe this family is in need for help?
            □ YES   □ NO   □ DON'T KNOW
In what specific areas?

Can you handle the problem?
□ on your own   □ with supervision   □ not at all
Should this family or any member be referred for:
□ family therapy   □ couple therapy   □ individual therapy
If individual, which one?

To whom?

Do you believe this family can change?

         ☐ YES   ☐ NO   ☐ DON'T KNOW

Does this family believe it should change?

         ☐ YES   ☐ NO   ☐ DON'T KNOW

Does this family believe it can change?

         ☐ YES   ☐ NO   ☐ DON'T KNOW

What is your evidence for this opinion?

REFERENCES

1. Balint M: *The Doctor, His Patient, and the Illness.* New York, International Universities Press, 1972.

2. Barnhill LR: Healthy family systems. *Fam Coordinator* 28:94, 1979.

3. Barrows HS, Tamblyn R: *Problem-Based Learning: An Approach to Medical Education.* New York, Springer Publishing Company, 1980.

4. Bateson G: *Steps to an Ecology of Mind.* New York, Ballantine Books, 1972.

5. Cronkite RE: The determinants of spouses' normative preference for family roles. *J Marr Fam* 39:575, 1977.

6. Dansak DA: On the tertiary gain of illness. *Comp Psychiatry* 14:523, 1973.

7. David HP: Healthy family functioning: A cross-cultural appraisal. *WHO Bulletin* 56:327, 1978.

8. Duvall EM: *Marriage and Family Development.* Philadelphia, J.B. Lippincott, 1977.

9. Eckert P: Beyond the statistics of adolescent smoking. *Am J Public Health* 73:4, 1983.

10. Epstein NB, Bishop DS, Levin S: The McMaster model of family functioning. *J Marr Fam Counseling* 4:19, 1978.

11. Gordon T: *P.E.T. Parent Effectiveness Training.* New York, North American Library, 1975.

12. Guttman HA: A guide to family function and structure. Unpublished manuscript, October, 1977.

13. Helvie CO: A proposed theory for nursing in community health. Part 1. The individual. *Can J Public Health* 70:41, 1979.

14. Haley J: *Uncommon Therapy. The Psychiatric Techniques of Milton H. Erickson.* New York, Norton, 1973.

15. Hinkle LE Jr, Plummer N: Life stress and industrial absenteeism: The concentration of illness and absenteeism in one segment of a working population. *Ind Med Surg* 21:363, 1952.

16. Huygen FJA: *Family Medicine. The Medical Life Histories of Families.* Holland, Dekker & Van de Vegt, 1978.

17. Madanes C: Marital therapy when a symptom is presented by a spouse. *Int J Fam Therapy* 2:120, 1980.
18. Marshall JR, Neill J: The removal of a psychosomatic symptom: Effects on the marriage. *Fam Process* 16:273, 1977.
19. McAlister A, Perry C, Maccoby N: Adolescent smoking and prevention. *Pediatrics* 63, 1979.
20. Minuchin S: *Families and Family Therapy.* Cambridge, Harvard University Press, 1974.
21. Minuchin S: Anorexia is a Greek Word (videotape). Philadelphia Child Guidance Clinic, Philadelphia, Pennsylvania.
22. Olson D, Sprenkle DH, Russell C: Circumplex model of marital and family systems. I. Cohesion and adaptability dimensions, family types and clinical applications. *Fam Process* 18:3, 1979.
23. Remen N: *The Human Patient.* New York, Anchor Press, 1980.
24. Satir V: *Conjoint Family Therapy.* Palo Alto, California, Science & Behavior Books, 1967.
25. Satir V: *Peoplemaking.* Palo Alto, California, Science & Behavior Books, 1972.
26. Smilkstein G: The family in trouble, how to tell. *J Fam Pract* 2:19, 1975.
27. Spitzer WO, Dobson AJ, Hall J, et al: Measuring the quality of life of cancer patients. A concise QL-index for use by physicians. *J Chron Dis* 34:585, 1981.
28. Steinglass P, Davis DI, Berenson D: Observations of conjointly hospitalized "alcoholic couples" during sobriety and intoxication: Implications for theory and therapy. *Fam Process* 16:1, 1977.
29. Strayhorn JM Jr: Social-exchange theory: Cognitive restructuring in marital therapy. *Fam Process* 17:437, 1978.
30. Tremblay J, Bibeau G: Les mécanismes d'initiation au tabac chez les jeunes du Québec. Une approche socio-culturelle. *Psychotrope* 1:1, 1983.
31. Watzlawick P, Weakland JH, Fisch JR: *Change: Principles of Problem Formation and Problem Resolution.* New York, Norton, 1974.

Chapter 15

Application of Family Assessment to Health Care Management and the Specific Skills of Working with Families

Yves Talbot
Janet Christie-Seely
Yvonne Steinert

The goal of family assessment in primary care is improved management of health problems. The assessment may point to a dysfunctional family pattern that is related to frequent stress-related minor illness; it may give clues to poor compliance; it may assist in clarifying a family's lifestyle that leads to disease; or it may identify the person whose cooperation is needed to change that lifestyle or whose health belief interferes with treatment. The acronym PRACTICE covers most areas of family functioning. However, for a given clinical management problem only one, two, or three of these areas may be relevant. Just as the clinician is aware of the full range of questions available for a functional inquiry, so he or she should be aware of the full range of a functional inquiry about a family. To use every question in the repertoire of inquiry into each of the body's many organ systems is characteristic only of the beginning medical student; such an approach would be hopelessly inefficient for the practicing clinician. Similarly, when first trying to understand family functioning, familiarity with all parts of PRACTICE must be developed. With further practice in family assessment and experience with family health problems, selecting the few appropriate areas necessary to manage a given problem will become second nature.

Hypothesis Generation

Familiarity with all aspects of family functioning and illness will, like familiarity with bodily function, enable the clinician to form hypotheses to direct questioning and observation. Teaching in medical school implies a mode of data collection that passes systematically from history of present illness through functional inquiry and physical examination to the generation of a differential diagnostic list based on all these data. However, this is not how physicians actually function. Studies have shown that the good clinician demonstrates an extremely efficient method of gathering data, labelled by Elstein[3] and Barrows[1] as the "clinical reasoning process." On contact with a patient, and often before contact, clues about the reason for the patient's visit, or the diagnosis, have generated a list of hypotheses ranked in order of probability in the clinician's mind. He or she has five to seven hypotheses ranked in order, and by 10 minutes after the onset of the interview, almost all relevant information has been obtained. If the interview continues it is because emergency treatment is not considered necessary immediately, and because the patient needs reassurance or information, or because negotiation is required for treatment.

Similarly, the family-oriented clinician generates hypotheses from experience with family function to explain problems in management, as in the following example:

An asthmatic 16-year-old boy, whose illness had been well controlled previously, is brought in by his mother because of an exacerbation of symptoms in the last 2 months. The mother speaks for her son, and is obviously in charge of all medication, prompting the hypothesis that age-appropriate autonomy is not occurring in this family. She may be having difficulties with the impending departure of her son, who is her last child; she has no outside interests or career, and the physician knows that her husband is frequently away on business.

However, the abrupt change 2 months ago should also prompt the question as to any recent changes, losses, or moves in the family. The death 3 months ago of the grandfather and a subsequent move into the house by the maternal grandmother suggests a change in family homeostasis. Hypotheses might then include rebellion by the boy against the authority of the grandmother, and hostility at losing his room to the grandmother, who displaced him to a smaller one; or, on the contrary, an alliance with the grandmother that allowed the boy for the first time to rebel against his over-protective authoritarian mother. Given that someone in the family had died, and that this family had a known tendency to avoid emotional expression, another hypothesis might be the displacement of the grieving process and the boy's acting out of family tension. These hypotheses directed the line of questioning and observation in the subsequent family interview.

Both an alliance between grandmother and grandson and repressed grieving proved to be the changes associated with the boy's poor compliance with asthma medication. In an interview with the family it was clear that the grandmother had a close relationship with the boy and covertly supported him when her daughter attempted discipline or control. No one had discussed the death or expressed the feelings associated with it. Two management strategies restored compliance. First, family sharing of sadness over the death was facilitated. Second, discussion of the grandmother's task of re-establishing ties with friends and outside activities relieved tension caused by both the death and the addition of a new household member. The grandmother's activity also encouraged the mother to begin to look for friends and experience outside the family and allowed the clinician to transfer control of medication to the patient after sufficient information about the disease was conveyed. Thus, the aspects of PRACTICE that were relevant to this family were family roles and structure (alliances), affect (repressed grief) and the time in the family life cycle (impending loss of the son). Not only was compliance with asthma medication restored, but possible sequelae of distorted grief and a disturbed family system were prevented by two sessions with the family.

A CONCEPTUAL FRAMEWORK

Like the medical student who may be overwhelmed by the amount of medical data that can be obtained from a patient, the clinician learning about family systems tends to be overwhelmed by data coming from many sources. The structure to organize these data provided by PRACTICE, and experience with families over time gradually increases the efficiency of generating hypotheses; a good clinician will have an idea of what is happening in a family with a health problem within the first 10 minutes of seeing the family.[3] Until such proficiency is achieved, the clinician can take comfort in the fact that families repeat their patterns of normal functioning every 5 to 10 minutes and their patterns of illness behavior over time, so that the clinician has plenty of time to develop an understanding of family dynamics. Some specific questions are helpful in eliciting the systems (tertiary) gain (see Chapter 20 on acute illness) of a given symptom, illness, or behavior (Table 15.1).

Table 15.1 **Questions to Elicit the Systems Gain (Tertiary Gain) from a Symptom**

---

1. What would be different for you and your family if your symptom/illness were miraculously cured?

2. In what way is a family member who complains of a symptom or behavior encouraging or facilitating the problem? What is the family "solution" to a problem that is keeping it going?

3. What were the family problems before a symptom developed that improved with the onset of the symptom? *or* What difficulties are present when the patient is well that disappear when he or she is sick (for example, poor marital communication in the "dry state" in alcoholism, compared with the increased physical contact and verbal communication during the "wet state")? Precipitating factors at the onset of illness, or in the exacerbation of a problem, often give a clue to its role in the system.

Source: Compiled by the authors.

THE GOAL OF ASSESSMENT: IMPROVED HEALTH CARE MANAGEMENT

Interventions by the health professional revolve around health maintenance and the correct diagnosis and management of disease. Thus the primary care clinician must develop several skills in working with families that are quite distinct from those of the family therapist. These skills include information-giving, education, anticipatory guidance, facilitation of a family's coping skills in the face of crisis or illness, and referral skills when the need arises for consultation or therapy (Table 15.2). Interventions may occur during a home visit, an office visit, or in the hospital or emergency room. Sometimes they take time, as when a clinician must convey a serious diagnosis to the family. Sometimes a sentence or two, if well timed, can be more effective than a long session, particularly if it comes from a clinician who knows the family well.

Table 15.2 **The Skills of Working with a Family**

Joining (see Chapter 12)

Data Gathering (family assessment, see Chapters 13 and 14)
    Mode: individual interview (genogram, open-ended questions about family as routine); family interview (PRACTICE)
    Goal: improved health care management
    Outcome: diagnostic impression (family hypotheses or systems formulation)

Integration and Negotiation
    Feedback of diagnostic impression to family; relabelling individual problem as a family problem
    Negotiation and contracting

Management
    Education: information giving
    Anticipatory guidance: before normative crises of family life cycle; before hospitalization or death of family member (if time permits)
    Crisis intervention
    Facilitation:
      Normalization
      Positive relabelling
      Support of family strengths
      Clarification
    Specific suggestions
    Referral (awareness of limits): for family therapy; to other resources (individual therapy, community resources)

Source: Compiled by the authors.

INTEGRATION AND NEGOTIATION

Feedback of Diagnostic Impression (Systems Formulation)

Once the clinician has assessed the family, an important step is feedback of hypotheses to the family, which is analogous to conveying a diagnostic impression at an organ systems level; as with a physical diagnosis, the diagnosis should be couched as a possibility or probability rather than as a dogmatic assertion: "Uncle Joe may have allowed his diabetes to go out of control because he felt the family would visit him more often if he was in the hospital." Or, "Your husband may still be smoking after his heart attack because he and the family are having such a hard time changing their view of him. It is so important for everyone to see him as the strong one and the only breadwinner that he has to pretend everything is o.k." Both these statements leave the possibility of change open to the family.

Often the essential step is relabelling as a family problem what is perceived by the family as a problem of one member. The family's response to such relabelling is an important indication of the degree of family dysfunction and of prognosis. If they react with interest or some members respond with data that support the idea that there are problems at the family level, prognosis is good. For these families such clarification may trigger a quick recovery. One family assessment interview in which feedback is given may be sufficient for the healthy or morphogenetic family to change its rules of communication so that the symptom becomes unnecessary.

However, there is a class of families, whose members come frequently to the physician's office, that is characterized by rigidity and conflict avoidance, and prone to produce physical illness. These are the "psychosomatic families" described by Minuchin,[10] and the maneuvers to clarify a problem described above would do little to improve their situation; nevertheless, responding with a diagnostic impression is always worthwhile and is a necessary first step in referral. In one psychosomatic family the parents persisted in symptomatic behavior and refused referral, but the children were able to understand that their difficulty in leaving home was because of the physical illness and the submerged conflict of their parents. Having recognized the problem, the children were able to deal with it.

Psychosomatic families are particularly difficult to refer, and a successful attempt to relable the problem as a family problem is the first step to enable such a referral to take place. In the case of a serious or fatal disease in one family member that is related to dysfunction, there is the same obligation to persuade the family to have treatment as there is in the individual patient with a perforated appendix.

Negotiation and Contracting

Contracting with the individual patient or with the family is an important step that is often forgotten. Good communication and clarity are only possible when both clinician and patient clearly outline their goals for treatment, as well as their expectations of how long it will take and the likelihood of success. When a hidden agenda, the "second diagnosis" or psychosocial problem behind the presenting symptom, is not elicited, clinician frustration and patient dissatisfaction result.

The clinician should openly express his or her expectations concerning treatment: use of other professionals only if referral is through the primary care clinician, necessity of involvement of other family members, punctuality, and rules concerning telephone calls from individual family members. The expectations of family and patient must also be elicited. It is important to ask for goals: each member can be asked "What would you like to change in how things are at home?" If a family expects rapid or total cure of a long-standing symptom the clinician should express pessimism and underline the fact that it is the family who has the power to cure. The clinician should be clear on issues of availability and limits to time, and then maintain both promises and rules. Although the goal of therapy may change over time, there will be no progress if goals differ and negotiation is omitted, and no direction to therapy if there is no goal in mind.

INFORMATION GIVING AND PATIENT EDUCATION

Information giving and patient education is part of the day-to-day work of the family physician and of the primary care nurse. This is often much more effective when given to the whole family or to the couple. It is very important that these processes be clear and simple, and meet the needs of the family members involved. Important occasions for convening the family for this purpose include the following:

the diagnosis of a new illness (rheumatoid arthritis, cancer, hypertension)
the description of complex treatment regimes (diabetes or coeliac disease)
illness with a genetic component (lipid disorder, glaucoma, cystic fibrosis)
health maintenance information (exercise, diet, smoking, alcohol consumption, stress management)

The family physician is the primary person providing information to the family even when specialists are involved in the care.

The physician or nurse may have been taught that jargon should be avoided, but may inadvertently use terms very familiar to the profession and forget to check whether they are understood. When information is emotion-laden, as with a serious or fatal illness, the ability to hear and to understand are greatly decreased by anxiety. Since the diagnosis in itself can represent a shock to the family, it is usually advisable for the clinician to limit information to the bare minimum at the beginning. A later appointment can then be set with the family to provide more details and allow the members more time to think of questions. This strategy prevents the need to repeat information later, when they are less bewildered by the problem and more responsive to factual data.

When the unpleasant news is first conveyed the clinician must be more attentive to feelings. For example, he or she might say the following: "It must be very difficult for you to hear that Jane has cystic fibrosis. You will have many questions to ask me and I will be available to answer these questions. However, I think at the moment it is important for you to be alone together and I can answer all of the questions that you have later on this evening or tomorrow morning."

Nurses are often much better trained than physicians in eliciting the family's understanding of a diagnosis, of a treatment regime, or of suggestions about diet or lifestyle. It is very important to ask the patient or the family how they perceive what they have heard and for them to repeat the instructions to ensure they are understood. Compliance is markedly altered when patients understand the reasons for medication and the relationship of this medication to their symptoms and to the disease process. If their belief system about a disease is very different from the clinician's, his or her credibility may be suspect (for example, if a "hot medication" is prescribed to a Caribbean patient with a "hot disease"—see Chapter 5). The professional's perceived expertise and belief that the treatment has a chance of altering the disease process clearly influence compliance. The clinician's enthusiasm for any treatment plan or medication is part of its healing power.

The opinion of family members is often even more important than that of the patient. Studies have shown that splints are used when family members believe them effective for rheumatoid arthritis,[11] and that mothers will give penicillin as prophylaxis for rheumatic fever when they understand the reason for the antibiotic and also when they feel that the clinician sees them as good mothers.[5] Hoebel[8] showed that wives were able to alter the lifestyle of their husbands following myocardial infarction when they understood and could apply the strategy suggested by a physician, whereas physicians had been unable to alter the men's behavior directly.

Knowledge of the family or family assessment will enable information to be given more effectively. For example, conveying the necessity for hospital-ization may be facilitated by a discussion of the resources available: a mother of six children, whose husband is frequently out of town and who was often left alone herself as a child because her mother was sick, may receive the news more calmly if the clinician has available the telephone numbers of agencies providing help at home or knows that there is a sister-in-law who might be invited to take over the family tasks. Awareness of a family's experience of illness may direct the type of information given. A family assessment interview or genogram may show that one family member (either of the extended or nuclear family) is the influential person concerning health problems and may contradict most information on illness or veto instructions. That person may be a nurse or grandmother or drug salesman. Under certain circumstances this person can be useful as an ally in the transmission of information and in management of the illness. It must always be kept in mind that any information given is conveyed to a family system, not just an individual.

ANTICIPATORY GUIDANCE

Anticipatory guidance is based on the awareness of the current developmental stage of a family and is aimed at preparing the family for the known tasks and potential stresses associated with the next stage. It can play a major preventive role in primary care. It is a specific type of information giving based on the clinician's broad experience of families and conceptual knowledge of their development. For the family each stage is a new experience for which there exists only minimal preparation, through memories of the same stage in the two families of origin and through observation of other families they know. Each stage requires a renegotiation and change in family functioning to allow family growth and individual differentiation.

For example, when a couple present themselves for a premarital examination, the practitioner has an excellent opportunity to extend preventive medicine to the new family unit. Quite apart from the opportunity to do the physical examination, the visit is a good time to raise such issues as independence from in-laws, division of responsibilities, work, feelings about sexuality, and contraception. By including these aspects in the evaluation, the family practitioner distinguishes his or her premarital examination from that of other practitioners. In addition, many family-oriented physicians find it beneficial to do the physical examination in the presence of the partner, which enhances the possibility for education. He or she also facilitates future questions from the couple in these areas.

Courtship and early marriage can be a precarious period, particularly when the couple has difficulty in separating from the two families of origin. Early problems with in-laws may present to the practitioner's office as headaches, abdominal pains, or other psychosomatic symptoms. One woman in the author's practice (J. C-S), presented with anxiety symptoms produced by the noise of a budgerigar! This bird belonged to the husband, who was inordinately attached to it. It was a symbol to the wife of her mother-in-law to whom the husband was greatly attached and who tended to chatter in a similar fashion.

Even greater stress is usually experienced by the family around the birth of the first baby. Anticipatory guidance for both husband and wife is crucial in the prenatal period. Attendance at prenatal classes by the husband is becoming the norm and probably prevents some of the estrangement during the birth process and with the newborn infant that can so easily lead to jealousy in the husband and subsequent family disruption:

Mrs. A. was pregnant for the second time, but it was the first such experience for her second husband. The first child, aged 7, had an apparently good relationship with her new father but the pregnancy aroused hostility as it destroyed all hope of reconciliation between her real father and her mother. This and the disparity of experience between the parents suggested a family at risk for difficulties over this new baby. Discussions with all three family members before its birth helped clarify expectations of the couple and of the daughter and prevented some disruption that would have been felt after the birth; the father said 3 months later, "Even though you said it would be tough, I had no idea how stormy a time it would be." He had carried out his plans to help his wife with cooking, feeding, and changing the baby so that they were equally tired but very united in the enterprise. The wife said she had forgotten what it had been like having a baby; 7 years was a long period between children. The daughter was very involved in the baby's care and had resolved her problem with her natural father. Her inclusion in discussions with the physician helped provide a role model for the parents in including her in baby care at home.

In contrast, other families have been seen with serious problems, particularly in the stressed young mother. Frequently, marital problems can be dated from the arrival of a child and the exclusion of the father from the bond between mother and baby. "Marrying" his work, returning to mother, or taking refuge with a mistress balances the alliance between mother and children. A few timely warnings to the couple with an infant and the suggestion of a weekly night out and time together as a couple may be remarkably effective in deflecting trouble in the future.

The arrival of subsequent children usually presents fewer problems but can also be a time of stress. The mother is often isolated and exhausted by the children's demands. The simple suggestion of exchanging days off with a friend with children whose ages are similar may prevent physical or mental breakdown—for which this group of women is at risk—or the beginning of a martyr syndrome.

Launching the first child into the school system can be a trial, particularly when the mother has no interests outside the family. In a brief discussion with the mother of a 3-year-old child the clinician may suggest that she should not lose touch with friends or hobbies, and prepare herself for the trauma of separation. School phobias are known to represent the difficulty of letting go in the mother rather than the child; when her anxiety is communicated, the child then experiences panic. If the father has felt left out of the mother-child relationship and has therefore devoted increasing time to his work, the mother will feel the new solitude even more. Difficulties between parents resulting from the stress of taking care of active young children can take the form of recurrent minor illnesses. When children of this age group present frequently with illness the possibility of family stress should be considered:

> A 5-year old child was brought several times to the office by her father, who believed she had asthma. No evidence could be found for this despite a strong family history, particularly in the father, of allergic illness. It became apparent that the parents were increasingly distant from one another and admitted to no sexual relations for the past 2 years. Ambivalence over having another child, dyspareunia resulting from a displaced IUD, and difficulties in communication had combined to produce the family's problem with sexuality. The father's tension was then projected as worry over the 5-year-old child, who might well have gone on to develop asthma had marital therapy not intervened. In this case it was the father who reacted most to school entry as a sign the child was growing up, and who wanted another child.

Perhaps the most stressful period in a person's life is when the turmoils of adolescence are combined with the parents' mid-life crisis and the looming departure of the children. (Gail Sheehy's *Passages*[13] did not pay much attention to the family unit as a whole.) The following is an example of the interplay of different individual stages within a family:

> A university professor found himself in a rut in his late 40s, and wanted a rural existence on a farm. He spent longer and longer periods on the family's vacation farm. His wife, angry at his success and her aborted education, sought a Ph.D. and spent every evening taking courses. Four children, close in age, were coping with adolescence and had very little parental contact and guidance. The 15-year-old daughter alerted the family physician to the chaotic home situation by her request to be given contraception; her father had apparently moved out of the parent's bedroom, and the wife had retaliated by providing no evening meal for the family because she was out studying. An escalation of the crisis was predictable. Preventing divorce and adolescent pregnancy and school failure in two other siblings involved referral for family therapy.

Most families with adolescents, however, handle their problems without needing therapy, and for many families adolescence proceeds smoothly and the departure of the children is seen as entailing a well-deserved rest by a couple looking forward to more time together. The clinician can often help the family recognize possible future difficulties by showing the parents how to give increasing age-appropriate autonomy to the younger adolescents and how to maintain flexibility. Parents often need a gentle reminder to keep up with their children's advancing abilities and responsibilities. Adolescents, on the other hand, when visiting the physician or nurse can be helped to recognize their parents as trying hard and struggling with their own problems and with a future on their own. Often the elderly grandparents are becoming an added burden to the parents just as freedom from the responsibilities of children is in sight. The sympathetic outsider who knows all family members can help each to understand the difficulties of the other.

It has recently been recognized by industry (through employee assistance programs) and by the public that pre-retirement counselling is an important preventive function. Both morbidity and mortality increase after retirement. The clinician can remind a man or woman in their fifties that anticipating the age of 65 and planning a second career, hobbies, or group interests is much preferable to the sudden shock of having nothing to do and no time to plan.

The role of the clinician is to help the family anticipate changes through nonthreatening, nonmoralizing questions or suggestions, and to prod the family into thinking ahead and preparing for the necessary adjustment. Very often crises brought to the practitioner's office, whether a behavioral problem in a child or an adolescent acting out, are related to transitional states that are normal parts of family development; these problems could have been anticipated and prevented. There is also increased incidence of illness at these crisis points, so that prevention of stress may mean prevention of illness.

CRISIS INTERVENTION

Puryear[12] defines a crisis as a state of panic or defeat when a person has tried every way possible to solve a problem and feels overwhelmed, inadequate, and helpless. The individual's normal or primary coping mechanisms (internal defenses such as rationalization and denial, and external responses such as turning to grandmother, praying, getting drunk) have been tried, as have some secondary coping mechanisms (ones less often used by that individual or family, such as asking help from a physician). They have failed because the problem is too great, perhaps because of its personal significance or because of the person's increased vulnerability during a series of crises. There may be inadequate perception of reality, inadequate social support network, or inadequate coping mechanisms. The problem may be a new one and the coping repertoire may be inappropriate, as when the adolescence of the first child is blocked by a parent who handles all family problems by taking charge and giving orders.

Such a crisis is of limited duration, but is characterized by lowered efficiency, decreased self-esteem, and a focus on relief of the symptoms of stress. Headache or depression become the targets for concern rather than the initial problem. Agitation or apathy compound the difficulty. If secondary coping mechanisms do resolve the crisis, a sense of competency and growth may result in improved functioning as compared to the precrisis level.

In parallel fashion, a family as a unit has primary and secondary coping mechanisms and a tendency to get sidetracked from problem-solving to focus on symptoms. The crisis may be the illness of the breadwinner, diagnosis of mental retardation in a child, or diagnosis of a terminal disease. The role of the clinician is to help the family define the primary problem(s) and decide on priorities; list attempted solutions that have not worked; and find alternative solutions. This process necessarily demands family communication. All members should be encouraged to express their perspectives and suggestions. The essential components of the process are facilitation of communication, support, positive relabelling, normalization, and specific suggestions. The goal is to develop new coping mechanisms and growth through crisis. Families are in a much more fluid adaptable state at a time of crisis; communication patterns long entrenched can change dramatically when a family is faced, for example, with the diagnosis of terminal cancer. A small push from a trusted clinician who is outside the system may help open channels long closed: "Why don't you talk about it, share what you're feeling."

Smilkstein's model of the cycle of family function (Figure 15-1) illustrates the disequilibrium that results following a stressful life event and points to the positive role of external resources such as the family clinician. Conversely, lack of resources can provoke a downwards spiral or development of symptoms that themselves may restabilize the system but at the expense of a state of chronic illness or psychologic dysfunction.

FACILITATION

Facilitation is a comprehensive term covering the ability of the clinician to help the family cope with crisis, particularly those associated with illness, and normative developmental crises. Family strengths, ability to function, and coping strategies may be temporarily frozen or distorted by shock, denial, anger, or other emotional reactions. It is important to recognize that during such a crisis families may appear dysfunctional but their past history will suggest otherwise. Facilitation of family communication and mutual understanding by a clinician may be an essential step before the family can move forward. Often it is a family's tendency to protect one another that blocks coping: in early marriage the tendency to avoid hurting the other's feelings is often a block to open expression of feelings or needs and leads to a pattern of conflict avoidance and poor negotiating skills. At this early stage the comment that anger between newlyweds is both normal and necessary can help the couple develop better communication. Families faced with terminal illness often protect the patient and each other by expressing grief alone, and putting a false front of bravado that convinces no one but effectively isolates each member from the others. The clinician can encourage sharing of emotion and allow important growth in the ability to communicate to take place.

The Cycle of Family Function:
A Model of Family Response to Stressful Life Events

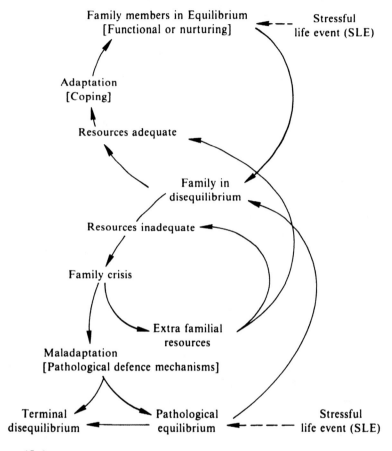

Figure 15-1

Source: Smilkstein G: The cycle of family function: A conceptual model for family medicine. *J Fam Pract* 11: 223, 1980.

The process of facilitation also includes normalization, support, clarification and specific suggestions to help adaptation to crisis, illness, or change:

"Normalization."   We have found it helpful to label this common form of reassurance in order to emphasize its usefulness: "normalization" is the simple statement that a given behavior or feeling is normal for its particular context. It is a statement that situates the event within the context of the normal life of a family: temper tantrums are commonplace in families with young children; it is normal to become depressed after the death of a family member, and normal to express this emotion with tears; masturbation after marriage is normal; it is normal for a female to take longer to reach orgasm (average, 15 minutes) than a male (average, 2 minutes) and for these times to be prolonged and shortened, respectively, by anxiety.

Clearly these statements are a form of information giving that places the reality experienced by the family in a perspective broader than their own experience. The family practitioner is saying, "You are not alone." Before making such a statement, however, the clinician should elicit from the family their own explanatory model of what they think of the situation and what is going on. Normalizing statements given too quickly by the physician may prevent the family from dealing with the family's real agenda or may give the impression the clinician is brushing the problem aside, in which case the statement will not have the expected effect of reassurance. It is also important to remember that the expression of anxiety and emotional content of a topic is always necessary before a family can hear any information or explanation.

Support of Family Strengths. If the clinician hopes to mobilize the family's own resources rather than develop its dependence on the health care profession, it is essential to focus on strengths on what the family can do, not on what it is unable to do. The research on coping with stress discussed in Section III emphasizes that failure begets failure, while success leads to further success. If the clinician can remind the family of present and past successes and strengths he or she will do much to increase current coping. Nurses tend to be better at this than physicians, who have a tendency to be concerned with "pathology" and disease rather than health.

Watzlawick[15] has pointed out that to help a family one must speak in its own language. This is another aspect of support as well as a good principle of communication. Discussing a problem using the family terminology conveys acceptance of their value system and emphasizes their strengths while subtly suggesting a change of direction: a wife who is overly solicitous of her husband's illness can be helped to be even more "helpful" by being pessimistic about his recovery. This pessimism may help him more than her previous optimistic efforts at encouragement if he tries to prove her wrong. A business executive can be encouraged to increase his family's efficiency and organization by decreasing negative feedback and increasing teamwork with his wife, and adding a vacation incentive as he would in his own office. Support of the family hierarchy, including support of family terminology, ways of thinking, and value systems, is usually important.

Positive relabelling is an art that distinguishes the therapeutic personality: the art of relabelling a person or action seen as negative by the family to facilitate change. Individuals or families feel respected and valued by a clinician who reframes their problems in a positive way; as attempts to be helpful or as ways of rescuing or protecting others: Lack of communication that is felt to be a lack of caring may be relabelled as fear of hurting feelings or of raising issues painful to the other person: the child staying home from school may be seen as helping his mother avoid her need for new activities; the delinquent can be considered protecting his parents from facing their conflict; and the depressed man can be thought of as providing someone for his wife, who has been trained as a nurse, to care for.

Clarification. The role of clarification is that of providing the family with the perception of an outsider to help the family make its own modifications. It means describing in understandable terms how the family's stage of development and way of functioning is influencing or provoking a symptom or illness. Clarification of a problem means helping family members to understand each other's positions and perceptions; it means enabling each to "stand in the other's shoes." By asking detailed questions about a conflict or illness situation, the clinician may clarify differences in perceptions previously unrecognized. For example, a wife's overconcern with her husband's recent mild cough may relate to her experience of a grandfather with lung cancer. Conflict over a husband's chauvinism may represent differing perceptions and means of conveying value messages; in the husband's family carrying a suitcase or moving furniture was considered a way of expressing caring and valuing of women; whereas in the wife's family doing such tasks scornfully implied that women are weak and incompetent (see communication in Chapter 15).

In general, clarification with a family systems orientation broadens the perspective of the patient and family, from the single symptom or the single patient to the family system as a whole. The family may have sensed confusion and ambiguity around the presenting problem, but is unclear about how this problem has developed, and why their solutions to correct it have failed. The family members bring the problem to the clinician as a plea for help. The more physical the symptom the more suitable it seems as an offering for the health professional, but the real wish of the family may be for the resolution of tension. The clinician can be a powerful teacher about how families and illness interact. With increased understanding many families can solve the problem themselves.

Often the underlying problem is a difficulty facing and solving a task in the family life cycle. When children reach their early teens, parents often find it very difficult to let go of a more authoritarian mode of relating to their children, which may be suited to the small child; changing to a style involving consultation and guidance, which is more productive for adolescents, is hard for parents to achieve. The parents' inability to allow increasing responsibility and autonomy is met with a rebellious attitude on the part of the adolescent; the parents then become unsure whether their parenting behavior is right:

A boy who presented with Osgood Schlatter's disease was the presenting problem in a family. The mother in this case focused exclusively on the swollen tibial tubercle of the boy's knee and the fact that the boy would not wear a protective pad in hockey; she felt that he was playing hockey far more often than was good for him. Close supervision of homework in this 14-year-old boy was not producing the desired grades in school, and hockey was largely blamed.

The clinician's assessment, which she conveyed to both parents and the son in a joint interview, was that there were two problems. The first was the parents' overconcern with their oldest child and only son and his scholastic achievement, a common and very normal mistake of most parents (normalization of the problem). The parents were giving their son the false impression that his success at school was for the parents' benefit and not for his own. He had therefore become dependent on the parents for supervision with homework and was being protected from the consequences normally provided by the outside world (school and later employment) for lack of self-discipline. This would become a greater problem for the son when he grew up and could no longer have his parents around to help with work assignments.

The second problem was that because he was their first experience of a fourteen-year-old, the parents did not understand that he had the ability to look after both his homework and his knee. He had no limp, and the knee was obviously not sufficiently painful to provoke the use of a pad; in this disease, pain was usually sufficient indication of severity and would prevent overuse of the knee, and consequently it would be safe to leave management of the knee to the son. The clinician stated that, like the parents, perhaps he had been remiss in underestimating the boy's ability to look after his own problem (thus the clinician is siding with the parents while complimenting the boy and role-modelling giving increased responsibility).

The clinician then explained at length to the boy (in front of his parents) about the disease process, reassuring the mother indirectly that no damage would result, particularly if her son were not given the opportunity to rebel through his disease. She also facilitated discussion by asking the boy whether his friends were able to do their homework alone, and made it apparent to the parents that their son both understood his problem with his knee and was concerned about his low grades.

If this discussion had been with the boy alone, or with his mother alone, much less would have been accomplished. The father was also present, and although relatively inactive in the discussion was the real source of the mother's authoritarianism; had he not been at the discussion he would have undermined the proposed changes. Finally, a brief and casual enquiry about the mother's interests outside the home led to a specific suggestion encouraging increased participation in an art group.

The session was no longer than the average visit (15 minutes), but contributed to a change in the parental attitude to school, sports, and to other areas of needed autonomy not covered in the discussion.

Thus, clarification includes relabelling of a problem so that it belongs to the family context rather than to the individual only. Since families are growing and adapting organic systems, often this clarification and broader perspective is all that is needed to give the family a gentle push along the path of its own development. Such flexibility is true of most families seen in practice, in contrast to families that are in serious trouble and seek psychiatric help, or who indirectly seek help through criminal behavior.

SPECIFIC SUGGESTIONS

Patients often come to a physician or nurse for advice. To respond to this request with a solution to the problem is at best to promote dependence on the health profession. At worst, trying to give advice is to fall into the trap of a resistant family system where the request for help is followed by a response that criticizes all suggestions as impractical (a "yes, but . . . " game); or if the advice is followed, it may prove to be a poor solution. The alcoholic is an expert at this game and can hook the clinician into the role of rescuer, only to later reject his help or show him up as overly gullible. Specific suggestions, therefore, should be aimed at helping the family develop its own solutions, rather than providing answers. Like other aspects of facilitation, the goal is to promote family coping, strength, and resources.

Resources other than the health profession in the community should be known to the clinician; referral to such resources and coaching in their use may be one specific course of action suggested. For example, a young adult having difficulty leaving home and finding a job may be directed to a career counselling service. This is far more appropriate than spending an hour with the young person discussing abilities and career options when more expert help is available. Similarly, a parent-training group in the community may be a more efficient resource with more expertise and support than could ever be provided by the clinician, even if time constraints permitted enough discussion of the subject.

Specific suggestions also include techniques for improving communication. Suggesting to a young couple with an infant to arrange babysitting so that they can spend a weekend together alone gives them permission to do something they would othewise feel too guilty to undertake. Also in this category are the techniques of active listening to improve couple communication, using "I" messages rather than "You" messages, (see section on communication in Chapter 14), setting aside specific time together for activities or discussion, behavioral methods for recording success in problem solving, and constructive ways of expressing anger.

When fixed triangulation is occurring in a family (when one child is constantly playing the role of scapegoat or is being called on to side with a parent; or when a parent is seen to be rescuing a child from the other parent's excess discipline) specific suggestions aimed as disrupting the triangle can be extremely helpful, particularly when the pattern has not been fixed over a long period. It can be pointed out to the "rescuer" that although it is the understandable human reaction to jump in protectively when two are in conflict (normalization); it also effectively prevents those two from ever resolving the problem alone. Support from the clinician can encourage the rescuer to stay out of the conflict and discover that dire results do not ensue. Obviously in severe situations such as child abuse or long-standing scapegoating the expertise of a family therapist is essential, and treatment of such problems ("detriangulation") should not be attempted by the less experienced clinician. Similarly when a couple is avoiding conflict by attacking a child, specific suggestions to focus the conflict more appropriately may help change the pattern, providing it is not fixed and long-term. Permission to express negative emotions such as anger or sadness or, just as often, to openly express affection may be the underlying message of such specific suggestions.

In summary, in facilitating a problem or helping a family resolve a crisis by a family-centered approach, the clinician can use normalization, support, facilitation of communication, clarification, or suggest a specific course of action to enhance the family's capacity to solve the problem. When the family cannot make use of such facilitation, the clinician may have to refer the family for therapy.

REFERRAL

Referral for Family Therapy

Rarely a family will need or request more intensive intervention. When there is a request for family therapy that appears warranted, and where family therapists are available in the community and cost is not a problem, referral is simple. The difficulty usually arises where a problem is seen by the clinician as a family problem but the family resists relabelling it as such. This problem becomes acute when the issue is a potentially fatal disease in one member. For example, anorexia nervosa has a 5% to 15% mortality rate. Although the disease may have an endocrinologic basis or predisposition, the evidence is overwhelming that this is a family illness.[10]

A psychosomatic family, because of its rigidity and avoidance of conflict, is both very difficult to treat and to refer. If the condition of the sick member is not acute, time may be the clinician's ally because repeated contact with the clinician allows repeated attempts at relabelling as a problem in the family system. When it is a child who is ill and the condition is serious, parental concern usually makes the process of relabelling and referral easier. When the problem patient is an adult, particularly when the spouse refuses to see the clinician and appears to have a vested interest in the maintenance of the illness, such relabelling may be impossible. If the patient accepts referral to a psychiatrist, change may be wrought in the family system through the individual parents. Often, however, the response of the family system to improvement in that patient is to have illness or dysfunction strike another family member or have serious marital difficulty ensue.

The clinician's belief in the referral and his or her confidence in the consultant usually convert family reluctance to the agreement to try family therapy. The clinician may need to accompany the family on the first visit, which decreases family anxiety and increases their hope of being understood by a stranger. Subsequently, the clinician should be in the role of monitoring the therapy and occasionally may need to try another route. He or she should obviously be aware of the problem of undermining the consultant by prematurely assuming that progress has not been made. Communication between professionals, particularly when several are involved, is often essential to prevent triangulation by the family (playing one professional off against another) and to fully understand each other's roles, approaches, and goals. In general, referral for family therapy is based on the same principles as referral for surgery or investigation by a specialist: The referring physician should have a knowledge of the field; he or she should have observed a family therapist in action, just as he has observed surgery in action, and should know something of the personality and practice of the specific therapist to whom he is referring the family. The clinician's confidence in the consultant and good communication between the two professionals will result in a good referral.

Many patients and families refuse, at least initially, to go to either a psychiatrist, marriage counsellor, or family therapist. The stigma of psychological help in our culture is great, and fear of labelling by the community is sometimes well founded. If a clinician is tactful, many families that need help can be referred if facilities are available. If resources are not available in a community, the clinician is faced with handling them alone, and further training is necessary. A maximum of three to six sessions should be sufficient to help families with resources to change their own system. If a family is more difficult and requires more time, and referral is not available or is refused, the clinician should attempt limited goals with the object of leading the family to a more experienced therapist later. Knowing which families will prove difficult and which can be helped in one or two sessions requires experience. Some warning signs can be helpful; the following were listed by Bullock[2] as indications for referral of difficult families:

1. history of repeated attempts at therapy;
2. missed appointments;
3. commitment to sessions as family unit but at no session does everyone attend;
4. long duration of dysfunction pattern;
5. refusal to pay prescribed fees (disrespect for counselling); applicable only in the United States. In Canada, psychotherapy is usually covered by the government medicare system.

6. no improvement after five or six sessions, the maximum number for the family physician or nurse (probably in most busy practices even six sessions is impractical).

Other indications could be added:

7. serious problems in more than one family member;
8. more than one serious problem in a child with behavioral difficulties;
9. changing doctors often and refusing to agree to drop all other physicians or health care contacts; and
10. when a physician has developed too strong an alliance with the patient or one family member and cannot be objective in assessment and intervention (compensatory alliance).

Another rule of thumb that indicates to the sensitive clinician that a problem is beyond his or her scope is simply a sense of discomfort.

Studies reported by Medalie[9] and Huygen[7] have demonstrated the benefit of referral and collaboration between family physician and family therapist. A significant decrease in the number of visits to the family doctor and a decrease in the number of prescriptions have been documented in both studies when families in difficulties were referred to a therapist (see Chapter 9). In addition, both professionals can learn from each other and benefit from the relationship. If the family therapist is available to observe some family interviews of the primary care clinician, support and coaching can be invaluable.

Referral to the consultant does not mean abandoning the family, and this message has to be clearly stated to the family. The primary care clinician continues to be the main provider of care for the family, and his role in monitoring the outcome of the intervention by the consultant is both important to the family and to the consultant; the clinician will incorporate in the continuous care management the increased understanding brought by the consultant.

> A young woman, 34 years old, came to the office for eight visits in 7 months with different complaints each time: cough, fatigue, epigastric pain, ecchymoses, hemorrhoids. Fatigue was the chief complaint. The physical exam was always normal except for hemorrhoids and, sometimes, one or two small blue spots on the legs, which she had intermittently since her children were born. She had mild anemia, and coagulation tests were normal.
>
> The woman was born in Sardinia. She now lived in Montreal with her Italian husband, two children (a 17-month-old girl and a 9-year-old boy), and her mother. She worked full-time as a college Spanish teacher; the family also owned an apartment building and a travel agency. This patient constantly claimed that there was no problem at home or work. She was also very resistant to the idea that she might be depressed.
>
> She was very demanding of the staff: she refused to be seen by the nurse

practitioner; and once the secretary had nightmares about her (which she never had about other patients).

On the ninth visit, complaining of fatigue, she burst into tears. She now admitted that she had had arguments and fights with her husband over the children and over her mother for a long time. The situation was bad at home and seemed always to get worse in March. The physician asked her to come with the entire family. She objected, saying that she didn't want the children to be involved because they were too young and also that her mother spoke neither English nor French. She agreed to come with her husband.

The couple were seen for three sessions. They talked about their fights, and the problems with the children and grandmother, who were involved in their conflicts through triangulation. The grandmother was siding with her daughter against her son-in-law. Mother and daughter were in a conflicting but symbiotic relationship; both had poor individuation. The couple didn't have any private life because of the over-involvement of both extended families; they had never had a holiday alone with their children, or as a couple since their wedding. They were clearly avoiding conflict, which followed the pattern of the wife's family of origin (her mother and father had never had a fight together).

One of the tasks they were given was to discuss and negotiate the coming Easter holiday; they were to reach an agreement on where they should go and with whom. At the third visit, on return from the vacation, they fought throughout the 1-hour interview, complaining about the holiday, and again repetitively arguing about the children, grandmother, and extended family.

The issue of divorce was broached, and once the husband accused the wife of wanting him to die of a heart attack as her father did; the husband blamed the wife's mother for the father's death.

At this interview, the decision to refer the couple to a family therapist was made for the following reasons:

1.   the chronicity of the problem
2.   fixed triangulation of children and grandmother with no response to attempts to detriangulate
3.   destructive fighting, which the therapist was unable to stop, and escalation of conflict with discussion of divorce
4.   the love that they still seemed to share
5.   their willingness to improve the situation
6.   the physician's lack of skills as a family therapist

The reasons and the process of referral were discussed with them, and a therapist was suggested. The physician was present at the first interview. She kept contact with the family therapist in order not to undermine treatment when the couple attempted to triangulate the professionals and maintained follow-up as the family physician.

In summary, when referring a family for treatment the family physician relabels the individual problems as a family problem, explores the benefit of treatment, establishes the relationship with the consultant, follows up on results, and integrates new information for future medical management. (The development of a practice in which a family therapist is practicing with a group of physicians represent an interesting way of providing this service.)

Referral to Other Resources

Referral for individual therapy may be indicated when one family member is in serious distress or is suicidal. However, the clinician with a family systems orientation will be aware of the great risk of escalating the family labelling process, or the extrusion process, in which one family member becomes the repository of the family "badness" or "madness." The "black sheep" (the delinquent, the alcoholic), the permanent patient, or the "crazy one" all serve the family system in maintaining a pathological homeostasis. The problem is isolated in one member like a tuberculous granuloma or abscess capable of reinfecting the whole body or producing a chronic malaise. Treatment of delinquency and even psychosis has been shown to be more effective in the family setting.[4]

Providing the patient referred is not labelled as *the* problem, individual therapy can be very effective in changing a part of the system and hence changing the whole family system. One individual may change a family, or, more frequently, will revert to his or her original behavior once the power of the family system is exerted; or the family may break up. There is evidence of increased incidence of divorce after individual therapy[4] and for marital problems after correction of an individual problem like obesity.[8]

Referral to community resources such as agencies, clubs, and organizations (Golden Age or senior citizen's clubs, mastectomy, colostomy, single parents, widow groups) should involve some of the same principles as referral for psychotherapy or to the medical specialties: knowledge of the resource, evaluation of its competence, communication with the resource when possible and within the clinician's mandate, and follow-up of outcome.

REFERENCES

1. Barrows HS, Tamblyn RM: *Problem-Based Learning. Approach to Medical Education.* New York, Springer Co., 1980.

2. Bullock D, Thompson B: Guidelines for family interviewing and brief therapy by the family physician. *J Fam Pract* 9:837, 1979.

3. Elstein AS, Shulman LS, Sprafka SA: *Medical Problem Solving. An Analysis of Clinical Reasoning.* Cambridge, Harvard University Press, 1978.

4. Gurman AS, Kniskern DP: Research on marital and family therapy: Perspective and prospect, in Garfield SL, Bergin AE (eds): *Handbook of Psychotherapy and Behavior Change: An Empirical Analysis.* New York, Wiley, 1978.

5. Heinzelman F, Bagley R: Response to physical activity programs and their effects on health behavior. *Pub Health Rep* 85:905, 1970.

6. Hoebel FC: Brief family-interactional therapy in the management of cardiac-related high-risk behaviors. *J Fam Pract* 3:613, 1976.

7. Huygen FJA: *Family Medicine: The Medical Life History of Families.* The Netherlands, Dekker & Van de Vegt, 1978.

8. Marshall JR, Neill J: The removal of a psychosomatic symptom: Effects on the marriage. *Fam Process* 16:273, 1977.

9. Medalie JH: *Family Medicine: Principles and Applications.* Baltimore, Williams & Wilkins, 1978.

10. Minuchin S, Baker L, Rosman BL, et al: A conceptual model of psychosomatic illness in children: Family organization and family therapy. *Arch Gen Psychiatry* 32:1031, 1975.

11. Oakes TW, Ward JR, Gray RM, et al: Family expectations and arthritis patient compliance to a hand resting splint regimen. *J Chron Dis* 22:757, 1970.

12. Puryear D: *Helping People in Crisis.* California, Jossey-Bass, 1979.

13. Sheehy G: *Passages: Predictable Crises in Adult Life.* New York, Bantam Books, 1976.

14. Smilkstein G: The cycle of family function: A conceptual model for family medicine. *J Fam Pract* 11:223, 1980.

15. Watzlawick P, Weakland JH, Fisch R: Change: *Principles of Problem Formulation and Problem Resolution.* New York, Norton, 1974.

Chapter 16

The Contrast Between Working with Families and Family Therapy

Janet Christie-Seely
Yves Talbot

Since the start of family medicine the discipline has relied on clinicians in other fields (obstetrics, internal medicine, and pediatrics) for the development of its knowledge base. Early recognition that the activity of the primary care physician is distinctly different has forced practitioners of family medicine to leave this dependency of its adolescent phase, to differentiate and redefine their activity. In the future, a more interdependent relationship of equals may occur in which primary and tertiary care professionals can learn from one another. Over the last 5 years, because the family is the focus as the unit of care, practitioners of family medicine have been very dependent on family sociology, anthropology, and family therapy for the elaboration of its knowledge base. Family therapy, with its clinical orientation and systems approach, has been the discipline from which family medicine has drawn the most knowledge. However, it has also been important to differentiate it from this second parental discipline; confusion of roles and expectations has resulted from the use of family therapy's theoretical base.

Primary care nursing has developed with a different emphasis. It is more concerned with health than illness, although equally focused on the family. Primary care nursing must differentiate from traditional nursing (which is primarily hospital based) and also from medicine. The old hierarchy must give way to egalitarian teamwork and division of responsibility.

Nature of the Activity

The community nurse or the family practitioner is above all a primary clinician: the first contact a patient makes within the health care system. The medical challenge is that of the "undifferentiated problem" and of health maintenance through continuous comprehensive, and preventive activities. In contrast, the family therapist's relationship with a family is episodic; he or she functions as a secondary or tertiary resource in the line of service. The family therapist's role is that of consultant whose involvement is limited to a specific clinical problem, in this case a dysfunctional family, and to a specific contract for change. In contrast, the family practitioner is concerned with health maintenance over time. These differences result in a very different clientele. The family practitioner is more likely to see individuals and families who adapt and change over time (morphogenetic systems), with increased illness incidence reflecting stress, whereas the family therapist primarily sees families with long-term difficulties in adaptation (morphostatic system), and chronic dysfunction. (An exception to this are the psychosomatic families in which family homeostasis is reorganized around chronic illness). Due to a different focus and therapeutic contract, working with families differs from family therapy in the nature of change that takes place. The chief target of interventions (*individual* and family versus family only), the time involved and the comprehensiveness of care are other major differences.

The conceptual model and the way of thinking about people (epistemology) are similar in both primary care and family therapy. Professionals in both fields use a systems concept, seeking to develop an understanding of the family and to intervene in such a way that the person and the context of the illness are taken into account. The goals, however, and the skills required are quite different. Family assessment, as done by a family practitioner, is similar to family assessment by a family therapist, although with more emphasis on illness and its role in the family and on coping, and with more knowledge of this family and probably the extended family over time. (The normal developmental tasks of the family are the focus rather than family dysfunction.) Prevention of illness is a primary goal, one that is not possible for a family therapist, who usually sees a family at a much later stage of problem formation. Missing from the family practitioner's interview is any contract for change in the family system (that is, the agreement that change is desired by the family and that change is *the* goal of visits to the practitioner). Time is used very differently by the family therapist and the family physician or nurse. Physical and psychological problems are equally the focus so that the mind/body separation present in the disciplines of social work, psychiatry, and the medical specialties is much less prevalent. In primary care, teamwork and use of community resources is an essential component, whereas the family therapist tends to work alone (these differences are listed in Table 16.1).

Change in the Family System

The difference between family therapy and working with families is highlighted by the source of change, which may be generated by the family itself or through interventions by a therapist. In primary care, clinicians work with the family as it is, with no contract for change. If change does occur, the source is from within the family. In contrast, the family in family therapy is requesting the therapist to initiate change. In working with families, the family physician or nurse assesses the family and then gives the family his or her view of the situation. This outside view may relabel the situation and put it in a new

Table 16.1 A Comparison of Family Medicine with Family Therapy

	Family Medicine (Working with Families)	Family Therapy
Thinking (Epistemology)	Family systems theory	Family systems theory
Type of Activity	Primary care Continuous (over years) comprehensive (includes crisis intervention) Health maintenance and prevention Case finding, risk assessment	Secondary/tertiary care Episodic or recurrent crises Prevention not a focus Contract for change
Clinician Role	Manager	Consultant
Predominant Family Type	Morphogenetic system (dynamic) Able to change from within	Morphostatic system (Static) Requiring external induction of change
Contacts with the Family	Frequently through individual Brief, spaced, fewer, (30 min every 2–4 weeks) 1–3 sessions Focus may be on physical symptoms or problems in relations	Primarily family unit Longer (1 hr), and more Sessions (weekly, 7–10 sessions minimum) Focus always on interaction (may be more threatening)
Limits of Expertise	Credibility primarily in medical areas	No medical expertise
Difficult Family Problems	Exceeding limits of training creates problems	Opportunity for change

Source: Compiled by the authors

light. Given the new information, the family may choose to modify its rules and change its behavior in the direction of better adaptation and coping. This change is initiated from within the system, indicating flexibility and no need for therapy. As with organic disease, the clinician is ethically entitled to give his diagnostic impression, but is not entitled to initiate therapy without adequate training in that modality and the patient's permission or request. (The family physician may diagnose appendicitis but not operate unless he has had surgical training.) The patient has the right to be fully informed of his condition and to refuse operation if he so chooses. If the family does not change and if the clinician feels that without change he or she can foresee a major difficulty, such as marital disruption, illness, death, or delinquency in a child, he or she is entitled to recommend further therapy. The success rate and complications of family therapy should be part of the information given to the family just as in the analogy of an operation, so that they can make an informed decision.

The Family within the Individual

In family medicine, in contrast to family therapy, most sessions are with individual patients and the family may not be immediately available. But an awareness of "the family *in* the patient" facilitates diagnosis, treatment, and prevention. This approach is different from the individual orientation even though the individual patient is still seen in the office:

A 36-year-old woman presented with fatigue, constipation, weight gain, hirsutism, headaches, and galactorrhea of several months' duration. A questionable double contour of the sella turcica added to the strong suspicion of a pituitary adenoma. However, all tests proved negative. At the next visit the physician repeated previous questions about tension related to her husband (institutionalized because of von Recklinghausen's disease) and unsympathetic parents (whom the physician had previously met). This time the questions produced a flood of tears. Tension that had been denied was admitted now that the diagnosis of tumor was ruled out.

The woman was referred for therapy and began to address the anger she felt at her controlling, rigidly religious parents and at her husband, who would not die despite psychosis, deafness, and blindness due to his disease. A session with the woman's son showed that she was exerting the same control on her son that she complained of from her parents. Age-appropriate, increased responsibility for this early adolescent was encouraged by the clinician. The woman was referred for individual therapy to help her take control of her life. Thus, knowledge of the woman's family and of the stage in this single-parent family life cycle helped the diagnosis and treatment of stress in the mother, and prevention of adolescent problems in the son. Had this not taken place, visits to the office for multiple physical symptoms might have continued.

The family therapist has the benefit of viewing interactions in the office; the family clinician must often infer such reactions but is very much aided in this task by family interviews when possible and by experience of family members over time.

Stress in a patient in the office may reflect stress in another part of the family system. Even when patients are living alone and far from their nuclear family, it is surprising how news of distress at home may produce a ripple effect. For example, members of one family in Canada, separated by a large distance, interact almost as if they were all under the same roof: When the first grandchild in the family arrived, this event was followed closely by distress in the marriage of another family member, which was in turn followed both by increased alcohol intake of the father in the next province and by acting out of a brother who had a delinquent history. (The telephone can be a powerful transmitter of anxiety in a family that is still enmeshed.)

The family in the patient can still be a powerful determinant of behavior, even when all other members are dead.

A woman in her 30s rather abruptly developed severe asthma. The family dog, which had been owned for some time, was held responsible. The husband was reluctant to part with the dog, which the wife had begun to feel he preferred to her. They had two children, a boy 7 years old and a girl 2 and one half years old. The wife became increasingly suspicious of her husband and accused him of extra-marital affairs. Eventually this man did have an affair—an apparent self-fulfilling prophecy. It was only when the divorce was well underway that the wife linked her suspiciousness to her past; her father had left her mother when the patient was 3 years old. Her daughter was now 3 years old, and it seemed that the mother needed to repeat her life history to help her solve unresolved emotions connected with her past. It was also true that the husband, who had spent a long period as a monk, had a life history he was repeating; his mother had been overbearing and rejecting.

Time: Problem or Advantage

The statement is often made, "There is no time in a busy practice to see families." This is a misconception. A family orientation is usually practical, even in a busy practice. Care with a family systems approach is a state of mind, rather than an entirely different mode of practice. Once a family has been introduced to the practice, it is rare that the whole family need be seen: 1 or 2 hours set aside per week for family interviews are all that is required. Many physicians have found it useful to set aside a half-day per week for half-hour visits for psychotherapy. This technique may eventually cut down on over-utilization of the office for minor complaints. With extension of the orientation to the whole family, time may be used partly to treat families and partly to treat groups of patients with related health problems such as obesity or alcohol abuse.

For the community nurse or the social worker, the individual is less likely to be seen alone and opportunity for observation of interrelationships are much more frequent. However, for both physician and nurse most encounters will be with individuals. It is the way that the health care practitioner sees the patient (with members of the family sitting invisibly around him or her) that distinguishes the family from the individual orientation. A single sentence of enquiry during a mother's visit with a child for immunization may reveal that the grandfather felt dizzy last week but did not think anything of it, that the mother's back has been hurting lately, and that things seem very tense at home. Suggesting that a family member visit may prevent later hospitalization or help vent feelings before they become explosive or are somatized. Concern for those family members not in the office aids in prevention of illness and anticipatory guidance and may, in the end, save time.

Time is more often the friend than the adversary of the primary care clinician. The family therapist, although spending more time over a shorter period with the family unit, does not have the benefit of an association with the family over years. As in physical illness where a tincture of time either cures or reveals the diagnosis, with families a broad understanding and a perspective over time aids enormously in family assessment and anticipating problems. Families who would never dream of visiting a marriage counsellor or family therapist gradually reveal their problems to a trusted family physician or community nurse, and allow interventions at intervals that will gradually transform a family system from one that focuses on physical illness to one that will solve problems.

The gradual acquisition of information over time from visits by different family members counterbalances the lack of time concentrated on the family unit, particularly if the clinician's thinking is focused on family interaction. Often the clinician does not focus on family problems or involve the entire family with therapy. Also, the family may revert to discussion of physical symptoms when resistant to dealing with problems of interaction. In this way, the family is able to stay with the family physician or nurse and at a later date may face the psychological issues. The social worker or psychologist who works in close association with a physician or primary care facility also derives this long-term association with families through the team. The individual or family may be seen by different members of a health care team depending on the particular need at any one time.

Mind and Body: A Unity for the Primary Care Clinician

The family therapist is not usually a physician or nurse and does not usually deal with problems of physical illness. Chronic illness and its relation to family function, acute illness, hospitalization and its effect on family function, recurrent minor illnesses, and the sickness-prone family are all considered the province of the family physician. (The evidence cited in Section III demonstrates the connection between family interaction and illness of almost every type.) This is not to say that all illness has its base in family interaction; however, all family interaction is affected in some way by illness.

Every illness is psychosomatic in that there is a somatic component and a psychic component whether the illness is physical, social, or psychiatric. The medical model has been shown to be an inadequate model to cope with the interactions between these components. Although the clinician may recognize that illness does not belong only to the mind or to the body, knowledge is often insufficient to bridge the gap between the two areas of emphasis. Endocrinal studies of the brain in depression, studies of isolation producing carcinogenesis in mice, and studies correlating stress with physical illness (see Section III) are often misinterpreted as evidence either that all disease is physical or that all disease has psychological origins. Both points of view are extreme and stem from an insistence on the mind/body split.

A knowledge of physical illness and of physical agents such as bacteria, carcinogens, and genetics related to physical illness is crucial for the social worker or a psychologist working in primary care. The physician or nurse must be convinced of the importance of family interaction in regard to illness, and the behavioral scientist also cannot afford to exclude the biomedical from the area of his or her expertise. The addition of behavioural scientists to the educational programs in family medicine in North America has been a great benefit; however, if it increases the division between patients seen to have "functional disorders" and those with "organic disorders", and between the clinicians oriented to the mind and those who focus on the body, this would be a major failure for family medicine.

In the area of diagnosis, the clinician should have sufficient knowledge of both domains and the ability to make a referral easily so that misdiagnosis is prevented. In the area of management more training is clearly required, and the manager appropriate for a given problem should be chosen. Knowledge of limits is essential for the untrained physician or nurse; attempts at family therapy are not appropriate without further training—usually of 3 years' duration. A great deal of mismanagement can occur in the hands of someone who feels he or she has expertise but is in fact ignorant of the field: family therapy, like any medical subspeciality, requires more than a 2-month elective to be handled adequately. However, with accurate assessment of families simple interventions for early problems may be well within the acceptable limits of family practice. Two rules of thumb may help: 1) the time needed to resolve a problem (if more than three sessions have taken place with little of no resolution of the problems, referral is probably indicated); and 2) be aware of the level of comfort in handling a problem (the feeling of being "out of one's depth" is often an accurate reflection of the situation. (See section on referral in Chapter 16.)

Teamwork and Use of the Community

In contrast to the family therapist, who often works alone, more and more family physicians and nurses in primary care work in a group with several health professionals who are often from different disciplines. Roles, remuneration, hierarchy, and decision-making have to be worked out; much has been written, particularly on the expanded or extended role of the nurse. Solutions to problems in these areas are sometimes poorly negotiated, with the advantages often going to the physicians in the group. Longer training, longer hours, and legal responsibility may be an added burden on the physician, but he or she is frequently poorly trained in teamwork and expects to be at the top of the hierarchy. In family medicine units, the nurse as team leader is often more appropriate, as he or she knows all families in the practice including those followed by the residents. In one practice in England the team leader is the receptionist. She has been encouraged to give feedback to the physician, for example, "The C family is worried about Mrs. C and I think you need to explain more about the hospitalization than you did, Peter". First name relationships may or may not be part of colleagial trust and does not negate the need for a leader and clear organization and for mutual respect. Working with the community is an aspect of teamwork that generally is not an aspect of family therapy (see Chapter 18).

Chapter 17

Prevention or Health Promotion

Janet Christie-Seely

Health promotion is considered an important function of the family physician. Yet it is rarely taught except in connection with immunization schedules and the "periodic health exam,"[31] which primarily deals with case finding rather than with preventing or promoting health. The medical world has focussed on disease and pathology rather than on health. Yet it is surprising to recognize that despite the many stressors, pathogens, and noxious agents in the world, we stay healthy much of the time.[1] Health, rather than disease, should be studied.

An emphasis on promotion of health and on the strengths of individuals and families has come largely from primary care nursing.[21] In an attempt to deemphasize the medical aspect of health, nurses have encouraged families to improve their own functioning and health practices.[16] Little has been done by the medical profession to study and improve family health practices. Some lay groups, notably the Catholic marriage-encounter movement, have tried to coach "normal" families to improve communication and prevent later breakdown of marriage. Few family therapists have dealt with the healthy family (a notable exception is Peggy Papp's description[26] of a project in which such families were invited to study and improve their own function with the use of sculpting and education on how families behave as a system).

What Is Prevention in Family Systems Medicine?

Prevention is not a topic of family therapists, nor is it often discussed by psychiatrists. But in family medicine it is a major *raison d'être*, a topic of much rhetoric, discussion and some research. In a linear model (the usual model in primary care) prevention is clear: the clinician simply blocks one of the steps in the linear chain of events leading to illness. In a systems model, prevention is much more difficult to discuss: the focus is on interaction in the present; causality and hence the concept of prevention tends to be seen as meaningless and irrelevant.

How do we reconcile the differences between these two professions which family systems medicine bridges? This is a particularly important question because a significant reason given for the acceptance of a family orientation is that a broader contextual approach to illness will help in the prevention of disease. There are three reasons for the differences between family therapy and family medicine in their approach to prevention:

1. Family therapy and psychiatry are both *concerned with treatment* of dysfunction. Rarely is the dysfunction in its early stages, and therefore great expertise and experience is required for treatment. A family system that has rigidified into dysfunctional patterns of communication and problem solving requires powerful and often dramatic maneuvers to shift it onto a new path. Change is the focus of family therapy, not prevention. Unlike family medicine, the families seen in family therapy tend to be incapable of initiating change in response to internal or external stresses. They require an external agent to stimulate change in behavior and relationship (induced morphogenesis).[33]

2. The principle of *equifinality* within a system implies that prevention of a particular behavior as a route to an outcome will only result in the use of a second behavior to produce the same outcome. In the case of illness, if the family's "need" for illness remains unchanged, treatment or prevention in one individual may simply result in a change in identified patient. There has been no real (second-order) change only superficial or temporary (first-order) change.[32] To a family therapist prevention is therefore a somewhat meaningless concept. (In circular thinking, at what point in the circle does one define a maneuver as prevention?)

3. Neither family therapists nor psychiatrists generally treat or even see *physical illness*. Families with admitted marital problems or behavioral problems in a child or psychiatric problems (depression, schizophrenia) tend not to be the ones who somatize.[3] Families that somatize conflict go to the internist or family physician. The internist rarely meets all family members and is unable therefore to develop a broader perspective on the disease. The family physician, however, is either trained to see or soon senses that families have something to do with illness. Aware of the literature on stress and illness,[4,7,28] he or she may recognize the role that families can play. Many family physicians begin to sense a complex interweaving of factors: the sickness role, secondary and tertiary (systems) gain, avoidance of unsatisfactory roles or relationships through illness, impact of relatives on treatment and compliance, and the physical symptoms themselves.

Taught to think in terms of prevention and wishing to improve the health of his clientele, the family physician needs help from those with expertise on the family. Working with illness inevitably raises the plea for better prevention: contact with the misery illness inflicts and experience with the irreversibility of illness once organic changes have taken place promote this concern. To ignore or deny the concept of prevention ignores the fact that time is linear: if one set of circumstances that is normally followed later in time by another set of circumstances consistently fails to occur whenever a particular maneuver is applied, then prevention is a perfectly legitimate word.

DEFINITION OF AN EFFECTIVE PREVENTIVE MEASURE

Notions of Prevention in the Medical Model

An effective preventive measure must be acceptable, do more good than harm, and should be directed at a defined disease or condition of sufficient prevalence or severity to warrant intervention. Prevention or early treatment should be more effective than treatment later in the course of the condition. Resources must be available to apply the maneuver, which should be relatively easy and cost effective.[13,6] Counselling for early family problems fulfills most of these criteria if the evidence for the stress-illness connection is accepted as indirect evidence of the family's role in causing illness. Evidence for effectiveness, and particularly cost-effectiveness, is sparse but there are at least three studies showing that utilization of medical care decreases when the psychosocial problems of patients are attended to.[10,14,20] The family physician has a major role in preventing illness through such counselling for stress and early dysfunction. The family feels no stigma in consulting a family physician who has had the role of trusted family confidant over long periods, and is available particularly at times of crisis when such counselling is both needed and more effective.

PRIMARY, SECONDARY, AND TERTIARY PREVENTION

Primary, secondary, and tertiary prevention is defined by epidemiology as prevention of the occurrence of disease, prevention of its development (early diagnosis and treatment), and rehabilitation or maintenance without deterioration of chronic disease. In the context of families, primary prevention includes recognition of high-risk stages in the normal family life cycle and anticipatory guidance and counselling to prevent the dysfunction or illness associated with stress. Counselling and facilitation of coping with medical crises, which are considered high-risk periods for the development of illness in other family members, could also be examples of primary prevention: in anticipation of the death of a patient with terminal illness, family interviews, support by the physician, and bereavement counselling may decrease the incidence of disease and death in relatives.[12]

Increased vigilance with high-risk families can improve secondary prevention or early diagnosis. High-risk families are those with frequent illness in the past or in which there is sufficient dysfunction suggesting increased likelihood of illness. Hinkle and Plummer[17] have shown that illness-prone families have both a high incidence of dysfunction (divorce, delinquency, imprisonment) and of disease and early death. Increased alertness to the symptoms of physical illness in such families and attempts to help in the area of dysfunction either by counselling or by sophisticated referral to a family therapist may prevent illness. It is for this group that studies of utilization of care indicate probable effectiveness of psychosocial interventions. A real change in the family system in the direction of improved communication and less need for scapegoating or the sickness role would be a good example of primary prevention of illness and secondary prevention of dysfunction.

In families with severe chronic dysfunction, tertiary prevention (maintenance and support) are all that can be achieved. In a fashion analogous to chronic congestive heart failure, the system (body or family) reorganizes around the symptoms in such a way that they have become an essential part of homeostasis.[23] Occasionally, family therapy may trigger second-order change and the need for symptoms will disappear. Primary prevention for the next generation in these families may be achieved by increased understanding of family processes.

HEALTH PROMOTION AND LIFESTYLE

Much attention has been paid in medicine and society to fitness programs and campaigns against smoking. It is apparent to most family physicians that including the family in advice about diet, counselling against smoking, alcohol control, and advice about exercise and recreation increases the efficacy of a patient's attempt to alter lifestyle. Many physicians are aware of the literature on family and compliance[30] and realize that compliance with a prescribed change in lifestyle as well as with taking medications is particularly enhanced by including the spouse.[18]

PAYMENT FOR TALK OR ACTION?

Funding may reflect the value assigned to prevention and the belief in the efficacy of counselling. Separation of the emotional (functional) and organic aspects of disease persists in medical circles and influences fees and funding. The physician is often uncomfortable in the role of psychotherapist, feeling that psychotherapy is outside the province of general medicine, particularly in the absence of somatic symptoms.[5] He or she is reluctant to charge for something so intangible as mere talk; the physician is someone who is active and feels incompetent when nothing is done. Even if such therapy appears to help or prevent further problems, the physician is unlikely to give the credit to the psychotherapy.[5] Conversely, in some areas where third-party payment is involved, the general physician often has financial considerations that will decide whether preventive counselling is done.

LIMITATIONS OF THE MEDICAL MODEL

Stress and Illness: Which Comes First?

The large body of research linking stress, family, and illness has been reviewed in Section III. Studies have either emphasized the impact of stress (or the family) on disease or the impact of disease on the family.[29] The scientific method, with its necessary isolation of variables, imposes such a format, so that researchers, though no doubt aware that the relation of stress and illness is bidirectional, often get caught up in circular arguments of which came first. They sometimes seem to forget that they are simply extrapolating from a highly complex series of interrelationships. For example, critics of the Holmes and Rahe's Social Readjustment Rating Scale have pointed out that 29 of the 43 events are events that may be symptoms or consequences of illness.[19] In his extensive review of stress and premorbid psychological factors and cancer incidence Fox[11] finds this to be "a fundamental problem." For Fox, causality of illness is complex: basic pathology $\longrightarrow$ stressful event $\longrightarrow$ illness, but is still a linear and unidirectional "chain of many links." In contrast, Michael Kerr[22] uses a systems view of cancer to describe a possible feedback system between cell and environment in which environmental stresses promote cellular growth, which in turn stimulates a defense response in the host that aggravates the cellular dysfunction, thus completing the circle. The concepts of feedback and homeostasis are the essential differences.

In a linear model of illness and stress, prevention clearly must be aimed at stress reduction or improvement of coping or defense mechanisms. This logical approach can at times lead to problems of first-order change.[32] The logical solution to a problem often does not work, yet a common response when it is not working is to assume one has not tried hard enough and that more of the same solution will work better. Inflexible families often persist with solutions that actually aggravate and maintain the problem.

For example, a man who has had a heart attack has a wife anxious to decrease his load of stress. Every time he lifts a shovel to the snow, or stays late at work she reminds him to slow down and take care of his heart. The more she attempts to decrease his stress, the more it increases and the less compliant he becomes.

The division into primary, secondary, and tertiary prevention may be useful in epidemiology but tends to simply add confusion to the concept of family prevention. It is arbitrary whether one assigns a primary, secondary, or tertiary preventive value to a given counselling session. Often the session may help at all three levels. "Health promotion" is a better term for this kind of care, but "health maintenance" may be a more appropriate term for some families (as in the case of the P. family in Chapter 20).

A SYSTEMS FORMULATION OF HEALTH PROMOTION

Family dysfunction and illness are interconnected and concurrently developing problems. Stress imposed from outside the system may exaggerate both dysfunction and illness, which in turn produce their own stress that can contribute to a downward spiral of progressive dysfunction and disease. Illness frequently reflects poor problem solving at a particular level—whether cellular, organ system, individual, family, community, or national.

A healthy system at any level is one in which there is flexible hierarchical control that allows sufficient individuation of the parts of the system with a healthy balance between the forces of individuation and separation and the forces of cohesion and togetherness. There is good communication within the system and with outside systems. Such a definition of health provides an appropriate goal or standard to guide intervention.

Families seen by the family physician, in contrast to those seen by the family therapist, tend to be less dysfunctional and rigid and are usually capable of constituting their own change. However, most families sometimes require an extra nudge from an outsider, be it a neighbor, an extended family member, or the family physician. The need for change in rules accelerates at certain periods in the family life cycle, the so-called "normal" life crises. These family tasks require second-order change, or change in rules or structure, for family members to grow and individuate.

At times of developmental crises, and when illness or death superimpose another type of crisis, family flexibility increases and the ability to find new solutions and different ways of doing things increases. The possibility for growth and change is greater, but so is the possibility for deterioration and further dysfunction. It is at these points that the family physician, particularly, can have a role in nudging a family in the direction of greater health.

Medical Labels and Health Promotion

A medical diagnosis results from the interplay of biomedical facts, the environment, and the doctor-patient relationship, but this diagnostic label, in turn, may become a potent factor in maintaining the role of illness in family dynamics. The family physician must have a broader understanding of illness, as opposed to disease. As Zola[34] has pointed out, patients in the hospital do not have a significantly different set of symptoms than those who are outside the hospital.

Approximately one fourth of patients with a given symptom visit a doctor. The patient's culture, family, personality, past experience with illness and health professionals, and the meaning of the symptom (to both patient and family) all help determine whether the symptom is ignored or emphasized, and whether action of some sort is taken (see Chapter 7). Balint[2] has indicated how the doctor and patient relationship is an essential part of the process of developing a disease: a person produces symptoms until the health professional reacts by labelling him as a patient with a disease.

A specific medical label may be picked up by the family system in a way many doctors are quite unaware. The concept of secondary gain is familiar: tertiary gain has been defined as the gain of the larger system. (As described in Section III, an asthmatic child may become the means of detouring parental conflict in a "psychosomatic family."[25])

Once labelled, the patient must want to be cured consciously and subconsciously and give the physician the mandate to intervene. The wish to get better is clearly influential in prognosis. Health promotion can only take place with the patient's cooperation. Society may grant certain mandates to clinicians, such as the right to tell a patient to stop smoking to advise recreation or rest, or to counsel about diet and lifestyle whether the patient wants to hear this or not.

In the area of family life the mandate is much less clear. Some studies have in fact shown that the public does not expect or wish their physician to advise them on marital difficulties.[24] However, once a trusting relationship has been developed, if advice is tactfully given it is almost always possible for the clinician to have some positive effect on the family context of health.

Interventions are aimed at improving communication within the system and communication with the outside systems (particularly with the health profession) and at increasing the family awareness of possible alternative behaviors. The clinician's diagnostic impressions and teaching a systems view of family functioning and illness allows the family to change if they so choose.

The Role of the Family Physician in Health Promotion

[*Editor's Note:* The following interventions are outlined in greater detail in Chapter 15. They are repeated here to emphasize the aspect of prevention or health promotion.]

Anticipatory guidance is a primarily preventive maneuver aimed at optimizing preparation for the normative crises of the family life cycle. Planning enhances problem solving, decreases tension, and may decrease the incidence of stress-related illness or dysfunction. If communication is encouraged by the clinician and early problems dealt with throughout the life cycle, adaptation and successful completion of the various tasks is more likely. High-risk families with a tendency to produce illness when under stress, or with obvious dysfunctional relationships, require close monitoring during times of stress and more rigorous efforts at anticipatory guidance. High-risk periods of increased stress occur during the preschool period of children, adolescence, the pending departure of the children, retirement, and the death of a spouse. There is evidence that help with anticipatory grief for a spouse's death and counselling during the bereavement period lead to a decrease in morbidity and mortality.[12,27]

Facilitation and Support

The main function of the family physician in helping high-risk families or families at high-risk stages in the life cycle is facilitation of coping and communication within the family. The physician should be skilled in family interview techniques when these are needed to help family members improve their own problem-solving abilities: a family meeting can be called when an elderly person living alone has just suffered a stroke that sufficiently alters functioning but does not necessarily imply placement in a nursing home. A solution reached by the entire family may help prevent further deterioration of the elderly person, hospitalization for a fractured hip from a fall over a loose carpet, or malnutrition resulting from inability to get meals. It may also promote health by preventing isolation; families often avoid a relative they would like to help but lack the necessary resources or knowledge. The physician can coach the family in working through the various problems. Home assessment can suggest how to avoid obvious dangers and what minor changes and equipment should be recommended that will make all the difference to long-term care in the home.

A family conference does not imply family dysfunction. However, it does imply the need for some change in family rules and habits and probably the need for improved communication to meet the crisis. The family may grow with the experience and be better able to handle another crisis alone in the future.

Chronic illness is often managed with total disregard for the family. Yet it is known that chronic illness puts extreme stress on the family that may result in divorce or illness in another family member.[9] Clinics often see the individual patient alone, discouraging the presence of the spouse or relative who sits anxiously in the waiting room. It is surprising how we can forget to recognize the family suffering in the midst of investigation and sophisticated maneuvers to relieve the patient's suffering.

The P. family were first seen by a family physician 4 years after Mr. P. received a kidney transplant. Within 10 minutes of the onset of the interview, three of the four children began to cry in response to the question, "How are things at home?" One year before the interview the mother had suddenly developed agoraphobia and had become unable to function, so that the two older girls had to do the grocery shopping and many other chores. Two main problems surfaced. First, the father's illness was seen as legitimizing his role as authoritarian and his abdication from any responsibility in the household; everything became the responsibility of his wife. Second, the family's rules of communication were that no anger, sadness, or worry should be expressed to protect family members from further hurt. Had emotional expression been facilitated and role changes and communication discussed with this family at the time of transplant (or, even better, when the diagnosis of chronic renal disease was made), and had the family been part of the management team, their distress might have been prevented.

Describing behavior or symptoms as normal for a given situation is reassuring; it may give people under stress permission to have emotions that they would rather not acknowledge, and it may prevent abrupt acting out of emotion. The clinician can say to a mother of a 2 and 1/2-year-old child, "Most mothers of children his age are ready to commit murder at times. It's o.k. to feel like throwing him on the floor, it's just not o.k. to do it." Normalizing statements about the common reactions to a terminal illness or the typical phases of mourning and all the dramatic symptoms that can accompany them can prevent serious negative labelling by the patient or others.

Information and Education

Giving information about illness (and the reaction to it), stress (and its ability to promote illness), disease, and the resources that can be used in treating disease can all improve family coping. Knowledge decreases the ambiguity and uncertainty of a situation and broadens an individual's or family's awareness of alternatives. This can help prevent a further downward spiral from increased stress and can enlarge the family's repertoire of coping behaviors in a crisis situation.

Specific Suggestions

Specific suggestions can indicate resources in the community or measures to reduce prolonged stress, or sources of information on illness or family function[26] or parenting and effective communication.[15] Often such suggestions are new alternatives for the family and promote second-order change. Suggesting that the couple communicate differently or that they spend a weekend alone may start a chain reaction of change.

Positive relabelling, reframing, and *insight therapy* all represent attempts to push the family out of their present frame of reference to a perspective outside its particular system. Relabelling the scapegoated child as the parental rescuer who helps the family to avoid conflict, or the sick person as the strong one who organizes the household (instead of the weak one as previously perceived) helps change the rules of the system and produce second-order change.

A woman in her early 40s had breast cancer. Her mother had died of breast cancer when she was 10 years old, and her greatest fear was that she would die when her youngest son, with whom she closely identified, was 10 years old. He was 9 years old at the time of diagnosis. The woman's father had been alcoholic and unable to cope as a widower. Her husband was now showing a strong tendency to the same problem. Her family history was repeating itself. None of these difficulties, however, were expressed in the family; "the problem" was the older son, 14 years old. He was getting into more and more trouble at school and was unruly at home.

A single family interview was able to relabel the problem as the son's attempt to deflect the family's anxiety away from the real issue. Every time the topic of the mother's illness was approached, the older son would draw attention to himself or the father would draw attention to the son's behavior. It was easy for the family to recognize this after the sequence of events had happened three or four times. It was also easy for the family to see the father's behavior and excessive drinking as a similar phenomenon.

The family-oriented physician suggested that they use the older son's behavior as an indication that the family was avoiding expression of emotion. Whenever he behaved badly, the family was asked to say aloud, "What are we all trying to avoid?" A lengthy and emotional discussion of the mother's illness and prognosis facilitated family communication, making it impossible for the family to go back to the point they were at before. Follow-up showed that the older son's behavior in school had improved and, in addition, that the father's drinking had decreased to the level of social drinking. The family was now solving the problem of care for their increasingly weak mother very well.

Referral

Referral for family therapy of a dysfunctional family may play a major role in health promotion. Huygen has shown the drop in health care visits following family therapy.[20] The ability to suggest family therapy in a way the family can accept is a skill needed by the family physician. Referral may require several family meetings to achieve. Similarly, referral to community agencies for support can be an important component of health maintenance by the family physician. There is an extensive literature showing that the degree of social support and the number of networks in which an individual or family play a meaningful role correlate with protection from disease.[8]

REFERENCES

1. Antonovsky A: *Health, Stress & Coping*. San Francisco, Jossey-Bass, 1979.
2. Balint M: *The Doctor, His Patient, and the Illness*. New York, International Universities Press, 1952.
3. Bowen M: *Family Therapy in Clinical Practice*. New York, Jason Aronson, 1978.
4. Cassel J: Physical illness in response to stress, in Levine S, Scoth N A (eds): *Social Stress*. Chicago, Aldine, 1978.

5. Castelnuovo-Tadesco P: *The Twenty-Minute Hour.* Boston, Little, Brown and Co., 1965.

6. Christie-Seely J: Preventive medicine and the family. *Can Fam Physician* 27: 449, 1981.

7. Christie-Seely J: Life stress and illness: A systems approach. *Can Fam Physician* 29:533, 1983.

8. Cobb S: Social support as moderator of life stress. *Psychsom Med* 38:300, 1976.

9. Downes J: Chronic disease among spouses. Milbank Memorial Fund Quarterly.

10. Follette W, Cummings NA: Psychiatric services and medical utilization in a prepaid health plan setting. *Med Care* 5:25, 1967.

11. Fox BH: Premorbid psychological factors as related to cancer incidence. *J Behav Med* 1:45, 1978.

12. Gerber I, Wiever A, Battin D, et al: Brief therapy to the aged bereaved, in Schoenberg B, et al (eds): *Bereavement: Its Psychosocial Aspects.* New York, Columbia University Press, 1975.

13. Geyman JP: Preventive medicine in family practice: A reassessment. *J Fam Pract* 9:35, 1979.

14. Goldberg ID, Krantz G, Locke BZ: Effects of a short-term outpatient psychiatric therapy benefit on the utilization of medical services in a prepaid group practice medicine program. *Med Care* 8:419, 1970.

15. Gordon T: *P.E.T. Parent Effectiveness Training.* New York, North American Library, 1975.

16. Gottlieb L: *Styles of Nursing as Practiced at the Workshop, a Health Resource.* Montreal, McGill School of Nursing, 1982, pp. 1-98.

17. Hinkle LE Jr, Plummer N: Life stress and industrial absenteeism: The concentration of illness and absenteeism in one segment of a working population. *Ind Med Surg* 21:363, 1952.

18. Hoebel FC: Brief family-interactional therapy in the management of cardiac-related high risk behaviors. *J Fam Pract* 3:613, 1976.

19. Hudgens RW: Personal catastrophe and depression: A consideration of the subject with respect to medically ill adolescents and a requiem for introspective life event studies, in Dohrenwend BP, Dohrenwend BS (eds): *Stressful Live Events: Their Nature and Effects.* New York, Wiley, 1974.

20. Huygen FJA: *Family Medicine: The Medical Life History of Families.* The Netherlands, Dekker & Van de Vegt, 1978.

21. Hymovitch D: *Family Health Care.* New York, McGraw-Hill, 1973.

22. Kerr M: Cancer and the family emotional system, in Goldberg J (ed): *Psychotherapeutic Treatment of Cancer.* New York, Free Press, 1981.

23. Kerr M: *Family systems theory and therapy,* in Gorman I, Kniskem DP (eds): *Handbook of Family Therapy.* New York, Brunner/Mazel, 1981.

24. Kiraly FA, Coulton CJ, Graham A: How family practice patients view their utilization of mental health services. *J Fam Pract* 15:317, 1982.

25. Minuchin S, Rosman BL, Baker L: *Psychosomatic Families. Anorexia Nervosa in Context.* Cambridge, Harvard University Press, 1978.

26. Papp P, Silverstein O, Carter E: Family sculpting in preventive work with well families. *Fam Process* 12:197, 1973.

27. Parkes CM: *Bereavement: Studies of Grief in Adult Life.* New York, International Universities Press, 1972.

28. Rahe RH, Mahan J, Arthur R: Prediction of near future health change from subjects preceding life changes. *J Psychosom Res* 14:401, 1970.

29. Ransom DC: The rise of family medicine: New roles for behavioral science. *Marr Fam Rev* 4:31, 1981.

30. Schmidt DD: The family as the unit of medical care. *J Fam Pract* 7:303, 1978.

31. Spitzer WO, et al: Periodic (vs. annual) health examination. *Can Med Assoc J* 121:1–38, 1979.

32. Watzlawick P, Weakland JJ, Frisch R: *Change: Problem Formation and Problem Resolution.* New York, W.W. Norton, 1974.

33. Wertheim E: Family unit therapy and the science and typology of family systems. *Fam Process* 12:343, 1973.

34. Zola IK: Culture and symptoms: An analysis of patients' presenting complaints. *Am Sociol Rev* 31:615, 1966.

Chapter 18
Working with the Community

Jacqueline McClaran

DEFINITION OF A COMMUNITY

The ability to conceptualize systems enhances efficiency of clinical judgement, whatever the system might be (organ systems, the total patient, the family system(s), the community(ies) in which the family lives). The community can be a source of health and of illness, and can in turn be influenced by those living in it. The health professional is an important agent for change, as well as for improving communication between community, subsystems, and resources. The clinician able to assess a community and use its resources can enhance patient care efficiently.

A community can be described in terms of its geography, topography, demography, epidemiology, and sociology. For example, where do people live, work, and spend leisure? How healthy and wealthy are they? How old is the population and what are the family structures? What are the institutions industries, and agencies which are a part of a community? One might describe one's own community in all these terms or qualities, and yet still not convey the full personality of, or the feel for a community.[19] Like a family, a community is more than the sum of its parts.

THE COMMUNITY AS THE CONTEXT
OF THE FAMILY

The clinician's diagnostic and therapeutic impact is strengthened when he or she understands health in the context of the family's or individual's community, as well as in the context of the family.[2] The community is a source of health to families and individuals. It provides cultural stimulation and job opportunities, which in turn influence the quality of life and health status.[3] For example, depression, immobility, and poor nutrition in the elderly may stem from isolation, and may be avoided through the use of community lunch clubs, day centers, and exercise classes.[18] The family influences habits of eating, exercise, and cultural values; in the same way, the community, the extended family, and neighboring cultures define systems and determine health behavior patterns.[19]

The Community as a Source of Health

The following are some examples of the community network as a source of health:

1.   Special transport for the handicapped allows the disabled family member to work outside the home. The availability of this service relieves other family members of some caretaking responsibilities, and allows them to pursue their own work and leisure outside the home. As a result, the disabled member is perceived as more capable, self-perception is enhanced, and quality of life for the entire family may be ameliorated.

2.   A community that provides child day care for preschoolers allows new mothers more choice about returning to work. Where no day care exists, the family may choose to hire help in the home, in which case only the well-paid female worker will return to work early. The results of day care can be very beneficial: the child is perceived by his family as more independent because he or she is learning things outside the home; the child may receive more and varied stimuli at day care; the mother's personal development and lifestyle may be ameliorated; the mother's income may increase the family's quality of life; the lifestyle of the entire family may be altered, since all members may now share home maintenance and parenting of the new member; the image of the role of "woman" and "mother" may be altered for growing children or husband or for the mother herself. Female children in such families may see themselves with more options because of mother's role-modelling; whereas male children may have a better chance of working well with future female co-workers, and of sharing household responsibilities.

3.   "Middle-generation" family members who have just finished raising their children, and who now may be required or inclined to adopt parenting roles towards their own now-aging parents, may have more freedom if day centers for the elderly exist in their own community. Without day centers and clubs for the elderly, the care-taking role of this generation may change the object of care from children, who are 21 years old, towards their parents who may be 75 years old and greater. The middle generation may not resist this new role, because in the short run it avoids the "empty nest" syndrome. In the long run, however, this change may make the grandparents too dependent and tie down the middle generation more than their children ever did. Twenty years later the now middle-aged generation may go from the "empty nest" to their own dependency, without a rewarding retirement phase.

4.   Day centers also prevent or delay institutionalization for the physically capable but forgetful elderly who can no longer stay at home unsupervised or unobserved.[18] These elderly living in our communities can be a valuable influence on family life and culture. Margaret Mead felt that children benefited from contact with grandparents, who were someone to run to or think of when the parents were angry. This safety valve is missing in our

single unit North American families, where budding egos have no defense or recourse.[17] Day centers also can help the elderly maintain self-esteem and improve confidence and independence. The entire family's perception of aging as a developmental maturing and adapting phenomenon evolves in their personal, family, and social lives.

5.   Rapid public transport brings working family members home less exhausted, and may allow for quiet family time before supper.

6.   "Corner stores," which make food shopping available near residential areas, allow various family members to do shopping on the way home from work during the week and to have weekends for leisure. Access to stores determines who shops when and affects family patterns (see Chapter 14 to see how the entire family is affected by role changes of one member).[8]

The Community as a Source of Sickness

What follows are some examples of the community as a source of health problems to individuals and families. Patterns of housing, industry, transportation, and economics affect individual and family health as surely as a sedentary lifestyle affects the epidemiology of cardiovascular disease.[12]

1.   The incidence and prevalence of depression and paranoia increase in the community during economically difficult times (such as the closing of a factory). Family health is affected throughout the community and so are doctors' practice patterns. Several studies have investigated the physiological effects of unemployment.[10]

2.   Community members speak with pride of their local industry, which may even provide their livelihood. However, individual workers may suffer industrial health hazards; chemicals wastes may be inflicted on the entire community.

3.   Increasing population density may lead to higher incidence and prevalence of stress and illness and their consequences. On the other hand, it may provide resources, such as neighbors close enough to help with meals, or to look in on a frail elderly person.

4.   Apartment buildings rising higher than two stories are associated with higher crime rates due to feelings of "depersonalization" experienced by people living in and near these settings.

The community thus influences family health; conversely, family and individual patterns influence community structure and resources.[15] If the nuclear family has no grandparent or other member nearby to help just after the birth of a new family member, the demand for community health workers increases. If an elderly member has no family member nearby to shop for groceries during the harsh winter, demands on home help will increase. If home help is not available, emergency room admissions for hypothermia, pneumonia, and other deteriorated states that follow on poor nutrition will increase among the frail elderly. Community self-help groups and pressure groups spring up where the need is identified and reinforce community awareness of local problems.[4]

THE CLINICIAN IN THE CONTEXT OF THE COMMUNITY

Most community nurses, doctors, and other health care workers expect to live in and serve the same community(ies) for a lifetime. Family doctors who do manage to stay in a given community usually express satisfaction with quality of life and lifestyle in both personal and professional spheres.[7,22] A satisfied community physician is likely to operate in a network with other physicians, other professionals, and nonprofessional helping groups. Generalists who are disenchanted with their role or who return for further training in another specialty complain of professional isolation and loneliness, feelings of incompetency in handling overwhelming problems, boredom, and "lack of pathology" in practice. "Helping people" (a category which includes all health care workers) risk "burn-out," the feeling that one's work cannot make any difference, or that he or she just cannot keep it up any longer.

Isolation merits a special mention.[22] The physician who does not work with or near other clinicians may avoid isolation by heavily using telephone consultation with other health care workers. On the other hand, working in a group is no guarantee against isolation for the clinician who sees the community reality reflected only by what he or she is able to perceive in patients that present episodically in the office.[9] The clinician may diagnose and treat the broken arm, and miss the family violence. He or she may trea' many pneumonias and not be aware of this year's influenza epidemic. Isolation may be caused by a fear of reaching out to the community, uncovering a huge number of health problems, or a type of problem; this is particularly true when the health problem is intimately related to the social milieu. Isolation may lead to inadequate management. Isolation breeds isolation.

For a successful "marriage" to community the clinician must take an extended role and needs a network to carry out this role. An extended role means taking a wide view of health issues. The term, "network," means that the clinician perceives himself or herself as one of many workers in a health system.[23] This orientation allows the now less crisis-oriented physician to see health in a wide definition and to think in terms of illness prevention. The network supports the health care worker as well as community members. The health care worker in this alternate role does not circumvent responsibility; to the contrary, he or she has a greater impact on health, and is thus more satisfied. The clinician can benefit from relationships with family, friends, neighbors, and other agencies in constructing the network necessary to every helping person.

Since the physician is seen as a helping person by the individuals, the family, and the community, he or she is often asked to sit on school boards, or to be an agent of social change (a role sometimes requested by local community groups). The difficulty is that the health care worker is neither necessarily educated nor necessarily equipped to deal with such issues. If the health care worker has been working in a team in practice he or she may feel trained to be a more effective group member. Understanding group dynamics is similar to understanding families and has theory backed by research, now taught by some medical and nursing schools.[1,23]

There are additional pay-offs for thinking in terms of interrelated systems in family and community. Clinicians whose philosophical frame of reference is that of interrelated family and community systems receive benefits in their own personal life; this concept is brought to their own cultural value system. They understand who helps whom, when, who asks, and how to ask; they are more effective and efficient in relating to friends, family, and in finding their own resources such as dentist, plumber, notary, and other helping people. This personal satisfaction, resulting from a comprehensive view of one's own culture, is also part of a system in that it feeds back into professional skills. The "participant-observer" obtaining first-hand knowledge in community systems is professionally satisfied because he or she is effective in understanding the system and efficient in making an impact on it.

A PRACTICAL GUIDE TO COMMUNITY ASSESSMENT

The clinician assesses the community in order to choose it, and in order to be therapeutically armed for systems crises anticipated in everyday practice. What follows is a practical guide to the rationale (the whys) and methodologies (the hows) of "canvassing a community." (Persons who have already selected a community or set up a practice should skip the first paragraph and go on to the section "Canvassing to build a therapeutic armamentarium—Why?")

How to Canvas to Seclect Your Community

The community(ies) in which you, the clinican, choose to live and work must suit you and each member of your family in regard to lifestyle and personal and professional development. Both the long- and short-term advantages of a particular community must be considered. For example, an isolated fishing village may have a stable population, low crime rate, and a beautiful environment to offer the clinician. While the quality of family and community social life is high, the leisure activities are limited for the most part to hunting and fishing. In another setting, the transient population would make establishing long-lasting friendships difficult for you and your family. It should be remembered that other professionals determine your referral pattern. For example, if you do not plan to deliver babies, you need, at minimum, an obstetrician, or hospital service within 30 miles of good road.

The professional climate must suit your particular style; perhaps you do not need a group practice to keep you interested in your work. If, however, you are completely on your own, you will need to get away periodically for educational refresher courses. What is the history of the previous health care workers in the same community or health care center? Will you accommodate their patterns or overcome them? For example, an experienced family practitioner was approached to move to a university family medicine training center in a high-powered, specialist-oriented university hospital; he became intimidated, stopped doing obstetrics within 2 years. Another example is a university-trained family practitioner who bought a practice in an isolated village. The previous doctor never took vacations, was on call 24 hours each day, and responded to all requests for house calls, treated most acute illnesses with penicillin injections, drank heavily, and died at the age of 54 of a heart attack. Five years passed before the new doctor had full community support, having re-educated the entire community to many new methods of operating, including tape-recorded telephone messages.

A home care nurse working for the public health system was assigned to a small, leftist community activist group. The integration of her skills in this milieu was extremely difficult because she found the group's methods unprofessional, and because the group was very suspicious of her professionalism. A productive working relationship was eventually established; however, the nurse left this post within 8 months due to burn-out.

When you assess a community where you may live and work for the rest of your life, visit community groups and schools at least 6 months in advance of your arrival. Write letters. Telephone people who have left the community. Obtain information from the local government and the Chamber of Commerce; learn the town history. The clinician and his or her family who learn about their community can avoid some pitfalls and be prepared to deal with others.[13]

Canvassing to Build a Therapeutic Armamentarium—Why?

Now that you have picked your community—why canvas? To "canvas" means to learn the problems of your community, to understand its resources, and its epidemiology.[18] This knowledge will reinforce your power to deal with systems crisis by compensating for your bias resulting from your hospital training by assisting functional working relationships, and by promoting prevention and professional satisfaction.

Today many hospital-trained health care workers have available to them innovative on-site training that matches educational objectives better than ever before.[6] However, most training is still based in large, prestigious university hospitals whose link to community and home care is tenuous at best. For in-patients, a hospital ward's connection to community services (including the primary care doctor) takes place only through the social worker, who must first receive a formal referral. The result is that the hospital-trained physician may perceive the community (all communities) as devoid of resources.

Formal family medicine training programs treat patients who are in the community. However, even in this setting, it is often the family medicine team nurse who has developed expertise in community services and resources, and who has a broad perspective on client needs that allow the selection of appropriate services and the connection of clients to these services. The nurse is often "delegated" to make house calls because the resident is "too busy." The nurse integrates the health-illness continuum with social and environmental problems, which results in excellent service with a wider scope than either the hospital social worker or the family doctor could have provided alone. However, the consequences are that clinicians training in this setting are not educated to assess community resources and do not relate to them easily. If this includes you, systematically canvassing your community is part of your remedial learning and recovery from training that is primarily (and perhaps necessarily) hospital-based.[21]

Trust, Contracts, and Efficiency and Effectiveness

Doctors and nurses are busy, and need to be efficient. When you are dealing with a multi-systems problem, you need to obtain help on your first phone call. Make it happen; learn the resources thoroughly and in advance. Go and meet the people you will be dealing with (social workers, clinical psychologists, community workers, and volunteers). Personal contact builds trust and keeps communication lines open. "Contract" with various agencies and helping groups—that is, find out who will respond to what, and under which circumstances. In this way, you will minimize loss of your valuable time and get the services to your distressed patient as quickly as possible. An example of the hazards of skipping preliminary community assessment is the following:

> In Quebec, the Ministry of Social Affairs allocated the budget for "home help" services to a private agency in the territory of a Montreal department of community health. This budget would normally be given to a local community service center if one existed in the given territory; in this

case, the private agency took the liberty of adding the criterion of "poverty" to eligibility for its sevices. Being unaware of the reasons for the organization's failure to respond to the needs of certain referred clients, community physicians subsequently did not refer other clients, and effectively delayed help for recognized needs.

Prevention

By definition, medical crises are distressing to you and your patient and are not predictable. In addition, they disrupt your office and interfere with your family life. Knowing the resources in your community in a personal and concrete way facilitates your ability and inclination to identify problems and risks early. You will be less afraid to face a difficult problem. Early recognition of risk factors allows you to *plan* intervention, rather than to wait for and to dread the need to respond to crises. You can structure your professional time more efficiently. For example, for an isolated, visually impaired, not so agile elderly patient who occasionally forgets to pay heating bills (and who is at risk to fall down the stairs and break her hip and then to be found dehydrated, hypothermic, and confused several days later) the community doctor might consider the following:

1. the "daily hello"—a daily phone service for the elderly that ameliorates their orientation and isolation, and alerts someone if the phone is not answered;
2. the community worker—who assesses the home environment, finds and corrects the slippery rug in a poorly lit hallway, and helps with bills, cleaning, cooking, and shopping; and
3. a senior's group—which may be a lunch club, day center, or community club. The physician's preventive interventions are especially useful in caring for the frail elderly who are often unwilling or unable to identify potential problems, and do not see the dangers of their environment and will not ask for help.

Knowing What to Expect

Satisfaction and management of time improve when the clinician knows what to expect. If he or she has canvassed the community, the epidemiology of the practice can be predicted. For example, inadequate psychiatric assistance may mean that you must allow for some 30- to 40-minute sessions in your office each week. Or, if you discover that there are many elderly persons in your rural, snow-laden town, you will have to organize your practice to make many housecalls. Thus, community canvassing contributes to access to appropriate resources and is efficient and effective chronologically, clinically, and economically.

Building the Therapeutic Armamentarium; How to Assess a Community

A method of community assessment should be defined that will arm you for systems crises. Reach out to existing resources to learn about their services and to build the alliances that form the basis of your future working relationships. Start by obtaining resource lists from local community groups such as Catholic family services, churches, local community health centers, and government and social service agencies. A wide range of agencies are capable of providing a wide range of potential assistance to you and your future patients, and include private nursing, home maintenance, women's shelters, self-help programs, companions, social service, grocers who deliver, day care for elderly and children, and police and fire departments. Other sources of information include licensing bodies for physicians, the hospital phone book, the hospital liaison nurse, the community health nurse coordinator, the post office, and the schools.

Look for clinical psychologists, pediatricians with special interests, and physicians with interests in sports injuries, etc. Contact public and community health agencies, the local department of health, the hospital medical director, and social service agencies. Special additional interest groups or resources may be appropriate for certain areas; consider for example, agricultural co-ops, the Ministry of Fisheries and Forests, or leaders of the minority community. Once you have compiled a list of resources, select the most appropriate groups and contact someone in each group. Phone; visit; ask questions. These are "helping people" just like you and will be only too glad to help.

Ask each group what services they provide. For example, if vaccines are supplied, are they free? How are they distributed? Who is eligible? Ask about catchment areas, eligibility, and hours of service. Obtain further information about the characteristics of the community from each group. For example, if you will be serving a particular community with a very low rate of alcoholism, you can expect to spend very little time identifying helping groups for future patients with this problem.

Make your assessment of services an ongoing task. Your personal contacts may change jobs or the agency itself may change, developing new services and terminating others. For example, a convalescent care hospital recently established a respite care program for families maintaining frail, dependent elderly at home. Each time you call to ask for something for any single client, check on the other services available.

In a small town, formal outreach to community resources is easy—you meet a few people, and that is sufficient. These persons may in fact be the same people you met when you were assessing the community for your own needs; there are just a few school principals, and there may be only one judge. The one and only community worker may come knocking on *your* door as you arrive! In a large town there may be three or more school boards and 30 to 50 schools. You cannot meet with them all. Start by identifying the community worker whose territory best matches your geographic office site. In the United Kingdom, this may be as simple as phoning the health visitor. Invite this person to your office; ask how the network operates.

When you are approaching agencies, groups, hospitals, and institutions, do not assume that workers in any given organization are unified. Goals, disciplines, and styles split them from each other. Even in the very integrated groups, no single person can truly represent or speak for the agency. When you evaluate fellow professionals and professional groups, remember that even the best community assessment does not always give the inside story on competency. Sometimes the informal telephone network will give more helpful practical information.

Feeling overwhelmed? Get help to do the outreach assessment. University students and study groups may make assessments for you which may be even more sensitive than the physician's more formal contact. In one case, students in a program offering a Master's of Nursing assessed the Notre Dame de Grâce community (in Canada) in 1980, covering such items as green spaces, transport, and access to health care services, and discovered in the process some of the more subtle network issues. They described one group of community workers as suspicious and militant, whereas community physicians could observe only the symptoms of trouble—two changes of leadership in an 18-month period.

THE COMMUNITY AS A RESOURCE FOR THE CLINICIAN

In the section above, why and how to canvas a community both for the purpose of choosing a community and for the purpose of enhancing one's therapeutic and diagnostic armamentarium have been outlined. The health care worker who has followed these working guidelines has achieved the following: he or she understands the sociology of the community, who calls on whom, when and for what reasons; has his or her own place in, and personal knowledge of the community; can identify problems early; knows the epidemiology of the community; relates to the microcultures, the social support and belief systems of the families in the practice; knows the transport system; knows the demographics of the community, the ethnic areas, and the economic map; and achieves a creative approach to problem solving and resolution.

What if the patient does not agree that the problem needs attention? For example, the grandmother who will not give up independence to receive shopping or cleaning help. What is early intervention? What is the decision-making process that predicts which resources are best applied to the problem, when to apply them, and at what stages of the problem's unfolding? The clinician can assure rational choice of resources by applying Donabedian's hierarchy of need identification[5] as a predictor of the ideal service required, and service identification as a predictor of optimum existing resources. If the clinician does not adopt some rigorous thought process, he or she may jump to resources without fully assessing needs. For example, the clinician who thinks, "Maybe I can get "Meals on Wheels" to go in to assist this elderly isolate," is suffering from fuzzy thinking. This is like giving iron for anemia or vitamins for fatigue; the result is not satisfying to the doctor or the patient, except when seen as the outcome of a therapeutic trial for diagnostic purposes.

More satisfactory results can be obtained by following Donabedian's system: if limited mobility is the patient's problem, the clinician asks himself what service would make the most impact on the patient's quality of life. In this particular case, he or she might choose a maintenance exercise program with intermittent reassessment by a physiotherapist. The ideal resource for such a patient would be the home care program from a rehabilitation institute. If that resource does not exist in the community, compromises can be considered; a bi-annual visit to a physiotherapy center might be arranged via public transport's special mini-bus for the disabled. A family member could go with the patient, in anticipation of supporting the patient's maintenance exercise program at home with weekly or monthly visits.

The risk of not matching resources to ideal services predicted by rigorous need assessment is illustrated by the clinician who has just discovered the women's center and who overprescribes at first. As a result, the center may be unable to support all of these clients, particularly when they eventually make their own assessment and discover that some cases are inappropriate. In these circumstances some patients will lose time, hope, and perhaps the faith required to comply with the clinician's next, hopefully more appropriate, regimen.

Identifying Needs

Difficulties in determining services and resources from needs stem most frequently from difficulty identifying specific needs. Maslow's hierarchy of needs provides a satisfactory schema reminding us that physiological needs such as food or shelter must be met before sociological and psychological needs, and that needs for self-esteem must be met before self-actualization is possible.[16]

Needs assessment must be specific and rigorous, and is most efficiently achieved via a formal functional assessment such as the O.A.R.S.[20] and those developed by Katz.[14] For example, at the basic physiologic level of need for food, a disabled person's ability to eat without assistance must be assessed. If he or she cannot eat independently, an assessment of functional level can help determine the specific assistance that the patient requires. For example, the patient may require assistance cutting meat, but be perfectly able to do the shopping (even if only by telephone) and to do most or all meal preparation. A daily mealtime visitor would solve this "disability." In contrast, "Meals on Wheels" is an inappropriate resource for such a patient who might, as a result, stop cooking altogether, feel "what is the use," and give in to a dependency level that he or she perceives to be related to his handicap.[11]

Identifying Resources

In contrast to needs assessment (where rigor and specificity are indicated), resource identification benefits from broad creative thinking. As part of management of an isolated elderly woman who is falling frequently, the clinician might ask the postman to phone a family member or community worker if she does not wave back to him on any given day. Other examples of resource identification include the following:

In one community, a handicapped girl with severely compromised lungs was given oxygen by the fireman next door while waiting for the ambulance and hospital treatment of a respiratory infection.

A pick-up and delivery diaper service helps incontinent elderly who wish to stay with their family but not to overburden them.

The pharmacist can help with patient education.

For the isolated elderly, the buddy system helps. Elderly may phone each other each day, or if they can see each other's apartment, may use a window blind system—if the window blind is not opened by a certain time each day, they telephone. If there is no response, they call the proprietor.

Young mothers can also benefit from a buddy system, using each other to babysit one day a week when sitters are expensive and unavailable.

Some communities have solved the problem of the isolated young mother in need of occasional babysitting, and the isolated but competent elderly, by developing a foster grandparent program. Such a mutually beneficial program may be triggered by the community nurse or physician, as may sexual health education programs in the school or local YMCA, or courses in lifesaving, sports programs, etc.

Exercise programs for the elderly seem to be more acceptable in the form of square dancing. This is a recommendation a doctor can make at an annual check-up long before the individual is experiencing any difficulty with mobility.

In certain communities the police will come to help an elderly person to get up when he has fallen. The elderly may have a buzzer or screamer to let someone know that they have fallen, but that person may be too elderly to help them and may phone the police.

THE COMMUNITY AS THE OBJECT OF CARE

Identification of needs, services, and resources is appropriate when they exist. But what happens if the resources do not exist or are unavailable to the client? For the clinician with a systems orientation, the community then becomes the patient. He or she may see a particular problem frequently and note a lack of the ideal resource, in this case bringing this need to the attention of the public health authorities or to a local church group. In some areas, family physicians obtain short-term contracts to set up a particular resource over a limited period of time under the aegis of the public health system. Where no formal system for building new resources exists related to the identified need, the clinician can approach volunteer groups. The socially responsible health care worker can be a very effective catalyst for community activists and an effective support to the health visitor or local authority in obtaining new resources.

Sometimes the resource exists but the agency is performing poorly. The health care worker/clinician can bring this problem to the attention of the public health authority, to the appropriate professional licensing body, or to the attention of the agency itself, providing a helpful approach is taken. Even with a very helpful attitude, however, the clinician is not always fully appreciated by the agency in question; "helping people" do not always like to be helped!

The clinician is also an epidemiologist, the vanguard of health of the individual, the family, and the community. Some health problems should be reported to departments of community health, and the physician must alert hospital emergency rooms of any recurring patterns that are noticed.

As the physician or community nurse, you are often in a position not only to work in and understand the network, but to make the network happen ("networking"). Here you are supporting and initiating other systems, alternate therapies, and demedicalizing therapy. For example, a busy physician whose practice included 1800 patients living in a wide area of northwest Scotland arranged for a daily team meeting after his morning's office hours. The two district nurses and the health visitor were daily participants, while the social worker, occupational therapist, physiotherapist, psychiatrist nurse, and consultants (en route to the next town 50 miles away) were frequent visitors to the meeting. Afternoon home visits were planned and the appropriate professional was designated. This guaranteed mutual consultation, and was satisfying to all.

The impact of a "link project" within a residential home for disabled people is another example of networking. At a home visit to a patient, the clinician suggested that there might be possibilities for successful interactions between residents, such as the blind person pushing the wheelchair of a physically disabled person, who could serve as the "eyes" for the blind person.

This sort of relationship was encouraged on subsequent visits (the clinician made the initial visit to check blood pressure) and eventually this impoverished milieu became a beehive of interaction, and seemed to be a much happier place.

A further example occurred in a department of community health where a private physician was asked by the community nurse to come to a private, protected residence for elderly in the community because she had noticed that residents there might benefit from assessment. The physician made a visit and, with the help of the nurse, set up a medication system for the home's proprietor. When the nurse and doctor brought this to the attention of the department of community health, the same medication system was instituted for all interested proprietors of private, protected residences in the area.

Police and fire departments are already functioning in a network and welcome liaison with the community clinician, particularly in high-risk areas. Not only do they respond to crises but also they are concerned with prevention and education, especially when supported by health professionals. The clinician using these resources will treat fewer cases of trauma, burns, and assault and spend more time educating people during "check-ups." The physician is in an ideal position to break down the insularity of a service. The doctor who frequently phones the home care nurse who changes dressings twice a week for the recently discharged patient can improve communication and help the nurse to feel a part of the team. Until the home care nurse feels secure in a working relationship with the doctor, he or she may feel caught in the "middle" between the patient and the physician.

The community nurse and physician with a nonthreatening approach can help institutions evolve by asking for expertise with optimistic and nonjudgmental attitudes to problem solving. This mode of working, enabling individual, family, and community care-related activities to continue to be cost effective in practice, takes a number of years to develop. Efficient systems set up in advance diminish the number of phone calls and interactions required in the long run. The clinician who understands the community as a system that influences and is influenced by the family and organizations within it can become an effective change agent.

REFERENCES

1. Bloom SW: *The Doctor and His Patient.* New York, Free Press, 1965.
2. Brody SJ, Paulshock SE, Masciocchi CF: The family caring unit: A major consideration in the long-term support system. *Gerontology* 18:556, 1978.
3. Brownlee AT: Community Culture and Care: A Cross-Cultural Guide for the Health Worker, in *How to Assess the Community.* St. Louis, C.V. Mosby, 1978.
4. Dever GEA: *Community Health Analysis: A Wholistic Approach.* Rockville, Maryland, Aspen Systems Corporation, 1970.

5. Donabedian A: *Aspects of Medical Care Administration: Specifying Requirements for Health Care.* Cambridge, Harvard University Press, 1973.

6. Fabb WE, Heffernan MW, Phillips WA, et al: *Focus on Learning in Family Practice.* Melbourne, Australia, Royal Australian College General Practice, Community Health Program, 1976.

7. Ferrier BM, Woodward CA: Career choices, work patterns, and preconceptions of undergraduate education of McMaster Medical graduates: Comparison between men and women. *Can Med Assoc J* 126:1411, 1982.

8. Freeman HE, Levine S, Reeder LG: *Handbook of Medical Sociology,* ed 2. Englewood Cliffs, New Jersey, Prentice-Hall, 1972.

9. Geyman JP: *The Modern Family Doctor and Changing Medical Practice.* New York, Meredith Corp., 1971.

10. Gordon D: *Health, Sickness and Society.* Australia, University of Queensland Press, 1976.

11. Hébert R: L'evaluation de l'autonomie fonctionnelle des personnes âgées. *Can Fam Phys* 28:754, 1982.

12. Hedinger FR: *The Systems Approach to Health Services: A Framework,* Ph.D. diss. University of Iowa, 1968.

13. Kark SL: *The Practice of Community-Oriented Primary Health Care.* New York, Appleton Century Crofts, 1981.

14. Katz S, Ford AB, Morkowitz RE, et al: Studies of illness in the aged index of ADL—standardized measure of biological and psychosocial function. *JAMA* 185:914, 1963.

15. Leigh H, Reiser MF: *The Patient: Biological and Social Dimensions of Medical Practice.* New York, Plenum Medical Book Co., 1980.

16. Maslow A: *Motivation and Personality,* ed 2. New York, Harper & Row, 1970.

17. Mead M: *Childhood in Contemporary Cultures.* Chicago, University of Chicago Press, 1963.

18. Moulthrop HE, Rohborough M: Know your community resources network support for the aged: The viable alternatives to institutionalization. *J Gerontol Nurs* 4:64, 1978.

19. Paul BD (ed): *Health Culture and Community: Case Studies of Public Reactions to Health Programs.* New York, Russell Sage Foundation, 1955.

20. Pfeiffer E (Ed): *Multidimensional Functional Assessment: The OARS Methodology, A Manual,* ed 2. Durham, North Carolina, Duke University, The Center for the Study of Aging and Human Development, 1978.

21. *The Rockefeller Foundation Study and Conference Center, Villa Serbellini: The Changing Roles and Education of Health Care Personnel Worldwide in View of the Increase of Basic Health Services.* Papers from a consultation sponsored by the Society for Health and Human Values, Bellergio, Italy 2-7 May, 1977.

22. Stewart MA, Bass MJ: Recruiting and retiring physicians in northern Canada. *Can Fam Phys* 28:1313, 1982.

23. Wise H, Beckhard R, Rubin I, et al: *Making Health Teams Work.* Cambridge, Ballinger Publishing Co., 1974.

Chapter 19
Cases Illustrating Working with the Family

Janet Christie-Seely
Gilles Paradis
Renée Turcotte

In this chapter eight families are described at greater length than the examples used in other chapters; they illustrate working with more complex families over time. These cases fall into the category of "illness-prone," "difficult," or "problem" patients or families who take up considerable time and attention in any practice. (When judging the time spent it is important to compare the time taken by a practitioner without a family orientation with a similar patient, or the time taken up by each member visiting a multitude of clinicians who each do tests, treat, operate, reassess, and give up in turn.) Healthier families require less time and may be better able to use our suggestions, anticipatory guidance, facilitation; such interventions for these dynamic (morphogenetic) families (see Chapter 2) are probably more potent.

Several physicians and nurses from McGill family medicine units provided the cases, demonstrating different styles of working with families. Since referral cases are not included here (except in Case 5, in which the multiple family therapy group was attended by the physician) social workers are not involved (this does not imply that social workers are nonessential members of the team and major contributors to the teaching of working with families). Each case is preceded by a genogram and followed by a summary of family assessment using the technique PRACTICE (see Chapter 14). Sometimes the genogram was elicited in detail, sometimes not.

In some of these cases knowledge of family dynamics comes too late. In Case 7, for example, little can be done but go with the family system. One might ask, however, if during a visit to that family when the daughter was 2, and when improved communication was still possible, whether facilitation by a clinician might have made a difference. The question of prevention is a pressing one, and it is hoped that working with families makes a difference. It must be done early, otherwise poor communication may lead to the problems shown in the following genogram:

CASE 1: AN ILLNESS-PRONE FAMILY

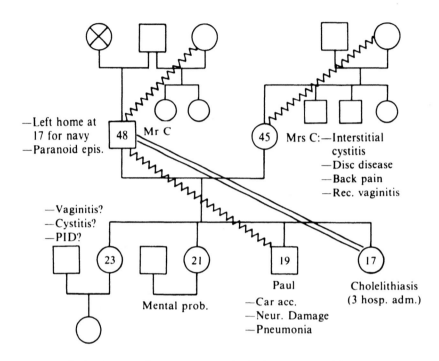

—Left home at
 17 for navy
—Paranoid epis.

Mr C

Mrs C:—Interstitial
        cystitis
     —Disc disease
     —Back pain
     —Rec. vaginitis

—Vaginitis?
—Cystitis?
—PID?

Mental prob.

Paul
—Car acc.
—Neur. Damage
—Pneumonia

Cholelithiasis
(3 hosp. adm.)

The C. family was first seen as a unit during a home visit. Every member had been known for some time before this visit. Mrs. C. had been followed for 2 years with interstitial cystitis and unremitting back pain that was poorly explained; the son, Paul, had been hit by a car 3 months previously and had finally recovered from severe concussion and a leg fracture; and Mr. C. had developed an acute psychotic breakdown, ostensibly related to work pressures. With the onset of his symptoms the wife's physical symptoms cleared abruptly! The home visit clarified for the physician (and therefore for the family) that the psychotic symptoms followed the disappointment of a cancelled visit by Mr. C.'s father and stepmother. The boss at work closely resembled his father and so became the conscious focus of anxiety. The father's cancelled visit was particularly upsetting because he had not even telephoned to enquire about his grandson, Paul, after the accident. Paul was 17, the same age the father left home to join the navy. It became apparent that Mr. C. had left home because he had felt unwanted by father and stepmother. This rejection was being replayed as a fear of rejection by his child, now adolescent.

Three changes were noted after this home visit: the incidence of visits by all family members to the office decreased; Mr. C. was dramatically improved (when he did have a symptom, primarily a numbness or pain in his right arm, he related this symptom to anxiety and told himself it was not a physical problem and it then would go away); and Mrs. C. gradually became aware of the marital conflict that had produced tension and physical symptoms. She obtained a job, which resulted in considerable relief and some role adjustments between the couple. Paul then developed a mysterious respiratory problem during a period when he was involved in litigation resulting from the car accident. Pulmonary function tests showed a clearly abnormal, restrictive pattern that later reverted to normal. Apart from visits in connection with this problem, the family remained well for a long period.

The second family interview occurred 4 years later. It was prompted by the recurrence of back pain, this time diagnosed as disc disease, in the wife. The two older daughters had, with difficulty, left home to get married. On each occasion the father particularly had been very depressed. The youngest, Marie, soon after deciding on a nursing career in another province, had developed severe cholelithiasis (we are unaware of literature suggesting cholelithiasis is linked to stress, although a surgeon of our acquaintance said he had noted a relationship). This girl's gall stones were very large, were located in the common bile duct and the right hepatic duct, and necessitated three operations. Her recovery after a year had re-opened the issue of her leaving home.

Paul, meanwhile, was close to leaving home, and had a girlfriend whom he visited frequently, but he stated openly that it was difficult to leave the family because he worried that marital conflict would ensue. Both younger son and daughter recognized because of increased awareness of family issues that their departure from home was the problem. Mrs. C. recognized her back pain as a response to role conflict. With a full-time job and housework and a husband who covertly undermined her efforts to delegate responsibility, she had no other way of solving her overload. Marie had come to the physician's office with complaints of fatigue. She had to do the extra housework in addition to her college courses and part-time job. Another function of the mother's back pain was to keep her daughter from leaving home. Mrs C., when asked the question, "What would be different if your pain miraculously disappeared?", admitted that her daughter might leave. When asked who benefited from her staying home, she said, "My husband—he's so attached to her."

This single session, in which back pain was relabelled as a solution rather than a problem, and in which it became evident that the father's distress with his own adolescent period was the cause of his difficulty in letting his own children go, resulted in a gradual change. The children were able to leave. The couple expressed more of the long-standing, unresolved conflict responsible for at least some of their illness.

Thus, contact with other members of the family was aided enormously by knowledge of the family system. When one of the older married daughters came in with apparent pelvic inflammatory disease but no fever, no organisms, and no response to antibiotics, the connection with an increase in the tension in the home was confirmed. Anxieties about her recent marriage were also related to her "illness," and were solved by only one session of information-giving in the area of sexuality.

This example illustrates the therapeutic role the physician played, without contract for family therapy and with only two sessions 4 years apart with the whole family. This family was clearly illness-prone and demonstrated the rotating patient pattern described in Section III. Much of the illness was serious and "organic." The physician learned to pay attention to phone calls in the middle of the night, despite the family's high anxiety level and frequent visits for "nonorganic" symptoms. Often the symptoms reflected serious underlying disease; a high index of suspicion is important in high-risk families since it aids secondary prevention. It may also be that the primary prevention occurred through facilitation of communication before a symptom turned into a manifest disease.

Assessment (PRACTICE)

Problems	Rotating patient with series of serious physical illnesses.
Roles	Housework role never resolved, back pain needed to avoid it, triangulation resulted from covert couple conflict.
Affect	Anger, particularly at families of origin, never expressed.
Communication	Indirect, through children or through illness
Time in life cycle	Great difficulty allowing children to leave because of parents' (especially father's) difficulty leaving their homes and because of covert couple conflict.
Illness history	Maternal grandmother chronically sick.
Coping strengths	Economically stable, work satisfying, sense of humor, strong bonds.
Environment/resources	Isolated family, hostility to extended family.

CASE 2:   THE PATHOGENESIS OF ARTHRITIS?

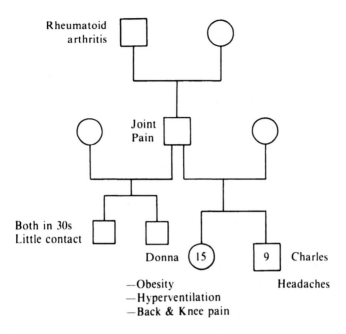

Donna, a 15-year-old girl, was the identified patient. She was referred from the emergency room where she has been seen on two occasions for hyperventilation. Her 9-year-old brother had been seen by a different physician at the same family medicine center for headaches that proved to be functional. Both parents were present at the interview with the patient. They were very anxious and pressured the physician to do tests and consult a specialist. The mechanism of hyperventilation and the circumstances under which it usually appears were thoroughly explained but the parents denied any stressful or conflictual situation at home. An electroencephalogram was done and results were normal. The parents were reassured that nothing was wrong. Shortly afterwards, the problem disappeared.

A couple of months later Donna came back to the clinic with the complaint of sore knees. Since the family physician was on vacation another physician examined her. This examination was negative and she was told that everything was normal. Two weeks later she was back to see the family physician complaining of pain in her thighs. On questioning she complained also of low back pain occurring intermittently during the past year. The pain was such that sometimes she couldn't walk and she had to be carried by her father to and from school. She was a moderately obese patient, who always smiled even when talking about the worst of her pain. A complete examination did not show any abnormality. A complete blood count with erythocyte sedimentation rate, basic biochemistry, and roentgenogram of the lumbosacral spine were all normal.

A follow-up appointment was planned 2 weeks later, but in the meantime Donna's parents phoned the clinic every other day, saying that Donna was in much pain and something had to be done. The family was invited in for another session. Again, everyone denied a stressful situation at home; the parents constantly returned the discussion to the girl's symptoms. Donna was silent throughout the meeting. It was noted that even though she was suffering, her parents did most of the complaining. When confronted with this, the father admitted his fear that Donna might have rheumatoid arthritis, which had killed his own father. He himself had vague complaints of occasional joint pain.

The suggestion was made to continue regular family meetings while the investigation was being pursued; and that only Donna would call when she had episodes of pain. This arrangement was readily agreed on by the family and afterwards the frequency of the phone calls decreased substantially. Further tests were done, including rheumatoid factor, antistreptolysine O, antinuclear antibodies, lupus erythematosis cells, and protein electrophoresis. All results were normal. Two or three family meetings were held; little happened except denial of conflict and inquiries about the test results, even though Donna's complaints had diminished. The father was the one most anxious about his daughter, who remained indifferent, but it was the mother who was clearly in charge of the family.

At the next appointment Donna was in more pain. Even though she had not called the office she had stayed home for the past week because of pain. The father was absent from this meeting. He often had to travel outside the city on business but had limited these trips since his daughter became sick and he had almost cancelled this one. Donna was asked what would happen if she weren't sick and in so much pain. She readily answered that "Dad would not be home as much."

At the next meeting, with father present, this issue was explored and it appeared that he was very frequently called outside of town for business. The mother revealed that she had considered separation because of this but instead decided to go back to work so she would feel less lonely at home. Donna's pain was then relabelled as a way of keeping her mother and father at home together. Further sessions emphasized this point and it was suggested later that the father and mother could use counselling, but they were still resistant. Further testing of Donna showed HLA B-27 to be positive, and two sacro-iliac roentgenograms, at 3-month intervals, showed the beginning of ankylosing spondylitis.

Assessment (PRACTICE)

Problems	Donna: hyperventilation, then pain in knees and back Charles: headaches.
Roles	Absent father drawn home by Donna's symptoms, mother dominant.
Affect	Anxiety ++. Strong resentment toward physician for not consulting specialist.
Communication	Poor. Little nonverbal or verbal between couple.
Time in life cycle	With poor couple relations, empty nest threatening illness.
Illness history	Grandfather died of rheumatoid arthritis. Father feared same in self and daughter. First wife died of ?
Coping strengths	Mother coped by getting job.
Environment/resources	Elderly predominate in area. Father from Europe—no contact, few friends.

CASE 3: FACILITATION OF VENTILATION AND COMMUNICATION

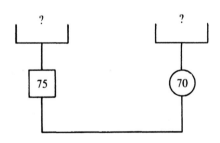

—Diabetes
—Alcoholism
—Angiopathy
—Bilateral amputation

—Osteoarthritis
—Anxiety
—Low back pain
—"Enabler" re drink, food, for Mr M.

Mr. M. was a 75-year-old Irishman. He had started smoking at age 10 and smoked two packs a day for most of his life. He had been an alcoholic and a diabetic for the past 30 to 40 years. He had been seen by many doctors who did not want to continue to care for him because of his uncooperativeness. Against all medical advice he had continued to smoke and drink, and he never followed a diet. Mrs. M., his 70-year-old wife, had a history of vague complaints, including osteoarthritis, anxiety, and occasional low back pain. Mr. M. developed diabetic angiopathy and ischemia in his right foot for which he was admitted to the hospital. When visiting her husband, Mrs. M. brought him cigarettes and doughnuts.

During that period Mrs. M. came to the clinic because of her osteoarthritis, but she spent most of the interview complaining about her husband's drinking, not following a diet, etc. The day before his leg was to be amputated, Mr. M. had a myocardial infarction; the doctors ordered 6 months rest at home and said they would operate on him thereafter.

Mr. M. was discharged but Mrs. M. refused to let him come back home because she said his leg smelled bad. The hospital staff were forced to keep him since he could only move in a wheelchair and since she did not come to see him for the next 2 weeks. The surgical team was putting pressure on the family physician and nurse to get Mrs. M. to accept her husband but she went to a local community service center where she was strongly supported and told to hold her ground. The family physician was triangled! He contacted Mrs. M. to break the triangulation and she came in to be seen individually. She was allowed to talk freely about her anger at her husband. Two or three sessions were necessary before she was able to talk about her own despair and her underlying depression because she felt she had not been a good wife. It was not until she was able to talk about her own depression that she could go to the hospital to see her husband. He had developed infection and had to be operated on, regardless of his recent myocardial infarction. He had a below-knee amputation of the right leg under spinal block.

The week Mr. M. was to be discharged and sent back home, Mrs. M developed an acute back strain. His discharge was postponed 1 more week because of this. A discussion was held in Mr. M.'s hospital room with his wife about what to expect on his return home. This session permitted them to voice concern about his rehabilitation. Home visits with his physician and visiting nurse were planned. Mr. M. was scheduled to attend a rehabilitation day-center to do some physiotherapy and learn how to use an artificial limb. During these home visits the husband was encouraged to talk about his frustration and anger over his situation; with support from the health care team and his wife, he cut down on his drinking and smoking and was able to follow his diet much more closely.

Mr. M.'s other leg then started developing ulcers and, later, gangrene when he refused to come to the hospital to be treated. Instead he used soaks of lanolin and sugar. A home visit to talk to them both was again necessary. Both started by saying that the leg looked bad but that there was nothing that could be done. Rather than discussing Mr. M.'s physical symptoms, the physician encouraged Mr. M. to talk about his feelings. His wife interrupted continuously and tried to bring the discussion back to his leg. The clinician interpreted this as her trying to rescue him from his depression (positive relabelling), and encouraged them to talk about their underlying depression. When Mrs. M. was able to admit to her own feelings of inadequacy in helping her husband he was able to talk about his diminished self-image. This resulted in lowering of the tension at home and Mr. M. was able to come to hospital for further treatment.

Assessment (PRACTICE)

Problems	Poor compliance with diet. Alcoholism. Bilateral leg amputation.
Roles	Wife acted as enabler, encouraging poor compliance, then caretaker.
Affect	Avoidance of guilt feelings and mourning for loss of limbs. Anger between couple expressed via symptoms.
Communication	Indirect. Wife's caring and husband's rebellion expressed through food and drink and illness.
Time in life cycle	No children.
Illness history	Not known. Reasons for poor compliance?
Coping strengths	Strong affectional bond between couple.
Environment/resources	Medical resources only.

CASE 4: LIMITED GOALS AND THE IMPORTANCE OF CONTRACTING

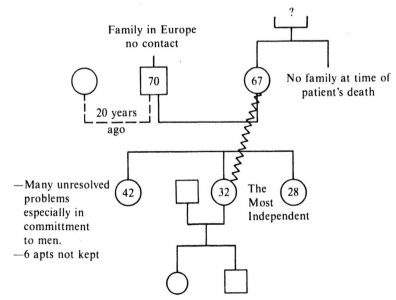

Mrs. T., 67-year-old mother of three, presented to a family doctor following visits to multiple doctors, whose investigations were negative. Her complaints included vague abdominal pains, joint pains, food intolerance, weight loss, irregular bowel movement (alternating diarrhea and constipation), sleeplessness, palpitations, headaches, and decreased energy. Her history included a cholecystectomy, hysterectomy, and appendectomy, but was very suggestive of stress-related, psychosomatic symptoms. The physician made a contract with the patient that it was doubtful he could help since so many experts had tried already, that he would be available to her on a long-term basis and would see her regularly as often as needed, and that there were to be no further laboratory investigations pending establishment of a family/psychosocial data base. This revealed the following:

1. husband's business failure;
2. change of living standard after the above;
3. unresolved extra-marital relationship that husband had 20 years ago, and which the wife had never confronted him with;
4. anxiety over husband's health (cardiac pacemaker);
5. children had not met expectations and did not go to church; and
6. tendency to internalize and be non-confronting.

With the above information obtained, a second contract was established, which included the following:

1. no additional lab investigations;
2. nightly sedation when needed;
3. short, weekly visits that were reality oriented, focussing on the relation between symptoms and stress;
4. occasional joint sessions with the husband; and
5. future consideration to possible tricyclic antidepressants.

On the issue of her husband's affair 20 years previously, the patient was adamant, refusing to discuss the problem. She said confrontation would open too many wounds, that she was afraid of the consequences of revealing her knowledge of the affair, and that she could "live with it anyway." Apart from this, there seemed little in the family system to explain an illness role. The husband was supportive but frustrated by his wife's symptoms. There was clearly avoidance of conflict, and the symptoms may have been indirect expression of anger at the past.

The patient was seen weekly, then biweekly, and finally monthly as symptoms decreased in frequency. This was over a period of approximately 2 years, with the patient showing better understanding of the relationship between life stress and symptoms. After this improvement, she developed new abdominal pain, diagnosed as adhesions by a surgeon to whom she had gone by herself. She developed postoperative complications, was admitted to the intensive care unit, and subsequently had four operations to stabilize complications. The patient died after 3 weeks in intensive care. The family doctor acted as a support system to the patient and family, and continues to see the family. He is still dealing with issues of bereavement.

Assessment (PRACTICE)

Problem	Abdominal pains. Doctor shopping.
Roles	Husband the strong one, resiliant; wife the weak one.
Affect	Husband supportive, but interviews tense. Anger at daughters, anger at husband's affair unexpressed.
Communication	Through children or illness. Family secret (affair 20 years ago).
Time in life cycle	One child married (the rebel). Single 28- and 42-year-old. Difficulty leaving nest/ individuating.
Illness history	Not known.
Coping strengths	Husband appeared to cope well.
Environment/resources	Religion very important but source of value conflict with daughters.

CASE 5: THE ORIGINS AND MAINTENANCE OF DEPRESSION

Mrs. S. was seen for several months before her husband came to the office. She was referred by another family physician who had treated her for years for arthritis. Her symptoms were of arthralgias in varying joints, myalgias, and chronic back pain. There was evidence of disc disease to a minor degree, but no biochemical or radiologic evidence of serious arthritis. Her visits to the office, however, were frequent.

When her husband came for a check-up it was found that he had suffered severe depression 1 year previously, following an attack of glaucoma that had turned out to be temporary and treatable. He was a railroad man as his father had been before him, and glaucoma had threatened early "retirement" to the yards rather than driving the train. Later an attack of chest pain, which he thought was angina, produced a similar depression. The man, though white-haired, looked young and always had a pleasant expression and a smile for everyone. Likeable and easygoing, his behavior contrasted somewhat with that of his wife, who had a chronically anxious expression on her thin face, and even a look of imminent tearfulness at times. When asked if she felt sad or felt like crying she reacted with great surprise and said no, she never cried. She

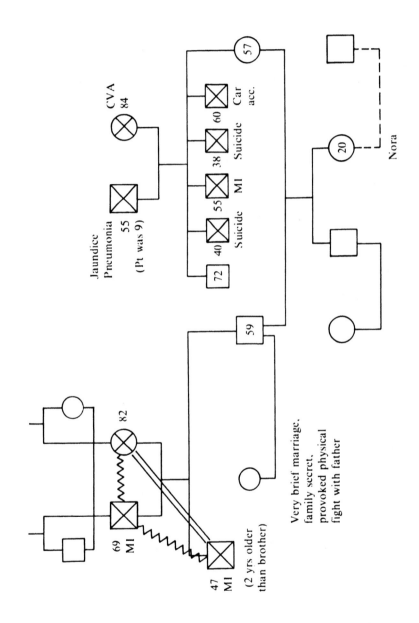

Jaundice
Pneumonia
55
(Pt was 9)

CVA
84

72 40 55 38 60
Suicide MI Suicide Car acc.

82

69
MI

47
MI
(2 yrs older than brother)

59

57

20

Nora

Very brief marriage, family secret, provoked physical fight with father

tended to follow his lead, and was quiet and unassuming and the less sociable member of the two.

They had two children: a son who had left home, and a daughter of 20, a very attractive, outgoing and friendly girl who was planning to leave soon for New Zealand. She was worried about her father's tendency to depression, but only the mother had ever spoken to her about it. It was an open secret and yet the father felt he could not bear for her to know that he tended to be depressed. No one had mentioned it to the son.

This couple then alternated in visiting the office over a period of 3 years: first the wife would visit frequently with arthritic complaints for a few months; then the husband would come with a depression, accompanied by the wife who would feel reasonably well when the husband was ill. The family physician and the nurse on the team pointed out each time this pattern of alternating symptoms but the couple vehemently denied any connection between arthralgias and depression and any problems in their relationship. Mr. S. was treated concurrently by a psychiatrist and treated with amitriptyline.

Two weeks after the daughter's departure for New Zealand (a location chosen perhaps purely because of its distance from the family problems; she knew no one there) the father developed a severe depression, was questionably suicidal, and was admitted to the hospital. He denied any connection with his daughter's departure, clinging to the psychiatric label of manic-depressive psychosis (*endogenous*) with which the psychiatrist had supplied him. The label seemed to fit; his mood between depressions was one of elation and hyperactivity. However, lithium did not help; large doses of amitriptyline were used with some success. After 6 weeks he was discharged from the hospital convinced that he had a life-long disorder that would keep on recurring. However, at this point he was told by the psychiatrists that it was a "neurotic depression" and that he would have to try and solve it himself.

The couple's clinicians continued to point out that they took turns being sick, and were perhaps having difficulties with the empty nest now that both children had left. Mr. S. and his wife then opted to join a multiple-family therapy group (which their physician attended). Mr. S. had begun to complain of his wife's overly placid unemotional, unexciting nature; Mrs. S. occasionally commented that Mr. S. was rather bossy. Mrs. S. tended to nag, and it appeared that when he was depressed he was unable to do the many things around the house that she gently suggested he do; when her back pains increased she was unable to do the painting and housework that he tended to leave her. Thus both symptoms appeared to have been adaptive in the marriage.

Mr. S. had been reared in a family where the father had an uncontrollable temper and his parents did not get on. He had been assigned (and volunteered for) the role of smoother and joker. Known for his even temperament, he was the family peacemaker and helper. He took up his father's railroad career although he secretly wanted to be a machinist. He was not allowed to experience normal mood swings, and followed the family belief that appearances and "what the neighbors think" are important. He grew up unable to say "No" and unable to be angry. In his community and church he was known as the one who always helped or volunteered. Again depression got him out of all these unwanted activities but imposed enormous shame when he had to say he was unable to socialize because of his illness. Admitting depression to his neighbors and his children, however, helped him to fear it less. Indeed, the paradoxical suggestion to stop running away from the depression and to become as depressed and immobile as possible, particularly with the help of Mrs. S., began to convert Mr. S.'s recurrent depressions into normal mood swings that were acceptable to him for the first time in his life.

The wife's role became increasingly clear. Her family history revealed that two of her three brothers had committed suicide, events she felt that had not greatly affected her. Yet she *never* spoke of her brothers. Her father had died when she was nine and she had become the family caretaker, playing the role of nurse, particularly for her mother who was chronically sick. As an adult she trained as a nurse and admitted some feelings of guilt at not having prevented the two suicides. She became aware of her nursing, protective role during her husband's depressions and gradually decreased her overconcern and attempts to joke him out of them. She was eventually able to allow him to go on vacations without her and to leave for a month herself with a friend. During these separations he was always remarkably well. Depressions began to decrease in frequency and in severity.

While away on a second trip, Mrs. S. fell and fractured a vertebra. Her history of back pain increased the significance of this injury, and she was able to admit for the first time to feelings of depression. Asked again about her brothers' suicides, she replied by recalling her father's death. In a vivid memory of the funeral parlor she found herself unable to locate either of the two brothers who later took their own lives, and she cried openly for the first time.

As Mrs. S.'s back improved she resisted further discussion of her father's death but began to express open anger at her husband's attempts to mold her personality. One episode of depression began after the couple had a muffled argument at home, but was aborted when they had their first open fight in the office. Mr. S.'s prediction, "If we fight we'll never stop," did not of course come true and a more open relationship with normal mood swings ensued. (The various factors contributing to Mrs. S.'s depression are discussed in more detail in Chapter 24, which outlines evidence that depression is a problem in the family system.)

Assessment (PRACTICE)

Problems	Mr. S., recurrent depressions; Mrs. S., arthritis, myalgias.
Roles	Mr. S., nice guy, "cheerer-upper." Mrs. S., caretaker.
Affect	Anger never expressed by either. Mrs. S. always looks close to tears/never cries. Repressed mourning for father and two brothers (both suicides).
Communication	Each avoid other's nagging and neighborhood duties through symptoms. Polite indirect communication. Depression a "secret."
Time in life cycle	Problems after last child left. Difficulty accepting both son and daughter-in-law.
Illness history	Mrs. S.'s mother depressed, father died young (patient, aged 9). Two brothers suicidal. Patient became a nurse. Mr. S.'s father and brother died young of myocardial infarctions.
Coping strengths	Strong bonds. Two delightful children. Sense of humor.
Environment/resources	Rich resource of neighbors/church—at times a burden.

CASE 6

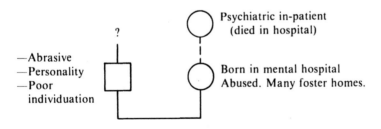

— Abrasive
— Personality
— Poor individuation

? Psychiatric in-patient (died in hospital)

Born in mental hospital
Abused. Many foster homes.

Mrs. E., a 48-year-old woman, presented to the family physician with multiple somatic complaints, a "hysterical personality," and behavior strongly suggesting that she used illness to organize her environment. A contract was made with the patient that no further laboratory investigations were to be made until all old medical records were reviewed. These records revealed that she was:

born in a psychiatric hospital to an in-patient;
between ages 1 to 3, lived in 12 foster homes;
at age 16 was raped by foster father;
at age 20, illegitimate pregnancy (1955); and
at 30 married a controlling, father figure, 15 years older.

Childhood illnesses included eczema, bronchitis, and asthma.

Hospital admissions
    1955—illegitimate pregnancy
    1963—recurrent ulcer (age 30), 60% gastrectomy and gastrojejunostomy,
        ? appropriate procedure
    1964—abdominal pain; cholecystectomy
    1965—phlebitis
        —post concussion syndrome
        —psychogenic vomiting
    1966—psychiatric admission: ? depression
    1967—abdominal pain; negative laparotomy
        —suicide attempt
        —abdominal pain; ? adhesions
    1968—pneumonia
    1969—menorrhagia; curettage negative
        —gastrectomy for retrocolic ulcer (Billroth II)
    1970—? dumping syndrome, ? psychogenic vomiting
        —weakness, ? demyelinating disease
    1975—Acute urinary retention secondary to medication abuse
        —right knee pain, normal investigation
    1976—dysfunctional uterine bleeding; curettage negative
    1977—hysterectomy
        —gingivitis
        —right knee pain, ?
    1978—tear right lateral meniscus
        —headaches
        —chest pain
        —polypharmacy
    1980—right knee pain, negative investigation
    1981—vertigo, negative investigation

The patient was found to have a low I.Q. and to have no psychological insight. With the above history, the primary objective of the family physician was to *maintain* the patient with the minimal number of laboratory investigations, decrease doctor-shopping, decrease polypharmacy, and eliminate surgical interventions.

Her husband was contacted by phone. He was a very beligerent man who came in on one occasion but usually refused. He tended to phone to confront the physician that his wife was not getting any better, and ask why he was preventing her from going to other doctors. Mr. E. clearly needed his little-girl wife (whose temper tantrums he encouraged) to be sick and dependent. His help was eventually enlisted in controlling his wife's medication, which maintained the family hierarchy but decreased the polypharmacy.

A second contract was made with Mrs. E. that included the following:

1. only one physician
2. no lab tests or consultations without approval
3. rapid availability of physician as necessary as symptoms arose
4. empathy/support relationship
5. behavior modification to control polypharmacy

This relationship was maintained for 3 and 1/2 years, at which time the patient self-referred herself to a new family doctor. However, the objectives of the first doctor were met: for the first time in 15 years, the patient went 3 and 1/2 years without a hospital admission, unnecessary surgical intervention, or excessive medication.

The principles of helping such unfortunate people are brief visits spaced at whatever interval will eliminate use of other resources (usually weekly at first, then biweekly or monthly, as the patient's sense of security increases); a focus on whatever strengths can be found, if only, "You're real tough, look at all you've had to go through"; and family assessment and use of family members as support for therapeutic goals. Family system change is probably not possible; in this family poor individuation of both partners would have boded ill for children had they existed. As in many such families, however, this was the end of the family line.

Assessment (PRACTICE)

Problems	Wife's frequent admission, many operations. Poor individuation.
Roles	Patient was the petulant child of caretaker husband.
Affect	No affection between them, angry outbursts. "Folie à deux."
Communication	None except through illness.
Time in life cycle	Patient was fixated in childhood. Luckily no children.
Illness history	Illness was only means of getting nurturance. Patient was born in mental hospital.
Coping strengths	Ability to manipulate environment and elicit caring.
Environment/resources	Few resources except medical—overused. Eccentric neighbors.

CASE 7: MAINTENANCE OF AN OLD FAMILY SYSTEM

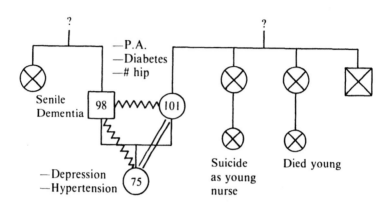

Mrs. R. is a very sweet old lady of 101 with pernicious anemia. She sits graciously fanning herself in her wheelchair while her daughter, aged 75, interprets for the nurse by yelling in the mother's ear. Mrs. R. is very deaf and had a broken hip 8 years ago, which confined her to bed or chair. Mr. R. has been senile for 10 years and been getting more so over the past year. He believes the nurse he has known for several years to be the hairdresser. A farmer in the past, he creates recurrent crises by thinking he lost his pigs and has been picked up looking for them by the police on many occasions. Miss R. is 75 years old and has always been their caretaker.

This precarious situation has been maintained for the past five years with the nurse from the family medicine unit visiting every 6 weeks to give injections of rubramin. She has the somewhat resistant back-up of two residents under staff supervision. When Mrs. R. had an episode of passing black stool the resident became more involved. The patient, it turned out, had been taking several tablets of acetylsalicylic acid and caffeine at least twice a day for 40 years. She generally popped pills of all descriptions. When these were stopped there was no further melena.

The daughter phones one to three times a week, almost always during office hours but always in a state of crisis: "He's about to go out the door, shall I call the police?", or "He leaned on Mum when he got out of bed and she's got a huge bruise again on her shoulder, and he's wetting himself again." Mrs. R. bruises easily, and the couple share a bed. Mr. R. may get violent when he's concerned about his pigs but he is not overtly abusive to his wife.

The abuse comes from the other direction. Mrs. R. is a tyrant under her delightful exterior and takes every opportunity to denigrate her husband. She is extraordinarily demanding and her daughter answers her every whim. There are no other living relatives. Mrs. R. speaks often of two nieces, one who was like a second daughter. This niece went to nursing school but then committed suicide. Mrs. R. often points to a picture of the niece in nursing uniform, saying "What a shame she had to end her own life." The second niece also died while young. Mr. R.'s sister, his last relative, died a year ago.

There is considerable affection expressed between mother and daughter: much propping of pillows, hand patting, and talk. Together they treat Mr. R. very badly. The daughter makes frequent comments making fun of his personal appearance and habits. The two women seem to be slowly extruding him from the system and his dysfunction is increasing; they have talked of placing him in a mental institution. Mr. R.'s behavior has improved since a particularly bad period just before the daughter's annual vacation (when the nurse arranges 2 weeks of respite care), when he regressed considerably and the phone calls multiplied. Miss R. has developed various tactics to prevent her father's excursions. He never goes out without his hat, so she hides his hat; she offers him a meal before going to look for his pigs and he forgets the pigs. She gives him postage stamps from the church to cut out, which effectively keeps him engrossed, although understimulated. Haloperidol is slipped in his juice. In all of these actions she is supported by the nurse.

It might be argued that in this geriatric "folie à trois" (terrible threesome), the nurse should be the advocate for this poor gentleman whose senility is at least partly a response to verbal abuse (as well as the current excuse for it). If the nurse chose to suggest a rehabilitation program for him she would be told to leave. Miss R. is a very determined woman. She received her B.A. in science, has a handbook on drugs at home, and regularly checks on medication. She has told the nurse, for example, that she found out that drug X increases gastric motility so that must be why her mother has diarrhea now. For herself, Miss R. believes in emergency medicine only. For example, she had some severe depressions during menopause, for which she would take two or three estrogen pills and then feel much better. She believed that pills should be taken rarely but always work. In contrast, her mother abuses medications of all sorts and has taken many daily for decades.

The choice of going with the system by keeping the daughter in charge but allowing the mother to think she is has kept the three out of institutions. Mrs. R.'s survival may be to give her daughter a role in life—when her mother dies the nurse is sure Miss R. will go to bed and die, with some disease as the excuse. Why Mr. R. has survived is less clear, but his senility probably insulates him from the barbs of the women who need him to diffuse any tension between them (see section on triangulation in Chapter 1). If he is placed in an institution it will be interesting to see the effect on mother and daughter.

Assessment (PRACTICE)

Problems	Pernicious anemia, immobility. Senility with incontinence and aggresivity.
Roles	Daughter in charge, but mother is queen. Father is scapegoat. Enmeshed family with triangulation.
Affect	Tension and anger focused on father.
Communication	Much of it around crises (father's activities) or dead relatives.
Time in life cycle	Fixated prior to empty nest.
Illness history	Pernicious anemia. Registered nurse visits. Medication abuse. Belief in "emergency" medication.
Coping strengths	Strong will of women. Ability to use the health care system (Family Medicine Unit, Emergency Room).
Environment/resources	Student neighbor comes in to bathe Mr R. Medical resources appropriately used. No relatives. Many friends (of daughter) who visit often for tea.

CASE 8: THE COMMUNITY IS THE PATIENT

Maria Pérez, a Mexican woman of 23, looks like a woman of 35. She lives with her family in precarious economic straights. She has not been married, but is living with her common-law husband and their children, who are 7, 5, and 2 years old. Five months ago, her husband started drinking and not coming home. Because of this situation she is working, (washing and ironing people's clothes) and leaving her children at home to take care of themselves. The entrance to the rundown building is even lower than is usual in that community, and health problems have started at home. The youngest one, Pedro, who is 2 years old, has measles; Maria, 5 years old, developed poliomyelitis.

Mrs. Pérez cannot cope with the situation because she needs to continue working to have enough money for her children's hospitalization. Also, her husband keeps returning drunk to physically abuse her and their children; he also takes away her money.

What is needed for this particular family? First, a complete program of vaccines should be given to these children. Second, Pedro and Maria must both receive help. Treatment will try to release the husband from his dysfunctional coping (his drinking daily); to keep him working and not

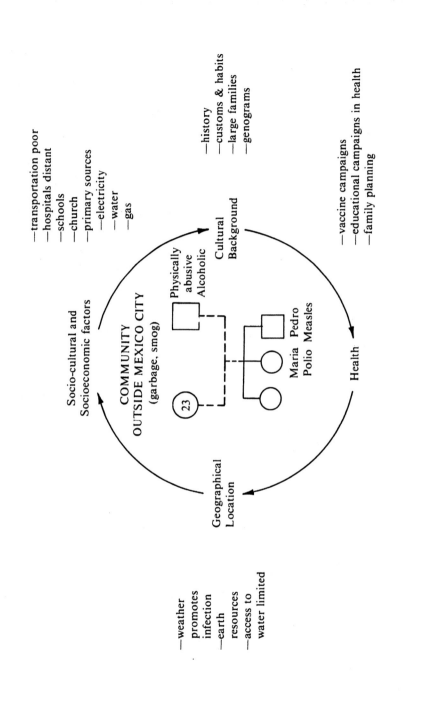

COMMUNITY
OUTSIDE MEXICO CITY
(garbage, smog)

Socio-cultural and
Socioeconomic factors

Cultural
Background

Geographical
Location

Health

Physically
abusive
Alcoholic

Maria Pedro Measles
Polio

23

—transportation poor
—hospitals distant
—schools
—church
—primary sources
    —electricity
    —water
    —gas

—history
—customs & habits
—large families
—genograms

—vaccine campaigns
—educational campaigns in health
—family planning

—weather
  promotes
  infection
—earth
  resources
—access to
  water limited

abusing his family will require the resources of Alcoholics Anonymous, community workers, and many interviews with the family and the husband himself.

This family's resources have been abruptly depleted in the face of a community replete with stress, pathogens, and readily available drugs including alcohol; its resources are low. The family's rapidly spiraling dysfunction is a reflection of community dysfunction. Treatment of this family is only symptomatic; the real ailing patient is the community. Discussion of this family's dysfunction and the patterns in the families of origin (which are no doubt repeating) would be to miss the point and to spin wheels fruitlessly.

This extreme case highlights what may also be true to some extent of other healthier North American environments. The family physician or nurse who can improve community health (for example, by starting an Alcoholics Anonymous program) is a much more potent agent of change than the one with a myopic focus on families. A healthy community has already done much of a health professional's job.

In the case of the Pérez family, the family physician involved decided on family planning as her focus of intervention. She studied other communities and their health programs, and in an effort to have an effective strategy for contraception she studied family systems. In Mexican culture one way men maintain authority and prestige is by frequently fathering children; a common response to a wife using contraception is physical abuse. Discussing the economic advantages of fewer children with the husband and addressing him as the head of the household while the wife is present would be more effective than an interview with the wife alone.

SPECIFIC HEALTH PROBLEMS

Chapter 20

Acute Illness and Hospitalization

Yves Talbot
Janet Christie-Seely

An acute illness is defined as a short episode of sickness or disease of sudden onset that alters the function of an individual and family for a brief period of time, after which the initial level of physiologic and social functioning is regained. Whenever a family member develops an acute illness, there is an impact on the family's organization and function. Conversely, the family organization and way of handling the crisis may have tremendous impact on the patient's course and recovery. Although an acute episode is usually self-limited by definition, it may be so perceived and managed that a more prolonged dysfunction of the individual may result. For example, an acute abdominal episode such as gastroenteritis in a 12-year-old child may, depending on how the family adapts to this child's sick role, resolve within a short period of time or immobilize and take the child away from school for the following 6 weeks.

Impact of illness on the family and that of the family on illness depend on the coping capacity of the family and individual involved. Coping, in general, reflects adaptability and the ability of a family system to use its own resources and outside resources to meet the challenge presented by the illness, minimize recovery time and negative effects on other family members, and prevent recurrence of the illness. Coping, therefore, depends on flexibility of roles and rules, direct and clear communication, economic resources, knowledge about disease processes, and use of community resources.

THE SICK ROLE

The concept of the sick role was first formulated by Parsons,[9] who considered the role to contain certain expectations by society: 1) The sick person is exempted from normal social responsibilities. This is both a right (which may be abused, as in malingering) and a duty or obligation: a sick person *ought* to stay in bed, stay home from work, etc. 2) The sick person cannot be expected to get well by an act of decision or will, by "pulling himself together." He cannot "help" his condition and must be "taken care of." 3) There is an obligation to want to become well since being ill is seen as undesirable. Unconsciously or consciously however, the privileges and exemptions of the sick role may provide secondary gain and decrease

316

motivation to improve. 4) Related to the desire to become well is the obligation to seek technically competent help, if the condition is serious enough to warrant it, and to cooperate with the professional in trying to get well. The professional may act as society's judge and policeman, and prescribe time off work and identify those who are abusing the privileges of the sick role.

Parson's formulation has been criticized as applying largely to modern industrialized societies, and as not being relevant to trivial illnesses, to incurable illnesses (when motivation for recovering is not relevant), to stigmatized illnesses, to various legitimate roles such as the handicapped (which may not involve the attention of a physician, exemption from normal activities, or a recovery motivation). His concept is taken from the professional perspective and fails to take into account variability due to context.[12] We believe it also fails to take into account the family's role.

Dansak[4] coined the interesting term "tertiary gain." "Primary gain" is a term for direct benefit to a person playing the sick role: the relief of lying in bed when one is feverish, the reassurance a cardiac monitoring device and hovering physicians and nurses give to a patient who is threatened with annihilation without them. "Secondary gain" is defined as the advantages the patient receives from the social environment, the social exemptions and privileges of being ill. "Tertiary gain," on the other hand, is the advantage of the illness to other people than the patient, in particular to the family. Although Dansak does not see secondary and tertiary gain from a systems orientation (that is, as two aspects of the same process), he nonetheless takes an important step towards recognizing the complexity of illness in context. Of particular note is tertiary gain involving health professionals; there is constant hazard that those who make a living from the care of the sick may at times unconsciously (or consciously) perpetrate illness or at least promote the activities and scope of health care institutions and professionals. Sometimes health professionals unwittingly take away the family's caretaker role and then fail to restore it.

IMPACT OF ACUTE ILLNESS ON FAMILY FUNCTION

The format: PRACTICE will be used to outline the aspects of family function that may need to be considered in acute illness.

P (Presenting Problem)

The problem may be the illness itself (which may be the presenting problem of family stress) or the need for hospitalization, or a consequence of illness, such as a child with behavioral problems responding to the illness of a parent.

R (Roles)

It is Monday; Mary, a 5-year-old attending a day care center, daughter of John and Andrea (both working as teachers), gets up with a rash that definitely looks like chicken pox. At this point a number of decisions have to be made rapidly; both parents have commitments at work and to their family. Someone must take the daughter to the physician. Arrangements have to be made for caretaking if it is possible or even for one of them to stay home. These parents, who share caring for the child and can also discuss the degree of accommodation of the two employers concerned, resolve the management of the acute illness episode relatively easily.

The same illness occurring in Tina, the 4-year-old daughter of a single mother who works in the neighborhood factory, will have a very different impact on the family. Role flexibility and availability of resources clearly are major assets in coping with an acute illness episode either in a child or an adult.

When Michael, a 46-year-old lawyer, had his first myocardial infarction, his wife Ann was able to find a job as a librarian. Despite the fact that Michael had good disability support from his work environment, his wife's added income minimized the loss encountered by the 4 months when he had to limit his regular work pace. When he recovered from his illness, Ann found her work rather interesting and decided to continue. In this specific case the illness episode precipitated a change that was almost ready to occur in that family, whose two teenagers had already left home for college. Communication during and after the crisis facilitated the change. The family's level of functioning was, in several ways, improved after the illness.

On the other hand, an episode of acute illness can reverse roles without changing them:

When John S., a 45-year-old mailman, had his first myocardial infarction, his wife returned to work. There were two young teenagers at home. Mr. S. was a rather assertive, domineering man who left little room for other people to take initiative. His wife complied with most of his demands and was considered less assertive and dependent on her husband. Immediately after her husband's infarct, she was rather insecure and would tend to rely on her older son to support her in many of the decisions. He reacted to this increased responsibility by daydreaming at school, and his school performance decreased. Just after Mr. S. returned home, his wife found a job. She slowly became more assertive and began to take some of the father's duties in handling the financial affairs of the family and making more decisions. To maintain such a situation, she encouraged her husband to remain in his dependent state.

This case is an example of the risks involved in role changes in which the lack of flexibility may simply reverse. The rigidity of this family adaptation hampered the recuperation of the patient.

Acute illness in the mother, who is usually the hub of family organization and activity, is usually the most stressful for the family. Particularly if the children are young and unprepared for the event, hospitalization of the mother can have a lasting effect. The clinician may have to provide help or advice in role reallocation and should try to minimize the period of separation.

The Health Care System and Family Roles

As mentioned earlier, the medical care system may take over major family roles. A premature infant, hooked onto multiple monitoring devices in an intensive care nursery, where all decision-making regarding the child is taken over by the medical institution, is deprived of contact with its mother. Mother-child bonding and all normal anticipated parenting roles are unable to be fulfilled. A child who is admitted with a severe episode of croup or bronchiolitis, or even gastroenteritis, may set up in the family feelings of incompetence in managing such a child. Long-term consequences of acute illness episodes have been well documented by Sigal and Gagnon,[13] who found out that over a 7-year follow-up parents had a different attitude to the index child compared to a sibling or a matched age group control. The family's tendancy towards such a child was more concern, more worry, overprotectiveness, and oversolicitiousness.

Even more obvious in our society is the impact on family roles of hospitalization of the elderly. Hip fractures are the classic marker event between home and institutionalized care. Lesser events, however, if sufficiently serious to warrant a visit to emergency, may result in family abdication of responsibility. An acute self-limited episode can rapidly convert to a chronic state of incapacity. In this case the hospital is the unwilling recipient, particularly in environments where beds for "chronic care" (that is, care for the elderly) are in short supply and paid for by the state. Frequently, however, a family finds itself unable to compete with the round-the-clock nursing care an institution offers, and in the hospital environment old persons may become so disoriented and deteriorated in all functions that they become impossible to look after. Prevention of hospitalization in the elderly is a major role of the family clinician.

A (Affect)

In a crisis situation there is often an initial period of stunned denial followed by some confusion, anxiety, and often resentment towards the sick member. Such a series of affective states are present whether the family is dealing with chicken pox or heart disease. It is very important for the family to be able to freely express the feelings of this transitional dysfunctional stage, and feel comfortable doing so; build-up of resentment impedes proper functioning of the family, which must deal effectively with the acute illness. A child's fears concerning hospitalization either of himself (or herself) or a parent or sibling must be addressed; it is important to be supportive.

C (Communication)

Communication among family members in times of crisis is essential to problem-solving. Whether the crisis is that of the couple whose child has just developed chicken pox, or whether it is the news that the mother has been rushed to the hospital with acute cholecystitis, communication that is open and direct facilitates the process of solving problems. On the other hand an indirect style of family communication that invites mind-reading and second guessing can make decision-making a much more laborious process and can increase the possibility of resentment and unexpressed feelings.

Clear communication is also very important with the medical care team. In the case of hospitalization the clarity of the information given to the family and expectations about the current illness episode will facilitate the family's coping. Often the many persons involved in situations like intensive care units or surgical wards may confuse the patient's family, which is already in a state of crisis. The family's dependence on health care professionals at this time is maximal; parents are very vulnerable to all forms of communication, especially the nonverbal ones such as rushing around the child's bed by the professionals, or gazing away when trying to explain something to parents. These messages often convey to the family that something worse might be going on and increase their feelings of uncertainty.

T (Time in the Life Cycle)

There are certain times in the family life cycle when acute illness is common. Clearly, young children, when they enter the school system, are at risk of infection until their immunity is built up. This is, therefore, a period of vulnerability for the working mother (or father) who must have contingency plans to cover care of a sick child. Acute illness also goes up in periods of stress (as shown by Huygen[6]), and there are times when the family is more vulnerable to the practical problems of illness. A young mother will often ignore symptoms of illness in herself as no mother substitute is available and someone must ensure that the one-year-old does not drink the varsol or fall down stairs or the three-year-old on his tricycle stays on the sidewalk. Hospitalization of a mother at this time is far more traumatic than the mother of teenagers who run their own lives and can share the cooking.

Acute illness may play a role in avoidance of the tasks of the life cycle or in maintaining family homeostasis; it may also be a way of expressing more serious problems. The young husband, whose wife is pregnant early in the marriage, who goes drinking and fractures an ankle may be indicating his lack of readiness for fatherhood. Many mothers with small children produce symptoms or stress diseases that effectively take them away from their job or force the partner to share roles. Competition for the sick role seems to be one of the most efficient ways of quieting a nagging spouse or spreading the work load. Acute illness may be seen as simply a sign of stress: in one family recurrent boils, eczema, and asthma were causes of repeated visits to the office until it became evident that the children were the go-betweens in a 10-year battle between the divorced spouses who lived one block apart. Family therapy eliminated physical symptoms and the frequent visits. The divorce, a task not completed, had to be finalized.

The mid-life crisis and the time of the children's departure is a period when illness often strikes in more serious form.[8] An acute infarction is the classic example; it may re-orient family roles and values, and sometimes allow retirement from an unpleasant job without stigma. It may also play a role in marital homeostasis and is always a test of spouse commitment and affection. It may help to keep children from leaving home.

In the elderly, acute illness may be a signal for help as waning capabilities and financial resources make living alone more and more intolerable. It may bring visits and signs of caring from relatives otherwise too busy to remember an elderly parent, grandparent, aunt, or uncle. Neighbors come in with food and help and social contact. Finally, it is illness that mobilizes the health profession that talks of prevention and health care but does little in this area.

I (Illness History)

The meaning of a given illness can vary greatly from one family to the next and will have an impact on coping with the acute episode. The family physician or nurse may have a very definite perception of what an episode of measles or "strep throat" or encephalitis may be, but all these entities are bound to have very different meanings for families with different levels of education, different health belief models, and different past experience of illness. For example, a family brought a 4-year-old child who presented with fever to the emergency room. The parents had monitored the child's fever for the last 2 weeks almost every four hours. The records of the hospital indicated that this was their fifth visit for the same complaint. Both mother and father looked anxious. On reviewing their records, the clinician noticed that the temperature variations were between 36° and 36.5° for a given day.

A thorough physical examination and enquiry showed no cause of the parents' concern. The parents were then asked what their fears were concerning the child's "fever". The mother immediately started crying, and the father explained that in the last few weeks they had heard a series on television that alluded to the fact that children with leukemia could present with a history of fever. At no time during previous encounters was the couple's view of the child's symptoms elicited. The clinician explained that although a recurrent, unexplained fever *could be* associated with neoplasm, there would be other associated symptoms and signs and reassured the parents that this was not the case with their child and suggested he confirm this impression by doing a routine blood count, which was normal. An explanation was given to the family about the normal variation of temperature in children during the day. The family left, apparently feeling very relieved that their child did not have cancer.

A family's understanding of an illness must never be assumed. Their system of information, cultural background, education, families of origin (or family member who acts as the medical interpreter) provide the family with a health belief model, often very different from the clinician's, and an understanding of what this particular illness may be. Clear communication and verification of perception allow the clinician to deal effectively with the meaning of an illness episode for a given family (see Chapter 7).

C (Coping)

In minor acute illness the very fact that the health professional is involved may indicate poor coping or that there is a broader problem for which the illness is the "ticket of admission". As Zola[16] has indicated many do not label symptoms as illness, and those who do often take the problem in stride or consult only family members. Families cope alone with most minor illness and often with more serious illness.[11] Depending on their level of medical knowledge they may recognize fever with a severe sore throat or frequency and dysuria as requiring an antibiotic. However, those who ignore urinary symptoms as a "cold in the kidneys" following an occasion when their feet got wet, may well, in the majority of cases, be coping well and not end up with chronic renal problems.

Huygen[6] noted regretfully in his study of three Dutch villages that the health of his patients seemed not to have improved over 30 years of practice despite his attitude favoring prevention. He found the incidence not only of psychological problems but also of otitis media, urinary tract infections, and other diagnoses had increased rather than decreased. He comments:

> If we define illness as a deviation of health for which medical help is called in, there can be little doubt that there is a substantial increase of illness in the population in the last 30 years. There can also be little doubt that in defining illness in this way the medical profession and health care in general have played an active role in this increase in unhealthiness.[6]

People turn to the doctor with problems that formerly were coped with at home. In their zeal not to miss serious illness, clinicians often overinvestigate, overhospitalize, and overtreat, resulting in the incredible figures for iatrogenic illness. Huygen's comments are to the point:

> Minor deviations from hypothetical "norms" and even physiological variations are apt to be regarded as "pathological" and to be treated as such, making healthy people patients, dependent upon health professionals. In my practice the hospital admission rate is only half the average of the country and still I suspect that about half the number of days my patients spend in hospital are not strictly indicated (ie. no procedures are undertaken which are not indicated and for which hospitalization of the patient is indispensable). . . . Peolple are expecting far too much from medical care nowadays. They think that medicine can take away from them almost all kinds of disease and discomfort, if medical advice is only called in betimes. . . . I have little doubt that the family plays an important role in the spreading of these expectations.[6]

Huygen concludes with the suggestion paralleling the old adage that physicians "cure sometimes, relieve often, and comfort always"; that the word comfort should be replaced by "helping to live with illness and disability."

Obviously, the converse may be true: ignoring symptoms of acute illness or lack of knowledge of their significance may be fatal. For example, the physician who recognized the fact that he had an acute coronary but insisted on concluding his afternoon office hours before leaving for the hospital was "coping" but hardly in an adaptive fashion. Denial may at times be a useful strategy, but its usefulness depends on the outcome. Families who cope by ignoring problems, blaming others, and masking feelings are the families who are illness-prone or dysfunctional. Poor coping in a family may therefore include both overreacting to minor problems and being unresponsive to major ones, or denying or being unable to problem solve (Section I, Chapter 2 describes coping styles in more detail). Clinicians tend to see families who cope poorly; this biased sample may make them overemphasize the impact of illness on the family.

E (Environment and Resources)

Like any other crisis, an acute illness requiring home care or hospitalization requires the family to develop an alternative coping strategy; more alternatives will be available if there is access to resources. Financial resources may allow the family to hire somebody to provide care to one of its members while the normal routine is maintained. This clearly facilitates adaptation. A family that is well informed about health and illness will put an illness episode in its proper perspective, deal appropriately with it, and prevent its recurrences. The presence of a network of support, whether the extended family, the community, or religious or lay organizations, may make all the difference between a family that copes well and one that disintegrates under stress.

The ability of a family to deal with an acute illness episode depends on its flexibility, its ability to mobilize its own strengths, and its use of available community resources to maintain the function of nurturance for each family member, as well as deal with the sick individual.

In the management of acute illness the household often becomes transformed: the bathroom becomes the dispensary, the kitchen the center of diet management, the bedroom the rest area where people take alternate shifts. In rural areas an efficient support network usually exists; in cities this will depend on previous work by the family to develop such a network. Neighbors may bring in meals, do the grocery shopping, or take shifts nursing if the family is at work. Greeting cards, flowers, and visits indicate awareness and support by the extended family, work colleagues, and school friends. Church groups are often vital in giving support and sometimes financial help. However, it is the extended family, who may travel some distance to help, who usually rally to the family in crisis. In the elderly the presence or absence of an extended family, or a community support group that acts as substitute family, often makes the difference between recovery or institutionalization or death.

HOSPITALIZATION

Anticipatory Guidance

Acute illness of a more serious nature may require hospitalization and possibly an operation. Hospitalization raises issues of serious outcomes even for a common problem like acute appendicitis. Hospitalization for a child is always a serious business and if possible should be well prepared for. Visits to the hospital, including frightening locations like the radiology department and the operating theatre, are now often organized by school groups, but a visit of a child who is to be hospitalized is essential. When there is no warning, time must be spent explaining procedures and answering questions. When at all possible facilities enabling the parent to stay with the child should be provided. Similarly, if a parent is to be hospitalized it is helpful to have a family interview in which young children as well as adults are encouraged to ask questions. Some hospitals are now relaxing their incredibly cruel rules against children visiting. For adults too, the need for prior discussion and explanation is essential.

The Family As Part Of The Team

The medical profession is often unaware of the extent to which it takes over the family's role in the care of illness. Families are often made to feel unwelcome intruders who can contribute nothing but germs, noise, and intrusive questions. A nurse or family physician may need to be a family advocate for the sake of both family and patient. Many studies show recovery from operation or illness to be dependent on emotional well-being.[7]

Long-term damage to families can be unwittingly done by hospital teams who find it easier to take over than to invite the family to be part of the team. In the case of a hospitalized child, parental authority is often totally disregarded, and the child may look to doctors and nurses as the only ones able to relieve misery. One child in pain at home, for instance, told his parents to leave once he was in the hospital. Only when the mother administered the pain medication did his trust in her return. For many families, dependency on the physician or hospital lasts far longer than it need because the professionals fail to give instructions and fail to return the task of caring to those best able to give it.

Prematurity—A Case Example of Hospitalization in Context

Although prematurity may not be considered an acute illness itself, it is often complicated with acute illness. (Pregnancy itself has been made into a disease: the mothers are called patients, and 90% of deliveries occur in the hospital. In the future, birthing rooms may provide both safety and a more homelike environment). Prematurity has the characteristics of a crisis situation and the potential for chronic ill effects. The premature infant is more at risk for failure to thrive, child abuse or neglect, behavioral problems, non-compliance with medical care, and frequent hospitalizations.[1,7] The reasons for this vulnerability lie partly in the interaction of infant, parents, and institution.

In the early 1900s, Budin, the father of neonatology, noticed that the parents of the infants in the "Child Hatchery," or premature nursery, did not behave as others did: they more often did not come back to pick up their child or more likely relinquished the baby for adoption.[2] Since that time, a great deal of research on the early behavior of infants, mainly between child and mother, has been generated. Is there a sensitive period for bonding? When is it? Until observation became an acceptable way to generate empirical data, the newborn was considered a very passive member of his or her environment. The observation of ethologists and pediatricians, such as Wolff,[15] Piaget,[10] Condom,[3] and De Chateau[5] showed that the infant was in fact a very active participant in the environment. The infant could hear, discriminate, smell, imitate, and see, which made him an active and interactive participant in the family and environment. These qualities were necessary for the infant to initiate caretaking in the parents ("Survival Kit"). Such knowledge has widened the scope on infant development and the infant at risk. He or she is no more a being who, in order to grow, has only to assume certain drives or be the sole passive victim of environmental stimuli; the infant can shape and be shaped by his environment.[14]

When a premature child is born, some major difficulties arise that prevent the parents from assuming their role in taking care of the child. Child care is taken over by the hospital, and the parents feel that they have been unable to produce a normal child and that they cannot assume its care. The sight of a small infant with a tube in most orifices and whose respiration is supported by a machine is very frightening; not only do the parents wonder about its survival but also about their ability to take care of such a child. Becoming emotionally attached to so frail an object seems hazardous. The physician has taken over the traditional decision-making of the father; the nurse may appear as a more expert and better mother. In short, the impact on the family is enormous. The parents become peripheral to the care of their own infant. The whole process of bonding is prolonged by early separation with an infant who does not respond with eye to eye contact or cuddling; the baby is more irritable, a tough cooky perhaps but not rewarding or lovable. The frequent geographic split of the couple (with father at work and the mother in the hospital) and their different styles of reacting to the situation can divide the family even more.

The extended family, which can be a source of support for the young couple, can also undermine confidence in the outcome. The financial burden on the family must also be contended with. (It is only recently that in Pennsylvania a law was proposed to make it mandatory that all insurance plans cover the first 28 days of life.) It is surprising that the vulnerable child syndrome is described but the vulnerable parent syndrome or the vulnerable family is not.

> Allen, premature by 4 weeks, was admitted to the ward with a low heart rate, cold extremities, and failure to gain weight. He had jaundice at birth, which required an exchange transfusion. Medical investigation was oriented to ruling out hypothyroidism. The father and mother were both in their second marriage, and Allen was the first child. The father, a university professor, was a specialist on the early development of primates. During the hospitalization, the father was very demanding, trying to ensure proper care. In contrast, the mother would go to the end of the room when a physician came to examine the child. Both parents had agreed the baby should be breast fed. The nurse assigned to that infant made the following observations: "This child is difficult to feed, arches his back, shakes his head on both sides, a typical "Mother Avoider." The mother looks tense and cannot get the child to take the breast. The father stands behind the mother and keeps giving advice. The mother then looks more exasperated and stops the feeding."

> After the nurse had reported the sequence, the physician decided to interview the family during feeding. He first examined the child with the parents present. During the assessment, it appeared that the infant had very short eye to eye contact and was difficult to soothe; the physician told the parents that this was not an unusual finding for a premature infant (normal-

ization) and that the baby would probably be more of a challenge for them. To break the cycle the clinician decided to become closer to the father by voicing an interest in child development. With the physician's encouragement the couple discussed ways in which the husband could make the mother feel more relaxed. During the interview, the infant took 1.5 ounces from the mother's breast, a much greater amount of milk than that taken during previous feedings.

How might this situation be prevented? How can the clinician give back to the parents the competence and confidence in caretaking of their infant? As early as possible the parents should become involved in the care of their infant; their fear escalates with time. Soon after the birth the team should orient the parents and show them the infant, letting them touch the child. While the mother is still recovering from the delivery, the father, who is the most mobile, should be encouraged to come to the hospital and be considered the main source of communication with the mother; mothers who want to breast feed are encouraged to send their breast milk to the medical center intensive care unit.

When the couple first visits the infant at the hospital, a physician, a nurse, and a social worker attached to the team should spend time with them in the unit explaining the function of all monitoring devices. Some fathers may have already explained the equipment to their wife. Progressively, the parents should assume more and more of the infant care. A flow sheet that is part of the infant's chart should monitor the parents' phone calls, visits, time spent with their infant, and their caretaking behavior. Other members of the family (including the extended family) should be invited to the hospital, giving the staff the opportunity to meet them and (perhaps) see their influence on the young couple.

The medical or nursing staff that works with premature infants is technically a very skilled and task-oriented staff. For them to recognize behavioral interactions and their importance is difficult and requires teachers who are competent in medical care and who are good role models in the care of the family. Family physicians have an important role in spreading a family orientation to other professionals involved with the acutely ill in emergency rooms, intensive care units, and hospital wards. It appears increasingly evident that the premature infant and parents (or any other sick person and family) are part of an ecosystem and that the primary clinician and hospital staff are part of the ecosystem as well. It is only by involving all persons connected with the infant that a rational preventive approach can be elaborated. In less technically advanced countries, responsibility for feeding and bathing of patients and for laundry is never removed from the family.

Intensive care units and emergency rooms are not only the most frightening environments for patients and family but also often the most impersonal; rooms are rarely available for discussion with families. Any family-oriented clinician should help modify the attitudes that perpetuate these negative aspects of acute care.

REFERENCES

1. Broussard E, et al: Maternal perception of the neonate as related to development. *Child Psychiatry Hum Dev* 1:16, 1970.

2. Budin P: *The Nursling*. London, Caxton Publishing Co., 1907.

3. Condom WS, Sanders LW: Neonate movements are synchronized with adult speech: Interactional participation and language acquisition. *Science* 183:99, 1974.

4. Dansak DA: On the tertiary gain of illness. *Comp Psychiatry* 14:523, 1973.

5. De Chateau P: *Neonatal Routines: Influences on Maternal, Infant Behavior and on Breast Feeding*, thesis. Umea, Sweden, Umea University Medical Dissertations NS 20, 1976.

6. Huygen FJA: *Family Medicine: The Medical Life History of Families*. The Netherlands, Dekker & Van de Vegt, 1978.

7. Leifer AD, et al: Effects of mother-infant separation on maternal attachment behavior. *Child Dev* 43:1203, 1972.

8. Lynch JL: *The Broken Heart: The Medical Consequences of Loneliness*. New York, Basic Books, 1977.

9. Parsons T: *The Social System*. New York, Free Press, 1951.

10. Piaget J: *The Origins of Intelligence in Children*. New York, International Universities, 1952.

11. Pratt L: *Family Structure and Effective Health Behavior: The Energized Family*. Boston, Houghton Mifflin, 1976.

12. Segall A: The sick role concept: Understanding illness and behavior. *J Health Soc Behav* 17:163, 1976.

13. Sigal J, Gagnon P: Effects of parents' and pediatricians' worry concerning severe gastroenteritis in early childhood on later disturbances in the child's behavior. *J Pediatr* 87:809, 1975.

14. Stern D: in Lewis M, Rosenblom LA (eds): *The Effect of the Infant on Its Caregivers*. New York, John Wiley and Sons, 1974.

15. Wolff PH: *The Causes, Controls, and Organization of Behavior in the Neonate*. New York, International Universities Press, 1965.

16. Zola IK: Studying the decision to see a doctor. *Adv Psychosom Med* 8:216, 1972.

Chapter 21
Chronic Illness

Marie Yaremko-Dolan

This chapter will examine methods of assessing a family's ability to cope with chronic illness, with the effects that chronic illness has on affected individuals and their family, and with the unique type of care which is required by the chronically ill patient. Chronic illness and family dynamics are inextricably interwoven co-evolving phenomena. Therefore, the influence of the family system on illness and on compliance with treatment will be also discussed.

Assessment: "The physician who treats illness as a family problem has the satisfaction of knowing that even though he cannot cure a disease, he can insure that its effects are limited to the patient and that it does not claim other emotional victims in the family."[8]

The concept of the family as a system with all parts being interrelated and interdependent was discussed earlier in the book and will not be further explored. It is well documented that illness is a potent agent of change for an individual, but when the disease is chronic, its "impact goes beyond the patient and touches all those who live with the affected patient"[8]:

The first step in providing the patient and the patient's family with care is the acknowledgment that disease engenders changes in the functioning of family members as a unit and as individuals. This step must be closely followed by an assessment of the family's response pattern to stresses in the past so that one can extrapolate to the present. The health professional can utilize multiple strategies to obtain data and identify the families that may have greater difficulties coping with a chronic illness. He or she can then provide them with particular attention and support.

The assessment of family function level by PRACTICE and SCREEM has been previously discussed, and is particularly well-suited to this context. Another framework similar to PRACTICE, but more specific for family assessment in chronic illness, is that of Hill and Hansen,[7] who have identified four interrelated but conceptually distinct factors:

1. Characteristics of the Event
   a. Nature of the pathology and system affected
   b. Type of disability

      c. Prognosis

      d. Potential for rehabilitation

      e. Family's perception of the illness

2. Perceived Threat to Family Relationships, Status, and Goals

      a. Past family roles, relations, and communication patterns

      b. Change in the above roles, relations, and patterns secondary to the illness (both real and perceived)

      c. Decision-making patterns before and after the illness

      d. Individual and family life goals, and changes in life goals secondary to the illness

      e. Feelings on the part of individual family members about the changes in relationships, status, and goals

3. Resources Available to the Family

      a. Demographic data: household composition, age, sex, educational background, ethnicity, religion, occupation, income, marital status, housing status, transportation available, insurance policies

      b. Persons: family members, friends, and community groups available to the client and family

4. Past Experience with the Same or Similar Situation

      a. Past crisis experienced by the family

      b. Decision-making patterns used during the crisis

      c. Individuals identified by the family as those who can be "counted on" in time of crisis

In addition, the clinician with a systems orientation is interested in stresses that antedated the illness. Factors precipitating, aggravating, and ameliorating illness and the family response to illness may provide important clues to the pathogenesis of the disease and may, on occasion, lead to more appropriate treatment and resolution of the problem. In the few illnesses that have been studied from a systems perspective (labile diabetes in childhood, asthma, anorexia nervosa[18]) it has become evident that understanding the family system early in the illness and providing family therapy may prevent the development of severe illness. The early symptoms of arthritis following the stress of unemployment[4] suggest that stress management and family assessment early in arthritis *might* alter the subsequent course of disease. The role of the illness in the family system is important to assess.[22] The question, "What would be different in your family if your illness were suddenly cured?", often elicits the role of the symptom or disease.

    Mrs. E. presented with incapacitating back pain of 2 years' duration. The pain originated from an acute disc that had not resolved, and for which, despite the lack of neurologic involvement, an operation had been done. A second operation followed, which again was not recommended by the orthopedists involved; arachnoiditis resulted. Chronic illness and poor compliance with pain medication resulted in hospitalization and a family assessment. The nurses who were trying to control this woman's pain found her very difficult to work with, she seemed to resist the pain relief. She was observed moving and sitting in positions that she had said produced pain.

This woman's reply to the question, "What difference would it make to the family if you were suddenly miraculously well?", was "Oh, I guess I would leave my husband." Before her illness she had attempted to leave her husband twice, but at that time he had been suffering from angina. She said that he "pulled a heart attack on me."

When the husband was asked the same question in a separate interview, he said, "Oh, I guess she would be back in control again." The wife was an artist and had students in the house regularly, some of whom had been young, good looking, and sexually attentive. The husband, the weaker member of the couple in many ways, had been unable to keep these students' visits to reasonable hours. Now that the wife was bedridden, he had some measure of control. He now assumed the role of breadwinner, after years of her denegration of his working ability that had produced the near collapse of his business. This couple's myth was that the woman was the stronger of the two and did not need her husband and would leave if she were not physically dependent on him, when one member of a relationship appears strong, and the other weak, this difference is usually on the surface only. The couple, through the issue of back pain, thus managed to maintain homeostasis, the myth, and the marriage and avoided confronting their real difficulties.

Prevention of further surgery contemplated by the wife was an important part of management, it was clear that without change in the marital relationship surgery would not remove the pain. A paradoxical intervention might be effective in this case but has not yet been tried: the clinician might see the couple together and adivse them that it was important that nothing be done about the pain, because without this symptom the man would go back to his subordinate position in the relationship, and the wife would be forced to realize that she needed to have him to feel strong and would in fact have great difficulty leaving the marriage.

Chloe Madanes[17] has described the politics in marriage that relate to illness or symptoms; for example, illness can reestablish a balance of power whereby the weak, submissive member gains a measure of control through symptoms, or the "strong" member is able to get pampering and care not otherwise permitted by the system. Physicians should be aware of the power in the sickness role that enables the patient to sabotage the helpfulness of a spouse or health professional, as well as the power of the healthy family member to undermine any attempt at recuperation. In this couple, the husband was very attentive and covered his anger at his wife's control by praising her as a marvelous woman, but any real attempts to improve the situation were discouraged by him.

Regardless of the framework used to assess and influence the family's ability to cope with the illness experience, the goals are the same. Data permit the health professional to construct a feasible clinical management plan that takes into consideration the psychosocial, financial, and cultural needs of the family, and that renders its success more likely. For example, in an Egyptian family, the brother of a patient with cancer was prepared to help with finances and decision making, whereas the wife, used to a sheltered position, could not be relied on either to organize family resources or get a job herself. Had she done so, moreover, she would have been rejected by her family for defying cultural norms. The presence of her brother-in-law in family interviews was therefore essential.

THE EFFECTS OF CHRONIC ILLNESS ON THE INDIVIDUAL AND HIS FAMILY

Role Changes for the Affected Individual and His Family

The ripple effect of chronic illness manifests itself in many ways, including changes in the roles of all family members. In the family system each individual has a role that prescribes appropriate behaviors, levels of responsibilities, duties, power, and type of relationship with other family members: "Family process and the general status of the family in society are intricately related to the successful enactment of multiple roles. . . . Illness is disruptive to the network of relationships which constitute the family system and to those which link the family to the community insofar as the specific role obligations can or cannot be met."[16]

> A 35-year-old patient, Mike, had a sudden cerebrovascular accident that resulted in a permanent right hemiparesis. Although Mike did not abdicate his role as husband and father of two children, it became rapidly obvious that he could no longer fulfill many of the duties associated with his roles. Most significantly, he could no longer be the family breadwinner as an airline mechanic. Mike had to adjust to this unexpected change in role and conversely his wife had to incorporate the duty of being family provider into her present role of wife and mother.

This brief example illustrates the necessary reallocation of tasks that is frequently the result of a chronic illness or handicap. (Chronic illness and handicap are considered to have similar effects on the family system.) An assessment of Mike's family would allow the health professional to determine the family's resources, strengths, coping patterns, and aid him in finding the meaning of this hemiparesis for all members of the family. Mike, while saddened by his hemiparesis, is deriving much personal satisfaction from his expanded role within the home and his augmented role as nurturer for the children. He had previously functioned as a workaholic in a job that necessitated much time away from home, and had often felt that he should consider an alternative life style. On the other hand, Mike was at times overwhelmed by a great sense of personal loss, low self-esteem, and depression at the probability of increased dependence on other family members. If such feelings were to proceed undetected by the health professional, Mike might completely withdraw from his family, and all members would suffer serious emotional trauma: "It may be that the value the person places on his various life activities helps to determine how the disability in one role affects his performance in others."[2] The health professional who possesses the knowledge of the family's value system, role adaptability, and how the family views the significance of illness can then attempt to minimize the deleterious effects of illness and assist the family in successfully attaining a new equilibrium in the family system.

Life Changes for the Spouse and the Children of a Person with a Chronic Disease

The presence of a chronically ill person in a family provokes a number of changes that vary depending on the role occupied by the patient within the family system. An illness in a parent or spouse engenders different shifts in responsibilities, lifestyle, and emotional well-being than would that same illness in a child.

The spouse who is confronted with the initial diagnosis of a chronic illness in his or her partner may experience a multitude of conflicting emotions. Most prominently featured is the threat of dissolution of the couple's original plans for their future together, which were built in part from shared dreams and in part from reality. Insecurity and disappointment replaces these plans. There is also the fear that the companion with whom many personal and family moments have been shared will be lost. There is apprehension at the increased family responsibilities and possible caretaker role that the healthy spouse may have to assume. Pity for the ill person or anger for having caused such an upheaval in the couple's lives may be manifested. These and other emotional responses to the illness can be tinged by sadness over the tangible and intangible losses that may ensue from the illness. The spouse may meticulously dissect events preceding the illness in his or her attempt to elicit the cause of the illness. Such an analysis may lead the spouse to consider his or her actions or thoughts—whether real or imagined—as blameworthy and to subsequently invoke an intense guilt reaction to illness. Guilt may in turn trigger certain behavioral responses that may be totally inappropriate. Conversely, there may be a total denial of the illness and its consequences, and the spouse may resume his or her regular routine.[5]

Mr. K. was diagnosed as having a malignant brain tumor 6 months before his death. His wife initially denied the implications of this diagnosis and proceeded with her annual "single vacation," leaving her husband behind. She later accepted his deteriorating condition and solicited "curing" medications, prayers, and other help from various less traditional health organizations. This behavior was closely enmeshed with anger at the medical profession for the late diagnosis and lack of proffered hope. Finally, Mrs. K. acknowledged her husband's impending death and was able to grieve with her husband and share their last few moments.

The emotional turmoil experienced by the spouse can be likened to a grief reaction, which undergoes a natural progression from denial and isolation to anger, bargaining, depression, and acceptance.[13] Armed with the knowledge that such a reaction is normal, the health professional can support the spouse in resolving these deeply conflicting feelings towards the illness and the patient and act as a facilitator for the couple and the family in exploring their feelings and behavior as they struggle together searching for an acceptable new balance. Intervention by the health professional at the outset of a chronic illness may reduce the potential for the development of emotional pathology in the family.

Practical Issues. Other issues that the family must confront are decision-making patterns, financial needs and resources, household duties, child nurturance, and lifestyle changes. It is not uncommon to encounter spouses who are unaware of routine family decisions or finances or who have rarely participated in the weekly activities of grocery shopping, cooking, and cleaning. The issues will vary depending on the type of chronic illness, its prognosis, and the potential for rehabilitation. An illness such as diabetes has different consequences on a person's lifestyle than does a patient's chronic renal disease necessitating dialysis three times weekly; also, an illness with an excellent prognosis such as asthma requires a different emotional adjustment than does a disease such as leukemia with a much poorer prognosis. Nevertheless, the family's lifestyle in asthma may be dramatically affected by multiple hospitalization and may in turn contribute to the illness and increase the frequency of hospitalization (see section III); the consequences regarding practical concerns may be as serious as those of leukemia. Financial resources can greatly determine the disruptive sequelae of a disease. Angina in a financially well-off professional will precipitate fewer lifestyle changes for the family than will a similar case of angina in a manual laborer with minimal financial resources. Income also affects the type of auxiliary care that a family can afford for the ill individual, thereby lessening the caretaker burden.

Resources. The extended family and neighbors can be a liability or an asset to a family coping with illness. They may inundate the caretaker with unwanted advice or with anecdotes with dire outcomes, or may actively interfere with management. On the other hand, family resources may make the difference between economic, emotional, and physical survival or collapse. Other community resources play a vital support role in many illnesses. For example, the Kidney Foundation, run by members of the community for families facing dialysis or transplants, gives information on the disease, treatments, and diet, and provides financial help and a forum for ventilating problems and for socializing with others similarly affected. Societies for multiple sclerosis, diabetes, and cancer, and organizations for those with colostomies, mastectomies, and other medical conditions supplement state financing and are most effective as self-help groups. A clinician must be aware these clubs exist and have some knowledge of government agencies and of groups providing financial support for the handicapped or chronically ill. Church groups and local cultural or community centers are other important resources.

Illness in Spouse.   Many studies have shown an increased incidence of illness in the spouse of a chronically ill person, but the cause of this increased incidence is not clear. Klein and associates observed that spouses reported "new and increased symptoms during the illnesses of their partners."[2] It has been suggested by Vincent[26] that there may be "familosomatic ailments" that "accidentally or purposefully, real or imagined, are developed to avoid certain tasks, since the illness of one spouse increases the tasks of the other." Lewis'[15] review of circumstances wherein the individual can be predisposed to illness applies strongly to the spouse of a chronically ill patient. These circumstances occur during periods that are perceived as stressful, or encompass a number of life changes, or include severe separation or object loss, or that follow a prolonged affective state of hopelessness or helplessness.[15]

Chronic illness may serve as a source of communication in the family: angina in a widow who does not want to be left alone, a slipped disc in a young mother who cannot cope with the burden of three children under 3 years of age, asthma in a child that diverts attention from parental conflict. Studies have shown that there is less sickness in families in which communication is open and direct, and that if sickness does occur such families cope better with the emotional and practical problems.

THE EFFECT OF ILLNESS ON CHILDREN

Children are greatly affected by illness in a parent. Their emotional anguish is very similar to that of their healthy parent, but with their limited life experience and minimal knowledge of how to seek help, their unresolved emotional turmoil can produce even greater deleterious long-term effects. One study showed that behavioral problems appeared or increased in 30% of children of a chronically ill parent.[2] This finding is similar to multiple other studies. Among the children of cancer patients, problems most frequently seen were school dysfunction, tearfulness, disturbed eating habits, and physical symptoms.[8]

The child's age and development and psychological maturity at the time of diagnosis of the parental illness influences the possible adaptive and maladaptive roles that may be assumed. The reallocation of tasks may result in children assuming responsibilities that are greater than their age and maturity would allow. In many ways, the health professional may have to act as the child's advocate in attempting to make other family members sensitive to the child's particular needs and also in minimizing the negative long-term effects.

In older children unresolved issues such as individuation and separation may become obvious at the time of parental disease:

> M.G., a highly successful, single 50-year-old executive lived with her mother, who was chronically ill and bed-ridden. As her mother's condition deteriorated, M.G. made increasingly inappropriate demands on the health professionals caring for her mother. She demanded weekly physical assessments, daily phone calls, etc. She interpreted all other helping gestures such as obtaining outside help as subtle accusations of her inadequacy in caring for her mother. She refused all help that was directed towards allowing her a few leisure hours a week.

The mounting demands that M.G. made for the care of her mother were totally unrealistic and inappropriate. An understandable response on the part of the health professional would have been frustration and anger towards her, but neither would alter the moving force behind these demands. On the other hand, the health professional could assist M.G. in separating from her mother and in exploring the motivation for her absolute dedication to her mother.

By viewing the family as the unit of care, the health professional can offer individual members the support and guidance they need and attempt to minimize interpersonal conflicts. By opening and clarifying communication within the family, a realistic assessment of the new situation engendered by chronic illness can be achieved, and a clinical management plan can be devised in both the family's and the physicians's expectations can be met. Such a clinical management plan has the least chance of sabotage by various family members and the greatest chance for success.

Life Changes for Children with Chronic Disease, Their Siblings and Parents

It has been reported by American and British surveys that 7% to 10% of all children under 18 years of age have chronic physical illnesses, including conditions such as asthma, cystic fibrosis, diabetes, hemophilia, leukemia, seizures, and sickle cell anemia. This figure results in an estimate of 4.3 to 4.8 million children affected by chronic illness.[9]

Isaacs and McElroy[9] surveyed the literature in an attempt to synthesize the effects of chronic illness on children, their families and teachers, and to provide the foundation for an "integrated and comprehensive approach to their care." They have classified the impact of illness on the child into the following categories:

1. fear of abandonment—hospitalizations and the feelings of helplessness heighten this fear;
2. misunderstanding the cause of illness—inappropriate or inadequate explanations of the illness may lead to distortions as to diagnosis and prognosis. A child may feel that illness is punishment for bad behavior or thoughts in the past;
3. feeling different—depending on the illness, the child may look different or need to behave differently from his peers;
4. disruptions in school attendance—school plays an important role in every child's maturation, and possibly an even greater role in the chronically ill child. It is the environment where the child comes into intimate contact with the world outside his or her family;
5. changes in activities and educational goals—depending on the illness, the child may need to reorient his or her activities and educational aspirations;
6. reactions of peers—peers and teachers who are uninformed or misinformed may subject the ill child to a multitude of emotional and physical indignities. A child with headaches and dreamy behavior was teased unmercifully by her peers and labelled a hypochondriac by teachers. Taunts increased when she had to spend time in the hospital for investigation. She later died of a brain tumor, leaving a legacy of guilt with her schoolmates.

Multiple factors determine the effects of a chronic illness for a child. These can be the age and stage of development at the time of diagnosis, the limitations of activities imposed by the illness, the external signs of disease and its treatment, and the prognosis. The chronically ill child must not only progress through the normal stages of development to attain maturity, but must also incorporate an adaptation to his or her illness and its consequences. The maturation process may be prone to greater difficulties for the ill child for several reasons:[2]

1. parents often protect the chronically ill child or adolescent from learning adult roles and responsibilities;
2. the chronically ill child may learn to use his illness to "get his way";
3. the chronically ill child is permitted by society to have more freedom

in the expression of feelings and behaviors regarding his or her illness than adults. When the child becomes an adult he or she may have to learn new and more socially acceptable ways of expression and behavior;

4. the chronically ill young person may not be able to adjust to illness as he or she wants to because his or her lifestyle may be controlled by adults.

The issues of parenting an ill child need to be raised and explored.[20] Parents have identified problems in the areas of everyday tasks, discipline, medical treatment, and worries about the child's social development. They question the appropriateness of the old rules and approaches to child rearing.

Marlena, a 12-year-old child, suffered from severe asthma attacks that frequently necessitated hospitalization. The nurse practitioner concerned with the negative effects of multiple hospitalizations went to the home to assess the child. Marlena's emotional development was felt to be markedly retarded to that of a 7-year-old child. Marlena was incapable of making any decisions for herself. The parents, on the other hand, were reluctant to exercise any discipline or to attempt to instill a sense of responsibility in Marlena, because every attempt was greeted by an asthma attack.

Louis, an 8-year-old boy had hemophilia and was classified as a "moderate bleeder." His family and school teachers expressed much concern about his behavioral maturation. Louis did not comply with any medical regimen, and was well aware that his behavior went unpunished. For instance, rather than use his crutches, he "rented" them to classmates and hobbled around himself.

Marlena's emotional development improved considerably when the parents reduced their protectiveness and guilt and permitted Marlena to express her feelings and mature. Louis' parents were given "permission" by the health professionals to scold and occasionally spank Louis for disciplinary problems. The health professional even attended the first spanking. As the parents' fear of making Louis bleed as a result of their discipline decreased, so did their feelings of anger and frustration at being held hostage by the child. Their need to spank him also diminished. The parents and the teachers remarked on Louis' behavioral improvements as he became more secure within their established limits. Both cases stress how vital it is for the health professional to elucidate the child's and the family's anxieties so that appropriate care can be provided.

Stein and Reissman[24] have described their preliminary findings while developing a scale that would quantify the impact of childhood illness on the family. They have focused on any change in the normative behavior of the family that is directly attributable to the child's illness. Four factors were elicited as requiring specific measurement in determining the impact of the child's illness on the family:

1. the economic burden—the extent to which the illness changes the economic status of the family and draws resources away from other areas;
2. the social impact on the quality and quantity of interaction with those outside the immediate household;
3. the familial impact—interaction within the family unit, including parental and sibling relationships;
4. subjective distress—the strain experienced by the primary caretaker that is directly related to the demands of the illness.

The effect of childhood illness on marital relations is not clearly defined. Studies have usually been cross-sectioned since longitudinal studies that assess family function before and after the onset of illness are difficult or impossible to do. The degree to which pre-existent dysfunction may have contributed to the occurrence of disease has rarely been considered, nor has the possibility that illness might play a role in family homeostasis and might be needed to keep the family together. Clearly, a disease like asthma has a greater possibility of being influenced by family dysfunction in comparison with genetic diseases like cystic fibrosis.

Begletder and associates[1] concluded that the prevalence of divorce or separation in families having a child with cystic fibrosis was no greater than that of the general population. Other studies tend to support the idea that the rate of breakdown in families with chronically ill children is high. The means by which chronic illnesses erode a marital couple's feeling of well-being can only be guessed at. The strain of coping with a sick child whose clinical course may be interspersed with exacerbations and remissions or a continuous decline of health may be cumulative over time. The child's increased dependence and need for nurturance may leave little time for couple activities. Reduced mobility and financial strain may also play a prominent part in explaining the effects of childhood illness on the couple.

Much of the burden and emotional strain falls on the mother, who is usually the caretaker. She is often chronically fatigued and feels she has no time for the other children, let alone herself. She may find it difficult to avoid feeling like a martyr, and may resent demands of the sick child and those of others in the family; she may also be angry at her husband who is trying to escape much of the work and worry. If the mother previously worked, she may have had to give up her career because of the child. Reliable babysitters are hard to find; it is all the more difficult to find someone capable of caring for a handicapped or sick child. The husband, on the other hand, may be suffering from lack of contact with his wife as well as having the often enormous financial burden of the sick child.

Siblings are important members of the family constellation. Children see them as significant persons in their environment. Relationships that enrich play and socialization and aid in psychosocial development are altered by illness in a sibling. The illness shifts the focus of family concern and creates a disequilibrium that may intensify rivalries and decrease the beneficial aspects of the sibling relationship.[14,25]

In a recent study, Taylor[25] interviewed siblings of children with asthma, congenital heart disease, or cystic fibrosis. She concluded that the reaction of a healthy child to living with a chronically ill sibling was a highly individualized and multifaceted process, and that the development of the healthy sibling was affected more negatively than positively. Two out of three of the children's statements showed that they experienced feelings of isolation, egocentricity, deprivation, inferiority, or inadequate knowledge about some aspect of their sibling's conditions. The largest single ill effect was the healthy siblings' feelings of isolation—they viewed the parents and the ill child as a unit that excluded them. These children also felt that there was a lack of parental time and attention, qualities necessary in fostering a good relationship between parent and child. All healthy children admitted that they occasionally wished their ill siblings were dead. Positive effects resulted when the healthy sibling participated in taking care of the sick sibling; empathy developed. Also noted was the association between increased development in healthy children and possession of more complete information about their sibling's illness. The health professional caring for the family again may take the stance of child advocate—but for the healthy siblings.

Coping with Illness

The occurrence of chronic illness in a family member can be regarded as a major life crisis for the family unit. An individual or family cannot remain in the ensuing state of disequilibrium for long periods; hence, this crisis is by definition self-limited. The new balance achieved may represent a healthy adaptation that promotes personal growth or maturation, or a maladaptive response that signifies psychological deterioration and decline.[19]

The pattern of coping skills used by a family is highly individualized. These patterns have been developed over time while the family adapted to various other problems. Generally, a coping skill cannot be considered adaptive or maladaptive without knowledge of the purpose it is serving and the duration of its use: "Emotional disturbance and equilibrium regaining behaviors can be indistinguishable at times."[10] For example, the denial of the presence of diabetes in one's child, accompanied by physician-shopping is not necessarily maladaptive at the outset of the disease, but may be considered so after a long period has elapsed. Such denial could be potentially life-threatening for the child.

Caring for the family as a unit should begin soon after the diagnosis of illness is made because the coping strategies, whether adaptive or maladaptive, begin within 2 to 4 weeks of diagnosis and become harder to change as the illness progresses.[8] Overprotection, overindulgence, smothering love, and total dependency must be balanced by appropriate levels of responsibility, discipline, trust, and caring. The established balance must be flexible and capable of shifting with the variable needs of the patient and other family members, as well as with the course of the disease.

Angela, an 8-year-old child, was admitted and treated for severe glomerulonephritis. She recovered well from her illness, but her care required close follow-up and strict adherence to a diet. The parents' compliance with the established regimen of care was excellent, but they proceeded to make all family activities reflect Angela's care: all siblings were on the same diet and had restricted activites; the reason given was "prevention." The parent's natural inclination was to overprotect Angela by prohibiting any participating in sports, parties, etc. They thwarted all her attempts to socialize and individuate. Angela then became very unhappy and was noncompliant with regard to treatment.

The family was presented to the health professional 1 year after the initial diagnosis and subsequent recovery from glomerulonephritis. Family members were all obviously unhappy and worried. The issues of medical compliance, the needs of Angela in maturing, and parental anxieties were explored, and a compromise was reached between the parents' overconcern with medically unwarranted restrictions and Angela's rebellious, depressed behavior.

Krulik[12] reported successful "normalizing" tactics used by 20 parents of chronically ill children to reduce their child's feelings of being different from his siblings and peers. The children suffered from cystic fibrosis, acute lymphocytic leukemia, and other forms of malignancies. In one family, everyone did the physical therapy required for the sick child as part of the family exercises. Other families gave out vitamin pills while the sick child took the prescribed medication so that "no one would feel left out." These and other strategies were directed towards strengthening the resources and coping abilities of the child and towards altering the environment to compensate and accept the child.[12]

Krulik identified several principles which underlined these "normalizing tactics."

1. Preparation, both of the ill child and his or her close environment for any changes in routine, function, or appearance.
2. Giving the child the opportunity to participate in decision-making and management of the regimens so that the child is a partner in performing the regimen.
3. The management of illness was a shared experience by the whole family; the ill child was not singled out.

4. The management of illness was a shared experience by the child's social environment; the illness ceased to be a "shameful secret."

5. Taking control—parents identified areas where control decreased the feelings of uncertainty, passivity and helplessness.

The community in which a chronically ill child lives can be the source of various kinds of support systems for the individual and his family. Kaplan and Mearig[10] describe an extensive community program that evolved to assist a family attempting to cope with three sons suffering from Duchenne muscular dystrophy. The original impetus for the community program was the projected need for adequate housing for the family when the three boys would be in wheelchairs. The community provided funding and labor in this endeavor. Local state university students developed an ongoing commitment (one generation of students replaced another) to assist the children with the day-to-day living requirements. The increased contact between the community and the family helped redefine the problem for both the community and the family. The community felt a responsibility for the family with three children who needed help to live effective lives; and the family felt less isolated by its emotional, financial, and medical burden.

Obviously, much ingenuity and thought is required to solve the ongoing problems confronted by the chronically ill person and his or her family. The greater the number of familial and community resources available, the greater the ability to cope with chronic illness.

The Role of the Health Professional

A thorough assessment of the family function level provides is a firm foundation on which a clinical management plan encompassing all aspects of the patient's life can be developed. The clinical management plan that is unique to each patient and family has a greater chance of success. A study by Steidl, Finkelstein and colleagues[23] of an adult population with chronic end-stage illness has identified a clear association between patient adherence to medical regimen and specific areas of effective family functioning. Whether illness begets dysfunction or dysfunction begets illness (or both) is difficult to assess. The three specific areas of family functioning that are found to correlate well with medical assessment are a strong parental coalition, respect for the individual in a context of closeness, and warm affectionate and optimistic interactions. The components of family functioning that correlate with adherence tend to be more task-oriented. The authors feel that these findings justify the evaluation of families of chronically ill patients who are either medically unstable or noncompliant and that if family dysfunction exists, family therapy may alter compliance or improve the medical condition. Possibly a "preventive" assessment of family function at the onset of management would identify families requiring greater support and intervention so that the problem of noncompliance and poor medical conditions could be averted.

The patient and his family may develop an expertise and sophistication in managing the patient's daily care, and may also become very knowledgeable about the particular disease process. The health professional when confronted with such a situation may experience discomfort and feel threatened, yet the family's expertise is an asset in providing the best care possible for them. Hospitalizations are frequently cited by patients and their families as being frustrating, humiliating, and anger-provoking.[3] Parents who have been monitoring care at home are often not allowed to give medications, do physical therapy, or handle routine care.[11] They are forced to abdicate all control to the hospital staff while being labelled as "over-protective," "bossy," and "neurotic." They are not involved in any decision-making and are rarely given the opportunity to choose their level of involvement in the care of their child during a particular hospital stay. Hence, it would benefit all parties involved if the role of the hospitalizations, the patient's and family's needs and expectations, and the needs of the hospital staff were clearly defined so that an effective working agreement could be attained.[6]

> Mrs. C., a 50-year-old paraplegic patient had over the years mastered bowel control by rectal touch. She required hospitalization for an elective cholecystectomy and was prohibited from performing her own bowel care while hospitalized. This experience proved to have negative emotional and medical sequelae: the patient felt humilated and totally dependent on the staff and developed a mild bowel obstruction. The patient was "cured" and returned home to resume her own appropriate daily routine care. Three years later, Mrs. C. now requires elective but necessary surgery for glaucoma. She expresses much reluctance to consent to the surgery for fear of loss of hard-earned independence once more.

This example illustrates the need for hospital staff to explore patient expectations, and to acknowledge and respect their ability to control their own care.

Generally the health professionals' role is to encourage and support the patient and the patient's family in becoming their own advocates. However, the health professional must remain sensitive to the fact that the family of chronically ill children or adults may simply "run out of physical and psychological steam to advocate steadily."[10] It may then become the health professional's role to advocte for the patient and family as they regain their depleted energy. The family and patient are also often afraid of retaliation for complaints to the hospital staff; they fear withdrawal of care and feel extemely vulnerable during hospitalization.

Open and effective lines of communication between the health professional and the patient and his family as well as between family members must be actively maintained and cherished. This communication plays a role in preventing much of the paranoia expressed by the ill patients, who are concerned about "what they aren't being told," and allows for appropriate alteration of roles and tasks as the disease changes. It also permits the ongoing sharing of anxieties, fears, and emotional upheavals as the patient and his family strive to live the most effective lives possible.

The family must be made to feel secure and confident that the care they are receiving is comprehensive. Many studies support the fact that parents of ill children are unclear about who is responsible for care, and this confusion may subsequently lead to a lack of understanding of the medical condition. The family and all care providers must know who is orchestrating the care.[21] Once the health professional responsible for the management of the patient care has been clearly defined, it then becomes imperative to synchronize the care offered by all other team members in their respective capacities. The team approach is most applicable in the setting of a chronically ill patient because of the many complex medical and psychosocial concerns that develop. Social workers, nurses, physiotherapists, clergy, and community volunteers can all be called on to assist and enrich the patient's and his family's life.

REFERENCES

1. Begleiter ML, et al: Prevalence of divorce among parents of children with cystic fibrosis and other chronic diseases. *Soc Biol* 23:260, 1976.

2. Bruhn JG: Effects of chronic illness on the family. *J Fam Pract* 4:1057, 1977.

3. Burch GE: Of the family of the sick. *Am Heart J* 92:405, 1976.

4. Cobb S: Social support as moderator of life stress. *Psychosom Med* 38:300, 1976.

5. Farkas SW: Impact of chronic illness on the patient's spouse. *Health Soc Work* 5:39, 1980.

6. Hibler M: The chronic patient: Perspectives from the 29th Institute on Hospital Community Psychiatry. The problems as seen by the patient's family (proceedings). *Hosp Community Psychiatry* 29:32, 1978.

7. Hill RA, Hansen DA: in Christensen HT (ed): *Families Under Stress: Handbook of Marriage and the Family*. Chicago, Rand McNally and Co., 1964.

8. Huth CM: Illness and the family. *Ann Intern Med* 89:132, 1978.

9. Isaacs J, et al: Psychosocial aspects of chronic illness in children. *J Sch Health* 50:318, 1980.

10. Kaplan D, et al: A community support system for a family coping with chronic illness. *Rehabil Lit* 38:79, 1977.

11. Kodadek S: Family-centered care of the chronically ill child. *AORN J* 30:635, 1979.

12. Krulik TJ: Successful 'normalizing' tactics of parents of chronically-ill children. *Adv Nursing* 5:573, 1980.

13. Kübler-Ross E: *On Death and Dying*. New York, Macmillan, 1969.

14. Lavigne JV, et al: Psychologic adjustment of siblings of children with chronic illness. *Pediatrics* 63:616, 1979.

15. Lewis JM: The family and physical illness. *Tex Med* 72:43, 1976.

16. MacVicar MG, et al: A framework for family assessment in chronic illness. *Nurs Forum* 15:180, 1976.

17. Madanes C: Marital therapy when a symptom is presented by a spouse. *J Fam Therapy* 2:120, 1980.

18. Minuchin S: *Psychosomatic Families.* Cambridge, Harvard University Press, 1978.

19. Moos RH: *Coping With Physical Illness.* New York, Plenum Medical Book Company, 1977.

20. Pond H: Parental attitudes toward children with a chronic medical disorder: Special reference to diabetes mellitus. *Diabetes Care* 2:425, 1979.

21. Satterwhite BB: Impact of chronic illness on child and family: An overview based on five surveys with implications for management. *Int J Rehabil Res* 1:7, 1978.

22. Shoemaker WH Jr, et al: Chronic invalidism in a young woman: A study of family dynamics. *J Fam Pract* 4:155, 1977.

23. Steidl JH, et al: Medical condition, adherence to treatment regimes, and family functioning. *Arch Gen Psychiat* 37:1025, 1980.

24. Stein RE, et al: The development of an impact-on-family scale: Preliminary findings. *Med Care* 18:465, 1980.

25. Taylor SC: The effect of chronic childhood illness upon well siblings. *Makin Child Nurs J* 9:109, 1980.

26. Vincent CE: The family in health and illness: Some neglected areas. *Am Acad Pol Soc Sci* 34:109, 1963.

Chapter 22

Terminal Illness and Death

Janet Christie-Seely

As sex was to the 19th century, so death has been to much of the 20th century—a subject not to be discussed and a phenomenon not to be acknowledged. This is still largely true; few physicians and nurses really feel comfortable with the dying patient.[17,26]

Literature on the impact of death on the family system is almost nonexistent in comparison with the impact on the individual. Despite the observation that family dysfunction often follows death, there has been little if any research into the effect of death on the family unit. Nevertheless, much has been written recently about the successive emotional stages experienced by patients and individual relatives when confronted by death. Dr. Kübler-Ross[17] has led a transition in the medical field, from a tendency to deny death to a conscious effort to deal more openly and thus more effectively with the end of life. Unfortunately, some health professionals have changed from hiding the facts about disease—"Patients really don't want to know the truth about their disease"—to an attitude characterized by abrupt and sometimes cruel "honesty," as in the following example:

> A woman admitted for suspected carcinoma of the pancreas had a brief encounter with a resident and his retinue of interns. He told her, "The ultrasound showed that you have a malignancy that probably has already extensively invaded." He then left the room without further discussion. Left alone in her room for 3 hours, the patient decided to pack her things to leave the hospital; having the operation clearly was not worthwhile. She was persuaded later by her husband and the surgeon to undergo the operation. A benign pancreatic cyst was found.

Many clinicians still join the family's "conspiracy of silence" and isolate the patient, despite the fact that the latter is in the vast majority of cases well aware of the diagnosis without being told. As a consequence, the family and the patient are deprived of the opportunity to share their reactions and help each other adapt to the current illness and the approaching death.

THE EMOTIONAL RESPONSE TO A FATAL ILLNESS

The Patient: Kübler-Ross observed a series of mental adjustments— denial, anger, bargaining, depression, and acceptance—commonly seen in those persons facing death. Further observations have made it apparent that her classic description of a dying person's "stages" may be combined, vary in sequence, or fail to appear in a particular situation. Dr. Kübler-Ross's work, however, is still a valuable guide for any family or health professional with a dying patient.

Health professionals who have come to know and care about a patient also go through the phases of denial of the prognosis, of bargaining over treatment, and of being angry at family members or other professionals (or at God) for mishandling the situation. They may also experience conscious or masked depression. Health professionals who take care of many such patients undergo particularly severe forms of stress requiring specific measures for its relief. In the hospice movement, the stress and "burnout" of staff members have usually been recognized earlier and managed better than the stress that occurs, for similar reasons, in the staff of intensive or coronary care units of hospitals.[12,32] Symptoms of such stress include depersonalized and inhumane medicine, absenteeism, ill health, rapid turnover of personnel, and scapegoating of patients, nurses, doctors, or administrators. More constructive responses include staff discussions,[27] efficient team work with distribution of the load of the seriously ill among several professionals, a strong support group with whom emotional ventilation can occur, time off for stress (a more honest practice than giving "sick leave") and, most important, recognition that the physician and nurse is human and should be allowed a human response to the suffering and pain that surrounds them.

The patient's family goes through similar emotional reactions. Family denial may impede transmission of information to the patient, who may be quite ready to accept what he or she recognizes must be a diagnosis of cancer while the family still refuses to believe it. Family anger is often directed at the medical profession. If the professionals fail to recognize that the anger directed at them is really anger at the disease and respond in kind, the care of the patient may suffer, and the family may then fixate its anger on the professional.

An elderly Italian woman was admitted because of abdominal pain but was discharged after laparotomy without being given a diagnosis. The family was told by the surgeon's answering service that he could no longer look after the patient. The family finally learned of the diagnosis of colonic carcinoma from a friend of the operating room nurse. The patient was subsequently admitted to another hospital because of uncontrolled pain. The family was overprotective and suspicious of the nursing staff, requested an overdose of morphine to prevent more pain, and hovered beside the patient 24 hours a day when allowed. The nurses felt that both their professional caring and their expertise were considered suspect. It was the *family's* fear of pain rather than the patient's, and the family's anger at the diagnosis, that produced a very hostile situation between the many family members and the nurses and doctors on the ward. Adequate pain control without sedation only became possible after discussion with the family allowed ventilation of anger and guilt.

In another example, the anger of the family was directed at a nurse who had given a very small dose of morphine to control the patient's severe pain. The family had stipulated, "Don't give him any pain killers or you might kill him." It became apparent that it was primarily the wife who was angry; her husband had never spent much of his time with her, took frequent business visits away from the home, and was now about to leave forever. Only after discussing her anger at the husband did the wife allow adequate pain control with morphine. It was postulated that her previously repressed anger was great, and that morphine represented her subconscious wish for his death.

The patient, the family, and the attending health care staff all react to the diagnosis and prognosis but may do so with varying degrees of denial, acceptance, anger, bargaining, and depression at different times and may be in conflict with one another. A new symptom may change the patient's attitude from accepting the illness and death to denying illness again because he or she is reminded by the symptom of the reality of approaching death. The family may realize that the new symptom means that it is time for the will to be written. The oncologist may also respond to the symptom by suggesting more chemotherapy, which may indicate that the oncologist is still bargaining and not accepting a fatal outcome, or that there is further chemotherapy of potential value that has not yet been tried. Recognition of reality factors and conflicting degrees of denial, acceptance, and bargaining help to prevent conflict.

LIFE THREATENING DISEASE: VALUE SYSTEMS AND CULTURE

The Role of the Clinician in the Meaning of Illness

As discussed in the sections on values and the meaning of illness, serious illness raises issues that go far beyond the medical problems of diagnosis and treatment. After the first shock of diagnosis, many patients with serious illness discover new ways of looking at life; indeed, they may experience a major reorientation of their value system. Family relationships often become central to what is valued in life. It has been said that there is no growth except through suffering and that all learning involves pain. During the crisis of life brought on by impending death, individuals and families gain an appreciation of what they truly value, and see and develop parts of themselves of whose existence they were unaware. An emaciated 22-year-old with terminal cancer said of his last 6 months that "they had been the happiest and most valued days of his life" (film: "The Last Days of the Living," Canadian Film Board, 1979).

An ethical question that has gained prominence recently, although it is as old as man's speculation about disease, is the problem of blame and responsibility for cancer. A series of studies demonstrating the relation between stress, personality, and cancer[4,15] has been brought to popular attention by LeShan[20] and the Simontons.[35] The effect of such studies (see Chapter 4) has been to refocus the problem of the cause of illness as retribution for faulty living. Whatever the truth may be regarding the many factors cited as playing a role in cancer causation, seeing it as the consequence of particular lifestyles adds a burden of guilt to families and patients. The same can be said of heart disease, with its known links to stress and lifestyle. The patient with a myocardial infarction must recognize the possibility that his or her type A personality, overwork, cigarette abuse, or other aspects of lifestyle have contributed to his predicament. The family may also blame the patient and be angry about the preventable crisis inflicted on them. The health professional can help by reminding the family that genetic factors and family patterns of diet and behavior built up over generations are hard to change, and by emphasizing the positive aspect of responsibility, that is, a change of behavior can help in the fight against cardiac disease. There is evidence that the outcome of heart disease and perhaps also of cancer is related to the patient's response to illness and to the workings of the family system.[13,39]

Questions and Denial—Conveying the Diagnosis or Prognosis

When the diagnosis of cancer, serious heart disease, renal disease, or other life-threatening illness first becomes known, the patient's immediate response is shock and usually denial: "Why me?", "What did I do to deserve this?", "Am I being punished, and for what?", and "If I'm a better patient/person, will I get better?" are questions that the medical or nursing professions are ill equipped to answer. Referral for pastoral counselling can be an important approach to dealing with this and subsequent phases of terminal illness for some patients. Other questions such as "Am I infectious?" or "Can this be passed on to my children?" can be answered by the health professional, but may often go unasked unless they are elicited.

The question "Should I tell my family or my children?" should usually be answered in the affirmative, unless there is a clear indication by the person concerned that he or she does not wish to know. Even then, it is probable that denial will be an effective defense and the patient or family member will not hear more than he or she is ready to assimilate at any given time. Frequently, a person who has been given certain facts quite clearly will deny having been told until ready to integrate it with his or her personality and experience.

The question "Should I tell. . .?" is most easily answered by questioning the person concerned. Patients can always be asked what they think is the matter with them, how they see the future, or whether they have any fears or specific worries. If the patient's answer is positive ("I have arthritis." or "I'm getting better and I'm going home soon."), the subject should probably be closed, at least for the time being. Patients' questions or comments indicate their willingness to discuss the subject. However, it is essential to recognize that lack of readiness indicates fear, which cannot be dealt with if not discussed. The question of prognosis must often be raised by the clinician so that the patient or family can voice anxieties that are worse if felt and not shared or expressed. Some fears, such as fear of pain or a dramatic demise ("I'll bleed to death like my friend's uncle." or "The tumor will make me burst.") can be relieved by the clinician's knowledge. Descriptions of death as peaceful by patients who have survived resuscitation[25] help many with the fear of the unknown, even if they have no religious faith in an afterlife.

Too often a clinician ignores an opportunity to help a family or a patient go beyond denial; this may be professional cowardice and self-protection rather than protection of the patient. One such physician's approach to ambivalence is illustrated by the following overheard conversation:

Patient: "I'm tired of doctors being evasive, they never tell you the truth."

Doctor: "Well, do you really want to know the truth?"

Patient: "Yes, of course, providing it's not bad news."

The doctor smiled and closed the conversation. He could have continued and sided with the part of the patient that wanted to know the truth, or he could have asked if the patient *really* wanted to convey the message that she only wanted good news, or he could have asked her what would be so fearful about bad news. Or he could have said, "Some of us don't want to think about possibilities that make us afraid, but often fears feel better when we talk to someone about them. Sometimes fears are worse than reality. Would you like to talk about what you're afraid of?" It is important to leave the option to pursue the subject with the patient.

The Conspiracy of Silence

Cultural background is a significant component of the "conspiracy of silence." Families of Mediterranean origin often say that if the patient were to know the diagnosis he or she would immediately become depressed and die. It is not natural for such families to break silence abruptly and inform the patient. The family's prediction may prove to be correct. Research into voodoo death supports the power of a belief system to cause death.[7] A clinician from a different culture may attempt to point out the advantages of the patient being made aware of the process of dying (affirmation of values, re-ordering of priorities, completion of unfinished business, making financial arrangements, emotional sharing and support instead of isolation, etc.) but should *not*, in most cases, ignore the family's wishes. Continuing to give gentle attention to the family's fear of death and denial often results in the agreement later on to break the conspiracy of silence. Such problems can be avoided by the policy of breaking the news of terminal illness to both patient and spouse at the same time. Clearly, both patient and spouse or family have a right to know, and each then can provide support to the other and maintain open communication and sharing. Choosing the appropriate time to give information or to embark on a discussion requires empathy and understanding of the workings of the family system and of the course of the patient's disease.

On the other hand, the *patient* may not be frank or open because of his or her participation in a "conspiracy of silence" to protect the *family*. Denial is an important and often useful protective mechanism because acceptance is a slow process. Questioning the patient in the presence of family members about his or her acceptance of the illness often reveals the patient's complete knowledge of the outcome of disease and relieves the family of the burden of breaking the news.

Sometimes there are fears for a person's state of health. For example: in one unfortunate family, the father was dying of cancer in one hospital while the daughter succumbed to histiocytic lymphoma in another hospital. Since the father had said he was waiting for his daughter's death, the family was very much afraid that they would lose a second member within days of the first if he were told. However, like the awareness of terminal illness, knowledge of death is often conveyed nonverbally. The man developed angina the morning after his daughter's death, before his relatives did in fact tell him; he may have guessed from the demeanor of nurses or family. When it was clear her death was an open secret, the family was encouraged to communicate freely; he was able to participate fully in a bedside service although unable to go to the funeral. The father was able to mourn without the dire circumstances the family had expected, and died several weeks later.

Understanding Other Cultures

Response to pain and the meaning of pain varies with culture (see Chapters 6 and 7). For example, Italians use dramatization as a defense against pain, where the Irish use denial.[41] The response to attempts to help is also culturally dependent. Ajemian and Mount[2] give some illuminating case examples to underline the importance of understanding cultural backgrounds. A patient from Pakistan who spoke only Urdu curled himself in blankets, responded negatively to music from Pakistan, and recoiled angrily to nonverbal attempts at reassurance such as touching his arm or shoulder. Through an interpreter it was later discovered that he was not pulling on the blankets because he was cold as first suspected but had wrapped himself up ritually to pray, that music has no place for a Muslim at such times, and that physical contact is seen as an invasion of privacy. Muslim laws concerning death dictate strict ritual; the body must be placed with the head towards Mecca and must be washed by relatives of the same sex immediately after death. Postmortem examinations, cremation, or cement graves or coffins are not allowed.

A Jewish woman who believed God took good men only on a Jewish high holy day was confused when her very sick husband did not die on Yom Kippur; she wondered if God was saving her husband for her or judging her for not fasting. She had never mourned an 18-year-old daughter lost in the Holocaust, and a father and brother were killed in Poland when she was very young. She showed profound guilt, and she had the insomnia, chronic depression and mistrust of Holocaust survivors. Health professionals should respect such a person's deeply entrenched way of coping and give support for the current event rather than attempting intensive therapy.

THE ROLE OF THE CLINICIAN—CURE OR PALLIATION: DEFINITIVE TREATMENT VERSUS SYMPTOM CONTROL

The concept that cancer is a death sentence is dated but is still unfortunately the average layman's belief. Some cancers—notably cervical, testicular, choriocarcinoma, Berkitt's, Wilm's, neuroblastoma, some skin cancers, and some leukemias and lymphomas—are now curable in most cases. Many other cancers are surgically resectable in their early stages. Chemotherapy and radiotherapy have had an impact on longevity but also have their own negative effects on the quality of life. When these are used indiscriminately or too late in the disease process by a physician who sees his role as fighting death at all costs, family and patient suffer unnecessarily. To admit that therapy is no longer effective is particularly difficult for physicians who may have entered medicine because of a great need to feel in control of disease and death. Stopping active therapy appears to be giving up. It is important to recognize there is still a great deal that can be done to relieve suffering and help the patient with the final challenge of life. Far from being useless, the clinician has a most important role in helping families at a time when they are highly vulnerable.

The Efficacy of Words. Most physicians have been taught that action counts not words. One cannot do a double blind, randomized control study of the efficacy of words in treatment. Yet this is the main ingredient of the drug "doctor" described by Balint.[5] The nonverbal messages and the emotional content, the "how" of communication, are even harder to measure. Two recent studies correlate patient understanding and satisfaction with the verbal and nonverbal content of doctor-patient communications.[14,18] At a time of crisis the need for adequate communication skills in the clinician is much greater than in the regular office visit.

Three crises occur in the family facing terminal illness: 1) the crisis of a fatal diagnosis—when, how and who to tell and the adaptation to such knowledge; 2) the crisis of a fatal prognosis when cure or long remission no longer appears possible; and 3) the crisis of death. At these times particularly communication within the family and with the clinician are of primary importance. The content and ease of such communication determine subsequent events and adaptation.

Without the help of someone outside the family system some families get stuck in a morass of emotions:

> David, a 22-year-old athlete and the son of a farmer, was diagnosed with a rare cerebral malignancy. The crisis occurred after an operation that relieved symptoms but did not magically restore normalcy as he had hoped. Three weeks later he was obsessed with the desperate wish to shoot himself (he was used to shooting animals in the hunt), and end his life "with a bang." He wanted to punch the intern who had told him his prognosis. He refused radiotherapy despite the probability of an excellent remission because he had been told there were "no guarantees" that it would give him at least 5 years of his old active life of hunting, fishing, cars, and girl friends. His reaction reflected that of his mother, the "emotional one" of the family, who cried continuously; she too was questioning therapy and wanted it "over with fast." Any limitation at all in David's activities was viewed as disaster and not to be contemplated. The father maintained a rational, nonemotional stance and was seen as noncaring by the son.
>
> The father was, however, anxious for therapy to continue and to optimize whatever time was left. A long discussion between clinician, father, and son ensued. With the encouragement of the clinician, the son cried for the first time in front of other people (which was triggered by the father when he expressed the wish to be able to cry like his wife). Gradually talk of guns was replaced by discussion of David's difficulty facing his six-year-old brother and two sisters. Preoccupation with his own plight turned to a focus on the effect on his family. A glimmer of hope that something more could be found in life, and in less active pursuits than in hunting and fishing, reversed the refusal for radiotherapy. The father, a highly intelligent man commented to the clinician afterwards, "I had no idea that just talk could do so much!" He requested a family meeting to help his wife and other children.
>
> The response of the 16-year-old sister had been to become pregnant within a month of her brother's diagnosis. Abortion was not possible in this strongly religious family. The baby boy that resulted was cared for by his grandmother and was at risk to be a replacement child for the family, who needed further counselling to facilitate grieving.

Pain control is central to the care of the terminally ill patient. In the above example, inadequate pain control added to the sense of desperation; once the pain was controlled the focus on suffering decreased and trust for the clinician facilitated her counselling role. Pain or fear of pain in patient or family can be so devastating and preoccupying that there is not time for the important communications and positive use of the remaining weeks of life. It is not appropriate here to elaborate on the clinical advances in the control of pain, and treatment of symptoms such as nausea and vomiting, dry mouth, constipation, and the medical treatment of intestinal obstruction. These procedures have been well described by Saunders,[34] and Ajemian and Mount.[2] All physicians and nurses should be knowledgeable about current use of oral analgesics, commonly morphine, given in round-the-clock, 4-hourly dosage sufficient to relieve pain and erase the memory of pain.

"Total pain" is a term coined by Saunders[34] to describe current awareness that pain is not just physical pain. A young man, who has a dependent wife with no marketable skills and several small children, may be in greater pain than the 80-year-old man who feels his time has come. Depression and anxiety add to pain and can be treated medically to provide greater pain relief. When the family is unable to accept the diagnosis and is unwilling to let the patient die, total pain may be increased. Thus, symptom control includes treating the family's pain. Some patients who appear ready to die seem to wait for family acceptance or for the conclusion of unfinished business. Drug-induced somnolence is not necessary (the threshold for pain relief is normally below that of central nervous system depression) and does not improve ability to communicate at this time. As in all areas of medicine, expertise in the appropriate pharmacology is essential.

Symptom control is important for quality of life in terminal diseases other than cancer. The control of symptoms in patients with renal failure by dialysis, or their elimination by kidney transplant, has been an enormous step forward in treatment. It is equally important to deal with the family's distress. The fear of death; the changes in roles that occurs because the patient must be given treatment three times a week; the effect of medical devices and the altered parental role or frequent hospital visits on children, and the altered self-image of patient and family can all be devastating and require professional support and understanding.

Much has been written recently about support and care for the cardiac patient after myocardial infarction. Considerably less attention has been paid to the family. Hoebel[13] has described how effectively wives can be enlisted as allies in the treatment regime, and Davidson,[9] in an article on the family system, has created an integrated program of cardiac rehabilitation in which the "unparalleled opportunity for increased awareness and growth of all members of the family" is emphasized. Symptom control is again important. In particular, careful instruction and advice concerning activities, including sex, graded exercise programs, and explanation of the disease process can give the patient and family a sense of control in regard to the illness. Sexual and marital problems may compound anxiety if the family is ignored.

Terminal neurologic disorders produce a complex and agonizing set of problems for the medical profession and the family. Gastrostomies and tracheostomies, although appropriate emergency measures when the prognosis is uncertain, may produce months or years of suffering and a very poor quality of life.[37] In some cases (as in cerebral carcinomas), the prognosis is sufficiently clear that such interventions are not in fact warranted. It requires courage for physicians or surgeons trained to save lives to abstain from action. The prevention and relief of suffering is our mandate but one we may forget. When it is clear that quality of life will be poor (as in a senile patient who develops a cerebral thrombosis) such interventions are inappropriate from the outset. The clinician's prior knowledge of the patient and family is often crucial for a correct decision. In the patient with progressive deterioration from disease such as amyotrophic lateral sclerosis, symptom control, and support for the family are essential. Explanation of symptoms and understanding of the probable cause, with the emphasis on living one day at a time and within current limitations, help give the persons involved a sense of control.

Clinician Support for Home Care

Home assessment, appropriate appliances, and aids, including home suction apparatus, an air mattress filled with water and sheep skins to prevent bed sores, physiotherapy and occupational therapy, and the use of community resources all help decrease stress and maintain care longer in the home. The impersonal and expensive hospital environment is thus avoided. The physician or community nurse willing to make home visits and help organize outside support should attempt to increase the use of home rather than institutions for terminal patients. A family interview including the children can help communication over the emotional and practical problems of home care. Death at home is not only often better for the patient if comfort and adequate care can be provided, it is also in many cases better for the family, providing sufficient resources are available and total exhaustion of care providers is avoided. In our generation, death, like birth, has been removed from the home environment. This isolation of death in hospital rooms has increased the sense that it is not a part of life and something to be denied and feared.

Sudden Death and Its Sequellae

Help is now available in some centers for patients facing terminal illness. In contrast, there is little help anywhere for the families of those who die in motor vehicle accidents, or of sudden pulmonary embolism or cardiac arrest. In addition, anticipatory mourning cannot occur and the acceptance of death is often much more difficult, frequently because of the young age of the patient. Parkes[30] has shown that widows in this category are particularly at risk for difficulties with bereavement.

THE DEATH OF CHILDREN AND THE ROLE OF CHILDREN

The Emotional Response of the Family and the Clinician

The rarity of pediatric death in a family clinician's practice makes it all the more difficult to cope with when it occurs. Avoidance of one's own emotions may be greater than when the clinician is faced with the death of adult patients, and for those clinicians who are parents themselves, empathy with the bereaved parents may be particularly threatening. Nevertheless, support for such a family before and after the death is essential.

Both parents should be present when the diagnosis of fatal illness is conveyed and this should be done in a quiet room away from the activity of the ward. Lescari[19] suggests that one should not stop after a statement such as "your child has leukemia" but should continue with a statement about plans and the likelihood of remissions and ability to control pain. The parents hear only a little of the details the first time, often distorting information, and will require more details later.

Grandparents or crucial relatives often do not accept the diagnosis and make the parents feel guilty that they are condemning the child. Close relatives should therefore be included in discussions, if not in the first disclosure of illness. Parents are usually inundated with advice and articles on alternative treatments, as are families with adult patients with cancer. Frank discussion about such views with the physician or nurse can be very helpful. If families are enthusiastic about nutritional or other approaches that are known to cause no harm the clinician should not condemn them because he believes otherwise. The problem, however, is that most quack remedies engender false hopes, are often followed by the family's feeling of being taken advantage of, financially and emotionally, when they fail to cure. Some putative cures are toxic and have caused death.

The Child's Response

It is now known that many children, aged 4 and older, are aware when they have a serious disease.[19] Most children, by asking direct questions or avoiding questions, will indicate desire to know the truth or to deny. If they are not told, they may learn of the diagnosis from a playmate. On the other hand, a young child may make it clear he or she does not want to know by ignoring the playmate.

Many dying children are incredibly open and honest about death. According to Kübler-Ross,[17] they develop an early sense of the meaning of life and a philosophical approach that may help their adult relatives who are struggling with bitterness or denial.

Fear of separation is potent in the healthy young and a fatal disease makes it terrifying. Reassurance that he or she will never be left alone and that someone will always be available to talk to are essential. A belief that the disease is a punishment may make the child passive and withdrawn. School phobia is common in such children partly because of separation anxiety, partly because the mother fears symptoms such as abdominal pains or headache. She may also fear that the child may die when away from her. The intense relationship between mother and child at home escalates in anxiety and irritability. The mother must be reassured and the child returned to school as soon as possible.

Effects on Siblings

Discipline may decrease and the child may suffer from insecurity brought about by unclear limits while siblings must still toe the line. Discipline may increase if the parent expresses irrational hostility. Siblings may feel, as may the parent, that they have caused the illness, particularly if normal sibling rivalry included subconscious wishes that the child be eliminated from the field. Those wishes may get even harder to handle now that the child is in reality taking up more parental time, money, and affection. Krell and Rabkin[16] have studied the effects of sibling deaths in the surviving child from a family perspective:

> Surviving siblings not infrequently become the focus of manoeuvres unconsciously designed to alleviate guilt and control fate through silence and efforts to maintain silence, through substitution for the lost child, and through endowing the survivor-child with qualities of the deceased. Three types of clinically identifiable types of survivor-children are described. Families that emphasize silence and focus on guilt, families in which the child becomes incomparably precious, and families in which substitution and replacement provide the major theme lead respectively to the "haunted," "bound" and "resurrected" child.

Guilt in each family member, for precautions not taken, for envy of attention or toys, for wishing the child dead in a moment of anger, can contribute to a tense atmosphere with hostility and vagueness and ambiguity surrounding the death. A new equilibrium may form around the surviving child. There may be extreme overprotectiveness, a shroud of mystery over the past (the dead sibling may not be spoken of), or a need to achieve on behalf of the dead child.

The death of an adolescent is particularly traumatic. Understanding the meaning of death and usually demanding absolute honesty, the teenager cannot accept the reality of personal death.[19,23] Striving for independence and self-sufficiency, he or she is suddenly faced with forced passivity and absolute dependence. MacDonald[23] described the horrendous experience for the family, the health professionals and the ill teenager himself, who expressed anguished rebellion by fighting the illness all the way.

Stillbirths and Neonatal Death

Perinatal death is common, about one in 100 deliveries, yet society shows great lack of understanding of the grief incurred. The suggestion that the baby can be replaced, that attachment cannot be the same as to an older child, that a grieving mother, or father, is "overreacting" may drive the grief underground. In some families the next child of the same sex will be given the name of the dead baby, a heavy burden to the child, whether or not the child is told who else had the name. Nonverbal communication can tell the "survivor" he or she has a special mission and expectations that come from something unconnected with him. When drawing a family tree, the clinician should always include stillbirths and miscarriages along with names if the baby was given one. The potency of such events is illustrated in the following example:

> Mrs. C. waited 6 years for her first live birth. Before this child was born, she had had two miscarriages (one of which had been an ectopic pregnancy), and one stillbirth caused by excessive anesthetic. The stillbirth was a baby girl they named Dorothy-Jane. The greatest trauma for Mrs. C. was when the minister refused a funeral for the baby, which was to be buried in the family grave, because the "soul entered on the first breath." Mrs. C.'s first live birth was a girl Janet who grew up aware of the death but apparently unaffected by it. Janet's first daughter was called Jane after a friend of the family; her second was named Dorothy because she "liked the name." Three months later an aunt congratulated her: "How nice you used your sister's two names." Angrily she defended this as coincidence, then later recognized she was giving back to her mother the sister she never had.

Advice on management of perinatal death was given by Speck and Kennell.[36] Parents seem to be helped in overcoming their grief when they are allowed to view or hold their dead child, to name it, to express grief along with all their hopes and dreams for the child, and to have a funeral. Tranquilizing medication for the parents should be avoided, and the physician should meet with the parents soon after the death to discuss the findings of the autopsy

3 or 4 days later and again 6 months after the death. It is unwise for parents to have another baby until grieving is completed.

Sudden Infant Death Syndrome (SIDS)

Crib death is still of unknown cause. It kills approximately 10,000 babies per year in the United States.[19] Sudden death devoid of warning is more devastating than death after illness, and in sudden infant death syndrome death is often made worse by misconceptions. Some clinicians still believe it is caused by suffocation or aspiration. Some communities even equate it with child abuse or neglect; parental guilt is then compounded and cruel and inhumane treatment received rather than compassion and consolation. It is most important to tell parents that their child died of a definite disease that could not be predicted or prevented, and that they are in no way responsible for the death. Siblings also suffer severely from guilt and grief and disbelief. May and Breme[24] have described a family assessment schema specifically for families who have had to cope with this trauma. This consists of ten items, each rated on a five-point continuum between poor and high levels of adaptation. Items included are open communication of feelings of grief within the family; resumption of usual individual and work activities; utilization/perception of community resources; receipt of actual factual data postmortem; cognitive belief in preventability (correlating with guilt); religious faith and spiritual values; physical and psychological morbidity; continued centrality of deceased (preoccupation, frequent grave visits, leaving deceased room "as it was"); and family solidarity. The impact of such a death on the family may remain for a long period. Family practitioners are often involved and can play an important role in facilitating resolution of the crisis. They can address the couple and siblings, and often the emergency room staff, who first receive the family. The clinician can also intervene with the police or other authorities who may still confuse sudden infant death syndrome with child abuse (suffocation) or neglect. He or she can play an important role in the family and community management of SIDS.

A family physician met Mrs. Smith and her 3-month infant with the police in the emergency room after she found John dead in his crib. Mrs. Smith appeared very nervous and asked many questions but she had no tears. She explained that her husband had not been notified and was currently flying from Vancouver to Montreal. She had arranged for a neighbor to take care of her two older children, aged 5 and 6, and came to the hospital with the police. She wanted to know what had to be done and was very preoccupied with the instrumental details. What would happen next? Would there be an autopsy and if so who would perform it? Throughout the discussion she kept her dead infant in her arms and refused to release him.

The police drew the clinician aside and asked what he thought had happened. He explained that he knew the family and what had happened was SIDS or "crib death." The police had never heard about it. A brief explanation seemed to satisfy the puzzled officer, who also had a 2-month-old child. They wrote their report and asked the mother if there was anything they could do; she thanked them and they left.

The mother then requested to speak to the pathologist. He was phoned and was made to understand that this mother was not going to release her child until she knew who would take care of him. This understandable request created a reaction amongst the nursing staff; the family physician had a further role to play in facilitating the process with the staff.

Mother and physician met the pathologist in his office, and only after she was reassured about what would be done did she give her infant to the pathologist while shedding tears. The physician offered to meet with the couple and their children if they so desired as soon as the autopsy was finished.

A few days later they met with the pathologist in the family physician's office. Mrs. Smith was still highly anxious and compulsively organized. She was also very protective of her husband, monopolizing most of the questions and trying to reassure him. The physician had known the couple for a long time and had known Mrs. Smith when she was a stewardess. Mrs. Smith recalled the time when her husband had been involved in a serious traffic accident and remembered he had almost lost a leg. He had recovered very well and his wife's nursing at home had been crucial to his recovery. Recognizing the couple's past coping helped mobilize their strengths for the current crisis. After the interview with the pathologist another meeting with the physician was scheduled 2 weeks later. On the second visit the same behavior was noted in Mrs. Smith, who tried to gloss over the issue of how the siblings were coping with the event. Because he knew the family, the physician was able to tell Mrs. Smith that she seemed to act like an air traffic controller; was her husband aware of that protection? The husband supported the statement and told his wife that he wanted to help her recall how nervous she was at home. She then allowed herself to cry on her husband's shoulder; he then showed himself to be a strong and warm person: "Let me take care of you for once; you have done your bit." The physician left the couple with the idea that they could use him as they saw fit. The follow-up showed that the family was doing very well. They dealt in a very open way with their two other children and their relatives.

An interesting sequel to this history was that 2 months later the physician received a phone call from the police chief asking him if he would address the officers one evening on the topic of sudden infant death. This contributed to education of the community.

Family practitioners can play very important roles as facilitators during such crises as SIDS with the family, their colleagues, and their communities.

THE DEATH OF A PARENT

Helping Children Cope

The presence of small children raises both the practical issues surrounding loss of a parent and the emotional issues of how the children are to be helped to deal with this loss. Many families mistakenly protect small children by never mentioning the illness or the possibility of death until the fact is obvious or the death has already occurred. Children are remarkably able to respond and adapt, provided the adults around them are being honest, are showing the emotion they clearly feel, and are caring. The sense of mystery, of things too terrible to speak about, that prevades the child's world when communication is avoided adds enormously to children's distress. Fertile imaginations often produce horrors worse than the reality, especially if the children are not allowed to visit the sick parent. When emotion cannot be easily expressed, distorted or abnormal grief reactions are produced and these can alter the child's adaptability and personality for life. Death of a parent is not easy for a child of any age but normal development is assisted if the child has an adequate parent substitute and is allowed full expression of his or her emotional response to the loss.

On the other hand, if the prognosis of a disease is several years it is probably unwise to tell young children too early of the fatal outcome, since this may be too much for them to live with on a day-to-day basis for months or years. Children who fear daily that they may come home from school to find a parent dead are not going to be able to live normal lives and deal with the normal stresses of childhood. In general, however, small children are much more aware of their emotional environment than adults give them credit for being. A 3-year-old child was observed in a terminal care ward reassuring her grandmother that "it would be very beautiful up there with all the angels." She also left her doll constantly at her grandmother's bedside as nurse. This child had an air of confidence, and proved to be the therapist not only for the grandmother, but for her parents who had at first been unable to talk about death openly. There was no evidence that this child was going to suffer unduly from her nursing role, and in fact was made to feel an important part of this life event, as children in the past normally did when death occurred at home.

A useful book for parents is Grollman's *Explaining Death to Children.*[11] For children aged 3 to 5 years death is separation rather than cessation. The child told about burial may ask, "Does the dirt get into their eyes when they open them?" The death of an animal can help them understand. For children older than 5 years, death becomes external, monstrous, and frightening; it is connected with ghosts and goblins and skeletons. Funerals help keep these away and may be reassuring as well as frightening. Death is something that happens if you are bad but that you can avoid "if you run fast enough." From 9 to 12 years of age a child develops the adult view of the abstract unbending nature of death. It is associated with old age and illness so children worry about family members in these categories.

Like adults, children take time to assimilate the concept of death: the topic should not be covered in a single discussion. Children (or adults!) at any age are prone to feel that it is somehow their fault that the person died and should be reassured about this. They should feel an important part of the family and be allowed to participate in the funeral if they wish.

Explanations should be given in the child's own language, and without sentimentality ("God wanted another angel so he took your mother.") Religious explanations should be congruent with the parent's beliefs. Parents should be warned that if children are told their sibling or parent was taken away by God, they will identify God with terrible death and loss. Mary Vachon[40] also points out that heaven can be made too attractive; one small child stated she wanted to jump off a roof so she could see what it looked like.

Another excellent book, *Learning to Say Good-Bye* by Eda LeShan[21] can be read by a parent or by a child as young as 10-years-old, and covers the range of normal and disturbed responses to this potentially crippling life crisis. The author offers practical strategies, based on real examples, for handling fears, fantasies, and stages of mourning. She indicates that the anger a child feels toward the dead parent or toward the one who remains may suddenly surface months after the funeral. She discusses guilt and idealization of the dead parent, difficulties with a new step-parent, the insensitivity of adults, and the unwitting cruelties of other children, but also the positive things death teaches us about life.

For a family at this stage in the life cycle, the death of one of the parents means death at a young age and all that early death encompasses. Loss of the breadwinner or of the nurturing role must be handled by the surviving spouse, with eventual replacement or redistribution of that role for both spouse and children. The "total pain" experienced by young people is often greater because of the vast implications of *their* death of which the pain is a reminder.

Helping the Family With Adolescents

The added stress of a terminal illness may produce total family disruption in the family facing the normal turmoil of adolescence. The mother may be experiencing menopause or the couple may be in a "mid-life crisis," may be considering retirement, or may be simply aware of the impending "empty nest," which will be much emptier if faced alone. The adolescent children must cope with emotional upheavals and dependence from parents made more dependent themselves by illness or impending bereavement. The clinician can be a stabilizing force and can facilitate communication in these already strained relationships. The adolescent's normal ambivalence becomes even more difficult when he or she is faced with the death of the parent. Expression of both positive and negative feelings, if these can be accepted by the parent, may diminish later problems with bereavement. The dependence of the surviving spouse on the children may subsequently add to the problems. Adolescents or young adults who have been ready to leave, or have in fact previously left, may feel drawn back to the home to help the surviving parent. Sometimes it is only with great difficulty that they can later pry themselves loose. Recognizing this possibility, the clinician should suggest counselling for the spouse before the patient's death, facilitate use of community resources, friends, and other relatives, and allow more appropriate support from peers.

Living With Uncertainty—How Can the Clinician Help

If angina is the presenting symptom of cardiac disease, or if the first myocardial infarction is not fatal, then the family must cope with the fear of sudden death. Similarly the cancer patient, even if "cured," can never be sure that the illness will not recurr. For humans the greatest source of stress is uncertainty: in Hitler's concentration camps it was the unpredictability and arbitrariness of the guards' decision as to who would live and who would die that caused more distress than starvation and physical pain.[10] Uncertainty is the basis for brainwashing techniques. It can produce neurosis or even psychosis in experimental animals, who have far less ability to think about their situation than humans and have less need to feel in control. Control is compromised when death can occur without warning at any time. Attempts to control lead to overprotection, avoidance of possible precipitants such as sexual activity or exercise, or total immobility and hopelessness. It is not surprising that other defenses such as denial can become extreme so that in fact the patient may tempt fate with excessive, high-risk behavior instead of leading a modified lifestyle.

It is the health professional's responsibility to guide patient and family between the extremes either of hopeless inertia with depression and over-protectiveness by the family, or hyperactivity and denial of any limitation or change in role and denial of nature's warning. The clinician can help give a sense of control after an infarct with reasonably concise instructions for all aspects of living that may influence cardiac activity. Open expression of fears, worries, and frustrations of both patient and family can assist the development of an ability to live with uncertainty and accept the eventual outcome. It may also decrease the emergency telephone calls or visits to panicky patient or relatives.

Strained family relationships increase the inability to cope. The uncertainty also increases tension and dysfunctional communication. Escalation of family problems can be prevented by improved communication with the health professional as catalyst (see Chapter 17).

Roles as well as communication may need adjusting. If the single breadwinner of the family is ill, the anticipation by another adult of the breadwinning role may necessitate planning ahead and months or even years of training. If denial is operative this planning will not occur. Financial stress added to the emotional stress can cause family disruption. Preexisting difficulties in relationships will be accentuated by any stress, and where roles have been rigid in the past conflict may break out. In patients on dialysis, for example, role strain may be considerable not only in the breadwinner (who may be the patient or the patient's caretaker) but also for the homemaker (whether patient or caretaker). Domestic roles will have to change, and in addition time must be available for the new roles of nurse and dialyzer if home dialysis is used or transporter if this is to be in the hospital.

Sometimes the needs of a family may be so great that the rigid adherence to old roles continues beyond expectations and beyond what is appropriate. For example, a young mother with chronic renal failure was observed dancing at a party with the energy of an adolescent despite hemoglobin of 6 g. She could have used that energy to cope with the demands of two small children but her husband had always needed her to play an outgoing and active social role. This family needed help to adjust that would not dampen optimism or seriously decrease the energy necessary for more important areas.

Children may begin misbehaving, fail in school, or take drugs in a family in which communication is difficult. Their role may be that of family distractor:

> A young mother, whose youngest and favorite son was 10 years old, was dying of breast cancer. Her mother had died when she was 10 years old, leaving her with an irresponsible father. Her husband was alcoholic and very anxious about his impending loss. Whenever the diagnosis or prognosis of the mother with breast cancer was hinted at, the father would draw attention to the current misbehavior of Jimmy, the older son who was 12 years old, or Jimmy would himself draw attention away from his mother by behaving badly. Jimmy was the "bad one," following the role of his father, who drank when the disease got worse. The whole family used alcohol or misbehavior to avoid the topic constantly on their minds. Only by pointing this out and facilitating communication of buried emotion is it possible to release the boy from his role as scapegoat and to emphasize the father's strengths.

Cancer, in contrast to heart disease has an inexorability that can destroy hope. At least, the disease contains less uncertainty. In fact, adaptation to the fact of certain death can produce extreme anxiety and family dysfunction if that fact is reversed. Caughill[8] reports a case of a man nursed for 5 years by his wife for glomerulonephritis. The wife, who was a nurse, gradually took over the nurturing, providing, and decision-making roles. When the husband received a successful kidney transplant, he expected to regain his old dominant role and make the decisions; they were unable to resolve these difficulties and divorced. Another phenomenon is involved here, "premortem dying"[38] or the tendency of families to gradually exclude the dying person from activities or decisions as if he or she were already dead. This is done in the name of protection but is actually part of anticipatory grief; withdrawal from the family is also a normal phenomenon in the patient anticipating actual death. Similar revised expectations occurred in the wives of war veterans. Anticipatory grief at the possible death of the husband led to acceptance of their loss and readjustment to life without them. When the soldiers returned home, their wives requested divorce.

The poet, Ted Rosenthal, in *How Could I Not Be Among You*[33] described his reaction to the possibility of a remission of his acute leukemia; "My whole world went crashing to the floor."

How Long, Doctor?

It is this uncertainty that is behind the frequent question, "How long?" Weary families often pressure doctors or nurses to give a date for the end of uncertainty. Patients have practical reasons to ask this question, but often the need for certainty and control are also behind the query. If the prognosis given proves wrong, anger at the clinician (or at the patient) may be extreme. This can be true whether the patient far outlives his prognosis or whether he or she dies short of it. The occasional family that is given a precise date by an inexperienced physician will be angry if death is not on or close to that date. The more anxious the family is, the more often they will ask for a date, but for such a family discussion of fears is more important than dates. The wise clinician will respond to pressure to prognosticate with, "I don't know anyone with the gift of prophecy." If the question is "Should I get my house in order?", the answer is "Yes, but that goes for all of us, and for all of us it is better to live day by day." If a range of time is given the questionner often hears a single date. As Kübler-Ross[17] points out, hope should never be destroyed, but for a family that is still largely denying the terminal nature of the disease and prefers to think death is years off, the statement that death may occur in months (or weeks) and not years may help adaptation to reality. Discussion about the anxiety produced by uncertainty helps relieve it.

Death is always "sudden," even when expected. The shock and disbelief seem to deny the preparation that has taken place. However, a follow-up of persons in bereavement shows that those who have gone through preparatory mourning have a briefer period of numbness (stage 1 of mourning), and have already done some of their "grief work" (Freud's term for the efforts required to successfully pass through the second painful stage of mourning and reach acceptance and adaptation to the loss (stage 3 of mourning). Relief that the ordeal is over may induce guilt, but can be normalized by a comment from the clinician.

BEREAVEMENT AND THE FAMILY-ORIENTED CLINICIAN

Recognizing and Understanding Physical Symptoms

As in the literature on death and dying, bereavement studies are of individuals not of the bereaved family as a unit. The process of grief of widows in London and Boston has been described by Parkes.[29,30] Symptoms that can occur in spouses and other family members after a death should be known to any clinician. Physical symptoms reflect the "alarm reaction" response of the organism: loss of appetite, dry mouth, weight loss, sleep disturbance, palpitations, headaches, and muscular aches and pains. Waves of somatic distress were described by Lindemann[22] in relatives of the Cocoanut Grove fire victims in 1944. They demonstrated a striking tendency to sighing respirations, shortness of breath with choking and a tightness in the throat, extreme exhaustion and lack of muscular power, and intense subjective distress or "mental pain." This syndrome was precipitated by mention or visual reminders of the deceased and there was a tendency to avoid the mental pain and physical symptoms at all costs. Anger was displayed at the clinician who raised the subject of the loss. Protective denial and the natural avoidance of this painful grief work can lead to delayed or distorted mourning.

A feeling of unreality and distance from others may lead to withdrawal from social contact particularly because the individual may be worried about the effect on others of his odd behavior. Irritability, memory loss, and inefficiency increases family tension. For example, Pincus[31] describes how in the first week after her own husband's death she was so absent-minded she deposited his important papers and will in a mail box.

Many bereaved people experience the same physical symptoms as the dead person, leading them to believe they will die of the same condition. They may also neglect their own health, as well as develop physical illness, particularly heart disease, cancer, ulcerative colitis, and asthma more frequently than those not grieving.[29,30] They should be advised, if possible before the patient's death, that symptoms are quite likely, but if persistent should occasion a medical check-up.

Some normal symptoms of mourning can be frightening to the bereaved and to observers. They experience pining (a persistent obtrusive wish for the person gone, preoccupation with painful thoughts), searching (restless activity focused on places linked with the lost person or familiar aspects of them, leading to "seeing" the person on the street, hearing their voice, or often frank hallucinations), irritability, or extreme anger (which may come in outbursts from previously mild people, and may be directed at God, the medical profession, family members, or the lost person).[22,30] Such symptoms can convince the bereaved person that they are "going crazy." Guilt and feelings of negligence before death are often extreme. When a relationship has been ambivalent, bereavement is even more difficult because of excessive guilt and the bereaved person is at greater risk for distorted or delayed grief. Overidealization of the dead person covers unconscious anger.

Gradually the part of the grieving person that has been invested in the dead person has to be reassimilated. For example, a wife who allowed her husband the decision-making role and financial knowledge may take pride in developing her own competence. A man whose wife had expressed the nurturing part of his personality may feel freer to become a nurturing father after her death. Lily Pincus[31] gives many such examples in her well-known book *Death and the Family*. However, her case studies deal with dyadic relationships rather than with families as systems.

Bereavement Outcome

Parkes[29] and Lindemann[22] studied the factors in individuals that influence the outcome of bereavement. Intensity of grieving pain is greater when the attachment to the person was strong (mothers of young children have particular difficulty), when there was emotional or financial dependence, and when the death was untimely or without warning. Potential difficulties are greater for the younger bereaved person (especially young widows), for those with a history of loss or separation particularly in childhood, or for those with previous mental illness especially depression. Intense ambivalence to the deceased is a potent risk factor; guilt and self reproach were present to a much greater degree in distorted mourning. Inhibition of feelings, the need to hide feelings to protect others or important tasks (for example, coping with the financial affairs of the deceased, work deadlines, exams, small children to care for), may result in delayed or distorted grieving. Other recent life crises or lack of social support may seriously curtail coping. Bereavement is made much easier by a supportive network of friends and relatives, especially if the bereaved person is able to communicate openly and ask appropriately for help. The availability of opportunities and interests for the future provides hope and challenge and less preoccupation with the past.

Religion is still a significant support to many people, particularly in some cultures and traditions. Many of the old rituals of different religious traditions that were based on sound understanding of the psychological needs of the bereaved have disappeared but the clinician should be aware of the potential support available through such practices. For instance, in the Jewish custom of shiva, visitors follow the lead of the family member in talking or not talking about the bereaved. There is prescribed "permission" to grieve and then to stop grieving, often an extremely helpful mechanism assisting grief work. The ritual time periods give a sense of control. Traditional American Indian customs respond to the needs of the early bereavement period when disbelief and numbness are the immediate response. A place is set for the dead person during the first ten days of the death, following which a feast is held in which all participants bring the favorite foods of the dead person. All food must be finished, or eaten subsequently at home, and with this and the clearing of the dead person's place, closure is reached. During this period communication with others is often minimal.

Mourning may be delayed for months or years, triggered sometimes by another death, an anniversary of the death, or even by the person reaching the age of the person who died. "Anniversary reactions" in which symptoms, actual illness, depression for no reason apparent to the patient, or accidents occur on or near the date of the relative's deaths. If a family physician is unaware of the frequency of these reactions, both he and the patient may remain unaware of the true diagnosis. For example:

> A woman was referred to a cardiologist because of repeated attacks of dizziness and weakness. Luckily, before the expense of a 24 hour Holter monitor to rule out a cardiac arrythmia was incurred, the primary physician asked some more questions. It was exactly a year after her mother's death that the symptoms began. These symptoms disappeared after discussion of the patient's anger at her father who was now dating another woman and the suggestion she bring out old letters and photos of her mother and allow herself to grieve openly.

Distorted mourning may be manifested by 1) overactivity without a sense of loss, particularly in areas in which the deceased was active; 2) development of symptoms of the dead person's illness, which may be labelled as hypochondriasis); 3) a recognized medical disease, predominantly angina, ulcerative colitis, rheumatoid arthritis, asthma and cancer; 4) alteration in relationships to friends and relatives with progressive social isolation; 5) hostility against specific persons, often health professionals; 6) emotional inhibition with wooden robot-like behavior as a defense particularly against anger; 7) a lasting loss of patterns of social interaction; 8) self-punishing behavior such as foolish economic dealings and "stupid acts" that alienate family and friends; 9) an agitated depression in which the person may be dangerously suicidal; and 10) prolonged mourning lasting for years or a lifetime.[22]

The response to bereavement of the family system as a whole has been poorly studied. It is a common observation, however, that family dysfunction can often be traced in origin to the period following a death, particularly if mourning is distorted or delayed. The family example used to illustrate systems theory in Chapter 1 shows the far-reaching effect of guilt and disrupted bereavement on a family years later.

If the family finds it difficult to communicate the feelings associated with the illness and the death, one family member may develop symptoms. A child may be scapegoated as an easy target for anger and the tension for unexpressed feelings may readily produce behavioral problems. One person in the family may be selected to express the family's feelings whether of sadness, anger or guilt. This was seen in a poignant interview of the family who had to face both the imminent death of the beautiful 18-year-old daughter from a disfiguring lymphoma and the death of the father, also from cancer. The oldest of the seven other children cried throughout the session, apparently ignored by the rest of the family, while another loudly expressed the family's anger at relatives who were providing no support. In a second family the 16-year-old daughter threatened suicide some months after the death of her father, an army colonel. When her mother, also the daughter of a soldier, was persuaded to drop her own stoicism and mourn for the first time, the girl lost her depression. An individual mourning response should be assessed in the context of the family; the assigned depression or anger will be resistant to treatment if the individual alone is seen but may respond readily to a single session with the family. In 3 years on a palliative care unit the author has been struck by how often the increased flexibility that occurs with crisis makes it possible for old family patterns to change dramatically with minimal facilitation interventions by someone outside the system. The simple comment that one person seems to be crying or angry on behalf of the whole family may alter the patterns and enable others to express their feelings. Sometimes family reunions complete unfinished emotions. For example, a father who had not seen his son for 18 years was reunited 10 days before his death as a result of the physician's efforts. The patient was too proud to tell his family of his illness but agreed to "routine" notification through a phone call from the physician. Communication between father and son led to a dramatic change in the father, from anxiety and a battle to survive to a very peaceful death, and a resolved sense of identity and kinship in the son.

Facilitation of Mourning by the Clinician

Communication and sharing of emotions appears to be one key to a good outcome. Anticipatory grieving is important. Before the death, the health care professional can play an important role in gently breaking the conspiracy of silence between family and patient and between family members. Certain remarks may help facilitate mourning: "In many families, people tend to protect each other by hiding their grief. If you share it, you'll actually make it much easier for each other to cope." Or, "Crying alone does much less good than crying together." For families from the more stoical cultures, a comment that crying is nature's way of preventing stomach ulcers and hypertension and not a sign of weakness may also help.

Faced with signs of delayed or distorted mourning the clinician should make a move to facilitate the process. Probably the most effective measure is to visit the family at home or request a family interview, and gently initiate discussion of how everyone is feeling. Sidetracking the issue to physical symptome or misbehaving children can be interpreted as representing the family's difficulty expressing painful feelings. One member will usually show some nonverbal response, and if this response is referred to rather than ignored by the clinician, it will usually trigger an emotional response in others.

If the mourner is alone or the family unavailable, asking the person to bring in photos or to describe memories of the dead person will usually trigger the needed emotional reaction. In this case, the clinician becomes the main support but should encourage communication with others.

There is now considerable evidence that for bereavement such talk is effective in promoting normal recovery. Barrett[3] demonstrated the effectiveness of widow's groups, and Cameron and Brings[6] in a controlled study of 40 subjects showed that bereavement counselling before and after the death resulted in much better outcomes 1 year later. There were fewer emotional signs (2.65 signs compared with 8.25) and less counterproductive coping strategies (coping score of 0.45 compared with 2.25 for controls).

A summary of relevant issues discussed in this chapter and that should be part of a family assessment is appended using the acronym PRACTICE.

APPENDIX

Practice

Presenting Problem (or reason for interview)

Physician's Role

Need to convey diagnosis or prognosis

Facilitation of communication between family members

Symptoms of distress (physical symptoms, scapegoated child)

Facilitate family's own coping skills/ problem solving abilities

Roles, Structure

Loss of sick person's role (breadwinner, homemaker, nurturer)

Help in defining substitution/communication with regard to role satisfaction

Caretaker role—role strain (e.g., patient on dialysis)

Facilitate/coach in use of community resources

Denial/overuse of sickness role (e.g., young mother with hemoglobin of 6 gm had to remain as social butterfly for husband)

Assess family system; facilitate communication

Affect

Predominant emotional tone: anger or jocularity masking sadness

Facilitate open expression of grief/sharing

Fear from previous experience with disease/death, from misconceptions

Normalization of tears as nature's protective mechanism

Denial of affect through hyperactivity

Elicit past experience, health-belief model

Excess/prolonged mourning

Assess its role in family system

Communication

"Conspiracy of Silence" re: diagnosis (Note effects of culture) re: prognosis

Note well: Remove blocks to communication Promote sharing. Label silence as "false protection." Encourage communication of reality to allow saying goodbye, unfinished business

Mutual protectiveness

Displaced anger instead of sharing vulnerability and sadness

Normalize, encourage laughter, music, making best of the time left

Excess guilt

Time in Life Cycle

Childhood death

Young parent

Bereavement F/U longer

Family with adolescents

Increased incidence of divorce. Morbidity and mortality in spouse high. Appropriate help for children.

Older patients

Encourage continuing individuation of children, facilitate widow(er) use of other resources

Illness

Health belief system

Explore health belief system/fears (especially specific fears with regard to mode of death) in both patient and family

Experience of cancer/death in past	Family history detailed
Past relationship with health profession	Reassure/education

Coping, Strengths

Coping in past, especially similar situations	Identify strengths with family
Strength of individuals and family; Values; Religion	Explore alternative coping strategies
Flexibility and capacity for change and growth in crisis	Crisis intervention principles
	Positive relabelling where possible

Environmental Resources

Social, cultural, religious, economic, educational, medical (SCREEM)	Facilitate communication with extended family
	Use of self-help groups (mastectomy clubs, widow-to-widow, etc.)
	Facilitate planning, execution of wills, etc.
	Advocacy in health care system
	Awareness of cultural/religious traditions—support these

REFERENCES

1. Ajemian I, Mount BM (eds): *The RVH Manual on Palliative/Hospice Care.* New York, Arno Press, 1980.

2. Ajemian I, Mount BM: Cultural considerations in palliative care, in Ajemian I, Mount BM (eds): *The RVH Manual on Palliative/Hospice Care.* New York, Arno Press, 1980.

3. Barrett CJ: Effectiveness of widows' groups in facilitating change. *J Consult Clin Psychol* 46:20, 1978.

4. Bahnson CB: Emotional and personality characteristics of cancer patients, in Sutnick AE, Engstrom PF (eds): *Oncologic Medicine, Clinical Topics and Practical Management.* Baltimore, University Park Press, 1976.

5. Balint M: *The Doctor, His Patient, and the Illness.* New York, International Universities Press, 1957.

6. Cameron J, Brings B: Bereavement outcome following preventive intervention: A controlled study, in Ajemian I, Mount BM (eds): *The RVH Manual on Palliative/Hospice Care.* New York, Arno Press, 1980.

7. Cannon WB: Voodoo death. *Am Anthropol* 44:169, 1942.

8. Caughill RE: *The Dying Patient: A Supportive Approach.* Boston, Little, Brown, 1976.

9. Davidson DM: The family and cardiac rehabilitation. *J Fam Pract* 8:253, 1979.

10. Frankl V: *Man's Search for Meaning*. New York, Pocket Books, 1963.

11. Grollman EA: *Explaining Death to Children*. Boston, Beacon Press, 1969.

12. Hay D, Oken D: The psychological stress of intensive care unit nursing. *Psychosom Med* 34:1972.

13. Hoebel FC: Brief family-interactional therapy in the management of cardiac-related high-risk behaviors. *J Fam Pract* 3:316, 1976.

14. Kent Smith C, Polis E, Madac RR: Characteristics of the initial medical interview associated with patient satisfaction and understanding. *J Fam Pract* 12:283, 1981.

15. Kissen DM, Brown RIF, Kissen MA: A further report on personality and psychosocial factors in lung cancer. *Ann NY Acad Sci* 164:535, 1969.

16. Krell R, Rabkin L: The effects of sibling death on the surviving child: A family perspective. *Fam Process* 18:471, 1979.

17. Kübler-Ross E: *On Death and Dying*. New York, MacMillan, 1969.

18. Larsen KM, Kent Smith C: Assessment of nonverbal communication in the patient physician interview. *J Fam Pract* 12:481, 1981.

19. Lescari AD: The dying child and the family. *J Fam Pract* 6:1279, 1978.

20. Le Shan E: *You Can Fight For Your Life*. New York, M. Evans & Co., 1977.

21. Le Sahn E: *Learning to Say Goodbye When a Parent Dies*. New York, Avon Books, 1976.

22. Lindemann E: Symptomatology and management of acute grief. *Am J Psychiatry* 101:141, 1944.

23. MacDonald F: Care of the dying adolescent. *Can Fam Physician* 25:1090, 1979.

24. May H, Breme FJ: SIDS family adjustment scale: a method of assessing family adjustment to sudden infant death syndrome. *Omega* 13:59, 1982.

25. Moody RA Jr: *Life After Life*. New York, Bantam Books, 1975.

26. Mount BM, Jones A, Patteson A: Death and dying: Attitudes in a teaching hospital. *Urology* 4:741, 1974.

27. Mount BM: Psychological impact of urologic cancer. *Cancer* 45:1985, 1980.

28. Mount BM: Staff stress in palliative hospice care, in Ajemian I, Mount BM (eds): *The RVH Manual on Palliative/Hospice Care*. New York, Arno Press, 1980.

29. Parkes CM, Brown RJ: Health after bereavement: A controlled study of Boston widows and widowers. *Psychosom Med* 34:449, 1972.

30. Parkes CM: *Bereavement: Studies of Grief in Adult Life*. London, Tavistock Publications, 1972.

31. Pincus L: Death and the Family: The Importance of Mourning. New York, Vintage Books, 1974.

32. Price TR, Bergen BJ: The relationship to death as a source of stress for nurses on a coronary care unit. *Omega* 8:229, 1977.

33. Rosenthal T: *How Could I Not Be Among You*. New York, Avon Books, 1973.

34. Saunders C: *The Management of Terminal Illness*. London, London Hospital Medical Publications, 1967.

35. Simonton OC, Matthews-Simonton S, Creighton JL: *Getting Well Again*. New York: Bantam Books, 1978.

36. Speck WT, Kennel JH: Management of perinatal death. *Paediatr Rev* 2:59, 1980.

37. Spitzer WO, Dobson AJ, Hall J, et al: Measuring the quality of life of cancer patients: A concise QL-index for use by physicians. *J Chronic Dis* 34:585, 1981.

38. Weisman AD, Hatchett TP: Predilections to death: Death and dying as psychiatric problems. *J Psychosom Med* 23:232, 1961.

39. Weisman AD, Worden JW: Psychosocial analysis of cancer deaths. *Omega* 6:61, 1975.

40. Vachon M: Personal communication.

41. Zborowski M: Cultural components in responses to pain. *J Soc Issues* 8:16, 1952.

Chapter 23
Behavior Problems in Children

Yves Talbot

The primary care clinician who deals with children and their families is likely to be presented with problems not encountered by a physician a few decades ago. Changes in infant mortality and a marked decrease in infectious diseases have brought child development, behavioral problems, and chronic illness to the forefront of the day-to-day care of children.[10,27,32]

Behavior labelled as a "problem" by the parent is often part of normal child development (crying, temper tantrums). On the other hand, a child with a constitutional vulnerability (asthma, enuresis, recurrent abdominal pain) may cause concern or conflict in a family, or the family may maintain the child's symptoms in such a way as to prevent the child's continuing development. For example, the maintenance of temper tantrum behavior in a 5-year-old may allow him to get everything he wants from his parents and siblings and will prevent the child from learning social skills like sharing, cooperation, or even classroom learning. A child with recurrent abdominal pain due to a relative lactose intolerance may maintain his symptomatic behavior when he becomes subconsciously aware that the symptoms can be used to prevent his parents from fighting, or can help the child avoid school.

In approaching a behavioral problem, the family practitioner or nurse will have to assess the role of genetic endowment, personality, and development as well as the role of parenting and the environment. Table 23.1 lists common behaviors and behavioral problems and their approximate age of occurrence. This is clearly not a normative chart; some behaviors are more common and more "normal" than others. For the reader interested in more detail about a given behavioral problem, references are indicated. Two important studies on common behavior in children, by Sheperd and Oppenheim[32] and by Achenback and Edelbroock,[1] provide the clinician with a frequency distribution of these behaviors from age four to sixteen years.

Table 23.1 **Child Behavior Timetable**

Behavior	Approximate Age Of Onset
Crying[6,7,8]	0–6 months
Feeding[22,32]	6 months
Recurrent vomiting (Rumination)[22,31]	6 months
Head rolling, banging, body rocking[28]	9 months–15 months
Temper tantrum[7,8,10,13,23,26]	18 months–36 months
Breath holding[7,8,13,23,26]	2 years
Toilet learning[5,8,33]	2½ years
Co-sleeping[17]	3 years
Resistance to bed time[13,23]	3 years
Fears (Animal, stranger, darkness)[8,12]	3–5 years
Sibling rivalry[8]	2½ years
Night terrors[17]	3–6 years
Sleep walking[17]	3 years
Thumb sucking[32]	3 years
Can't control[8,23,24]	2½ years
Soiling[19]	3½ years
Recurrent abdominal pain[3,4,16]	5 years
Bed wetting[15,18]	6 years
Fighting[13]	5 years
Stealing[13,23]	5 years
Shyness, no friend[11,12]	5 years
School avoidance[7,30]	5–6 years
Lying[23,24]	5 years
Somatization[12]	7 years
School problem (restlessness, learning) Asthma[20,21]	
Food fads[13,31]	8 years
Brittle diabetes[20,21]	8–9 years
Moodiness[32]	10–12 years
Drugs	12 years
Depression	14 years
Anorexia[21]	13–14 years
Nail biting[32]	13–14 years
Truancy	15 years

ASSESSMENT

When parents seek help for a child with a problem behavior it is usually because the behavior is a cause of concern or conflict in the family rather than to one member. It is therefore very important in assessing such a problem to see all the family members involved in it, not only to provide a better understanding but also to increase the possibility of effective management. The clinician must obtain the following information: a brief developmental history of the child and relevant family history; the type of temperament of the child; a precise description of the behavioral problem and of the parents' attempted solutions.

Based on the assessment of the problem and its role in the family system, management may then consist of: reassurance, education, anticipatory guidance; specific suggestions; facilitation; and referral (to a social worker, psychologist, family therapist, psychiatrist).

Developmental History

A review of the principle developmental stages of the child and the child's current abilities establishes the chronological sequence and the appropriateness of the current behavior. For example, retarded sphincter control can explain the frustration of parents in some cases of enuresis or encopresis. A family history of late development in the same area can be elicited.

Important family events in the recent or remote past may have a bearing on a behavior. For example, it is well known that a move or the arrival of a new sibling produces regression in the older children and the return of temper tantrums or enuresis. Clearly if a problem has recurred after a period of normalcy or greater development, the most important question to ask is what happened to the child or family immediately prior to the recurrence.

Temperament

The important work of Chess and Thomas in the area of child temperament have brought two main contributions to the understanding of behavior problems.[11,12] First, these investigators have stressed the innate differences between children in activity levels, biological regularity (sleep and appetite), sensory thresholds, mood, approach to a new situation, adaptability, intensity of response, ability to be distracted, and attention span. These qualities demonstrated in newborn children help explain the behavioral style of children. Second, these authors highlighted the interaction between a particular child and a particular set of parents. A docile child, for example, may be less acceptable to energetic, active parents than an active and aggressive child, who might be labelled as "hyperactive" by a quieter set of parents.

This approach has beneficial effects on the parent-child relationship when the clinician can indicate to the parents the particular personality of the child, often removing guilt of failed or inadequate parenting. A typical example, described by Chess and Thomas, is the slow-to-warm-up child, who tends to be timid and adapts very gradually to any new situation (new food, new people). Such a child may create anxiety in parents eager to see their child develop, and they may feel that they are doing something wrong as parents. By pointing out the particular style of their child the clinician can prevent the problem from escalating and help the family find alternative ways of managing. For example, a normally active boy in a family used to quieter girls may be labelled as "hyperactive," and the situation may be made worse in a nursery school with little space for activity, where quieter pursuits and quieter personalities are favored by the teachers for practical reasons. A nursery environment encouraging more activity and with more space may prevent frustration in child, teacher, and parents. The slow-to-warm-up child will be helped by gradual introduction of new situations, and limited contact with visitors.

Description of the Problem

A full description of the problem and a recognition of who is defining it as a problem often clarify reasons for the problem's development and indicate a management strategy. Such data gathering begins on the first telephone call or a visit and should continue in a family interview in which all relevant members are present.

Who Defines the Problem?

It is important to identify the person for whom the behavior is a problem, and with whom it is occurring. This will allow a better definition of who should be present at the initial interview. For example, if grandmother defines a 2-month-old's crying as resulting from a lack of food or as an abnormality because her children never cried, it is better to include her in the discussion since she has an important role in this family system's child-rearing support. If behavior is defined as a problem by one parent and not by the other, this may indicate lack of support or undermining by the second parent, or a plea for help with a broader family problem by the first parent.

Exact Description of the Problem

Vague expressions (such as "My child is nervous, hyperactive, anxious.") often represent concepts that are very different for the clinician and for the parent. Specific descriptions of what happens and when, its intensity, and its frequency are necessary. For example, a 2-month-old child who cries for 20 minutes every evening after supper is not abnormal. This is usually the period of the day when infant crying occurs. Questions should be specific. For example, with a bedtime problem in an older child it is preferable to ask what time bedtime commences with the child and when it is finally accomplished, rather than asking parents whether they have difficulty with this task.

Are There Any Other Problems?

It is important to know for prognosis and management whether this is the only behavioral problem of this child and whether other children in the family show the same behavior or other problems. Some behavioral problems tend to cluster, indicating more general problems or difficulty parenting. It is also important for the family to specify, when many behaviors are creating concern, which one specifically they want to deal with. There is evidence that when one problem is successfully solved, learning generalizes to other areas of problem-solving, and increased self-confidence may allow the parents to proceed on their own.

What Is the Context and Sequence of the Behavior?

This line of questioning is aimed at eliciting the family's solution or adaptation to the behavior, which can often be seen as contributing to its maintenance. A sequence of behavior, who does what and when, is important to find out: "What happens first . . . What happens next . . . What then. . . ." By identifying the sequence of behavior the clinician can see how the behavior is reinforced. For example, when dealing with a temper tantrum, a classic sequence between parent and child would be as follows: (1) parent asks child to do something (pick up toys); (2) child resists; (3) parent insists and may use threats, sometimes only unrealistic ones ("You will go to your room for the rest of the day."); (4) child resists; (5) mother insists; (6) child resists; (7) mother takes child to his or her room; (8) tantrum occurs. Depending on the intensity of the child and the behavior, he or she is asked out of the room or stays in the room until calm. He or she may then come out but is not asked to pick up the toys. In any event, the child ends up winning. A different sequence may occur when father is home: after two attempts from mother, he may intervene and successfully have the child pick up the toys, avoiding a temper tantrum. This makes his wife feel incompetent and even less able to deal with the problem when it occurs the next day when the child is alone with the mother again. The child will continue to misbehave when dad is not at home.

Behavior sequences can be obtained by doing the following:

1. taking a history during the family interview;
2. utilizing a daily record on which parents note their interventions before and after the occurrence of the behavior. This record, like any record used in behavioral therapy, can be a useful adjunct to chart progress, timing of behaviors, associated events, as well as sequence; and
3. by directly observing during the interview the way the behavioral problem is expressed and dealt with. This is termed "enactment."

The second and third methods are particularly useful as they take little time. The observation necessary in enactment is rarely more than 5 minutes in the course of the regular examination. We have found that the same behavior for which the parents consult will often happen during the interview. For example, temper tantrums are almost automatic or very easy to provoke. This is not the case, fortunately, for enuresis or encopresis. If it does happen, however, it is important for the clinician to allow it to continue since it is an important source of data about the ways in which the family handles the problem.

Why Is the Behavior a Problem?

As in other areas of health care, a behavioral problem is a symptom that may disappear with reassurance and education. At present, there is a lack of training and role modelling in good parenting, and there is insecurity as to which of many experts to follow; guidance by the clinician over one to three sessions may be necessary. At the other end of the spectrum the behavioral problem may be the tip of a submerged iceberg of family conflict and dysfunction which requires referral. The underlying reason for the problem must be elicited. It is important to understand the family's explanatory model of the behavior. For example, recurrent abdominal pain may represent the family's worry about cancer or gastrointestinal disease that is prevalent in this family or to its culture. Any folkloric or cultural explanations may be the key to effective communication as in other areas of health care, and if left untouched may result in the family seeking help from other providers. Lack of experience with normal child development, together with fear of inherited illness, may produce marked anxiety. For example, if the child is slow in development in the first year in comparison with the neighbors' child, or if the child is given to head banging or body rocking (activities not necessarily abnormal in a 5- to 15-month-old child) a family with a history of mental retardation may experience panic. In one family the mother recognized the normalcy of supper time crying in the first-born child, but for the husband this crying was intolerable because he remembered as a young child listening to a baby's continuous crying next door and later learned that the baby had died. In this case discussion of the problem with the mother alone would simply aggravate the couple's conflict over the definition of this as a problem.

If the reason for the child's misbehavior is a problem at the spouses' level, it may need to be eventually relabelled as a marital problem. To do so before helping the couple with the problem as they experience it is to be seen as irrelevant, judgmental, and unhelpful. Usually by focussing on parenting skills around the behavioral problem, the couple will either improve their competency as a team, which may have beneficial effects on the marriage, or be able to recognize for themselves that conflict in the parenting arena represents more serious underlying marital conflict. As in other areas of health care, simple explanations or diagnoses should come first, as should simpler and shorter interventions.

What Solutions Has the Family Tried to Relieve the Problem?

Assessment of how the family has approached the problem gives information on family consistency, flexibility, and ingenuity, and the ability of the parents to work together. For a problem of any duration, the typical solution used by the family will often, in fact, be the mechanism for its maintenance. For example, the parent may have developed the habit of rewarding the child for stopping the undesired behavior; the child quickly seizes on the fact that if he or she wants the rewards he must present the behavior. A candy for stopping a temper tantrum will clearly increase the incidence of tantrums. A parent who uses coercion or violence to stop violence doubly reinforces the behavior: Peter hits Marie so that she will stop doing something he dislikes. He then is hit by a parent, and his use of violence not only is reinforced by his sister stopping the behavior but also by role modelling by the parent using the same tactic. The parent who makes threats that are never carried out teaches a child to never take the parental demands seriously and reinforces bad behavior. The instruction, "Say no three times a day but mean it.", helps some of these parents, as does the guiding phrase "firm but friendly."

Finally, there are the parents who would like the professional to be a substitute parent and are asking in effect, "Please fix our child." Here the solution is up to the professional; if this bait is accepted, the prognosis is poor. It is often a temptation when children are misbehaving for the professional to step in and provide proper discipline. This has some benefits if done sparingly, but has the danger of making the parents feel incompetent or of suggesting the professional is willing to take over for them.

Family Styles

Observation of family interaction has led to the identification of certain family styles that are often related to the maintenance of behavior problems. Allmond and colleagues have identified five family types: the uproars, the reasonables, the silent, the blamers, and the intellectualizers.[2] (Satir describes similar stances of individuals: the distractor, the super-reasonable, the blamer, and the placator.)[29] Each configuration will be briefly described.

The Uproar Family

This family given to uproar is best described by disorganization, often requiring many phone calls for scheduling their first visit. On entry to the office children are out of control, running around or playing with the medical equipment. Everyone talks at once and the clinician may have the feeling of being in a disaster. The situation is best dealt with by politely establishing the rules of office behavior and asking the parents to have them observed. This enactment of discipline allows observation of their compliance with the request and ability to perform as a team.

The Reasonable Family

The reasonable family often presents as a model of togetherness, always finding a way to keep the peace. They will avoid talking *to* anybody, but will talk about everybody. This sense of togetherness may often erroneously lead the physician or nurse to see them as a family without problems. The conflict avoidance in the reasonable family often translates into inconsistencies and undermining by one of the parents. After seeking the clinician's advice this family will often not act upon it and give good reasons for not doing so. The best strategy is to teach better communication skills by insisting members talk to each other, not about each other, to encourage use of the pronoun "I," and not "we," and to support any expression of discord. This encourages individuation and owning of opinions and statements. Early good advice should be avoided in favor of encouraging decision-making by the family.

The Silent Family

This silent family is the monosyllabic family. Heavy silence often makes initiating the interview very difficult. The behavioral problem is often maintained by lack of communication. The first task of the clinician is to deal with the family silence and sense of discomfort. To challenge the silence leads to even more withdrawal; it is better to deal with the family's expectations of the sessions and to normalize their anxiety by stating that most families find it difficult to come to a professional's office to discuss a problem as a family. Starting with "Is your family as private as mine?", or with a suggestion that the children draw a family picture or talk about a picture of a family scene may help to warm up the discussion. Joining with every member of the family at the beginning of the interview is particularly essential for this type of family, and must convey the impression that everyone's opinion and perspective is important and needed. As comfort increases, communication with the professional may open areas that have never been discussed at home.

The Blaming Family

Families that blame argue almost from the moment they enter the office, or the moment you enter their home. Problems are always someone else's fault. A family member is always under attack and this person is expert in his or her own defense; they do not listen to one another. The escalation of blame may make them similar to an uproar family. It is very difficult to establish a relationship with such families without siding with one member in the discussion. But for the family to communicate effectively and manage a behavioral problem, they need to learn to talk without explaining and defending. A neutral outsider who refuses the role of judge can be extremely helpful in pointing out how blame becomes an avoidance of responsibility and change and prevents problem-solving.

The Intellectualizing Family

The intellectualizing family keeps the physician or nurse up to date on journals and books on child care if their style is not recognized for what it is: an intellectual evasion of feelings. The family members limit themselves to the facts, as if taking part in a professional case discussion, and sound as though they are talking about a child from someone else's family. This pattern can, as in the reasonable family, lead to undermining and inconsistency about the child's problem. The task of the clinician is to open a crack in this intellectual barrier to enable the family to express how the situation makes them feel. If Danny is having temper tantrums, the family members need to describe their own feelings of helplessness or anger when unable to control him. The tantrums may be Danny's way of expressing bottled-up family emotions. If a trusting relationship has developed between the clinician and the family, the suggestion that Danny has a particular role in family dynamics, and that spreading the expression of emotion to other family members may help him give it up, may act as a catalyst for change in this family. It will also help Danny's parents to act as a team in controlling his outbursts.

MANAGEMENT

In managing families with a child with behavioral problems, the role of the family physician or nurse is threefold. He or she can provide information and anticipatory guidance; give specific suggestions to the family about how to react to a given behavior or to improve communication; or refer families in need of more intensive involvement and family therapy or requiring some instrumental assistance (babysitting, daycare) to handle the current problem of their child.

Education and Anticipatory Guidance

The goal of educational counselling is to "normalize" age-appropriate behavior of a child and to put the behavior in its developmental context. The clinician can also play a preventive role by anticipating such problems before they occur, and by preventing their maintenance by appropriate suggestions. For example, when giving instructions and advice to a mother leaving the hospital with her newborn child, the clinician can mention the typical pattern of bedtime crying in a 6- to 12-week-old infant. Through no fault of the parents, this pattern may persist for a longer period in a child with greater excitability or sensitivity to environmental stimuli, and is a normal phenomenon in the North American baby (cultures that maintain constant physical contact with the infant, such as the Eskimos, do not have this pattern.)

Crying infants ("colicky" babies) often reflect tension in the mother or the family system by crying or being difficult to feed; maternal anxiety may occur and manifest itself by a lack of milk if the mother is breast feeding; and the demands of other children, of in-laws, and of outside work pressures are all interrelated. For example:

> Mr. and Mrs. P. came to see their family physician because of their new baby's constant crying. There were two other preschool children in the house. The mother described this baby as more irritable and a light sleeper who reacted more to noise. He seemed not to be as cuddly as the older two had been and when held would sometimes arch his back. During feeding he would often swallow greedily and then choke and stop feeding, only to be hungry 2 hours later. When the baby slept the mother was preoccupied with the demands of the two toddlers, and as soon as they were settled the baby would wake up. The repeated cycle, left the mother exhausted. The father was a hard worker who had been recently promoted, and who was trying to make the mortgage payment on the new house. He was not very supportive when he came home in the evening. They had recently moved to a new community near Mrs. P.'s parents but they were rarely available and the family knew no neighbors or other resources. The family's coping abilities were now stretched to the breaking point by the crying baby.
>
> During the interview the clinician noted that the child was very calm and relaxed. He enquired whether he could also be relaxed at home. The mother admitted that at night the baby would nurse perfectly when everyone else was asleep and they were both relaxed. The clinician recognized that the parents were dealing with the type of child whose temperament made him highly sensitive to his environment, which in this case was a very stimulating one. The crying was part of a chain of events for this family, but there was a need for an immediate solution. Knowing that the grandmother had accompanied Mr. and Mrs. P. he asked them if they thought she could take the other children during the day for a period. They felt this would be a good idea and the grandmother joined the interview and agreed to their request.
>
> One week after the interview the mother phoned and said that the baby was feeding well and was more relaxed. He had increased his time between feedings, and when the two little girls returned for supper, both the mother and father spent time with them. The mother had also resumed some community activities because more time was available between feedings. Thus, the clinician had addressed the feelings of inadequate

parenting that resulted from a crying child, had put the child's behavior in the context of his own temperament and that of the family, and had acted as a catalyst to allow use of resources and the family's solution to the problem.

Anticipatory guidance can easily be incorporated in the child's regular visits for immunization and physical examination. Changes such as the decreased appetite of the infant around the age of 1 year, the development of temper tantrums common at 18 months, issues around toilet training at 2 and a half years, and sibling rivalry after the birth of an infant can be described as part of normal development. The usual sequence of bladder control, dry by day and then dry by night, is established for most children by 3 years old, but 15% of 4- and 5-year-olds still are enuretic. It is important for the parents to avoid giving excessive negative attention to this problem, which will encourage persistence of enuresis and lower the child's self-esteem. Temper tantrums, although normal, require firmness and consistency to prevent their continuation as a useful means of controlling the environment. Sibling rivaly against a newborn baby is expressed in a stronger way when the child is over the age of 18 months once an increased independence has occurred.

Entry into the school system, particularly for the first child, can be traumatic for both child and family. It heralds an opening up of the new family's boundaries to include more contact with the outside world around the child. Anticipating this event, the clinician can suggest that the mother avoid cutting herself off from friends and interest groups, and that she introduce her child gradually into play groups or a nursery school in preparation for school. School phobia, when it does occur, can be a serious problem. It is important if it does occur not to allow it to continue for long, but to treat it as an emergency situation, the child must go to school as soon as possible, and should have the support of the teachers. The anxiety felt by the mother both for the child and for herself left alone at home must be dealt with seriously. Awareness by the clinician of the couple relationship may increase his preventive role through suggestions to increase the couple's time together if this is not occurring, and through recognition of warning signs such as increasing absence of the father at work.

School problems tend to present again during the time of adolescence, as in the following case:

> Mr. and Mrs. T. brought their 14-year-old son because of truancy. He had been suspended because he had not shown up in class, but the school had not had any previous complaint although he had been away frequently.
>
> Jack was the youngest son in a family of three boys; the older two were currently doing well in school. The father, a member of the school board, was a self-made man and very active in his community. Mrs. T. felt quite desperate about Jack's poor school achievement.
>
> The family physician enquired about the problem, eliciting the

sequence that typically occurred, and kept the discussion to a very factual level—what happens first, next . . . , what then. . . . He rapidly discovered that when Jack decided not to go to school he was allowed to sleep in until 11:00, watch television during the day, and go out with his friends in the evening. Apart from the school problem he was a cooperative boy and when asked what he wanted to do instead of school he said he wanted to work. The physician took this opportunity to use the father's expertise as a person who had also learned to work at a young age; the father planned with his son a regular day with pay if Jack elected to stay home. Father and mother as employer decided what had to be done. Jack had to get up at 6:30 a.m. After breakfast he was to work all day with a brief break mid-morning and at lunch. This lasted 2 days.

Jack has now been attending school all day, and his father has a built-in checking system with the school to confirm Jack's attendance. As a reward, father and son have planned a trip together for the summer.

Although there are many reasons for a child to wish to avoid school, something must be happening to allow these wishes to be acted on. A concrete investigation of the sequence of events usually gives a very good picture of how the behavior is handled. Recognition that this boy was repeating the father's own adolescent history facilitated a rapid solution in which parental teamwork was involved. Had the couple not been able to function as a team, and had conflict between them surfaced as the reason for the truancy, the clinician's role would have been to steer the couple to seek counselling for themselves.

Anticipatory guidance in adolescents is often in the area of discipline and setting limits. The clinician's awareness of age-appropriate autonomy can help in educating parents as to cultural norms, and the need to gradually increase autonomy but at the same time increase the expectations and responsibility of the growing adolescent. For the mother whose main preoccupation has been watching the child, some nudges in the direction of her own growth and autonomy and interests can be helpful preventive maneuvers. Such mothers may otherwise undermine the children's attempts at independence, and be overly affected by adolescent mood swings and derogatory comments about the parent's abilities. Support from the clinician in expanding horizons and increasing couple time and vacations may prevent the problems of the "empty nest."

Specific Suggestions

The two cases cited above are both examples of prompting by the clinician, who wishes to help the family devise a plan of management; he or she acts as a coach, giving occasional specific suggestions when the parents are at a loss. These suggestions should be based on several practical principles:

Positive Enforcement

Verbal and nonverbal support by the parent for good behavior or appropriate attitude in the child is defined as positive reinforcement. As in the previous cases cited, parents often unwittingly reinforce the negative aspects of behavior. For example, it has been noted that parents often pay attention to their children only when their attention is drawn by a fight. Such parents would do well to note when children are happily playing together and either comment on it or reward such behavior nonverbally (candies at this time would be more appropriate than after bad behavior). Excessive fighting in children may be a result of excessive attention to the fighting, or may at times represent a fight between the parents that cannot be expressed otherwise.

Shared Information

The child should be included in discussions of the behavioral problem and in discussions of the solutions planned: negotiation, particularly once the child has reached adolescence, is a better basis for discipline than dictated authority. Rewards and punishments are much more effective when set according to the child's preference or dislike.

Parental Agreement

Parents must agree on the definition of the problem and on the methods of solving it. Persistent disagreement effectively blocks problem solving and may suggest the need for referral for family therapy.

Avoid Attention Being Given to Negative Behaviors

The visit to a health professional is, itself, a focus of attention on the "problem child." As soon as possible this attention should lead to a solution, with the parents again in control, and the child seen as no different from his siblings. The parents must learn to turn their attention to the child's positive behavior.

Progressive Desensitization

The principles of progressive desensitization can be applied not only to fears and phobias of childhood but also to problem-solving skills of parents: just as in patients with phobias mild fears are dealt with first, and the sense of mastery and decreased anxiety then is extended to more difficult areas, so in parents of patients with behavioral problems success in easier areas installs confidence and competence for more difficult areas.

The Adolescent as Problem Solver

Some problems are more appropriately dealt with by the child rather than by the parent, particularly if the child is adolescent. Overinvolvement and too much watching of the child beyond an appropriate age can produce problems in school or of difficulty with peers. When parents give the impression that it is for their sake that the child must make good grades, eat a hearty meal, have a certain number of a type of friends, or wear a sweater, they are inviting rebellion. Once the parents perceive that their efforts are counterproductive the child's own desire to succeed and make friends (or his own physiologic needs in the case of eating) and his or her fear of the consequences of poor work at school will take over. For example, a child should be responsible for getting to school on time in the morning; he or she can be given an alarm clock and should not be "bailed out" by being driven to school if he or she is too late to walk or take the bus. The cooperation of the teacher often facilitates a change in increased responsibility.

Intervention Models

For certain very common behavioral problems, intervention models have been described in detail by Christopherson.[13,14] These have been reproduced with permission at the end of this chapter for: (1) bedtime problems, and (2) the child who will not listen or develops temper tantrums. These suggestions can be used by the family clinician; compliance with the "prescription" is increased if instructions are written. A telephone follow-up or clinician availability if the parent's first attempts do not succeed will markedly decrease the incidence of failure.

Use of Graph Analysis

K-Lynn Paul[25] has described a technique to be used by the family physician for counselling in child-rearing problems. The method is simple and has been devised to graphically depict a family's interactions and behavior. The objective is to identify on a graph the patterns of the relationship between parents and children during times of stress and to illustrate faulty child-rearing habits and poor teamwork during such stresses.

The parents are asked to describe their problems so the physician can distinguish the cases that require special treatment techniques (enuresis, stuttering). Then, they must label their basic disciplinary technique as being strict, moderate, or permissive and put a mark on the bottom of the graph where they feel it is most appropriate (see Figure 23-1). Each parent must determine if they maintain the same position under increased stress (from work, from the child's own misbehavior or from couple conflict), or if their attitude becomes more permissive or strict. Lines are drawn to represent these changes of attitude during stress and even during very high tension.

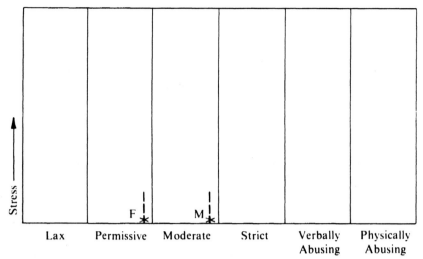

| Lax | Permissive | Moderate | Strict | Verbally Abusing | Physically Abusing |

Figure 23-1. Graph for analyzing parents' position in disciplining children. Here the father described himself as more permissive than his wife; in both their attitudes did not change with low level of stress.

Father's and mother's basic position and stress patterns may be similar. In one example, the disciplinary attitude of parents of an 8-year-old child are slightly different: the mother's position is moderate, and the father's position is more permissive. Both become verbally aggressive as stress increases significantly but finally always capitulate (Figure 23-2). Their child tolerates their verbal abuse because he knows he will be rewarded in the end by getting his own way. The parents are helped by recognizing this shift to the lax position and accepting that this behavior must cease.

Most of the time parents have different patterns. The interaction may be one of a triangle. When one parent feels that under stress he or she may become physically aggressive, he or she may choose to shift abruptly to a more permissive position, forcing the other parent to take the strict role (Figure 23-3). The contrary is also true: the shift to the permissive role may be necessary in one parent's mind to antagonize the strictness of the other (Figure 23-3). Conflicts between parents may arise at some points, usually when lines are diverging. The arguments between parents help the child to win if they prevent them from following through on discipline; or they may cause one parent to lose control due to the excessive stress. If mother becomes more severe it may relieve the tension of discipline on the father. This togetherness benefits parents and children. Parents must be aware that eliminating verbal and physical abuse increases the child's self-esteem and discontinuing overindulgence helps the child feel more loved and secure.

Charting of behavior and reporting on when behaviors occur and the parental response before and after help record progress and link parental

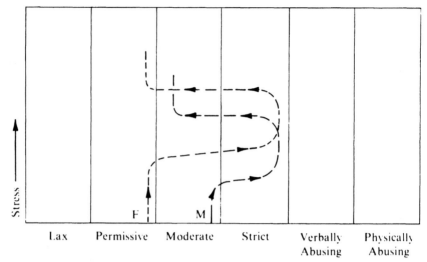

| Lax | Permissive | Moderate | Strict | Verbally Abusing | Physically Abusing |

Figure 23-2. Same parents as in Fig. 22-1. With more stress they become very strict but do not keep this position for a long time. Mother is the first to give in, followed soon after by her husband.

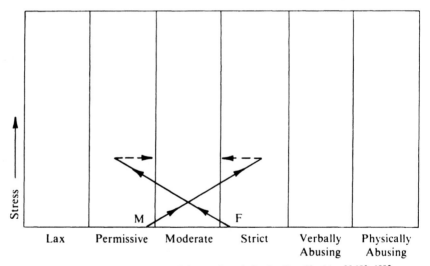

| Lax | Permissive | Moderate | Strict | Verbally Abusing | Physically Abusing |

From: Paul K-Lynn: Brief family therapy utilising graph analysis. *Am Fam Physician* 25:183, 1982.

Figure 23-3. When parents antagonize each other, two possibilities can happen: the mother becomes abusive to make up for the father's laxity at the system's limit of tolerance of violence. Father acts to modify her behavior and becomes more strict. At points where the parents' lines cross, negotiation and teamwork is possible. If father becomes more strict under tension, mother may be able to relax (*dotted lines*).

factors in maintenance of the child's behaviors. One should allow for two to three meetings with the family before change occurs and can be maintained. Meetings can be scheduled for half an hour at 2- to 3-week intervals. After the first visit, parents should be warned that the child's behavior will worsen before it improves. The classic punishment of isolating the child for a short period of time has to be applied consistently to young children (between the ages of 4 and 6 years) to be successful. For older children, rewards or punishments have to be set according to preference or dislike (see cases given above).

REFERRAL

There are certain situations in which referral for more intensive or expert guidance is indicated. If parents need more support and ongoing discussion than time permits, parenting groups in the community are often extremely helpful. If problems are more complex or of long duration, as in many problems of adolescents, or if one or two sessions reveal parental conflict or need to maintain the problem for other reasons, then referral is a service to the whole family. A dysfunctional family, such as a psychosomatic family in which conflict between the parents is detoured through a child's asthmatic attack or delinquent behavior, is difficult to treat even in the hands of a family therapist. The challenge to the primary care clinician is to reframe the problem presented as a family problem. This may take a long time and can often only be done by a trusted clinician with ongoing contact with the family. Too abrupt a restatement of the problem simply prompts family disbelief and doctor-shopping or individual therapy for the child.

Referral carries with it the family's trust in the primary clinician and should be monitored without interfering with the relationship between family and therapist. If the therapist is in the same practice location, communication is particularly easy and awareness of the consultant's goals allows the primary care clinician to support interventions.

APPENDIX A[13,14]

Guidelines for Parents: Bedtime Problem—Getting out of Bed

1. Establish a reasonable bedtime or naptime for normal day-to-day circumstances, and put your child to bed at that time *every* night.
2. About 30 minutes before bedtime, start "quiet time," during which your child should engage in quiet activities rather than roughhousing.

3. Go through your regular bedtime routine (bedtime story, kisses, drinks, bathroom, etc.).

4. At the established bedtime have your child in bed—tell him goodnight, turn off the light and close the door (optional).

5. Monitor your child *very closely* the first few nights to catch him getting out of bed the instant he gets up.

6. When your child gets up, give him one spank (the first spank is for the child, all others are for you)—DO NOT TALK TO THE CHILD. Put him back in the bed—DO NOT TUCK THE CHILD IN—make this as matter-of-fact as possible.

7. Continue this routine each time your child gets up. You may be surprised how often your child will get up the first night or two; don't become discouraged—he or she is testing you to find out whether you really mean it—and don't give up.

8. In the morning, if your child has remained in bed praise him or her verbally and offer a reward, like a choice between two different favored foods for breakfast.

APPENDIX B

Guidelines for Parents: Bedtime Problem—Crying

1. Establish a reasonable time for bedtime or naptime, and under normal day-to-day circumstances put your child to bed at that time.

2. About 30 minutes before bedtime, start "quiet time," during which your child should engage in quiet activities rather than roughhousing.

3. Go through your regular bedtime routine (bedtime story, drinks, kisses, etc.).

4. Tell your child good night and that you will see him in the morning.

5. Turn off the light, leave the room and close the door (optional).

6. Do *not* go back into the room. Your child may cry for a very long time but if after 1 or 2 hours you go in and pick him up, you will teach him or her that all he or she has to do is cry for a long time—then mommy will come back in. Your child may also try a variety of different noises, calls, etc. in an effort to get you to give in— don't fall for these. Stay out of the room.

7. Don't get discouraged—it only takes a few nights.

8. After your child is regularly going to bed without crying for more than a minute or two, it is alright to check on him if he continues to cry to make sure he is alright.

Follow these suggestions for any bedtime crying to avoid having the bedtime problem recur:

1. Do not talk to your child after he is down for the night.

2. Check diapers, etc. as quickly as possible.

3. If everything is okay, leave the room without saying a word or holding your child.

APPENDIX C

Guidelines for Parents: Temper Problems/Noncompliance

If you are having problems getting your child to follow instructions the first time or if your child has tantrums if you tell him or her "No," the following procedures can help you teach your child how to follow instructions appropriately.

1. *Praise* your child every time he or she follows instructions.

2. Only give instructions once.

3. If your child does not comply with your instructions the first time that you give it, then place the child in "time-out" (kitchen chair, steps, etc.—NO CLOSETS OR DARK ROOMS).

   a. Carry the child (if needed) to the chair in such a way that he or she cannot look at you.

   b. State the rule, "Whenever you don't follow instructions, you have to sit in the chair."

   c. Place the child on the chair.

   d. After the child is quiet, set a timer (a portable kitchen timer is best) for 2 (toddler) or 5 (schoolage) minutes. Never more than 5 minutes.

   e. If the child gets up, give him one spank and put him or her back in the chair. As soon as he is quiet, reset the timer for 2 or 5 minutes.

   f. When the timer rings, ask the child if he wants to get up.

   g. If the child says "No" or starts fussing or crying, wait for him or her to be quiet, then reset the timer.

   h. When the child is through with "time-out," encourage him to engage in a pleasant and/or acceptable activity.

EXAMPLES:

Temper Tantrums. Practice the situation again while prompting the child to say "OK" and not throw a tantrum. PRAISE him or her during the practice situation.

Noncompliance. Have the child then carry out the instruction. PRAISE him or her for carrying out the instructions. If he or she does not comply, replace him in "time-out." This may be necessary several times when you first start using the procedure.

Fighting. When the children play together nicely or share, etc. PRAISE them.

REFERENCES

1. Achenback T, Edelbroock C: Behavioral problems and competencies reported by parents of normal and disturbed children aged four through sixteen. *Monogr Soc Res Child Dev* 46(1):1, 1981.

2. Allmond B, Buckman W, Gofman H: *The Family is the Patient.* St. Louis, C.V. Mosby Co., 1979.

3. Apley J: *The Child with Abdominal Pains.* Oxford, Blackwell Scientific, 1975.

4. Barr RE: Recurrent abdominal pain in childhood due to lactose intolerance. *N Engl J Med* 300:1449, 1978.

5. Brazelton T: Toilet training. *Pediatrics* 129:121, 1962.

6. Brazelton T: Crying in infancy. *Pediatrics* 29:579, 1963.

7. Brazelton T: Anticipatory guidance. *Pediatr Clin North Am* 22:3, 1975.

8. Brazelton T: *Doctor and Child.* New York, Seymour Laurence, 1979.

9. Burger H: Somatic Pain and School Avoidance. *Clin Pediatr* October, 1974.

10. Chamberlain R: Behavioral problems in pre-school age children, in Haggerty RJ, et al (eds): *Child Health and the Community.* New York, John Wiley and Son, 1975.

11. Chess S, et al: *Behavioral Individuality in Early Childhood.* New York, New York University Press, 1963.

12. Chess S, et al: *Your Child is a Person: A Psychological Approach to Parenthood Without Guilt.* New York, Viking Press, 1972.

13. Christophersen E, Barnard J: Prevention, Detection and Treatment of Commonly Encountered Pediatric Behavior Problems. Presented at an advanced ambulatory pediatric association workshop, Washington D.C., September, 1976.

14. Christophersen E: *Behavioral Pediatrics. Am Fam Physician* 17:3, 1978.

15. Cohen M: Eneuresis. *Pediatr Clin North Am* 22:3, 1975.

16. Green M: A developmental approach to symptoms based on age groups. *Pediatr Clin North Am* 22:3, 1975.

17. Guille M, Anders T: Sleep disorders in children (Part II). *Adv Pediatr* 22:151, 1976.

18. Kolvin I, MacKeith R, Meadows R: *Bladder Control and Eneuresis.* Philadelphia, J.B. Lippincott, 1975.

19. Levine M: Children with encopresis—a descriptive analysis. *Pediatrics* 156:3, 1975.

20. Mitchell K, Berenson B: Differential use of confrontation by high and low facilitative therapies. *J Nerv Ment Dis* 153:165, 1971.

21. Minuchin S, et al: A conceptual model of psychosomatic illness in children. *Arch Gen Psychiatry* 32:1031, 1975.

22. Murray M, et al: Behavioral treatment of rumination. *Clin Pediatr* July 1976.

23. Patterson G: Champaign, Illinois, *Families.* Research Press, 1971.

24. Patterson G: *A Social Learning Approach to Family Intervention. Families With Aggressive Children; I.* Eugene, Oregon, Castaglia Publishing Company, 1975.

25. Paul K-Lynn: Brief family therapy utilising graph analysis. *Am Fam Physician* 25:183, 1982.

26. Reid JB, et al: *A Social Learning Approach to Family Intervention: Observation in Home Setting, II.* Eugene, Oregon, Castaglia Publishing Company, 1978.

27. Rogers D, et al: Some observation on pediatrics: Its past, present and future. *Pediatrics* (Suppl) 87:5, 1981.

28. Sallusto J: Body rocking, head banging, head rolling in normal children. *J Pediatr* 193:704, 1978.

29. Satir V: *People Making.* California, Science and Behavior Books, 1972.

30. Schmitt B: School phobia—the great imitator—a pediatrician's viewpoint. *Pediatrics* 48:433, 1971.

31. Schwartz A: Eating problems. *Pediatr Clin North Am* 5:595, 1958.

32. Sheperd M, Oppenhein B, Mitchel J: *Childhood Behavior and Mental Health.* London, Grune & Stratton, 1971.

33. Stehbens JA: Toilet training. *Pediatrics* 54:493, 1974.

Chapter 24

Psychological Problems of Adults: "Individual" Problems

Janet Christie-Seely

The primary care clinician is on the receiving line for problems defined since Freud as neuroses and psychoses. These are perceived by patients and families and many professionals as psychological problems residing in an individual family member. The attitude and perspective of the health professional consulted may determine the subsequent course. The symptomatic member may become permanently labelled, perhaps rejected by the family as sick or insane, and may be delivered to a mental health professional for treatment, or the identified patient may be the ticket of admission for family help. The family or patient may improve their coping strategies with some support from the clinician and resolve the problems.

Obviously hospitalization of those who are a danger to themselves or others may be essential; medications, individual psychotherapy, shock treatment, and other treatments have caused major changes in the outcome of mental illness. However, it is important to recognize the impact of these professional interventions on the family system. Therapy for the individual is often necessary, and if done with full awareness of the family system it may be the best means of producing change in that system. Unfortunately such awareness is not the norm and disastrous courses can be taken that aggravate the problems and perpetuate family dysfunction and dependence on the health professions in future generations.

There is a vast literature on psychological problems of the individual and on the etiologic contribution of genetics, personality characteristics, childhood experiences, and recent losses. In comparison, the literature on the family system's role in generating and maintaining such problems is sparse. This chapter deals only briefly with the psychoses (references can be consulted for those interested in this area) and in more detail with the common problems of practice: depression and anxiety.

SCHIZOPHRENIA

In the area of schizophrenia considerable work has been done demonstrating that family dysfunction can contribute to psychosis, particularly in the genetically predisposed individual, and that family therapy can be effective in curing early schizophrenia and preventing a recurrence after discharge from the hospital.[6] The origins of family therapy in the 1950s were based largely on work with schizophrenics; Bateson's studies of communication showing the complexity of levels of communication between family members.[2] The degree of sophistication increased from the earliest recognition that the mother-child relationship was distorted in schizophrenia and progressed through Laing's concepts[17] of the schizophrenogenic family, in which the schizophrenic child was seen as the victim of the parental distorted communication. In families with schizophrenics particularly, the verbal content of a message and the nonverbal or emotional meta-message (the message about the message) may contradict each other. This produces a double bind[3] for the receiver who is unsure which message to comply with. For example, a mother requests a hug from her son, complaining he is never affectionate, but responds to his hug by cringing or pushing him away. When such confused communication is the norm in a relationship the other may respond in kind by confusion, withdrawal from reality and psychotic behavior as self-protective adaptation. Clearly, the problem of the double bind occurs to some extent in all families and is by no means the entire explanation for schizophrenia.

In the systems view, which considers all family members to be equally involved, the schizophrenic child may be as much the persecutor of the parents as their victim; he or she may be the rescuer, drawing attention away from marital conflict. The whole family is caught up in a process transmitted through generations of decreasing individuation and increasing enmeshment and symbiosis.[5] To treat these families requires professional and experienced family therapists, preferably two per family to allow one therapist, as Whittaker puts it, "to join the family craziness"[20] while the other can remain outside the family system in safety. Multiple family therapy groups have been used with considerable success by Lacqueur and others.[16] The primary care clinician should be aware of the efficacy of family therapy, particularly for early psychosis. Unless trained in family therapy, he or she should not undertake dealing with these difficult families without psychiatric back-up. However, the family physician can play an important supportive role for both family and psychiatric patient. If medication is required it can often be monitored by the primary care clinician, and facilitation of communication and problem resolution will decrease the conflict known to exacerbate the patient's symptoms.

NEUROSES

The neuroses have had scant attention in the family literature. Much greater attention has been paid to behavioral problems of adolescents, particularly delinquency, to marital problems, and to some psychosomatic problems.

Anxiety Reaction

Anxiety is a term that covers such a wide variety of clinical situations that it is often merely a descriptive term of use only as a label for charts and forms. Anxiety may disguise depression; it may represent an acute reaction to environmental stressors (exams, death, or illness in a relation) or internal stressors (elevated thyroxin, chest pains of dire significance, subconscious reminders of past stress); or it may be a chronic state caused by the pile up of chronic strains, daily difficulties, and unresolved emotional issues. Understanding the environmental situation and the individual's way of coping are essential to improving problem solving. Beyond this level of understanding is recognition that the anxious individual is but the tip of the iceberg of a disturbed family. The disturbed family may be *within* the patient in the case of the lonely person whose family has died or otherwise disappeared. The problem usually lies in interpersonal relationships, or the lack of them.

It is usually more effective to deal with the problem of anxiety at the level of the family system, if the family is available. If not, working with the family genogram (see Chapter 11) is an excellent way to assess the family and help facilitate insight in the patient. Clarifying current stresses and coping strategies, and coaching in the use of resources can be supplemented with relaxation techniques, yoga, or meditation, etc.

Phobias

There is considerable evidence that phobias, particularly agarophobia, do not exist in an environmental vacuum: antecedents in the individual patient's history cannot continue to produce conditioned symptoms without maintenance by feedback from the present environment. Otherwise extinction would occur. The problem is usually maintained or aggravated by a family system that needs the symptom. For example, if the spouse of an agarophobic person is included in therapy it is often found that he or she generally encourages the behavior unwittingly by consciously disparaging or attempting to cure it.

In a childless couple in which the husband was a prominent and successful business executive, the wife's agarophobia was the factor that maintained the balance of power in the relationship. While he was the apparently successful one, his wife was clearly dominant in the relationship, but prevented from dominating his work environment by the fear of leaving home. Her illness was both a means of power to control her husband's movements, and a labelled weakness to compensate for her strength. (see Chloe Madanes' work[19] in power relationships in couples in Chapter 20).

Thus individual therapy, whether behavioral modification or uncovering of the basic anxiety and remote historical associations that produced the phobia, may fail or have only short-lived success if the environment that undermines therapy is ignored.

Hysteria

An excellent article on the marital system of the hysterical individual[4] is particularly interesting as it elucidates a marital pattern that is an exaggeration of the typical North American marriage. A super-reasonable unemotional male marries a dependent emotional and increasingly irresponsible female. Sixteen such couples were studied; in 15 the wife was diagnosed as hysteric, in one the husband was the hysteric. The authors describe how each partner plays a role in setting up and maintaining a chaotic marriage in which the "hysteric" may end up labelled "insane" by herself and by her husband.

If the clinician is misled by the apparent health and reasonableness of the spouse he will feed the dysfunction of the system, particularly if he or she hospitalizes the "patient." The characteristic type of individual who selects and is selected by the hysterical person is one willing to take the "helper" role, is calm and detached even in the face of emotional crises or life crises, but is not a strong, demanding male who will threaten the hysterical individual's precarious sense of autonomy. Unsure of himself as a man, the wife's exaggerated caricature of the traditional North American female role (emotional, labile, helpless, irresponsible) makes such a man feel masculine and adds excitement to his colorless emotional life. As the marriage goes on, however, the wife's selfish demands and increasingly strident attempts to get an emotional reaction from him (overspending, affairs, eventually suicide threats) produce increasing anger expressed obliquely by withdrawal and greater emotional detachment. She in turn becomes aware of his inability to give any real help with her behavior that she feels unable to control. She is also aware of his avoidance of emotional involvement, and of his lack of practical involvement with any responsibility other than his wage-earning role. His emotional distance and poor contribution to family life make the wife feel unloved, and she becomes desperate for attention from her "nice guy" husband and feels she is a "crazy bitch."

The essential role for any professional with such a family, and particularly for the family physician or nurse whom the family trusts, is that of educator. The premise that one partner is the problem must be changed to the systems perspective and understanding of the vicious cycles set up between them. Though neither is to blame, both are responsible for their own behavior and for change. The pattern of alternating rage at the partner and severe self-condemnation must be replaced by a joint effort to correct the three major areas of imbalance in the relationship. These are 1) allocation of family responsibilities: the woman, although helpless in other ways, has generally assumed almost all family responsibilities in response to the man's abdication in these areas; he in turn feels useless and valued only for his paycheck; 2) helper—helped role mutuality: the husband's sense of exploitation and hers of helplessness and selfishness can be alleviated if she can have a turn at giving and he at asking for help; and 3) rationality—emotionalism: overemphasis on one aspect of life in each member of the couple is a natural result of partnership with the other: extreme behaviors become more extreme to compensate for their absence or the contrary behavior in the partner; instead, each partner can become the teacher of the other in developing their underdeveloped function.

Some couples will not contemplate referral to a therapist but will in fact be able to change their own relationship if the clinician consistently behaves as well as speaks as though the problem is *between* them. Accurate family assessment of imbalances such as are listed above may, after even a single session, provide the couple with enough information to produce change and a stabilization of the relationship (see Chapter 27).

Many such families require therapy and go willingly, but only after it has become clear to them that making one member the patient will not solve the problem. Thus an understanding of the systems orientation in the couple is an essential first step to referral and to a rational ongoing relationship with the family for other medical or life-cycle problems.

DEPRESSION

Depression is one of the most frequently seen psychological states in general practice. When visits for depressive equivalents such as headache, low back pain, and abdominal pain are included the significance of depression in the primary care clinician's clientele is enormous. Anxiety and depression often blend or co-exist and the anxiety may be found to mask an underlying depression. Physical symptoms, whether "functional" or already linked with organic changes, may be easier for the patient to accept than the recognition of depression (our culture is particularly afraid of emotional illness). In fact it is often the fear of depression that results in defenses against it that themselves produce the problems (see Section III on mechanisms of disease). A case of apparent anxiety and marital conflict was poorly handled by a physician who failed to assess the family system.

Maria M. was a strong-willed, obese lady in her 50s who was treated for some years for somewhat labile diabetes, hypertension, and headaches. As trust in her physician grew she admitted to being constantly anxious and unable to relax and had severe insomnia. Methods such as meditation, yoga and self-hypnosis were tried to no avail. Her anxiety was focused on her ailing, inadequate husband and an apparently unrewarding and hostile relationship. Following discussions of the marriage the patient decided to leave her husband, who the physician barely knew. A few days after making this decision, the patient took an overdose of diazepam and was admitted to the hospital for several weeks. In the hospital she told the psychiatrist that Dr. X. had suggested she leave her husband.

Later, it became apparent that the physical symptom of headaches, hypertension, and poor diabetic control had masked an underlying depression. This depression stemmed partly from her loss, at age 9, of a younger sister and a total absence of mourning for the sister with whom she had had a poor relationship. Subconscious attempts to work through this death and the death 20 years later of her mother had resulted in a counterphobic close association with elderly people and those with serious illness. Each death renewed her anxiety and when her husband developed symptoms of a neurologic disorder, which ran in his family, her anxiety had become acute. Repressing the reason, she had focused on the difficult relationship. The husband, seen briefly at this point, was a small, weak, and ineffectual man beside his wife's large, imposing, and powerful presence. Her physical symptoms and psychological disability was the couple's solution to the unequal balance of power.

The Etiology of Depression

Only recently has depression been seen as a disease state; until the turn of the century it was termed "depression of spirits," a mood caused by black bile ("melancholia"), not an entity. Views of causation have varied widely, from the humoral (now monoamines rather than bile) or structural (lesion is the brain or genes) to the environmental (weather, bad winds, poverty, family stress).

Linear View of Depression

An overview of recent research in depression by Akiskal and McKinney (1975) listed 10 different models of depression.[1] The psychoanalytic school has viewed it as aggression turned inward, as object loss (disrupted attachment bond), as loss of self-esteem, or as a negative cognitive set (helplessness-hopelessness).[12] The behavioral schools see depression as learned helplessness or loss of reinforcement for coping and positive mood (with rewards for the "sick role" as substitute).[18] The sociologists perceive loss of role status; the existentialists, loss of a meaning of existence. The biologists have focused on the role in depression of biogenic amines with impaired monoaminergic neurotransmission or on neurophysiologic phenomena such as hyperarousal secondary to intraneuronal sodium accumulation, cholinergic dominance, or a reversible derangement of diencephalic mechanisms of reinforcement.[9]

Clearly, there is evidence for each of these etiologic factors. Genetic vulnerability has been shown for bipolar and recurrent unipolar depression.[13] Developmental events such as loss of a parent in early childhood may sensitize a person to depression later;[6] the occurrence of recent life events categorized as "exits" (death, divorce, separation, departure of a child) occurred in the 6 months before depression in 46 of 185 patients, compared to 9 of 185 controls ($p > .01$).[21] Individual personality traits and low self-esteem can predispose a person to depression. Physiologic stressors such as reserpine, viral infections, childbirth, and hypothyroidism effect diencephalic function and can cause depression. The professional should always be alert to depression as a side effect of drug or disease. A recent article[15] listed drugs and nonpsychiatric disorders associated with depression and found one or more present in 47.8% of 157 family practice patients with depression. Since the drugs include antihistamines, many antibiotics, caffeine and alcohol as well as anti-inflammatory agents and minor tranquilizers, while the illnesses include many infections and endocrine disorders, including menopause, this figure is not surprising! In the absence of a control group this study does little more than remind the physician to look for contributing drugs or illnesses. It also illustrates the linear approach of most medical research and the reification of depression as entity rather than a symptom of one part of a system.

Each of Akiskal's ten models focuses on a different systems level—cellular, societal, individual—but until recently nothing was written about the prime context of most depressed individuals, the family. In another review of the biological, psychoanalytic, cognitive and behavioral theories of depression, L. B. Feldman found that almost all theories focused exlusively on the individual depressed person's biological or intrapsychic functioning, and ignored the interpersonal context in which the depression arises and is maintained.[11] Behavioral theorists may have paid some attention to this context but have not dealt with the system properties of the depressed person's interpersonal world. For example, some cognitive restructuring therapies, such as rational emotive therapy,[10] have recognized the power of a spouse in maintaining the depressed person's self-blaming and self-denigrating thinking that contributes to the ongoing depression. However, the spouse, who is not seen in therapy, may then very easily be viewed by therapist and patient as responsible for the depression. Instead the depression is part of a feedback system produced conjointly by the couple.

Systems View of Depression

The systemic thinker views the depression as part of a feedback system produced conjointly by the couple. Feldman describes a positive and negative feedback system between husband and wife with depression-triggering and depression-maintaining feedback loops. A circular rather than linear process is conceptualized, implying mutual causality. The intimate associate or marital partner of the depressed person tends also to have an underlying depression and low self-esteem that go unrecognized. The spouse who is not depressed triggers the depression by an "innocent" remark or act that "just happens to strike at a particularly sensitive spot in the depressed spouse's shaky sense of self-worth." The self-depreciation, sadness, and guilt of the depressed person stimulates the spouse who is not depressed into overprotectiveness and omnipotence, which reinforces the depression. The oversolicitousness eventually results in withdrawal, passive-aggressive, hostile, or self-assertive behavior by the depressed spouse. This behavior in turn triggers self-depreciation in the spouse who is not depressed, he or she then defensively reacts with further depression-triggering behavior. This is shown in his diagram, reproduced as Figure 24-1.

In a recent book, *The Melancholy Marriage and Psychosocial Approaches to Therapy*, Hinchcliffe and colleagues point out that depression is a rarity in the unmarried, particularly in the woman who has never married.[14] Persons most at risk in a study of Brown and colleagues in London were the married women of lower class whose youngest child was under 6 years.[7] The arrival of young children was postulated to cause depression primarily through isolation and removal of all outside supports except the husband. Withdrawal from the wife's excessive dependency and demands for attention, conversation, and affection was particularly marked in the husbands (who were noted for communication in monosyllabic grunts), thus supporting a downward spiral in the wife. The authors suggest that the female/male preponderance of persons suffering from depression (2 to 2.5:1) may reflect not only the social isolation of the wife but also the fact that in society it is more acceptable for females to express affective disorders; that alcoholism may be the male equivalent of depression in our culture.

The extreme dependency of the depressed person, which parallels the dependency of the alcoholic, was noted in an early study of 12 manic-depressive persons.[8] This study also described a common pattern in the families of origin of the patient. Those families felt singled out or "different" (e.g., by minority status or social status change) and selected one child, destined to be the depressed patient, as the chief carrier of the burden of raising the family's prestige and image. This child's value was measured by good grades and other achievements; he or she was the instrument of the family and was not valued as a person in his own right; self-esteem was low and dependent on achievement. The mother in these 12 families tended to be the more determined parent; the father tended to be the weak one, and was blamed by the mother for family failure. The father, however, was the warm, lovable one, and blamed the mother for cold contemptuousness. (How many of the 12 families displayed this pattern is not mentioned, nor was there any attempt at a study of controls.)

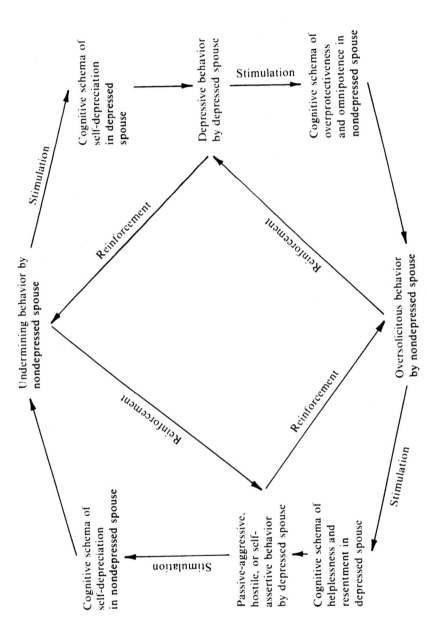

Figure 24-1. Patterns of Reciprocal Stimulation and Reinforcement in Depression.

Source: Feldman, I.B: Depression and marital interaction. *Fam Process* 14:389, 1976.

Hinchcliffe, in contrast, did a careful, controlled study of depressed couples to test his hypothesis that it was the interaction specific to the couples that stimulated and maintained a depression in the spouse who was depression prone.[14] Twenty couples with a hospitalized, depressed member were compared with 20 couples with a member hospitalized for minor surgery. The depressed patient's behavior with the marital partner was also compared with his or her behavior with a stranger of the opposite sex. A final comparison was made between the couple during hospitalization and the couple after recovery. For each of these comparisons the index patient or control, with spouse or stranger, were videotaped alone in a room. Each couple was asked to discuss differences of opinion revealed by a questionnaire given to them individually. Their 20-minute interaction was divided into communicative acts (28,000 in all!) and each was coded as to expressiveness, responsiveness, disruption, and locus of power.

Results confirmed the hypothesis that a depressive mode of communication specific to the couple distinguished these couples from the control group; the depressed member did *not* display this mode with a stranger of the opposite sex. This mode consisted of verbal or more often nonverbal expression of hostility, and orderly, formal style of "turn-taking"; high levels of tension produced negative emotional outbursts, and personalization of issues which were dealt with more objectively by the controls. This mode disappeared in the male patients on recovery but did not in the female patients. The authors suggest that the role shift to dependent, depressed partner was easier to reverse in the men, whose normal role was instrumental (work-related) rather than affective or emotional. In contrast, control couples and the patient interacting with a stranger were relaxed and mutually supportive with conciliatory techniques of agreement, laughter, and joking when their arguments became too difficult.

Eye contact was high in the depressed couple during hospitalization—as high as for the controls. It was on recovery that it dropped to much lower levels, perhaps indicating the poorer intimacy level of these marriages. The results are reminiscent of studies of alcoholic couples whose behavior becomes more stereotyped but also shows much more contact with each other during alcohol consumption than in the dry periods[23]; perhaps depression, like alcohol, serves as a symptom complex around which greater contact can be made. Physical contact was unfortunately not assessed in the study by Hinchcliffe. Hinchcliffe summarizes the process of depression in couples with the following description:

> Two individuals who maintain distance between themselves and do not allow a reciprocally intimate relationship to develop create long-term problems. The resulting insecurities, misunderstandings and jealousies generate endless incomprehensible mutual rejections which become a stereotyped pattern of need and hostile rejection. This pathological system leads very frequently, we suggest, to the ultimate disturbance of depression.[14]

Past experience (e.g., early parental loss), low self-esteem, and hence low capacity to cope with conflict and threatened withdrawal of spouse affection result in a vulnerable state. Denial of conflict and negative emotions become a mutually defensive maneuver. Intense stimulation of feelings of inadequacy in one spouse through job loss (or promotion with an attendant loss of old support systems), illness, retirement, or the departure of children trigger the depression. The partner's response is ambivalent, with a pattern of care, concern, rejection, and hostility followed by a sense of despair and guilt.

If the response of the partner of the depressed person is ineffectual in altering the depression the feeling of hopelessness increases and leads to the "depressive premise": that this is an illness state rather than an interactional problem. This premise prompts a move towards the health profession with further stabilizing of a sick role. Sometimes dependence on the health professional or dependence on medication or hospitalization produces temporary relief of the excessive dependency on the spouse; this may decrease spouse rejection and help re-establish the old relationship. On the other hand, if the sick role totally eclipses the old marital role, permanent patient status with hospitalization or dependency on the physician may result.

Management of Depression

As in other individual manifestations of a disturbed system, the depressed person may be the target of therapy and the system will in turn be altered. The danger, however, lies in the possibility of a permanent label or sick role for that individual and in removing the responsibility for change from family to health professional. The possibility of change becomes remote once the conflict at the relationship level is relabelled as a problem within a particular spouse who may willingly accept all the blame. The longer the sick role remains the more the system will stabilize around it, and once a health professional is consulted the need to wrestle with interpersonal problems is replaced by giving the clinician the responsibility for cure.

Anti-depressant medications are an important part of therapy, but must be used with recognition of their impact on the system and on the sick role. They can be described to the patient as symptom relief, like aspirin for a headache, while work is proceeding to get at the cause within the relationship and the depressed person's life history. For many it is helpful to give a biomedical explanation that neural hormones are altered by stressors in the environment and in turn may add to the depression; these neurohumoral changes can be reversed by anti-depressants. Origins of the depression can relate to early childhood experiences that may be better dealt with in individual therapy, but their ongoing maintenance in a marital or family system must be understood to produce lasting relief.

The complexity and interplay of individual and system components is illustrated in the case of a recurrent depression in a man whose wife alternated with him in visiting the physician with complaints of myalgias and back pain. This case (Mr. and Mrs. S., presented in Chapter 19) was followed by the author for a period of 8 years. The personality of the patient, the dynamics in the family of origin, several feedback loops with the spouse in the current family, the stage in the family life cycle, and the stage in the individual patient's life cycle were all interrelated and contributing factors.

These factors contributing to the depression can be grouped by system level:

1. *Individual*

    Meaning of illness: glaucoma and later one episode of chest pain suggesting angina made the patient aware of his age, and impending retirement reminded the patient of his thwarted desire to be a machinist and repressed anger at his father.

    Family of origin: as in the families described by Cohen,[8] the patient's role was special compared to that of his brother, and involved keeping the peace and maintaining cheerfulness and presenting a good image for the neighbors. Normal mood swings became unacceptable and were denied.

    Death of both parents and a brother occurred shortly before the onset of depression. Mourning particularly for the father was incomplete because of repressed anger.

2. *Marital*

    Underlying depression of the patient's wife caused by delayed mourning for her father and repression of the memory of two fraternal suicides was defended against by assuming the nursing role for his depression. The wife helped to trigger depression by increasing the pressure on him to perform in house and community.

    Role assignment problems were solved by her physical symptoms and by his depression rather than through open negotiation.

    Conflict avoidance in the couple resulted in anger converted to depression and physical symptoms.

3. *Family and Stage of Life Cycle*

    The empty nest threw the couple together, with their problems, particularly because of Mr. S.'s retirement.

    The departure of the couple's daughter to New Zealand may have reminded them of past losses, especially Mrs. S.'s father and brother, but also Mr. S.'s parents and brother.

    Mr. S.'s need to hide depression from his son and daugher and the genetic fears, expressed by the daughter to the physician, repeated the old need to keep up appearances.

4. *Work and Community*

    Early retirement precipitated by depression deprived Mr. S. of congenial colleagues and forced him into his wife's company. Achievement oriented, he no longer had a sense of purpose.

Community demands resulting from Mr. S.'s sociable and agreeable nature became excessive and avoidable only through depression.

SUICIDE

In any clinician's practice, actual suicide is a rare event but concern about suicidal thoughts or threats in the depressed is very familiar. Suicide is an act determined by numerous factors; family tensions and patterns of interaction are prominent. In a study by Richman,[22] family conflicts and arguments were a major precipitant of suicide in 94% of patients under 40 years old, and in 70% over 40 years old. Loss was a factor in 28% under 40 years old; in 60% over 40 years old; illness in 30% under 40 years old; and in 55% over 40 years old; and work problems in 34% under 40 years old and in 10% over 40 years old. As Richman points out, however, too few practitioners are skilled in both the management of suicidal patients and a family approach to the problem. The family physician or nurse should clearly refer patients who are assessed as a definite suicidal risk. However, the clinician may have an important preventive role if able to recognize and help redirect family patterns that are destructive and capable of causing suicides.

Richman believes these patterns are based on intense symbiotic ties and inordinate fears of separation and change. Suicide is a psychosocial event in which the self-destructive act may be needed by the family to maintain a specific pattern of relationships; the family must therefore be regarded as the patient. Family crisis intervention is the treatment of choice when a person is actually suicidal. Such intervention is combined with individual interviews in which the suicidal person is assessed for decompensating defenses, feelings of despair, problems in impulse control, tendency for dissociation and psychotic features (many patients were found to be prone to psychosis or borderline), organic signs, and specific suicidal ideation.

As Richman points out, "The treatment of the patient who has attempted suicide and his family is not for (psychiatric) residents or trainees." Neither is the treatment therefore for family physicians or nurses. However, as in other areas of working with families, understanding of the family interaction around suicide allows preventive maneuvers and anticipatory guidance to be focused on families at higher risk (an enmeshed family facing the departure of the children), facilitate family interaction in a less destructive manner, and facilitate referral to an appropriate therapist. If the family already trusts the clinician a major and very difficult first step has been achieved, since such families generally forbid close relationships with anyone outside the family. This relationship will be a necessary tool in sufficiently opening the closed family boundary and family secretiveness to allow in another outsider. Conversely, once it does occur the dependence on a therapist makes that person prone to suicide threats or acts if he or she cannot sustain such a dependence. Self-awareness, the understanding of the countertransference, is necessary to a degree not usual in the untrained clinician.

The family is threatened by the suicidal person's dependence on outsiders. Improvement in the patient may cause less dependence on and confiding in the family, which may in turn provoke *increased* hostility and suicidogenic behavior by the family. Incredibly, such families often overtly or covertly suggest suicide to the patient. In one family known to the author, a young woman previously extruded by her family went home after her husband's death. As her depression deepened, family empathy was not forthcoming. (Richman comments that empathy implies a knowledge of separateness and differentness that does not occur in these symbiotic families). She became increasingly dependent on a therapist. With beginning efforts at differentiation from her family of origin the mother in particular became more punitive. Finally the patient picked up a large handful of pills and swallowed them while the mother sat calmly watching.

Paradoxically, suicide, like a family "cut-off" or like extrusion of a member to a mental hospital or institution, seals off the family pain so that it can be denied. Like a repressed memory or a skeleton in the closet, such an event will become a "toxic issue" for subsequent generations. Not all families of suicidal patients are malevolently inclined. Richman also describes "benevolent families" whose members feel hopeless and helpless, who are accepting of help and respond to help, and who can be relieved of their anxieties after a relatively brief intervention. Fewer of these families require hospitalization of their depressed members.

Prevention lies not only with the family therapist but, earlier, with the family clinician. Visits to the office may be used to encourage individuation attempts of growing children; awareness of family enmeshment can prompt the occasional home visit (usually on the basis of a physical illness) during which family communication can be observed and facilitated. Symptoms of disturbed homeostasis as developing adolescents threaten the enmeshment will usually occur well before suicide or severe depression and can alert the clinician to the need for a family session. His role then is to remove the "barriers to process," or blocks to communication, and "to rely on the healing forces of the family itself."[22] Giving permission for the airing of grievances and angry feelings leads eventually to the sharing of positive feelings. If more than one or two such sessions are needed, referral for family therapy may be necessary. The role of a trusted outsider as an influence on family process over time should not be underestimated. Research to evaluate whether the anecdotal impression that facilitation of communication has prophylactic value is not yet available and will be difficult. As in other areas of working with families in primary care, such research is a crucial next step.

REFERENCES

1. Akiskal H, McKinney WJ Jr: Overview of recent research in depression. *Arch Gen Psychiatry* 33:285, 1975.

2. Bateson G, Jackson D, Haley J, Weakland J: Toward a theory of schizophrenia. *Behav Sci* 1:241, 1956.

3. Bateson G, Jackson D, Haley J, Weakland J: A note on the double bind. *Fam Proc* 2:54, 1963.

4. Berger RM: The marital system of the hysterical individual. *Fam Process* 85, 1975.

5. Bowen M: *Family Therapy in Clinical Practice.* New York, Jason Aronson, 1978.

6. Brown GW, Birley JLT, Wing JK: Influence of family life on the course of schizophrenic disorders: A replication. *Br J Psychiatry* 121:241, 1972.

7. Brown GW, Bhrolchain MN, Harris T: Social class and psychiatric disturbance among women in an urban population. *Soc* 9:225, 1975.

8. Cohen MB, Baker G, Cohen RA, et al: An intensive study of 12 cases of manic depressive psychosis. *Psychiatry* 17:103, 1954.

9. Coppen A: The biochemistry of affective disorders. *Br J Psychiatry* 113:1237, 1967.

10. Ellis A, Harper RA: *A New Guide to Rational Living.* California, Wilshire Books, 1978.

11. Feldman, LB: Depression and marital interaction. *Fam Process* 14:389, 1976.

12. Freud S: Mourning and melancholia, in *Collected Papers.* New York, Basic Books, 1959.

13. Geshwinn E, Dunner D, Goodwin F: Towards a biology of affective disorders: Genetic distributions. *Arch Gen Psychiatry* 25:1, 1971.

14. Hinchcliffe MK, Hooper: *The Melancholy Marriage and Psychosocial Approaches to Therapy.* New York, John Wiley, 1978.

15. Katerndahl DA: Nonpsychiatric disorders associated with depression. *J Fam Pract* 13:619, 1981.

16. Lacqueur HP: Multiple family therapy, in Guerin PJ Jr (ed): *Therapy— Theory and Practice.* New York, 1976.

17. Laing RD: *Sanity, Madness and the Family.* New York, Basic Books, 1976.

18. Liberman RP, Raskin DE: Depression: A behavioral formulation. *Arch Gen Psychiatry* 24:515, 1971.

19. Madanes C: Marital therapy when a symptom is presented by a spouse. *Int J Fam Therapy* 2:120–136, 1980.

20. Napier A, Whitaker C: *The Family Crucible.* New York, Harper & Row, 1978.

21. Paykel E, Myers J, Drenelt M, et al: Life events and depression. *Arch Gen Psychiatry* 21:753, 1970.

22. Richman J: The family therapy of attempted suicide. *Fam Process* 18:139, 1979.

23. Steinglass P, Davis DL, Berenson D: Observations of conjointly hospitalized 'alcoholic couples' during sobriety and intoxication: Implications for therapy. *Fam Process* 16:1, 1977.

Chapter 25

Psychological Problems in Adults: Violence in the Family

Gilles Paradis

SCOPE OF THE PROBLEM

Violence in the family has only recently become an issue for the public and the social and health professionals. To the concepts of child abuse and wife battering one must now add husband abuse, violence between siblings, and parental and elderly abuse. Early research in this field concentrated on easy targets. The "beater-psychopath" was first identified and then the "masochistic-wife."[7,16] Both these concepts gave a very incomplete and inaccurate portrait of the actual problem.

A systems approach is needed for considering this phenomenon. It is not just the person who does the actual beating that must be considered but the entire family system. The father, the mother, the children, and the environment all play a role. No system (family or other) exists in a vacuum. An understanding of the different components of the family system and its interlocking relationship with the wider systems of community and society at large is mandatory for effective intervention to treat and prevent abuse in the family.

Violence is as old as the family. References to child abuse are found from ancient Greek mythology to the Old Testament. "Spare the rod and spoil the child" goes the dictum. Indeed, in the Roman Empire the child was the father's property, and he could do whatever he wanted with him or her. Destruction of children considered undesirable because they were female or defective was approved in ancient Greece. For many centuries women were not believed to have a soul, and in colonial times men were allowed to beat their wives as long as the stick was not wider than their thumbs.

The first legal interference on behalf of an abused child in the United States was in 1874, when the American Society for Prevention of Cruelty to Animals intervened for a 9-year-old girl found chained to her bed in New York City.[11] The child, who had been malnourished and was regularly beaten, was given legal protection on the grounds that she belonged to the animal kingdom.

The problem of family violence is not limited to the western hemisphere; family violence exists irrespective of culture or race; it is prevalent in Africa and Asia as well as in Europe and the Americas. In fact, people are more likely to be beaten or killed in their homes by a family member than anywhere else and by anyone else.

Even though data on family violence is becoming more reliable, the true dimensions of the problem are still unknown. The cases reported in incidence studies may represent the tip of the iceberg; they do not include cases not treated by the physician, cases not identified as being abused, or cases identified but not reported. Furthermore, the diagnostic standards and the methods of documentation vary from one center to another.

It is estimated that the incidence of child abuse in the United States is 10 per 1000 live births. Two million children are abused each year, and of these, 2000 to 5000 die. The mortality rate from child abuse until the child reaches 6 months of age is second only to the incidence of sudden infant death syndrome. In children 1 to 5 years of age, mortality from violence is second to death from true accidents.[11] Violence is not limited to children only; some studies have shown that even college students are physically injured by their parents. Overall, three out of five households with children are the scene of child abuse.[15]

Three quarters of abusive acts are done by biological parents. When the father is present in the family system (the father is absent in 30% of cases), he seems to be using violence slightly more than the mother. But it is the mother who is more prone to use severe violence against children. Abusing parents tend to marry young, have financial difficulties, and a high rate of unemployment; they live in crowded homes, and have a high degree of geographic mobility.[4,14,15] Social isolation, income, and education are factors that have not consistently been associated with abuse.[1] The high incidence of child abuse in lower socioeconomic classes may also be a reflection of underreporting of cases in higher socioeconomic classes.

Mrs. L. was a 24-year-old single mother, born in northern Ontario but who had moved to Quebec in the last 5 years. She had no family here, and her closest relatives lived some 300 miles away. Her second baby had been delivered 4 months previously. He had been given away to her mother in Ontario soon after birth. Her first child (from a previous relationship) was being taken care of by her current boyfriend's mother.

Both she and her boyfriend were illiterate, unemployed, and on welfare. They rarely lived for more than 4 to 6 months at the same home because they did not pay the rent and left before being evicted. At the time they lived in a rural area 40 to 60 miles north of Montreal. Since the only time they could come to the hospital was when the boyfriend could borrow a friend's car, Mrs. L. was irregularly followed throughout pregnancy. She had not been seen since her discharge from the maternity ward. Their current house had no phone and no electricity.

They appeared without an appointment at the end of a Friday evening clinic. The boyfriend's mother had been sick and her first child, now 3 years old, had been with them for 2 weeks. The presenting problem was that she felt nervous and desired "nerve pills." On questioning, it became apparent that the cause of this nervousness was her child and she had hit him and thrown him on the ground on several occasions when he wasn't quiet.

The child had only minor bruises but the mother stated that she did not know if she was going to be able to control herself during the weekend as her boyfriend was leaving the next day for a week's work as a laborer.

After careful explanations to the mother, she readily accepted hospitalization for the child for a few days, and that a social worker would get in contact with her to arrange visits for the child.

Marital violence is as pervasive. In the course of their marriage, 28% of couples will engage in violence and in any given year one out of six couples will use violence against each other. Some studies have shown that approximately the same percentage of men and women are victims of violent acts. It should not be forgotten though that these studies do not tell us what the percentage is of violent acts done by the wife in response to her husband's violence. Men are stronger and perpetrate more dangerous and injurious forms of violence, and they tend to repeat their violent behavior more often than women.[15]

These data have not led to the establishment of widespread programs of detection and treatment for cases of abuse. This is due in part to the lack of validated and reliable diagnostic instruments and to ongoing litigation between advocates of parents' rights to privacy and proponents of "children's rights,"[10] an example of the intense involvement and the strong but ambivalent feelings of the community system to violence in the family. Gelles has identified six subsystems within the community that are all involved in identifying, labeling, treating and preventing abuse[4]: the medical system, the social service system, the criminal justice system, the neighborhood and friends system, and the family system. These systems are not just simple reactors to social problems; they play a major and active role in producing the problem and in defining its scope and its nature. These definitions in turn determine which cases are found or missed. Our current knowledge about child abuse is affected directly by the processes and interactions both within each system and between each other.

CHILD ABUSE

Physical punishment is used by 84% to 97% of all parents at some time in their child's life.[15] It is nearly impossible to draw a clear line between discipline and abuse since our society is committed to the belief that children are the parents' property and that physical punishment is a legitimate form of child rearing. Child abuse, outside the immediate threat of physical injury, has enduring societal consequences. It establishes the moral justification to hit other people, whether they are family members or not. The pattern of interaction between persons it promotes is that violence is permissible and can even be an end in itself.

The concept of the "battered child syndrome" introduced in 1962 by Kempe[9] was the starting point for a decade of research and rising public interest culminating in public policies designed to protect children from abuse. Early research, quite understandably, focused on the violent individual and looked for something wrong with him or her; someone who would beat a child had to be sick. Hence the linear models were developed. As our comprehension of the phenomenon improved it was understood that abuse and violence were a problem of the family system and that irrespective of who did the actual beating, all members were actively involved in the dysfunction of the system.

Linear Model

It has become common to describe the abusing parent as a psychopath. Research has portrayed him or her as impulsive, immature, depressed, sadomasochistic, dependent, narcissistic, insecure, with poor emotional control, and self-centered. This mental defect model is but one of many linear models that were suggested to explain the behavior of the abuser. Other models include the environmental stress model, which emphasizes the outside factors with which a family has to deal. Social position, geographic mobility, and unemployment are examples of such stresses. The social learning model points to the fact that 30% to 60% of abusers were themselves abused as children. They argue that abusers have learned their behavior by their own parental role models.

Gelles[4] has put forth a social-psychological model of child abuse. In this model, frustration and stress from marital disputes, too many children, unemployment, an unwanted or problem child (handicapped, retarded, etc.) are important factors for child abuse. These stresses combined with values from the community sanctioning violence and with role modelling from parents contribute to the potential for abuse. The spark necessary to the outburst of violence can be an argument or the child's misbehavior.

The common problem with these models is that they account for only a fraction of the total problem. Their discussion of the causes of abuse is therefore contradictory and inconsistent. Child abuse is not the product of some mental aberration of the individual abuser but grows out of the nature of the family and the community. From a systems view it is understandable that the child abuser would be seen as a scapegoat for blame. It prevents the system from admitting its role in the origin of the violence, which could be very threatening for a community.

The Systems Model

To fully understand child abuse the clinician must consider the dynamic interactions within the family (father, mother, child) and with the community system and the society at large. What affects one affects the others. The focus is not put on who hits the child; both parents are equally involved in the systems process. The child plays a role as well as the spouses, the environment, and the culture in the system.[5]

Poor Individuation

Justice and Justice[8] developed a "psychosocial system" model for child abuse based on Bowen's differentiation concept.[3] The abusing family's system is characterized by emotional intensity and fusion. Either the spouses are tightly bound to one another, one parent is fused with the child, or one or both parents are intensely tied to his or her family of origin. These people are poorly differentiated and have little sense of self.[3]

There is intense competition within the family over who will be taken care of by the other. When one member loses and has to care for the spouse, he or she looks to the child to act as mother in a last ditch effort to be nurtured. When the child cannot deliver sufficient emotional support, the parent's frustrations caused by unmet dependency needs are expressed in violent behavior.

The child is an easy target for the parents to express their frustration in violence. The stressful condition of helplessness and need that the child represents is the necessary precipitating event for abuse. When the child makes unusually great demands or represents exceptional stress (is illegitimate, premature, etc.) he or she is in even greater danger. As a result of parents too needy to give, members in the next generation fail to learn how to individuate and to meet their own needs. Child abuse is thus perpetuated in one generation after another.

Triangulation

Children are often caught in the middle of covert conflicts or power struggles between the parents. In triangulation a parent, rather than openly expressing his or her anger or resentment at the other spouse, transfers these feelings to a child, who is now the scapegoat. A father, for example, resenting his wife's long hours at work may reprimand his daughter for always coming in late for supper.

Another possibility is using a child to prevent separation of the spouses. A mother may subtly encourage a behavior in her child that she knows will provoke a strong reaction from a distant father and thus bring him closer to her. A child can also be put in an alliance or coalition that one spouse resents and be subject to his or her anger, which normally would be directed to the other spouse. Scapegoating or triangulation can often result in child abuse. This abuse can be physical injury, psychological abuse or deprivation, or even incest.

Incest

Incest is also a problem of the family system rather than the result of a disorder of the character of an individual member. In the commonest form, father-daughter incest, the father is aided and abetted in his liaison by conscious or unconscious seduction by his daughter and by his wife's collusion. Both spouses in this type of family are usually dependent and infantile. The father and daughter feel abandoned as the mother distances herself from the unwanted maternal role and as she sexually deserts her husband. The mother displaces her own unresolved conflicts to the daughter and unconsciously pushes her to assume the role of wife and lover with her own father. The mother's denial then freezes role relations and keeps them from changing. As a result of unresolved conflicts in his own family of origin, the father is unable to achieve a stable heterosexual orientation.

MARITAL VIOLENCE

In a survey done by the United States Violence Commission, 25% of the people questionned said they could think of circumstances when hitting the spouse was appropriate. It has been shown that people react less at seeing a man beat a woman if they think the man is her husband. It is estimated that 2 million women are victims of severe physical violence each year.

Why is the family such a violence prone setting? Gelles has identified characteristics of the family system that can help build a warm supportive climate or can be used to attack intimates and lead to conflict.[4] These are age and sex differences; the time spent with one another; the wide spectrum of possibilities in interaction; the great intensity of involvement; conflicting desires and decision-making; ascribed roles; the right to influence other members of the family; the stress related to life cycle changes on individual stress that reverberates to the other family members; and the extensive knowledge of other members' strengths, weaknesses, and fears.

Young age, low income, unemployment, exposure as a child to severe conflict, and violence in the family of origin are all strong predictors of spouse abuse. Mental illness in one of the spouses explains only a small proportion of marital violence, as is the case for child abuse. The gentle husband who loses control and becomes violent under the influence of alcohol seems to be as much as a myth as the wife who stays with him because of her masochistic need to be punished. Indeed research indicates that husbands who get drunk and start beating their wives are fully aware of what they are doing and use alcohol as an excuse for their behavior.

Strauss and colleagues[15] reported that men were at least as likely as women to be battered. Furthermore, men and women tend to use the same type of violence against each other, and as many women kill their husbands as men their wives. Women, however, are seven times more likely to murder in self-defense, and it is also true that by sheer physical strength men will cause more damage than women by using the same form of violence.

The violent act committed by the husband or the wife is an equally strong message of frustration and despair. This occurs when the system sees itself in a dead end, its known coping mechanisms exhausted or ineffectual. The conflict cannot be solved without one of the participants having the feeling that he or she loses too much. The loss can be that of power, of control, or, as discussed earlier, of who will nurture the other. When the tension gets too high, one spouse may trigger the other one to act violently. The nonviolent spouse remains in control and can convey the negative message afterwards: "I didn't lose my temper, you're a beast," etc.

> Mrs. X. was 27 years old and pregnant. She had been married less than 6 months to a man 20 years her elder. They both had a background of violence in their families of origin, and she complained to her physician that they could not communicate. At the couple interview done on the physician's insistence, it was disclosed that the pregnancy was unwanted, that the couple would fight over it and frequently came to blows. The sequence usually occurred as follows: the husband would come in late; the wife would then start asking him over and over where had he been, what had he done, etc.; he would get irritated and tell her to shut up; this would aggravate the conflict and she would attack him verbally; and then the husband would tell her that he doubted if he really was the father of the unborn child. The effect of this statement was automatic: she would slap him in the face and he would respond by hitting her back.

The problem of violence during pregnancy should not be overlooked; 25% of assaulted wives are also beaten during pregnancy. Moreover the blows that the woman then receives are often redirected from the face to the abdomen. The additional strain and stresses associated with pregnancy are possible explanatory factors for the violence. This behavior has also been described as prenatal child abuse.

Rape

It is generally assumed that rape victims are typically assaulted in dark alleys by strangers; however, Amir[2] has shown that up to 48% of rape victims know their aggressor. Of 250 rape victims studied at the Philadelphia General

Hospital,[12] 58% of the victims under 18 were assaulted by a relative or acquaintance. When the victim was a child she was likely to have been assaulted by her father (six out of thirteen victims).

PARENT ABUSE

The phenomenon of parents being physically abused by their children is becoming increasingly recognized. The assaillant most often lives with the parents and is economically dependent on them. The assaults normally occur inside the home and are not related to alcohol or drug abuse.

The child, usually going through an adolescent crisis, is involved in triangulation between the parents; he or she becomes the symptom of their covert conflicts. Often one parent will disapprove of a certain behavior, while the other subtly encourages it. Caught in a double-bind situation where he or she is bound to feel rejected whatever he or she does, he or she reacts with violence. Most cases involve a male child (rescuing the father from having to express his anger at the mother) and a female parent. Some children have even called the police themselves when their parents failed to react to their violent incidents.[17]

Elderly Abuse

The most recent area of concern in the field of violence is the elderly family member, who is being increasingly recognized as a victim of abuse, neglect, and exploitation. The most frequent types of abuse include physical assault, verbal and psychological assault, misuse of money or property or theft, forced entry into a home or a nursing home, misuse and abuse of drugs, financial dependence and exploitation, withholding basic life resources, and not providing care to the physically dependent.[13] Usually the abuser has some care-giving function, and if it is a family member the family system is involved in direct or indirect ways. Since the abused elderly rarely reports acts of aggression by those they are close to or depend on for fulfillment of their basic needs, most cases are unnoticed. The lack of prevalence and incidence data and the paucity of clinical studies make it difficult to describe adequately the phenomenon and determine the forms of family dysfunctions associated with abuse.[6]

The abusing child may have an undifferentiated self[3] and may be closely bonded with his or her parent. This could be an unconscious reason to have the elderly father or mother still living with him or her. The child may turn to the older, frail, and dependent person to be nurtured and cared for, which results in a frustrating experience for the child that can be expressed through violent behavior. The vulnerability of the elderly also identifies him or her as with the case of children as a prime target for triangulation by conflicting spouses.

A very common occurrence is the verbal abuse of baby talk. The primary care clinician's attitude is important in dealing with people who use child-like language to their elderly parents, remove their right to discuss a problem, and take away all decision-making responsibilities from them. By role modeling respect for the elderly, the health professional may help alleviate the additional burden the humiliation of baby talk and lack of responsibility puts on growing old.

Many different professionals are presented daily with cases of abuse of the elderly. Unfortunately, there exists as yet no established procedures for dealing with or following up mistreatment. Again, as in child abuse and marital violence the community system views neglect of the elderly as a somewhat inevitable and therefore "normal" phenomenon.

TREATMENT AND PREVENTION

When confronted with a case of abuse, the health professional should not be expected, under usual circumstances, to manage it alone. The problem is determined by a number of interacting variables, and it is best dealt with by a multidisciplinary approach. The characteristics of the health professional system are such that the primary care physician or nurse is more likely to see certain types of abuse more than others. Furthermore, the primary clinician's degree of involvement is limited by a variety of factors (interest, time, type of practice, type of community).

At the community level, the ways the different elements of the system interact, and each system's particular characteristics determine which type of abuse is identified, treated, and treated successfully. Services are client specific. The health professional system has nonetheless the specific responsibility of protecting an identified victim against further harm that could hinder physical or psychological well-being. This can mean hospitalization of a child, even against the parents' will. Abuse has been shown to recur in approximately 50% of cases when intervention is not instituted, and in 35% of these a child will be severely injured or killed. Referring patients to shelters, crisis nurseries, and day-care centers if available are other possible interventions. Many communities have developed emergency social services that can be contacted 24 hours a day for such cases.

Once the immediate protection of the victim has been insured, the professional has the legal obligation in most regions to report the case to the appropriate agency. Referral of both spouses either together or separately for therapy should be the next step. Family therapy, behavior modification groups, and impulse control training are some of the methods of treatment available for abusing parents or spouse. Moreover, there exists self-help groups such as Parents Anonymous to which abusing parents can turn during periods of crisis and stress.

Prevention

As part of the larger system of the community, the primary care physician or nurse can work effectively towards a reduction of violence in families. The prevention of abuse in the family by concentrating on individual families is doomed to failure. We must recognize that family, community, and society are all parts of a single system and that what affects one will affect the others. As long as cultural norms continue to promote violence as a reasonable and sensible way to deal with interpersonal relationships, efforts to reduce violence and abuse in the family system will be severely hindered. Violence on television, physical punishment in schools, and the death penalty are all parts of such cultural norms.

Other authors[4,8,15] have suggested societal measures to enhance primary prevention of abuse: reduction of the violence-provoking stresses created by the community; combating isolation by integrating families into a network of kin and community; eliminating the sex-patterned allocation of roles and tasks in the family; limiting access to weapons; and producing programs to sensitize the population to the problem of violence. It is not until this cycle of violence in family, community, and society is broken that we can expect a significant improvement to the problem of abusing families.

REFERENCES

1. Altermeier WA: Antecedents of child abuse. *J Pediatr* 100:823, 1982.
2. Amir M: Patterns of forcible rape. Chicago, University of Chicago Press, 1971.
3. Bowen M: The use of family theory in clinical practice. *Compr Psychiatry,* Oct. 7, 345, 1966.
4. Gelles RJ: Family Violence, vol. 84. Sage Library of Social Research, Beverly Hills, 1979.
5. Goodwin J: Cinderella syndrome: Children who stimulate neglect. *Am J Psychiatry.* 137:1223, 1980.
6. Hickey T, Douglass RL: Mistreatment of the elderly in the domestic setting: An exploratory study. *Am J Public Health* 71:500, 1981.
7. Hilberman E: Overview: The "wife-beater's wife" reconsidered. *Am J Psychiatry* 137:1336, 1980.
8. Justice B, Justice R: *The Abusing Family.* New York, Human Sciences Press, 1976.
9. Kempe CH, Silverman FN, Brandt FS, et al: The battered-child syndrome. *JAMA* 181:17, 1962.
10. Markham B: Child abuse intervention: Conflicts in current practice and legal theory. *Pediatrics* 65:180, 1980.
11. McNeese MC, Hebeler JR: The abused child. *Clin Symp,* 31, 1979.
12. Peters J: The Philadelphia rape victim study, in Draphin I, Viano E (eds): *Victimology: A New Focus, III.* Lexington, Lexington Books, 1975.

13. Rathbone-McCuan E, Voyles B: Case detection of abused elderly parents. *Am J Psychiatry* 139:189, 1982.

14. Solomon T: History and demography of child abuse. *Pediatrics* 51:775, 1973.

15. Strauss MA, Gelles RJ, Steinmetz SK: *Behind Closed Doors: Violence in the American Family.* New York, Anchor Press/Doubleday, 1980.

16. Symonds A: Violence against women—the myth of masochism. *Am J Psychother* 33:161, 1979.

17. Viken RM: Family violence, aids to recognition. *Postgrad Med* 71:115, 1982.

Chapter 26

Alcohol and Drug Abuse in the Family

Michael Liepman

Alcohol dependence is one of the commonest health risks in the western hemisphere.[19,32,40] Family physicians can have a crucial role in prevention or treatment of this condition when dependence is involved.[24] Alcohol abuse and dependence are a family and community disorder, as well as a disorder within a person; alcoholism adversely affects the family and community, and dependence cannot be treated without affecting or involving the family and community.[24] This chapter will prepare the clinician to understand a family dynamic model of alcohol dependence in order to aid clinical decision-making and to provide appropriate care and guidance to families suffering from this or other substance abuse. Also addressed are the more general issues of psychoactive substances in families that do not necessarily suffer from dependence.

ETIOLOGY

Although there is evidence of a genetic role in alcoholism,[15] family and social systems play an important role in developing and maintaining this disorder. In alcoholic families, the drinker's drinking serves as a permanent recurring solution, at an increasingly high cost, to unresolved family conflict and stress. It maintains some harmony, predictability, and homeostasis. Costs to individual family members include, for instance, depression and suicide attempts, psychosis, enuresis, phobias, psychosomatic illness, hysteria, sociopathy, etc. Social costs to the family may be extremely high because solutions that work in the nuclear and extended family may not necessarily be tolerated so well by the surrounding community. Removal of a child to foster care, teenage pregnancy, juvenile delinquency, financial ruin, alienation of support systems (church, friends, and extended family) all commonly occur in alcoholic families at some point in the downhill progression of the disorder. As alcoholism is known to run in families[15] one should not be surprised to see other substance abuse and dependency in members of the extended family.

The psychological damage of alcoholism in the family can be rather extensive. All members of the family are affected by the alcoholism, sometimes with overt emotional symptomology, other times more subtly. In the physiologic realm, one frequently sees psychosomatic flares of illnesses such as diabetes, rheumatoid arthritis, asthma, or peptic ulcer disease in the family members of an alcoholic. Visits to the doctor or hospitalizations may reflect ways in which family members cope with the alcoholic problem, that is, by escaping from home into hospital, by forcing a parent to sober up to visit the hospital, by attracting outside attention to the state of things at home, etc. Physiologic and anatomic damage can also occur as a result of victimization in an auto accident, domestic violence, or child neglect, all of which are common within alcoholic families or may occasionally be associated with an isolated episode of acute alcohol abuse.[27] Both the psychosomatic illnesses and the domestic violence may vary in a cyclical fashion; flares of illness or violence may be associated in time with either flares or remissions of the overdrinking behavior, depending on the family. Sometimes the adolescent (and even younger) children may begin to ingest alcohol or drugs "lying around the house" with adverse health consequences.

A family in which alcoholism plays a role will adjust itself to the oscillations between the "wet" and the "dry" states.[49] One sees a dramatic "Jekyll-Hyde" transformation in family behavior and mood, depending on whether the drinker is drinking or sober. By analogy, the family is like a group of performing square dancers who have previously agreed to a repertoire of dance steps cued by the music. The dancers have complementary roles that are beautifully choreographed to maintain family homeostasis and to minimize uncertainty. The "wet" state serves as a "solution" for certain family needs such as achieving the appearance of greater intimacy, escaping conflict, expressing emotions, or coping with stress. While initially the "wet" state may serve the family well, eventually side effects of this solution occur (family members begin to be hurt by or during the "wet" state). The "wet" state becomes a permanent part of family function that the family members cannot easily control or limit.

While individual family members all have input on whether or not the drinker drinks, no single individual determines this outcome. Vernon Johnson[20] introduced the term "enabler" to identify those persons whose behavior supports the continuance of the substance-dependent behavior. This may consist of overt support such as that offered by a drinking buddy or inadvertently may be provoked by attempts to discourage overdrinking in which one undermines one's own authority, that of another person with similar goals, or that of the drinkers. For instance, pouring the vodka down the drain may provide an angry scene followed by the father's leaving the house to get something to drink. The other family members may take sides. Liquor reserves may also be hidden in the future.

The specific mechanisms by which alcoholism is created and maintained by the family, and in turn harms the family, are complex and multi-faceted. In the emotional area, however, one discovers a rather stereotyped mechanism for feelings management. Interpersonal communication and interaction frequently produce conflicts between various family members and result in conflicting feelings.

Persons within the family who utilize a chemical substance as a means of suppressing their perception of feelings will at times become singularly unresponsive to interpersonal communications. At other times in the wet-dry cycle, the drinker may overreact. The so-called "enablers" become victims: they must either satisfy themselves alternatively with no response or an explosive one. They may "walk on eggs" or escalate the affective stages of their communications, or both. For example, the alcoholic father of 14-year-old Lisa has not resolved his disagreements with his wife about the age at which to permit her to date, so whenever it comes up in conversation, he retreats to his drinking and becomes oblivious to Lisa's anxiety over the lack of clarity of the dating policy. Her mother gives permission by proxy and conceals her dating to protect Lisa from her father's "rages" and to protect him from "stress." When he does assert his stand, he must "fortify" himself with a few drinks so he can more easily "speak his mind." However, the father's authority is discounted by the family and his statements are ignored since he was "drunk." The next day he either cannot recall the event or he is unable to defend his authority without a "few drinks." Lisa escalates matters by staying out all night. This pattern becomes another family stress and another instance in which the family may not be able to resolve conflict, hence renewing the cycle.

Ordinarily, when a family is stressed it will initially try to use internal resources as a means of coping.[48] Alcoholic families rely on various substances and other techniques of conflict avoidance that may not reduce the overall stress for the family though insulate certain family members from a personal perception of stress. To make a change, someone within the family must rebel before help from outside authorities is sought. A stressed family in disequilibrium may move from inadequate internal resources towards the family physician, community authorities, or other supports.[48] It may be that substance-dependent families are more rigid and have less effective mechanisms for using internal resources, and attract and accumulate more trouble and stress.

Identification of families with or at risk of developing alcoholism (or other substance dependencies) may be accomplished by looking among the families who are frequent users of external supports. For instance, one quarter to one half of all mental health cases involve alcoholic families.[25,34,35,38] In addition, 20% to 30% of patients in general hospitals are alcohol-related cases.[40] A large portion of criminal justice and social welfare cases also involve alcoholic families. In a clinical practice, it should be expected to find alcoholism in at least 10% of adult patients. Except in unusual populations, the clinician should be alerted by a lesser prevalence that he or she is not looking hard enough.

The distinction between alcohol abuse and alcoholism lies in the chronicity and loss of control over ingestion such that repeated harm is not avoided. The drinker under certain circumstances drinks beyond a safe level despite an awareness that trouble may ensue. During the "wet" state, the drinker may appear unconcerned about this, while other family members may become quite vocal, angrily or sadly reminding the alcoholic of "dry" state promises that are being broken or warning that harm may ensue. Sometimes during the "wet" state, family members may blame each other for provoking the onset or continuance of drinking and its consequences. From an individual orientation, it might be posited that the loss of control over drinking is an individual-centered phenomenon over which the family has no control. However, from a systems perspective a state of unresolved conflict demands a solution, for which the drinking and family "wet" behavior has been used in the past. In this instance, the individual drinker is merely playing a role for the mutual benefit of the entire family. (Paradoxically, the drinker may be chastised by the health professional who understands the system for kind acts of self-sacrifice that "solve" the family problems or at least avoid "rocking the boat" but that may lead to serious illness if continued).

Clinical Course

The clinical course of alcoholism is insidiously progressive, chronic, and relapsing. Usually, many years of heavy intake, leading to many years of harmful consequences, occur before attempts at recovery begin. The gradual worsening of symptoms is often misinterpreted by the alcoholic and the "enablers" as external and unrelated to the drinking or drug use. Alcohol is seen as an aid to coping with the "hard knocks" life seems to be dealing them. Eventually, the alcoholic may make amateur attempts at quitting or cutting down the ingestion, often at the urging of a doctor, friend, or relative. But the so-called "will-power quit" has only a 5% to 10% chance of permanent elimination of the harmful drinking pattern.[54]

Eventually the family may request help from a community resource or the family's problems may come to the attention of a community authority. This may lead the family to ineffective treatments, unless the agency recognizes alcoholism and then provides or demands high-quality alcoholism treatment as part of the help they offer. Following quality treatment, the recovery rate may be as high as 75% to 85%.[53]

Brief relapses are quite common as a part of the recovery process, in some instances playing a therapeutic role of identifying family "enabling" and other resistances to treatment. Alcoholism is a disorder that leads to progressive loss of valuable resources as the drinking and enabling continues. The family becomes progressively more compromised by its behavioral adjustment to drinking and wet/dry cycling. This process is insidious because the loss of resources and increased dysfunction may occur in almost imperceptible increments. Initially, the family may not be able to distinguish itself from any other family. As the family becomes more involved, it may replace parts of its support group with other alcoholic families. It may also isolate itself from the community out of embarrassment and fear of stigmatization. Children often refrain from bringing home their classmates or friends.

As the family problems become more severe, individuals within the family may practice denial, rationalization, and wishful thinking in an attempt to normalize their attitude about their family. They may even angrily fend off outsiders who question the family health. Some families convince themselves that the drinking is "not a problem." Hence, the alcoholism becomes a family secret that is never discussed openly. In other families, the alcoholism or drinking problem is a central theme of lively, but never resolved, family conflict. Eventually, if recovery does not occur, the family may disintegrate through death, suicide, divorce, institutionalization, or the exit of children from the home (through foster care, running away, juvenile delinquency, teen pregnancy, and military school).

RECOGNITION AND DIAGNOSIS

The family physician or nurse, with an interest in community and health, has the responsibility to recognize health risks as they are developing in their patients and the community. Alcohol dependence is a chronic, progressive, and insidious disorder that may enormously damage the host and his or her family and community if not corrected. The clinician should be aware of the prevalence of this disorder in the community in order to institute appropriate measures. Methods of screening or early recognition provide tools for identifying hosts of the dependencies early in the clinical course of their disorder, providing an opportunity for early intervention. In addition, the physician is often faced with patients (or families) at high risk of developing or who are concerned that they might develop dependence. The family physician must be prepared to respond to these situations in an educational and constructive manner.

EPIDEMIOLOGY

There has been much speculation about the prevalence of substance dependencies in the general population without much evidence.[32,40] Reasons for this are in part related to the difficulty of obtaining social survey data on a stigmatized condition and failure to recognize this disorder in health care settings. Cahalan and colleagues[10] did an extensive survey of the population in the United States that resulted in knowledge about factors that influence prevalence of increased alcohol consumption such as ethnicity, religion, religiousity, family income, gender, age, urbanicity, region, etc. They only reported frequency and quantity of consumption of alcohol, and did not address individual factors in alcoholism.

Prevalence in Medical Settings

Several studies of medical settings have revealed a surprisingly high prevalence of alcoholism and related illness and injury.[32,40] Markedly increased prevalence of alcohol-related cases in the medical setting is expected because of the excess morbidity and mortality that has been well documented in heavy drinkers.[37,43] The same has been shown for tobacco smokers. There is less evidence for users and abusers of a variety of other drugs. While estimates indicating that 5% to 10% of the population in the United States suffers from alcoholism, and another 5% to 10% have problems with drinking are weakly supported, there is good evidence that 20% to 30% of all hospital admissions are alcohol-related.[46,52] In Veterans Administration hospitals in the United States, roughly 55% of patients are admitted for problems related to alcoholism. In the Providence Veterans Administration hospital, Johnston and Lex[21] found that alcoholics comprised 47% of consecutive admissions. Just before hospitalization only a minority were in total or partial remission.

Another study of men in Scotland[44] showed that 26% of admissions and 52% of those patients aged 21 to 40 years had an "alcohol problem." Likewise, Funkhouser[14] reports that 55% of elderly hospitalized patients present with alcoholism. However, despite the apparent high prevalence of alcohol problems in hospital patients, when examined with the alcoholism screening instruments of experts alcoholism appears to be rare when hospital records are examined.[13,25] Patient and physician denial conspire to minimize the prevalence of recognized alcohol problems. In addition, even when clinicians recognize a case, they may conceal the diagnosis from the medical record, allegedly to "protect" the patient from stigma. When the diagnosis of alcoholism is in the medical record, physician ignorance about resources and pessimism about recovery seem to deny treatment of alcoholism.[7,25] Only a fraction of cases are detected or addressed by most physicians.[25,34,35,38] Alcoholism seems to be more easily recognized as it progresses to its end-stage; however, the prognosis and reversibility of damages are severely reduced.[25] Furthermore, clinician expectations may block perceptions of women and young people as having alcoholism.[25]

Frequent Clinical Attenders

There is a tendency for persons with chemical dependence and their immediate family members to use the health-care system more often than others in their age cohorts. They sometimes use the system just to obtain drugs from the doctor, but usually seek care for the excess morbidity that is the heritage of substance-dependent families.[32,40] A wide variety of illnesses and problems are known to be associated with excessive alcohol intake: gastrointestinal (especially hepatic), musculoskeletal, cardiovascular, cutaneous, metabolic, respiratory, genitourinary, and behavioral or psychological. Numerous health problems are associated with other drug abuse problems as well, such as the dirty needle complications of intravenous drug abusers (e.g., hepatitis, arterial emboli, phlebitis, pulmonary foreign bodies), those problems arising from uncertainty about the identity of the street drug ingested (causing "bad trips," accidental overdosage, drug-drug interactions) or complications of prescription or over-the-counter drugs (causing insomnia, mood disturbances, withdrawal syndromes). In addition, there are a variety of psychosocial concerns that arise in families with substance dependency, such as worry about whether the user will get caught or be medically harmed, whether the user will harm someone else, whether the family is being financially drained by the habit, etc.

One way to utilize this information is as a clue about who among one's practice is from a substance-dependent family. Like a game of hide-and-seek, the clinician has the responsibility to find those patients who are concealing problems related to substance ingestion in themselves or in close family members. In all cases, the clinician should maintain a relatively high index of suspicion just because dependencies are so common.

CLINICAL CUES

When the clinician is perplexed by:

1. clinical entities that do not make sense,
2. multiple illnesses that all could be tied together by a chemical toxicity or dependence problem,
3. failure of an illness to respond to the usual correct treatments for that diagnosis,
4. social or family problems, stresses or crises, or
5. repeated unexplained office visits or cancellations,

he or she benefits from looking harder for a substance dependency in the family. The clinician must be cautious about avoiding the all too common pitfalls of stereotyping patients. This practice leads to premature exclusion of a diagnosis without data to back it up (for example, the statements that "she is too young," or "he still works," or "they are too successful to be suffering from chemical dependence"). This is reinforced by most medical training, especially clinical experiences in hospitals where "private" patients are "protected" from being labelled alcoholic or addict more than the indigent patients, and where patients must be hospitalized many times with substantial loss of resources before a diagnosis of alcohol or drug dependence will be made.[25] In some cases, the dependence was known, but clinician therapeutic nihilism or ignorance led to no referral[7] or to an unsuccessful one. The use of stereotypes for early recognition is hopelessly inadequate, undermines family efforts to get help, and may contribute to serious diagnostic and treatment delays, which increase risk of family resource loss and morbidity.

Family members of a person with substance dependence visit a clinician frequently for vague complaints that may be indirectly related to alcoholism or drug abuse (for example, insomnia in spouse due to worry while waiting for husband to come home late at night; excessive bruising due to domestic violence; genital concerns related to marital and sexual problems in the alcoholic marriage). This person may be called the "emissary" from the sick family[24] who comes in hoping the clinician will do something to help the family. Often the emissary is a child who misbehaves or has psychosomatic complaints ("hyperactivity," stomach aches, drug experimentation, falling grades). If the child has a chronic illness or disability (hemophilia, diabetes, allergies, asthma, mental retardation, etc.), the case is often particularly difficult to manage. In other cases, the child is labelled "accident-prone" or "incorrigible" but is actually suffering physical, sexual, or emotional abuse. Sometimes the emissary comes to physician attention through law enforcement or other community agents of social control. Often the family, school, or employer sends the drinker or drug abuser or emissary to the doctor for a "check up" with a medical excuse, hoping that this will uncover the dependence and lead to treatment. The police sometimes bring intoxicated "emissaries" to the emergency clinic. However, the patient usually does not know the true purpose of the visit or denies it; hence the clinician usually has to take the initiative and discover the ingestion problem.

SCREENING TECHNIQUES

There are screening approaches, aside from taking a complete history, which may be used to identify the patient with a substance dependency in self or significant others. Waiting room health screening questionnaires often include some questions about alcohol, drug, and tobacco use (rather than problems) that may alert the clinician. There are more elaborate questionnaires that concentrate on drinking information, such as the Michigan Alcoholism Screening Test (MAST)[45] or the SAAST[50] and others.[18] One may also screen briefly with the use of simple mnemonics, such as John Ewing's[33] CAGE:

C: Have you ever *C*ut down on your drinking?
A: Are you ever *A*nnoyed by complaints from people around you?
G: Do you ever feel *G*uilty about your drinking?
E: Do you ever drink in the morning as an *E*ye-opener?

Two laboratory tests may prove very useful in identifying alcoholics. Elevated serum glutamic-oxaloacetic transaminase (SGOT) or mean red corpuscular volume (MCV), or both suggest alcoholism; these tests have 85% accuracy in hospitalized patients.[13] For ambulatory populations, serum gamma-glutamyl transpeptidase (SGGT) may be a more sensitive measure of alcoholism, although it has not gained wide acceptance in the United States because of its lower specificity, especially as used in tertiary care research centers.

THE ALCOHOL/DRUG HISTORY

In taking a thorough alcohol/drug history from a patient, one must first consider the impact of probing into personal habits, family problems, or lifestyle. To do this without generating shame or hostility, the clinician must maintain a nonjudgmental stance. This requires care and attention paid to choice of words, timing, facial expressions, gestures, and personal reactions. The patient may wonder why the area is being explored. A statement of relevance at the onset may be helpful. For example, the clinician might say, "As part of my routine questioning, I like to make myself aware of the various habits and aspects of lifestyle that may affect a patient's health, as well as the drugs I prescribe and the illnesses that I treat. Perhaps we could begin by looking at your consumption of beverages containing caffeine." It is crucial that the clinician put the patient at ease during this inquiry to receive reliable information. Patients generally want to please their doctors and are afraid that the physician may not understand, endorse, accept, or even comprehend. Furthermore, if there is substance abuse or dependence, the person may suffer from shame and strong denial. In such a case, the patient would not be able to tell the doctor accurately what is happening.

The family emissary may have similar feelings of shame and guilt and may deny to himself or herself that substance ingestion is a family problem. Therefore, it is important to extend the same gentle courtesy of a nonjudgmental approach to the emissary that is offered to the dependent patient. The clinician must try initially to avoid alerting the patient that the outcome of the diagnostic evaluation will be the confrontation of the problem, until he or she has had the opportunity to obtain as much data as possible.

A good sign of patient fibbing is inconsistency. As one asks questions about this stigmatized area, watch for inconsistencies of data. For example, after asking for a typical intake of alcohol, the clinician may ask for the most the person ever drank in one episode. Then he or she can assess maximum dosage with the report of neurologic competence after the episode (pharmacologic tolerance). The clinician may also ask for the minimum dose it takes to have any effect. If this turns out to be more than the typical intake dose mentioned earlier, this indicates inconsistency, since most drinkers do not drink if they will not get an effect.

The clinician might also worry about the veracity of the history if the patient responds with defensive remarks, hostility, vagueness, or attempts to change the subject. The patient is telling you that he or she is uncomfortable with the area being explored. A good approach avoids patient discomfort but obtains factual information.

There are nine major areas of potential inquiry within an alcohol/drug history. These can be handily recalled by using the mnemonic formed from the letters of the word CHEMICALS.[26]

C: Consequences or Complications
H: Help sought
E: Effects on others/Enablers/Environment/Ecology
M: Maximum dose ever/Minimum dose to have an effect
I: Intake
C: Concern over one's own use
A: Abstinence
L: Loss if quit/Loss of control/Loss of memory
S: Synergism

Each of these areas will be discussed. The order is mnemonic rather than to suggest the best sequence for asking the questions. Optimally, the flow of the interview will suggest this.

Intake

Intake information is often the first logical step in taking a patient's alcohol/drug history because it helps orient the clinician to patient use. In routine preventive health interviews, the clinician might begin with the less stigmatized drugs like caffeine and tobacco. When drug intake seems relevant, the clinician would more likely begin with intake information: Which drugs have ever been used and which are currently used? What frequency of use of each drug and all drugs combined is characteristic for this patient? How does the frequency and dosage vary? What are the routes of administration? What are the sources of drugs? What is known about their identity and purity? What are the contexts of drug ingestion?

In taking a drinking history, the clinician might be able to estimate blood levels to correlate with breath sample data from police or medical settings. A typical drink is roughly equivalent in alcohol content if taken at the usual doses: a 12 oz can of beer at 5% alcohol has 0.6 oz (18 cc) of pure ethanol; a 4 oz goblet of 12% wine has 0.5 oz (14 cc); a 1.5 oz shot of 50% (or 46% or 40%) liquor contains 0.75 (or 0.69 or 0.6) oz. A dose of 1 cc/pound of lean body weight usually is sufficient to bring blood levels to 150 mg/100 cc. Hence, a 120-pound woman who drank a liter of wine (120 cc of ethanol) on an empty stomach could be expected to reach blood levels of the order of 150 mg/100 cc. within 90 minutes. Food and liquid diluents (mixers) slow absorption, which decreases effect. The perception of effects is related less to the blood level than to its rate of change. This is why most people think that the peak effect occurs within 5 minutes after ingestion. They are perceiving the initial rapid absorption of small amounts through the gastric mucosa, which by-passes the liver.

The clinician might get inaccurate information about the frequency and dosage, and even possibly an incomplete listing of the drugs used. But one will begin to communicate acceptance to the patient, which will engender trust in the relationship, and make future information more likely to be accurate and complete. The clinician must always exert skepticism about all information that is obtained while taking a patient's history. In cases of inconsistencies, the clinician might either confront disparities at this time, or wait further in the history.

In cases of multiple-drug intake, it may be easiest to combine inquiry about various drugs by categories of pharmacologic action: sedative-hypnotic, including alcohol; stimulants, both strong and weak; opioids; hallucinogens, including cannabis; major tranquilizers (anti-psychotic neuroleptics); antidepressants; solvents; and tobacco. Patients generally stick to one or two classes of drugs for intake, but may experiment with many classes. However, there are some persons whose use seem indiscriminate: children, prisoners, the poor, and certain borderline personalities are more likely to use whatever is accessible. When a polydrug abuser has an extensive intake history with variable intake patterns, history may be truncated in the interest of time.

The goals of this section of the history are to get oriented and to assess how much further the history should be pursued. The clinician may be alerted by intake information of a potential drug-drug interaction, of potential drug dependence, and of a withdrawal syndrome or patient reluctance.

Minimum/Maximum

This section is designed to explore dosage ranges and to assess pharmacologic tolerance. Most people are less reluctant to report their greatest amount of drug intake because almost everyone has at least one outrageous episode to report. Once the episode has been recounted, the clinician should follow with an inquiry about neurologic competence and consistence, as outlined earlier.

The minimum dose to get an effect is also often more easily admitted by patients than daily intake. The patient may ask for clarification of what is meant by "effect." It is important to determine the reasons why the person drinks and outline inconsistencies between minimum dose and daily intake.

Loss

There are three separate subsegments to loss: Loss of memory, loss of control, and losses if the patient were to quit using a substance.

Loss of memory, or "alcoholic blackout," is an important clue to the diagnosis. It is a period of retrograde amnesia during waking activity such that the person cannot later recall actions or context for short or extended periods of time. This condition is not to be confused with an acute episode of Wernicke's encephalopathy, during which anterograde amnesia occurs along with nystagmus, extraocular ophthalomoplegia, and ataxia. Behavior that occurs during blackouts may or may not appear intoxicated or impaired. Amnesia is sometimes partial; sometimes the person can recall part of the period. On the one hand, emotionally charged activities such as violent or sexual acts may be repressed. Memories could be recalled under amytal interview ("truth serum"), hypnosis, dreams, or psychotherapy. On the other hand, when the forgotten events were not emotionally charged, and blood levels quite high (usually over 200 mg/100 cc), amnesia is believed to be related to some biochemical effect on brain memory function.[5] Occasionally, a patient may report that memory returned on the next binge. Presumably this represents state-dependent learning, or may reflect a "truth-serum"-like effect of alcohol on repressed memory.

Loss of control represents the inability to reliably modulate the dosage of a drug when using the drug, or to reliably choose times for use that are not potentially troublesome. In Western culture, loss of control is stigmatized. Consequently, many patients deny loss of control, despite the evidence. One helpful question is "Have you ever thought of quitting or cutting?" Any quick response to this question usually reflects familiarity with the concept and indicates conscious or unconscious struggling with an inability to control intake. Some patients may answer, "I can take it or leave it." Such a reply probably means limitation to the extremes of total abstinence or excessive intake, and inability to modulate intake.

Patients or family members who respond to questioning by reporting rituals that are being used to "control" drinking or drug use may help the physician to identify earlier signs of loss of control.[55] Family members may be employed in the control rituals (*enabling or co-alcoholism*).[20] The danger of this is that the person has succeeded in transferring responsibility for self-control to another person. If the enabler tries to escape from this role, the ingestion may escalate, which would be blamed on the enabler. If the enabler remains in this role, the substance abuser may try to find clever ways to defeat external controls and frustrate the enabler.

Loss if quit refers to the purpose of the ingestion. If a person ceases for a period of time, it becomes painfully obvious what functions ingestion has been serving. This information is essential in preventing relapse or side effects of abstinence. The realm of such functions may include the physiological, psychologic, and social well-being of a person or family (for example, to ward off the physical withdrawal syndrome, to help the person to behave assertively towards authority figures, to make loving easier, to keep the person alert for long hours, to make dishonesty easier at work, to decrease competition between family members, etc.). These functions may be discovered by asking what triggered a relapse or what were the major problems during periods of abstinence that were not present or bothersome during periods of drinking or drug ingestion. These functions may need attention during the treatment process, which ideally finds new alternative solutions to the problems of abstinence (medically controlled detoxification, assertiveness training, learning to feel comfortable with sober loving, finding a different job, helping the family tolerate intrafamily competition, etc.). It is not unusual for the patient to deny or be unaware of the function of drinking, but often the family can supply some answers to this question. In an individually oriented treatment, the function of drinking may be ignored as irrelevant, since this line of reasoning could be used as an excuse to continue to drink. Yet failure to address the absence of functions within the sober family context during treatment or recovery generally leads to treatment failure and relapse in the patient or other family members.[28]

Consequences or Complications

There are an endless variety of medical, psychological, and social complications from substance dependence or abuse, some of which were listed before.[31,37] The array of complications discovered during the past medical history and systems review may be augmented by specific inquiry into more common consequences (asking about drunk driving, getting caught smoking "pot" at school, nervousness and insomnia in caffeine abuse, etc.).

The data gathered from such an inquiry usually provide assistance in judging severity and stage of the disorder. It also suggests levers to motivate the patient or family to consider treatment. The clinician must be careful not to scare patients or family. It is known from the health behavior literature that scare tactics often result in greater denial rather than constructive behavioral change.[23] Alcoholics often respond to frightening news from the doctor by increasing their drinking. Consequences may take the form of escalation. With the development of tolerance and increased escalation of dosage, the desire for analgesia from emotional pain evolves into the desire for anesthesia. The patient becomes insensitive to usual emotional signals from the environment (especially family) and his or her behavior becomes much more self-centered. In a way, it is as though the person loses touch with reality in the realm of emotional communication.

Effects on Others/Enablers/
Environment/Ecology

In looking for consequences of dependence or abuse, it is wise to look for trouble in relationships as an early sign. Since this is usually a major part of family practice, it provides the family physician with a sensitive diagnostic instrument for recognizing the onset of dependency. Recognition of dependency may be done through the drinker or drug user by asking if anyone in his or her life complains or worries about ingestion or its consequences. It may be assessed by talking with emissaries or family members who do not spontaneously come forward seeking care for the drug user. The clinician may look for nonspecific trouble in relationships, such as marital or sexual problems, parent-child problems ("hyperactivity," discipline problems), problems between the family and the community or the extended family. If the nature of this trouble is not directly related to drug use and its consequences, look for failure of the user to heed appropriate warnings of the need to respond or change. Also look for a tendency for enablers to protect the user from usual environmental stresses and demands by family isolation (for example, a teenager not bringing friends home), concealment of trouble within the family, and covering up for the drug-dependent person's malfunction in the community (for example, lying to the employer about father's absence from work).

Synergism

When looking for consequences of alcohol or drug intake, the clinician should be alert for *synergistic* effects of drugs with one another and of interactions between drugs and pathologic states. For instance, a person taking tolbutamide may experience nausea and vomiting after drinking alcohol because tolbutamide blocks acetaldehyde dehydrogenase, just like disulfiram or citrated calcium carbamide.[4] In addition to drug-drug interaction, ethanol interacts with diabetes in the following manner: 1) ethanol is a calorie source; 2) heavy ethanol ingestion interferes with glycogen storage and glucose catabolism, leading often to hypoglycemia; and 3) extreme drinking may cause pancreatitis, which in turn may increase the severity of diabetes. It is important to be aware of physiological implications of drug ingestion.

Personal Concern over Use

Most patients will deny that their drinking or drug use is a "problem," but they will have some regrets, at least about the consequences. Persons who have tried to control their drinking or drug use often fear loss of control of intake. This line of questioning may serve to initiate a therapeutic contract between the clinician and the patient.

Abstinence

The patient may report several periods of abstinence which can provide useful information about what concerns led to quitting; what it is like being abstinent initially (withdrawal syndrome?) and subsequently (which essential functions were lost?); and what triggered the relapse. It is important to determine whether the patient was truly abstinent and not switched to another drug (for example, stopped drinking while on diazepam). It is also important to inquire about the exact circumstances of the period of abstinence to determine the degree to which the patient voluntarily began and maintained abstinence (a measure of motivation). In the case of involuntary abstinence, the clinician can determine which part of the environment had influenced the patient to temporarily quit.

Help Sought

This line of inquiry aids in assessing the severity of the disorder and the stage of the recovery process. It also helps in planning treatment to be aware of what treatment has been previously tried and why it did not work. The patient or family may report attempts at quitting or cutting down without help from anyone (the so-called "will-power" quitting). This should be recorded with information about the attempt's degree of success or failure, its duration, and what interfered with final success. Others may report professional help via a physician, counselor, or mental health worker who was not specifically trained in working with substance-abuse problems. The clinician should inquire as to the degree to which this help was focused on substance abuse behavior. Most mental health professionals may have overemphasized psychopathology and may not adequately exploit the value in self-help programs that are available.[11,25] They may inadvertently support or even stimulate the feelings of stigma that must be reduced in order for recovery to proceed.

Some patients may report that they have attended a self-help group such as Alcoholics Anonymous (AA) and its groups for cohorts (Al-Anon and Alateens), Women for Sobriety, Narcotics Anonymous, Pills Anonymous, etc. Inquiry about these experiences should focus on the extent of effort that was put into this approach and the nature of any reduction in progress. Some patients may have had formal treatment for substance abuse by trained professionals. It is then useful to ask about the educational exposure to basic concepts, discover the major thrusts of the prior treatment, and find why a permanent recovery track could not be followed.

Often the involvement of family in treatment is insufficient. For example, AA and Al-Anon put emphasis on the individual taking responsibility for personal behavior. However, neither program addresses the alcohol- or drug-related interactive patterns such as the so-called "wet" and "dry" behavioral patterns described by Steinglass.[49] This gap has been filled in part by the spawning of new self-help groups known as Families Anonymous or Ala-Fam, which meet as groups of families. They focus on interactive changes that they have determined are important for recovery. Usually members also attend AA or Al-Anon meetings separately.

DATA FROM OTHER SOURCES

It is very helpful to obtain information from a variety of sources so as to verify validity. So much of the information gathered about substance abusers is prone to inaccuracies that this becomes crucial in some cases. For a start, gathering information from other family members, the employer, friends and neighbors in the community, and agencies of social control (police, courts, child protective services) can help to augment what is obtained from the patient. Reviewing the prior medical record at the hospital and in the clinic or office is frequently helpful in suggesting complications and help seeking that have occurred in the past.

Laboratory data may be useful in refuting or confirming historical information. Qualitative urine drug screens, especially on admission to the hospital, provide positive evidence of drugs that have recently been ingested. This may alert the physician to a potential for the development of a serious withdrawal syndrome. Quantitative blood alcohol levels are easily obtainable by a hand-held breath alcohol analyzer, which can provide evidence of marked tolerance to sedatives and can corroborate intake histories. The use of a breath analyzer also permits confrontation of the patient who falsifies intake history for that day; if a confrontation exists, it should be supportive in nature, addressing the clinician's need to have accurate information for proper patient care and the patient's perceived need to avoid being stigmatized by the clinician. Emergency room data suggest that in some communities nearly half of the care is delivered to persons with alcohol in their bodies.[47]

A blood level over 150 mg/100 cc without accompanying signs of gross intoxication suggests marked tolerance that could only occur in persons accustomed to large intakes. A blood level over 300 mg/100 cc is considered diagnostic of alcoholism except in extraordinary circumstances of ingestion. One must beware of two exceptions to the usual neurologic and behavioral manifestations of intoxication: the person who is concurrently taking other synergistic drugs (for example, diazepam) may demonstrate less tolerance than he or she has if the effect were presumed to represent that of alcohol alone; the person with portal venous congestion and variceal rerouting of gut blood efflux will appear to have lower tolerance in terms of dosage ingested but not in terms of blood levels, because the ingested alcohol goes directly into the systemic circulation.

Ethanol catabolism occurs at a rate of approximately 30 mg/100 cc per hour in the experienced drinker who takes no competing drugs. The rate is half as fast in inexperienced drinkers (one drink per hour).

DIAGNOSTIC CRITERIA

The National Council on Alcoholism has devised a set of criteria for diagnosing alcoholism.[39] The criteria were recently converted into a more practical tool by Brown and Lyons.[9] This instrument gathers complications from the history and scores them. A simpler but perhaps less standardized method of diagnosis is to look for trouble that can be associated with intake and look for loss of control of intake. If both occur, substance dependence can be diagnosed. Tolerance is usually high in dependence,[1] but is not necessary because it may decrease as the liver deteriorates, or it may appear lower if the patient combines synergistic drugs. Loss of control over intake may take the form of high dosage or episodic abuse or both. It can occur only some of the time or under certain specific circumstances (when feeling depressed, when other people are buying drinks, during the time of menstrual flow, or only after three drinks have been consumed within an hour).

The patient who has repeated episodes of troublesome use probably has at least some difficulty with loss of control. Many persons will have tried various methods of controlling their intake in an effort to regain the lost control and to continue drinking or drug use without trouble. Those persons who fail at these efforts are dependent and will need to abstain in order to reliably avoid trouble. One diagnostic trick known as the "acid test" for alcoholism challenges the patient to hold drinking at two or three standard sized drinks for a duration of 3 months. Unless the person characteristically had days of abstinence interspersed between drinking days, no days of abstinence are prescribed. Much attention is paid to the rapport with the patient and family to ensure honest reporting. Some skepticism is to be expected from the family. Most victims of alcoholism do not find this challenge easy. Many quit drinking altogether once they reduce it this far.

TREATMENT: CONFRONTATION

When it becomes evident that a patient is suffering from substance dependence, a clinician begins to feel ethically bound to report this to the patient and family, just as he or she would feel obligated to report cancer. This is hopefully done in a constructive and supportive way. The best way is to gather as much information before reporting the diagnosis. If possible, attempt to involve the family in this data collection phase or at least in the diagnostic reporting. Inform patient and family that treatment can increase chances of recovery. Families can produce an 85% chance of recovery, when the patient is unwilling with a family constructive coercive confrontation of their dependent loved one.[20,22,27,28,30,36]

Smilkstein[48] suggests that the family is much more pliable when in disequilibrium or crisis, and when it discovers that the usual solutions do not work. Hence, stressful times become the most likely times for change. Medical crises are an excellent time for the physician to intervene in an alcoholic family. Medical illness frightens the family; it interrupts their daily routine and stimulates an interest in change. They should have the opportunity to learn about family contribution through enabling behaviors (also known as co-alcoholism) and how they can get help for this. Confronting family-enabling behavior is one way to begin to change the behavioral interaction pattern of the alcoholic family. Children of alcoholics often find it enlightening to meet other children of alcoholics and to share experiences and feelings.[6,8,12,17] Children also get caught in the enabling web and may present with problems related to their roles in the family alcoholism.

Some families respond to confrontation and treatment quickly and easily. But other alcoholic families resist help and continue to relapse. Careful study of many such families[28] has revealed that the drinking behavior is embedded in a sequence of routine behaviors that comprise an essential element in the overall repertoire of family behaviors. The immediate consequences of treatment may then be traumatic (divorce, running away from home, suicide), because these families cannot live comfortably without all their essential functions. Family treatment should replace the drinking or other drug ingestion with healthier ways to retain their essential functions.

TREATMENT MOTIVATION

It is often difficult to motivate a person to accept treatment for alcoholism or substance abuse, even when the patient-clinician relationship is excellent. This is largely due to several factors indiginous to the disorder: 1) denial of a problem; 2) denial that help is needed; 3) shame and embarrassment from stigma; and 4) support from others (enablers) in the environment to resist change.

Denial

It is possible in many cases to overcome denial in the alcoholic patient or family by showing the damage. Trust in the clinician is crucial in this process. Optimistic and supportive confrontation of the denial often convinces the person to seek help. However, if the family does not begin treatment immediately, the denial may return. Paradoxically, alcohol or substance abuse may serve this denial through its pharmacologic action (sedative, anxiolytic). It may be helpful to use educational material, such as pamphlets or films. Overcoming denial is also extremely important for the family members, and can be accomplished with the introduction to another similar substance-dependent family several years further in the recovery process.

Those persons who believe the myth that alcoholism is treatable merely by cutting the dose of intake may encounter problems in treatment or recovery. Since loss of control of intake is a keystone in diagnosis, cutting the dose would comprise an insurmountable task (at least if it was to be 100% effective) for a person suffering from alcoholism. These periods of reduced dosage are usually short enough that tolerance does not decrease significantly. However, if dosage were controlled long enough to reduce tolerance, it is conceivable that long-term control might be achieved by this strategy.[16]

Denial makes the alcoholic appear to be doing something about the drinking problem while heavy drinking is still occurring. This tends to quiet those who are expressing their concern about the untreated alcoholism. It is important to realize that in formal treatment by experts it is unlikely that the notion that a person can achieve control of drinking will be supported. Alcoholics Anonymous considers this a harmful myth to the alcoholic because it delays acceptance of alcoholism and onset of true sobriety. Such an attitude sometimes drives the alcoholic who wishes to recover without abstinence away from AA or treatment.[41] Although realizing the low probability of recovery without abstinence, the scientific community is not as rigid about this notion because of scientific optimism that someday we will learn how to "cure" loss of control of drinking.

Stigma

The patient and family who suffer from alcoholism also suffer from social stigma. Cultural attitudes in North America derive largely from a mixture of various and sometimes conflicting attitudes towards drinking and drunkenness. Some groups do not distinguish between use and excess (southern Baptists, Mormons) while others may encourage drinking but shun drunkenness (Italian-Americans). Some drinkers or their family members may feel anxious when they associate with a person who does not drink because of some concerns they have about alcohol in their own life. This may with time reduce the extent of their socialization processes.

Most family members are at least subliminally aware of their role in this process and hence tend to feel some guilt, shame, and remorse over their involvement. These feelings may motivate their interest in Al-Anon or in obtaining help for their alcoholic loved one (that is, playing the role of emissary from their sick family). In reacting defensively to these feelings, family members may paradoxically alternate between heaping stigma on the alcoholic person or defending him or her from others who do the same. This two-faced behavior produces difficulties in self-esteem and family relations for family members who begin to feel dishonest, isolated, crazy, and angry about their own behavior. The whole family may try to deny, project, and rationalize these problems to avoid stigma.

Normalization

In motivating the family to act constructively, the clinician may first need to decrease some of the stigma so that they can listen without defensive protestation. It usually helps to describe what the clinician perceives to be their experience (this enhances physician credibility) as typical of family alcoholism. Grief/adjustment counselling will help the family members accept their "diminished status" as people and their life-choice restrictions will help in the early phases of recovery.[3] Introducing the family to another family later in the recovery process is a good strategy to reduce stigma, instill optimism, and facilitate links with the recovering community (e.g., AA, Al-Anon).

Environmental Enablers

Enablers can escape from the enabling role only if they refuse to rescue or rescue under strictly enforceable conditions that lead to treatment. Al-Anon is helpful in teaching enablers to be honest with themselves. This supports constructive action in the form of refusing to rescue the drinker from the consequences of behavior (called "tough love" by Al-Anon members). If all of the family members simultaneously avail themselves of this kind of help, they may be able to avoid mutual undermining or transfer of enabling around the family circle.

A procedure called "Intervention" by some[20,30,36] and "Family Constructive Coercive Confrontation" by others[27,28] is an approach based on social and ecological treatment. The emissary brings together other enablers from the family and extended environment to work as a team towards the goal of supportively confronting denial of the need for treatment.[27,30] Even if the alcoholic initially refuses treatment after such a confrontation, the team can collectively refuse to enable drinking and other associated behavior. With their newly organized team cohesion, they can avoid mutual undermining and withstand pressure from the alcoholic to rescue him or her. The team may also support one another emotionally from suffering undo anxiety or guilt during this difficult period.

The probable causes for failure of the procedure are incomplete team composition or lack of team cohesion, or both. If the team failed to approach the alcoholic respectfully, compassionately, and supportively, the failure can be interpreted as an attack. There have been cases of suicide. This procedure is not altogether benign and should be done carefully by trained experts. For more details the reader can refer elsewhere.[20,22,29,30] The Johnson Institute in Minneapolis provides training courses and excellent films about this procedure. Clinicians can either refer these cases to experts in the community, participate as a member of the ecological network of ex-enablers, or play a leadership role. The latter has been part of one family practice residency program.[2] It may be easier to play the leading role as a stranger who is relatively uninvolved in the process.

The myth that alcoholism or other substance dependence is untreatable has been widespread until recently. Many patients and professionals believe that lack of motivation has prevented most victims of alcoholism from recovery. Denial and stigma coupled with enabling social support make it very unlikely that even a well-trained clinician will encounter many co-operative and self-motivated patients volunteering for treatment. Tennant and colleagues[51] have written that a physician's advice motivated 70% of patients to enter treatment. Clinicians can have significant impact on motivation and mobilization of social support (ex-enablers) for treatment success.

REFERRAL

If a patient asks for or agrees to alcoholism treatment, the clinician needs to develop a treatment plan that will meet the needs of the patient and family. An essay on how to properly match the needs of the family to the available resources can be found elsewhere.[27] If the clinician believes that referral to an expert is necessary or optimal, it is important to prepare the family for this referral by explaining to whom they are being referred, the nature of that expertise, the expected services they should receive, the costs (financial and otherwise) they will incur, the reason for the referral, and their clinician's continuing role in this referral and future family care. This will prevent misconceptions about the referral, and it will relieve any concerns that the family may have that they are being abandoned by their clinician because they have alcoholism or drug dependence. Each clinician must decide the degree to which personal interests, skill, experience, and costs (for example, time) mesh with patient needs and available community resources. Some clinicians who work in areas where there are insufficient resources may find themselves filling a gap by learning quite a lot about effective approaches to treatment of substance abuse. Others may take a leadership or supportive role in community development of the needed resources.

TREATMENT DETOXIFICATION

The inpatient or outpatient detoxification process may be medically assisted, when necessary, by providing sedation in sufficient amount to substitute for the alcohol that is no longer available, and to account for the high tolerance to sedation in most abusers. The basic principle is to adequately sedate the patient to eliminate withdrawal symptoms during the first 24 to 48 hours. Then, sedation is tapered by 20% per day. The patient should be able to sleep during the first 2 days without additional sedation at night. I have had to give as much as 1600 mg of chlordiazepoxide in one day to a severe case of withdrawal. Only one sedative drug should be used to avoid medical confusion. If there is liver disease, oxazepam is better. If oral sedation cannot be administered, intravenous diazepam or lorazepam may be used. The inpatient should be drug free for several days (and comfortable) before discharge. The commonest error is to underdose initially and then to overdose at the end of the detoxification. Home detoxification is possible if responsible family cooperation is elicited in conjunction with daily visits for vital sign checks and obtaining the prescription for the next day.[42] More complete information on detoxification can be obtained from several other sources.

REHABILITATION

The process of recovery for the person with alcoholism involves several phases: acceptance of alcoholism, abstinence, relearning how to cope with feelings without substance use, developing a new lifestyle and social set, maintaining the progress that is made, and adjusting to stresses and life-stage changes without relapse. Participation in the AA program provides ongoing support for growth by the recovering person at his or her own pace. If a person cannot grow past a certain issue, the clinician may explore this issue with the person to help overcome barriers to progress, or may refer this patient to an expert. It is rarely beneficial for a recovering person to enter insight-oriented individual psychotherapy before 2 years of sobriety have elapsed. Most issues that appeared important earlier than this have usually disappeared without therapy, and such treatment usually precipitates relapse until patients have strengthened their defense patterns to maintain sobriety. The removal of defenses by a psychotherapist is therefore contraindicated. The therapist with expertise in alcoholism knows this and only does supportive therapy in the early phases of treatment.

The roles of all family members in the recovery process also vary considerably. The family and close friends react differently to a person who does not consume alcohol or other drugs in the usual contexts and situations. They may find themselves less comfortable with the dry alcoholic, creating a temptation to provoke drinking and to suffer ensuing guilt if they succeed.

Most alcoholic families do not realize the degree to which drinking has become integrated with essential family functions. They assume that drinking is an isolated behavior that can be stopped anytime without negative consequences. Clinicians realize that treatments seem always to have side effects, and behavioral change is no exception. It is more realistic to counsel the patient and family that once the drinking stops, they will discover some changes in the family that may be unpleasant. The clinician can offer to help the family to discover ways to solve these problems when they arise in order to avoid relapse or chronic dissatisfaction with sober family life. He or she can empathize with the alcoholic, saying that after the early enthusiasm wears off, the abstinence may not be easy because some family members may seem to wish the person would begin to drink again. In addition, one should prepare the person who expects his or her family or friends to appreciate the efforts and results of the recovery for disappointment. Despite initial support for quitting from family and significant others, the AA program often becomes a major source of reliable support for abstinence during the early phases of recovery.

The oversimplification of the recovery process, which has been a myth among the lay public, has suggested that no treatment is necessary for alcoholism recovery. This oversimplification probably explains the high relapse rates among those who indulge in home remedies for their alcoholism, and may also explain the high rates of family relapse (other members start abusing chemicals when one member quits) when only the drinker gets help.

The intricate balance of complementary behaviors within the family dynamically changing over time makes it difficult to predict with precision how each change will affect the overall pattern of interactions. The clinician must always be aware of the context of the nuclear family and consider those influences. Extended family, friends, employers, neighbors, and the larger cultural community all have influences on the choices that are made at points of change.

FOLLOW-UP

After initial treatment has been started, there is always the risk that the patient and family will quit treatment and relapse. The clinician who ensures continuity of care would build communication links with the family and experts to provide early notification. Immediate exploration of reasons should be undertaken, so that appropriate strategies of response can be devised. If there is a problem with the quality or appropriateness of the treatment, this problem may be resolved by a different referral. However, the problem is often that the treatment has become too intense or rapid, frightening the family with the rate of change. The family should also realize that this is their problem, so that they can either speed up their pace or accept that it will take longer than they hoped to make the necessary changes.

The family may come to the clinician with other problems that are responsible for failed treatment or relapse of drinking by the alcoholic. Nevertheless, these problems should be approached as though they might be related to the recovery, at least until that has been ruled out, especially if these problems are social, psychological, psychosomatic, or behavioral.

The clinician also has a role after the bulk of treatment and change is over. Families continue to evolve over time as they go through life-cycle developmental phases. At each step there is stress and new problems may become important to the family members. It is helpful to anticipate some of these periods of high risk, and to check with the family members whether they are preparing themselves for some of the inevitable stresses and strains that usually occur. If their recovery program is adequate, they will already be working on these issues. If not, the clinician may stimulate their attendance to these issues. It is also wise to be sure that they know to ask for help on problems as they arise during these transitions so that they do not end up going to less aware professionals.

SUMMARY

Alcohol and substance abuse is a chronic family disorder that can best be treated by involving the whole family in the recovery. Failure to do so puts the patient at greater risk of relapse, and the family at greater risk of disruption. Treatment involves several phases: becoming aware of the problem, accepting the problem, and motivating the family to seek help. The clinician has an extremely important role to play in these phases. Formal treatment is usually done by specialists, although the clinician may develop this special expertise with additional training. Nevertheless, the referral and collaboration with experts is also extremely important for the success of the treatment and for the quality of the primary care that is being delivered. The earlier this disorder is treated, the more effective the treatment will be in halting the progression and deterioration of the family and patient.

REFERENCES

1. American Psychiatric Association Task Force on Nomenclature and Statistics: *DSM-III: Diagnostic and Statistical Manual of Mental Disorders, III.*

2. Anderson R: Personal communication, 1979.

3. Bean M: Presentation at the Boston Area Alcohol Interest Group, 21 April, 1982.

4. Becker CE, Roe RL, Scott RA: *Alcohol as a Drug: A Curriculum on Pharmacology, Neurology and Toxicology.* New York, Medcom Press, 1974.

5. Birnbaum IM, Parker ES (eds): *Alcohol and Human Memory.* Hinsdale, NG, Lawrence Erlbaum Associates, 1977.

6. Black C: Innocent bystanders at risk: The children of alcoholics. *Alcoholism* 1:22, 1981.

7. Breitenbucher RB: The routine administration of the Michigan Alcoholic Screening Test to ambulatory patients. *Minn Med* 59:425, 1976.

8. Brooks C: *The Secret Everyone Knows.* San Diego, The Kroc Foundation, 1981.

9. Brown J, Lyons JP: A progressive diagnostic schema for alcoholism with evidence of clinical efficacy. *Alcoholism: Clin Exp Res* 5:17, 1981.

10. Cahalan D, Cisin IH, Crossley HM: *American Drinking Practices: A National Study of Drinking Behavior and Attitudes,* Monograph #6. New Brunswick, New Jersey, Rutgers Center of Alcohol Studies, 1969.

11. Curlee J: Combined use of Alcoholics Anonymous and outpatient psychotherapy. *Bull Menninger Clin* 35:368, 1971.

12. Deutsch C: *Broken Bottles, Broken Dreams: Understanding and Helping the Children of Alcoholics.* New York, Teachers College Press, 1982.

13. Drum DE, Jankowski C: Diagnostic algorithms for detection of alcoholism in general hospitals. *Curr Alcohol* 1:361, 1977.

14. Funkhouser MJ: Identifying alcohol problems among elderly hospital patients. *Alcohol Health Res World* 2:27, 1977/1978.

15. Goodwin D: *Is Alcoholism Hereditary?* New York, Oxford University Press, 1976.

16. Heather N, Robertson I: Controlled Drinking, 1982.

17. Hornik EL: *Your and Your Alcoholic Parent.* New York, Association Press, 1974.

18. Jacobson, GR: *The Alcoholisms: Detection, Diagnosis and Assessment.* New York, Human Sciences Press, 1976.

19. Jarvik ME, Cullen JW, Gritz ER, Vogt TM, West LJ: *Research on Smoking Behavior.* NIDA Research Monograph 17, Rockville, MD, U.S. DHEW Publication 3 (ADM) 78–581, 1977.

20. Johnson V: *I'll Quit Tomorrow.* New York, Harper & Row, 1973.

21. Johnston RGM, Lex B: Alcoholism in consecutive hospital admissions to the Providence Veterans Hospital. Unpublished manuscript, personal communication, 1981.

22. Koppel F, Stimmler L, Perone F: The enabler: A motivational tool in treating the alcoholic. *Soc Casework* 61:577, 1980.

23. Leventhal H: Fear appeals and persuasion: The differentiation of a motivational construct. *Am J Public Health* 61:1208, 1971.

24. Liepman MR: Recognizing and managing the family at high risk for alcoholism, in Hess JW, Lipeman MR, Ruane TH (eds): *Family Practice and Preventive Medicine: Health Promotion in Primary Care.* New York, Human Sciences Press, 1982.

25. Leipman MR, Maiorana R: Staff denial of alcoholism in psychiatric inpatients. *Alcoholism: Clin Exp Res* 3:184, 1979.

26. Liepman MR, Spurgat T: A mnemonic for the nine essential elements of an alcoholic/drug history. Unpublished but copyrighted, 1981.

27. Liepman MR, Tauriainen M: Factors contributing to success or failure of family coercive interventions on alcoholics. *Alcoholism: Clin Exp Res* 4:79, 1980.

28. Liepman MR, Tauriainen M, Boblitt V: Outcomes of family constructive coercive confrontation training for alcoholic families. Manuscript in preparation, 1982.

29. Liepman MR, Wolper B, Vazquez J: An ecological approach for motivating women to accept treatment for chemical dependency, in Reed BG, Mondanaro J, Beschner GM (eds): *Treatment Services for Drug Dependent Women, II.* Rockville, Maryland, Treatment Research Monograph Series, National Institute on Drug Abuse, 1982.

30. Logan DG: Getting alcoholics to treatment through intervention. Unpublished manuscript, personal communication, 1982.

31. Lowenfels AB, Rohman M, Shibutani K: Surgical consequences of alcoholism. *Surg Gynecol Obstet* 131:129, 1970.

32. Marvin MW, Garland B, Hackland S, MacLean B: *Alcohol Problems in Canada: A Summary of Current Knowledge.* Technical Report Series #2, Health and Welfare, Canada, 1976.

33. Mayfield D, McLeod G, Hall P: The CAGE questionnaire: Validation of a new alcoholism screening instrument. *Am J Psychiatry* 131:1121, 1974.

34. McCourt WF, Williams AF, Schneider L: Incidence of alcoholism in a state mental hospital population. *Q J Stud Alcohol* 32:1085, 1971

35. McLellan AT, Druley KA, Carson JE: Evaluation of substance abuse problems in a psychiatric hospital. *J Clin Psychiatry* 39:425, 1978.

36. Meagher MD, Scripps Memorial Hospital Alcohol Treatment Center, P.O. Box 28, LaJolla, California, 92038, (714) 457-6573. Personal communication in 1982 revealed a listing of 75 programs or professionals in the U.S. who claim to do coercive interventions.

37. Mezey E: Medical problems associated with alcoholism. *Primary Care* 1:293, 1974.

38. Moore RA: The diagnosis of alcoholism in a psychiatric hospital: A trial of the Michigan Alcoholism Screening Test (MAST). *Am J Psychiatry* 128:115, 1972.

39. National Council on Alcoholism (NCA) Criteria Committee: Criteria for the diagnosis of alcoholism. *Am J Psychiatry* 129:127, 1972.

40. Noble EP (ed): *Third Special Report to the U.S. Congress on Alcohol and Health.* U.S. DHEW Publication # (ADM) 78-569, 1978 and the support document (ADM) 79-932, 1979.

41. Orford J, Oppenheimer E, Edwards G: Abstinence or control: The outcome for excessive drinkers two years after consultation. *Behav Res Ther* 14:409, 1976.

42. Palmen MA: Personal communication, 1979.

43. Pell S, D'Alonzo CA: The prevalence of chronic disease among problem drinkers. *Arch Environ Health* 16:679, 1968.

44. Quinn MA, Johnston RV: Alcohol problems in acute male medical admissions. *Health Bull (Edinb)* 34:253, 1976.

45. Selzer ML: The Michigan Alcoholism Screening Test (MAST): The quest for a new diagnostic instrument. *Am J Psychiatry* 127:1653, 1971.

46. Selzer ML: Study of alcoholism prevalence on a general medical ward of a midwestern teaching hospital. Unpublished study, personal communication, 1972.

47. Senior JR, Sloan BP: Emergency measurement of stat, timed, serum ethanol levels for medical management. *Alcoholism: Clin Exp Res* 5:6, 1981

48. Smilkstein G: The cycle of family function: A conceptual model for family medicine. *J Fam Pract* 11:223, 1980.

49. Steinglass P: The alcoholic family at home: Patterns of interaction in dry, wet, and transitional stages of alcoholism. *Arch Gen Psychiatry,* in press.

50. Swenson WM, Morse RM: The use of a self-administered alcoholism screening test (SAAST) in a medical center. *Mayo Clin Proc* 50:204, 1975.

51. Tennant FS, Day CM, Ungerleider JT: Screening for drug and alcohol abuse in a general medical population. *JAMA* 242:533, 1979.

52. Westermeyer J, Doheny S, Stone B: An assessment of hospital care for the alcoholic patient. *Alcoholism: Clin Exp Res* 2:53, 1978.

53. Whitfield CL, Williams KG: The Disease Alcoholism, in Whitfield CL, Williams KH, Liepman MR (eds): *The Patient with Alcoholism or Other Drug Problems.* Chicago, Year Book Medical Publishers, 1982.

54. Whitfield CL, Williams KH, Liepman MR: *The Patient with Alcoholism or Other Drug Problems.* Chicago, Year Book Medical Publishers, 1982.

55. Zinberg NE, Jacobson RC: The natural history of 'chipping'. *Am J Psychiatry* 133:37, 1976.

Chapter 27
Working with Couples: Marital Problems

Yvonne Steinert

Mrs. M., 46 years of age, comes to her family physician for her annual "check-up." When asked how things are at home, she tells her physician that her major concern at the moment is her relationship with her husband. Mrs. M. has been married for 26 years, but for the past year she has been feeling increasingly unhappy in her marriage. She does not describe any change in the marriage; rather, she feels that the change is in her. As she says, she now wants a "slice of the pie."

How can the physician best help in this situation? What should be his role? Should he see Mr. and Mrs. M. together or separately?

Mrs. A., a 28-year-old mother of two preschool children, returns to her nurse with recurrent complaints of palpitations and weakness. Although Mrs. A.'s nurse has discussed the possible connections between her symptoms and the current stresses in her life, Mrs. A. does not see this connection and she fears that she has "heart problems." During today's interview, however, Mrs. A. reports that her last "attack" occurred on Saturday, following a disagreement she had with her husband because he had forgotten their anniversary on Friday.

Mrs. A.'s nurse questions how she can best use this new information.

Mr. R., a patient of Dr. B. for 5 years, calls Dr. B. to tell him that he wants to divorce his wife, but is very worried about how she will react. He does not know what to do and is asking Dr. B. for his help. Dr. B. is wondering what the best move would be.

The goal of this chapter is to focus specifically on the role of the family physician or nurse in working with couples who are experiencing difficulties in their relationship. Given that the couple is the "architect" of the family,[19] it is important to explore the couple system in more detail.

The family physician and the primary care nurse are in ideal positions to work with couples and families. They are able to observe the couple's relationship and functioning over time, and they are able to use their knowledge of the family's structure, development, and functioning to more effectively treat and prevent biomedical and psychological problems.

449

Moreover, there is generally no stigma attached to confiding in a physician or nurse; in contrast, marriage counsellors or psychiatrists are often considered only when problems are "severe."

Clinicians may find themselves working with couples at various moments in clinical practice: during key life cycle stages; at the onset of a serious, acute illness; during the management of a chronic illness; or when the couple presents with relationship difficulties. This chapter will focus primarily on couples* who are experiencing marital problems; strategies for working with couples in other clinical situations are described in more detail in other chapters.

People with marital difficulties often turn for help to their physicians, either directly or indirectly, by presenting with a variety of physical or psychological symptoms. Although the practitioner cannot attempt to solve a couple's problems, he or she may provide a forum for the clarification and assessment of their conflicts.

Working with a couple's problems implies that the family physician or nurse has the ability to assess and clarify marital difficulties, to provide information and support to couples in distress, to facilitate couple interaction, and to refer appropriately. Working with couples does not imply couple therapy. Rather, this form of intervention generally takes place within the context of other visits, is short term in nature, and focuses on circumscribed marital difficulties. Early assessment of couple problems—and appropriate referral—*is* considered a major form of intervention.† As with families, understanding the couple as a system is essential to effective management.‡

MARRIAGE

Marriage is a complex, vulnerable relationship, currently in a state of rapid transition: the rate of divorce is increasing, people are getting married at an older age, both members of more couples are working, and the extended family network is disappearing. Yet, despite these transitions and many dire

---

*Although the major emphasis in this discussion is on the marital relationship, the authors recognize that many couples are not legally married; what is described here applies to couples, whether married or unmarried, as long as the relationship is one in which each partner has made a commitment to the other.

---

†Please see Chapter 16 for a more complete discussion of the distinction between working with couples families and couple family therapy. Table 16-1 provides a good summary of this distinction.

---

‡Please see Section. IV Chapter 5.

predictions about marriage and divorce, couple relationships persist.[3] Indeed, most adults over 30 years old are married.[5] Why? What is marriage and why do people marry? Clinicians should have a "theory of marriage," and be aware of the reasons people get married, because knowledge of these basic motivating factors and their apparent relationship to the "success" of the marriage is an essential ingredient in effective premarital counselling, as well as in the accurate assessment and comprehension of a couple's problems.

> Lorraine L., a lonely 18-year-old, unemployed woman, came to see Dr. T., whom she had known for the last 10 years, for a renewal of her birth control pills. During the visit, she mentioned that she was planning to get married in the following month, to a man she had only recently met.
>
> Although Lorraine was initially reluctant to elaborate on her decision to marry, it soon became apparent that her major reason for getting married was that she wanted to leave her parents' home. She was hoping that marrying an "older man"—he was 26 years old—"with a job" would get her "out of the rut" in which she found herself. Given that Dr. T. had developed a relationship of confidence and trust with Lorraine, he felt that he could help her to re-evaluate her decision to get married.

Factors that influence people's decisions to marry[10,11,16,17] include the following:

1. the romantic notion of love;
2. societal expectations;
3. parental pressures;
4. the fear of loneliness;
5. the desire to escape from the family of origin or the current living situation;
6. the need for emotional or economic security, enhanced self-esteem, perceived social worth, prestige, or status;
7. the desire for an intimate relationship with another adult, and for sexual intimacy; and
8. the desire to have children.

People's reasons for getting married are not always "conscious" or deliberate; neither is their "choice" of partner. Although the concept of romantic love with its implicit notion of individual freedom in mate selection has always been depicted as the norm in American society,[6] the choice of partner, usually occurs within significant social, economic, and cultural constraints. It is also influenced by a person's developmental history: by his or her past experiences within the family of origin as well as with peers.

In choosing a partner, people may repeat, or try to avoid a pattern experienced in their family of origin. For example, the daughter of an alcoholic may marry a young man with a tendency to drink, believing that she can help him change. A man dominated by his mother may choose a subservient wife, but may later complain that she lacks initiative. A close assessment of many marriages from a systems orientation may reveal a neat coupling not only of personalities, but also of past histories. It is wise to remember that most marriages are not accidental—people have picked each other for a reason.

The belief that "love" is necessary for a satisfactory marriage and that most married people love each other has been labelled as a "myth" by Lederer and Jackson.[16] Indeed, mutual trust, caring, commitment to the marriage, and respect for oneself and one's partner are key factors in its successful outcome.

Once marriage has been entered into, there are as many reasons for remaining married as there were for marrying in the first place. Conversely, marriages may fail or be dissolved because the very characteristics that were so appealing, initially, later become sources of irritation.[1]

> An organized, careful provider seemed to be the ideal husband for a girl who had difficulties in curbing her spending impulses and keeping a steady job. Her sociable nature, impulsiveness, and "joie de vivre" seemed like the "spark of life" this shy man had always needed. Her talkativeness allowed his shyness to go unnoticed. However, as the years went by and the arrival of children demanded better teamwork, the characteristics that helped this couple fall in love became liabilities. The more she spent his hard-earned money, the "stingier" he became. The more he chided her for spending, the more she resented him. The more she talked, the less necessary it was for him to talk. The more she pressed him to talk, the more he withdrew. Eventually, they separated for the same reasons they married.

COMMON STRESSES IN MARRIAGE

Marriages are often troubled—or fail—because of unfulfilled expectations.[11,16] Many individuals enter marriage with unrealistic expectations based on false romanticisms rather than on reality: that marriage will dispel loneliness, that time will enhance intimacy, that one must always be loved by one's spouse in particular ways. And once it becomes apparent that the "romantic" notion of marriage is a "myth," disappointment and disillusionment may set in.[9] The marital relationship generally proceeds from an intensive romantic infatuation to an extensive problem-solving relationship that is based on the needs and expectations of each partner.[18] Within this progression lies one of marriage's main difficulties.

> Mr. P., a 34-year-old business executive, married for 3 years, came to his physician for "help" with his marriage because he was feeling increasingly dissatisfied with his wife. Although Mr. P. was unable to specify

particular problems or conflicts, he did state that he and his wife were not as "happy" as married couples should be; they were not communicating as openly as they should.

This disappointment with the marriage was, in part, a result of Mr. P.'s initial expectations of married life. Unfulfilled expectations may also arise from the failure to communicate these expectations to the partner. Good communication is a vital ingredient to satisfaction in marriage. Proficiency in communication ensures mutual awareness of needs and expectations, and makes it possible for the partners in a marriage to discuss, negotiate, and resolve their problems.

Personal problems and turmoil also affect a marriage. Low self-esteem in one or both partners is a common theme in marital difficulties. Persons who enter a relationship to bolster their low self-esteem usually encounter disappointment or dissatisfaction. In fact, as Satir[19] has pointed out, most marriages are of people with equal self-esteem; and when one partner with apparently low self-esteem marries someone with greater self-confidence or strength, this difference may, in fact, be superficial. The "stronger" partner may depend on the other's "weakness" to hide his or her own vulnerability. Individuals with low self-esteem also have considerable difficulty in handling differences of opinion, and frequently believe that marriage should be a state of "perfect" togetherness.[11]

The marital relationship may also become a "dumping ground" for unresolved personal problems that may stem from past experiences in the family of origin, previous relationships, or individual psychopathology. Anger at the past, or at parents with whom relationships were hard to change, may often influence the marital relationship.

Differences in the partners' rates of maturation or growth can impose similar strains. For example, when John and Jane C. first married, she was happy to be directed and dominated by her husband. She wanted him to be the "decision-maker." Over time, however, her needs to be directed changed, but her partner's need to dominate still persisted. The current state of rapid change in various aspects of Western society constitutes an additional source of external stress. Few marriages have been unaffected by the advent of the "Women's Liberation Movement," which has brought more women into the labor force, altered the roles of husbands and wives, and presented people, generally, with more options.

Although unfulfilled needs or expectations may be the underlying cause of conflict, marital problems are more often expressed in terms of difficulties with relationships with the extended family or friends, children, sex, recreaction, finance, work, or religion. These are the areas in which the themes of power and dependency first emerge, and in which couples must first negotiate their rules for living together. Major life events, or the usual developmental crises encountered as the family life cycle unfolds, may also provoke marital problems or discord, dispite the fact that the marital relationship can be a source of support or fulfillment during these particular times.

In summary, people generally get married, and stay married, because their basic needs are met within marriage. The need for security is strong; people often stay in an otherwise unsatisfactory marriage because security exists. Marital stability is therefore not a reliable indicator of marital happiness, nor is marital happiness an accurate reflection of marital stability. In essence, it is not the presence or absence of problems, but the ability to solve problems that distinguishes successful from unsuccessful marriages.[11] Conflict is inherent in marriage because marriage is a difficult business[1]: how conflict is dealt with is the critical factor in success or failure.

WORKING WITH COUPLE PROBLEMS

Working *with* couple problems refers to the assessment and clarification of marital difficulties, the provision of information and support to couples in distress, the facilitation of couple interaction, and referral when appropriate; it does not imply couple therapy.

When To See Couples

Although some physicians or nurses choose to see couples during routine office visits, certain "moments" in clinical practice seem to be more critical. Such moments include the following:

1. during pivotal life cycle events such as pregnancy, the birth of the first child, the departure of children from the home, pre-retirement, and post-retirement;
2. at the diagnosis of a serious, acute illness;
3. during the management of a chronic illness;
4. following the onset of symptoms in one partner that relate to couple problems revealed during routine inquiry;
5. at the direct request of one of the partners because of couple problems, sexual dissatisfaction, or impending separation; and
6. at times of acute stress, such as the death of a family member.

As the reader will note, these moments for working with couples closely resemble those outlined in an earlier chapter on working with families.

When working with couples who are experiencing problems in their relationship, clinicians often wonder whether they should work with the entire family or only with the couple. If the presenting problem relates directly to the marriage (for example, a communication or a sexual problem), it is generally preferable to work with the couple, at least initially, even though the clinician may wish to see the entire family once, to assess the impact of the couple's problem on the family. If the problems are being expressed in a child, it is important to see the whole family.

Because the family is a system, problems between the partners may manifest themselves directly, or in another family member such as a vulnerable child. This is not simply the result of stress on the child, but rather an active involvement of the child in the parental problem. The child may feel the parents' distress, express it for them, or he or she may subconsciously try to protect them from their conflict by detouring attention to himself or herself. Children may unwittingly, or sometimes consciously, maintain couple problems by acting as a buffer or a means of conflict avoidance. If this is suspected, a family session is advisable. For older children, it is often a great relief to experience parental conflict *and* resolution of conflict with a third party present so that they can be relieved of their role as "go-between" or "family therapist." Often children in an interview will give nonverbal information about the couple that is invaluable. For example, a 6-year-old child reading a comic book suddenly got up to go and sit on her mother's lap in response to a profoundly sad look that the clinician would not otherwise have noticed. In another example, two young children contradicted their parents' statement of a peaceful week by staging a fight between two puppets resembling their parents.

Whenever a couple problem is expressed, it is preferable to see both partners at the same time rather than seeing either one, or both, of them individually. One partner, seen alone, tends to elicit sympathy with his or her position although the other partner's position, when heard, may seem equally justified. Seeing the partners together helps preclude the premature development of an alliance with either one, and allows the physician to discover patterns of interaction that may differ significantly from what either partner has described individually. In addition, simultaneous interviewing provides the physician with an opportunity to observe how the partners deal with each other, and reduces the risk of the physician being handicapped by being made privy to "confidential" information. Although individual interviews may, at times, be justified, to discuss an "affair" or one partner's desire to leave the marriage, an initial couple interview is best, whenever possible.

Enlisting the Other Partner

Although the physician or nurse may wish to see the couple, or the other spouse, it is not always easy to do so (see Chapter 13). For example, when Mrs. D. came to her physician complaining of dissatisfaction with her marriage, he expressed a willingness to explore the problem with her, and invited the husband to come in. Mrs. D. responded by saying that her husband would not come in. Given that it is usually the woman in the couple relationship who first alerts the clinician to the need for help, the difficulties involved in bringing the male partner in for a couple interview will be discussed, although the reverse situation also occurs.

When Mrs. D. stated that her husband would not come in, it may have meant that Mr. D. really did not want to come in, or that Mrs. D. did not want him to come in. The husband may have refused or been reluctant to come in because he was apprehensive about criticism, feared being blamed, did not see a couple "problem," did not want to concede anything to his wife, feared the possibility that certain family conflicts might surface, or thought that he might be asked to change his ways. The wife's reluctance to have her husband come in may have stemmed from the same fear of criticism or blame, from reluctance to change the marriage because of the attendant risk of rejection or continued failure, or from anxiety that she might lose the physician as her "ally" if both sides of the problem became known to him.

Thus, telling the physician that her husband does not want to come in may be a projection of Mrs. D.'s own fears or resistance onto her husband rather than an indication of his unwillingness to cooperate. The clinician must, therefore, assess where the resistance is coming from, and deal with it accordingly. If the main problem revolves around the wife's fears, the physician can help her to deal with them by exploring the roots of her concerns and by helping her to examine whether she actually wants to work on her marital relationship. The clinician may also explain that he is asking her husband to come in, not to judge or assign blame, but to more fully comprehend the total situation. If necessary, the clinician should also tell the wife that he will not be able to help her with her marital problems unless her husband participates, and that increased marital conflict may be more likely if he does not come in eventually.[13]

The physician can also help the wife to explore strategies for encouraging her reluctant husband to come in for an interview. Reviewing how she should explain the need for her partner's presence and suggesting alternative approaches can be very helpful. For example, when Mrs. D. was asked how she had explained the need for a conjoint interview to her husband, she replied that she had told her husband that "The doctor wants to see you to find out what you are doing to upset me so much." Clearly, this is not the way to encourage a spouse to come in for a joint interview. Working with Mrs. D. to develop a more tactful and constructive approach was helpful in finally encouraging Mr. D. to cooperate.

Clinicians often offer to telephone and invite the husband in when the wife is unable or hesitant to ask him herself. Making such a move as a first step may give the impression that the clinician is siding with the wife, is rescuing her, or is picking up the couple's burden, any or all of which may convey messages that he does not wish to send. On the other hand, if the wife is really unable to persuade her husband to come in, a phone call from the physician or nurse may be helpful. In the course of making the call, the clinician should attempt to "join" with the spouse on the telephone, and might ask how he is coping with the situation at home.

Occasionally, a separate appointment with the "reluctant spouse" may be a prerequisite to a conjoint interview. The physician has the distinct advantage of being able to use his or her ongoing relationship with the husband to encourage him to come in, or to make the husband's next medical visit into an opportunity to discuss the couple's problems. As a general rule, however, a couple interview should be arranged at the outset.

When the reluctant spouse finally appears, it is imperative that the physician "join" with him in a way that will decrease his anxiety and make the usefulness of the couple interview readily apparent to him. The husband will need some time to become accustomed to the couple interview and to give his perspective of the current situation. Rules about the confidentiality surrounding any of the topics already discussed with the other spouse should also have been established.

The persistent reluctance or refusal of one spouse to participate in a joint interview requires careful analysis. Clinicians may be able to work with an individual concerning couple problems, but the outcome under such circumstances is frequently not in favor of the marriage; it is well that the practitioner be fully aware of this consequence before planning to follow the "individual" route.

The Couple Interview

Given that couples are subsystems of families, most of the principles governing the interviewing of families as described in Section IV remain applicable. Nevertheless, a review of these general principles and the addition of some that apply specifically to couple interviews are appropriate.

1. Clarify What the Couple Wants

Although one member of the couple may complain about the marital relationship, or may have consulted the clinician because of such difficulties, it cannot be assumed that either the troubled spouse or the couple wants to do something about the problem; that is, the complaint may be neither a "cry for help" nor an indication of "motivation for change."

Similarly, even though the couple has sought help, they may not wish to have the clinician take charge. When working with couples, individuals, or families, the clinician must remember that the responsibility for change lies with the patient(s) and not with the health professional. Consequently, a deliberate effort must be made to clarify the individual's, couple's, or family's expectations and goals.

2. *Remain Neutral*

One of the key challenges in interviewing couples is the ability to remain neutral: not to form an alliance or even appear to side with one of the spouses. Identifying with, or sympathizing with the position of, one member of the couple may not only impair the professionals's subsequent ability to help the couple, but may, indeed, aggravate the existing dysfunction of the couple system.

The clinician and the partners of a couple form a triangle and, as Stahmann and Hiebert[22] have stated, three interactional combinations are possible: mediation, alliance, and collusion. Constant awareness of these three possible interactions on the part of the physician or nurse is essential to success in avoiding them.

In addition to recognizing the need to remain neutral and monitoring his or her own reactions to the couple's interactions, the adoption of certain interviewing techniques can help the physician or nurse maintain a position of neutrality. He or she should ensure that both partners get a chance to talk about each issue; elicit the other partner's feedback on a particular topic under review by asking "What do you think about this?"; observe and reflect the other partner's reactions; and resist any tendency to get pulled into an "individual interview." The mere act of pushing one's chair back or looking at one spouse when the other is talking can also help the clinician to remain, and appear to remain, neutral.

3. *Attempt to Decrease Anxiety*

Couples, like individuals, often feel shame or embarrassment about their problems. It behooves the physician or nurse to be sensitive to this issue and to attempt to create an atmosphere in which both members of the couple will feel comfortable.

A number of strategies to decrease the anxiety of couples can be followed. The first, and most important, is constant vigilance against "blaming" during the couple interview. Progressing from individual blaming and fault-finding to the mutual exploration of goals and decisions is a definite challenge in working with couples. The interviewer will often have to intervene actively, and even interrupt an unproductive style of communication, by pointing out to the couple exactly what they are doing and why it will lead nowhere.

Maintaining a "systems" view during the interview, and sharing this perspective with the couple, can also contribute to the avoidance of a "blaming" stance. For example, asking one partner how he or she contributes to the problem voiced by the other can serve the dual function of detracting from initial fault-finding and helping to educate the couple to think of their relationship in terms of an interacting system.

In the earlier example of the "spendthrift wife" and the "withdrawn husband," each partner's "problem behaviors" may have become exaggerated by the response of the other partner. If the clinician is aware of these vicious cycles, the couple can also become aware of them by answering questions such as the following: "What do you do when your husband is silent? Does pushing him to talk more make him talk more or less? Does your wife nag you more or less when you withdraw?"

Finally, the clinician should allow each person to tell his or her own story, should not "push" the couple to disclose its secrets, should not encourage continuation of circular, repetitive fighting, and should not interpret or "feedback" all observed behaviors and sequences at the beginning of the interview.

4. *Encourage the Couple to Talk to Each Other*

Although people usually feel that they have to talk to the interviewer, the partners in a couple should be encouraged to talk to each other. This strategy helps the clinician to avoid the role of "go-between" or mediator, and provides useful insight into how the spouses communicate. Once again, simple maneuvers like pushing one's chair back or suggesting that the couple face each other and use the word "You" rather than "He" or "She" will facilitate direct communication.

5. *Focus on the Positive as well as the Negative*

When patients present with problems, the strengths of their situation are often overlooked. Accordingly, particular care should be taken in focusing on the positive aspects of a couple's relationship. At times, it is helpful to asks the couple to recount their courtship and early years of marriage to reactivate their original sense of couplehood, and to dispel some of the current tensions. The clinician should not, however, dwell on past mistakes, for an emphasis on the present and the future will more easily promote a sense of optimism and hope.

The Couple Assessment

In working with couples, clinicians must consciously separate their own ideal concepts of marriage from the couple's concept of what constitutes a functional marriage for them; "idealism" and "health" must not be confused. Clinicians who deal with illness and endeavor to promote health are frequently inclined to seek a definition for a "healthy" marriage. It is more constructive, however, to abandon this approach and to concentrate on discovering whether the couple is able to meet its own needs and provide for the growth of the members of the nuclear family.*

To assess the couple's relationship accurately, the answers to the following key questions must be routinely sought:

1. What is the couple's commitment, both to each other and to making the marriage work? Couples often present with problems and appear to be asking for help despite the fact that they do not want to remain together. Consequently, it must not be assumed that a request for help implies a commitment to the marriage or that it is the clinician's role to keep the couple together at "any cost."

2. What is the couple's motivation for change?

3. What are the couple's goals? What changes in the marriage does each partner desire in order to feel more satisfied? The first step in working with couples frequently involves helping them to negotiate what they would like to work on together. A written description of the desired behavioral changes can facilitate this process, and can also be used at a later date to assess progress.

4. What is the couple's history?

The acronym PRACTICE denotes one systematic approach to family assessment; it is equally applicable to couples. Given that most of the characteristics requiring assessment for families overlap with those for couples, only a brief review is required to point out the particular emphasis appropriate to each category when dealing with couples rather than families.

P (The Problem)

The couple's problems may be expressed directly or indirectly to the practitioner. That is, a spouse may come in complaining of marital problems or a variety of psychosomatic complaints that relate to the couple relationship. In the latter situation, the astute clinician will aim to discern the real problem and help the patient to see the link between his or her symptoms and marital concerns. Couple problems generally occur in three areas:† in the area of couple "tasks", or activities, such as finances, recreation, child rearing, relationships with in-laws and friends, religion, or sex; in the couple's ability to communicate with each other and to solve problems effectively; and in the area of need satisfaction and the fulfillment of expectations.

---

*Please see Chapter 2 for a discussion of family characteristics that tend to promote need satisfaction and mutual growth.

---

†For a more detailed discussion of couple problems, refer to "Common Stresses im Marriage", an earlier section in this chapter.

A good history of the couple's presenting problem(s) usually includes the following data. Who identifies the problem? Do both partners agree on what the problem is? Is it an individual, couple or family problem? How long has the problem existed? Under what conditions did it arise, and what solutions have been tried? Often, the solution can become a problem in itself.

> As Mrs. G.'s four teenage children were growing up, she began to feel more and more "unproductive" and socially isolated. Although she had a few friends, she felt that she did not have enough activities to keep her busy.
>
> In an attempt to be helpful, Mr. G. called his wife once a day with an "idea": "Why don't you go to Jennifer's today?" or "Why don't you go to the Shopping Plaza?" In the evening, he brought home newspaper clippings describing local community activities.
>
> When Mrs. G. finally came to talk to her nurse about her recent problems, she described her husband's "pushing" her as more troublesome than her social isolation.

If a couple comes in and says, "We are unhappy," the exact meaning of that statement must be defined and the underlying problem must be clearly specified. Are the partners not communicating? Are they not able to show affection to each other? Are they not able to meet each other's needs?

A complete inventory of the couple's problems and strengths, and an estimate of the priority and severity of each problem, are basic requirements for the development of any effective intervention strategy. Completing the "PRACTICE" form or utilizing a standardized questionnaire are useful methods of collecting and assembling this information.[24]

Use of the family tree (see Chapter 11) can also be extended to couple problems in order to increase insight and decrease blaming.

R (Roles and Structures)

Family roles are the repetitive patterns of behavior by which individuals fulfill family functions.[12] Accordingly, questions like those that follow form an integral part of couple assessments. Who has what role in the couple relationship? Who makes decisions? Who nurtures? Who takes care of the house? Who earns the family livelihood? Are both the husband and wife satisfied with their roles, or would they like to see them changed? What kind of change would each partner like? What happens when one partner becomes ill? Are the partners able to alter their roles according to need? Is there room for individual growth and development?

Role flexibility and satisfaction are significant dimensions of healthy family functioning while the distribution of power and its correlation with role distribution, role expectations, and negotiations around power may be a source of dissatisfaction.[14]

A (Affect)

How a couple expresses emotion is a variable of such importance that it warrants specific assessment. Are the partners able to express feelings of joy and happiness, or anger and sadness, without feelings of guilt or remorse? What consequences follow the expression of such emotions? Are the spouses satisfied with their ability to share feelings?

How is affection expressed? How is anger expressed? Is each member of the couple able to accept the differences in their modes of expressing emotions? Is there evidence of mutual support in the couple system? Couples who present with difficulties are often dissatisfied with the expression and sharing of emotions in their relationship, as well as with the opposite partner's ability to fulfill his or her needs for dependency, intimacy, security, or self-esteem.

The degree of involvement of each partner in couple and family life is another important affective dimension. How "involved" do the partners feel? How do they spend their time together? Are they able to have fun together? Do they share common interests? How satisfactory is their sex life?

C (Communication)

Communication refers to the process by which the couple exchanges information about feelings (Affect) and ideas. Assessment of the couple's communication skills requires evaluation of each partner's ability both to express his or her ideas to the other and to listen to the other. Does each partner feel "heard"? Couples often blur the distinction between being heard and being accepted. Is the couple able to accept differences in their individual modes of communicating? One partner may be more verbal than the other; one partner may be more emotional.

Communication difficulties may express themselves in a variety of ways. Couples may complain that they do not have anything to talk about, that they do not spend enough time talking to each other, that they do not feel listened to, or that they cannot express themselves. Observing the couple's style of communication in the office is one of the best ways of assessing their strengths and weaknesses in this area.

Satir[20] has described four styles of communication that can lead to dysfunction in the couple system: blaming, placating, leveling, and distracting. Each of these styles impedes the resolution of problems and generally reinforces the feeling of individual dissatisfaction and couple unhappiness. Identification of each couple's particular style of communication is a helpful first step. This should be followed by an assessment of the couple's ability to solve problems and reach decisions. How do the partners arrive at everyday practical decisions? How do they resolve affective problems? Do they deal with issues or avoid them? Do they jump from one problem to the other, or do they meaningfully attempt to solve one problem at a time? Once again, observing the spouses' problem solving behaviors in the office can provide the most helpful clues about how they function as a couple.

T (Time in the Life Cycle)

The couple's position in the marital life cycle adds a particular dimension to the couple's functioning. On the one hand, the developmental tasks required at each life cycle stage may evoke certain stresses on the couple system. For example, the birth of a child necessitates a readjustment in the couple's roles and relationships with the extended families and friends. If the couple has been experiencing problems in these areas prior to the arrival of the baby, this additional stress may tip the precarious equilibrium achieved to date. Although some couples decide to have a child in order to improve their marital relationship, the advent of children usually aggravates existing tensions.

On the other hand, couple problems present themselves differently at different stages of the life cycle. During the first few years of marriage, conflicts usually center on the couple's relationships with the extended family and friends, money management, the use of time, sex, and careers. Issues of power and dependency and the task of negotiating rules around these issues are themes that run throughout the first few years of marriage.

With the advent of children, new issues emerge. Pressures and limitations on the couple system increase, and dissatisfaction will inevitably ensue if the couple is unable to deal with these new demands. With the arrival of the first child, a triangle is set up; at times, the newly formed closeness between mother and child may lead to a felt or real exclusion of the father. The father, however, may not be able to express his feelings of exclusion or jealousy; instead he may start a common paternal pattern of increased involvement at work. Early recognition of this type of problem by the family physician is an important ingredient in effective counselling.

The children's entrance into adolescence often coincides with the parents' own midlife transitions. At this stage, they may be questioning their achievements in life, and they may wonder what the coming years have to offer. As a couple, they may have to readjust and find a new equilibrium, and concerns around finances, occupation, and sex may again become prominent.

I (Illness)

Illness may stress the couple's ability to function as a unit, provoke anxiety or fear in one or both of the spouses, or dictate a change in the partners' roles.* It may also be a way of expressing needs for dependency, attention, or power. Interestingly, although the person who is ill is apparently weak, illness can also confer power.

> Mrs. K., a 46-year-old patient of Dr. C., had been asking her husband, 50 years of age, to participate in household tasks for many months. Although Mr. K. accepted the principle of "shared responsibilities," he felt that his responsibilities at work did not allow him the necessary time. Nevertheless, whenever Mrs. K. became ill, he left his work responsibilities and took care of the house. Indeed, Mrs. K.'s illness behavior seemed to give her the control that she could not gain otherwise.

In couples who have difficulty expressing or accepting the expression of emotions, illness may be more readily accepted than unhappiness or depression. Consequently, the couple's "rules of communication" can precipitate illness behavior just as illness can enhance or decrease communication.

C (Coping with Stress)

How a couple copes with change and stress provides an indication of its strengths as a unit. Troll[25] has identified three ways in which the family system can react to the changes that accompany normal development: it can compensate in a manner that seeks to maintain the system's existing state; it can accept and incorporate change as part of the desirable growth and development of the system; or it can break up.

The couple's response to change, therefore, requires evaluation. Does the couple see change as a threat or as an opportunity for growth? Are the partners able to provide mutual support or do their different styles of coping with stress increase their marital tensions?

E (Ecology)

The couple's social, cultural, educational, and economic environment,[21] and their interactions with it, deserve inclusion in any thorough couple assessment. What are the couple's relationships with their extended families? Do they have friends? Are they involved in community activities? Do they have the educational and economic resources necessary to meet their needs? Although enmeshment with either family of origin can cause problems in the couple system, harmonious relationships can facilitate the development of a good support system and a smoother transition into marriage. The

---

*See Chapter 20 for a complete discussion of the effects of illness on the couple family system.

availability of resources and an adequate support system is an important index of the couple's ability to cope with and adapt to stress.

CLINICAL MANAGEMENT OF COUPLE PROBLEMS

Following the initial assessment of the couple, which may occur in one or several interviews, the clinician will generally share his or her perceptions and impressions with the couple. In doing so, it is helpful to combine this feedback with the couple's own perceptions of their difficulties. The greater the congruence between the clinician's and the couple's impressions, the easier it is for feedback to flow in both directions.*

Occasionally, the physician or nurse may be in the more difficult position of identifying other problems not perceived by the couple. In this situation, the clinician often wonders whether it is appropriate or constructive to share such impressions with the couple. As a general rule, the clinician should discuss his or her perceptions or systems formulation of the problem, as this discussion is helpful in clarifying the basic problem and how each partner plays a role in maintaining it. This may increase the couple's willingness and motivation to seek help when it is needed. It must be remembered, however, that it is the couple's responsibility to decide what they will do with such information once it has been given to them.

To return to the first two cases described in the introduction to this chapter:

> When Mrs. A. was seen by her nurse because of recurrent palpitations and weakness, it was important for the nurse to help Mrs. A. to draw the link between her symptoms and her marital stress. As part of the process, the nurse invited Mr. A. to come in for an interview with his wife—which he did willingly. During the conjoint interview, a number of couple problems were identified, including Mr. A.'s non-demonstration of his affection for his wife in a way that she desired, and Mrs. A.'s silence about her dissatisfactions. When the nurse discussed her perceptions of these difficulties and outlined possible ways of modifying each partner's behavior, the couple responded by stating their unwillingness to work on these problems at that time. The decision was theirs. Several months later, however, the couple returned to see the nurse with other manifestations of the same problems, and this time they expressed the desire to seek help. The couple was then seen for eight sessions in short-term counselling. The focus of the interventions was on how Mr. and Mrs. A. had each learned to express, and to interpret the expression of, affection; how they currently demonstrated and received the expression of affection (for example, Mrs. A. felt that bringing home a

---

*Please see Chapter 15 for a detailed discussion of how to give feedback or clarification to couples and families.

steady income was a sign of his "love" for his wife; Mrs. A. felt that physical touch was an indication of caring); and how they might learn new ways of communicating their feelings to each other.

Airing their problems in the presence of a third person not only helps a couple to clarify and to understand their concerns, but often has a therapeutic effect in itself. Following Mrs. M.'s expression of her desire to have a "slice of the pie," her physician suggested a joint interview with her husband. During this interview, Mrs. M. openly voiced her dissatisfaction with her more traditional role of wife and mother, and she went on to say that this was the first time she had felt comfortable in doing so. She was also able to explain to her husband what she wanted out of the marriage in a way that enabled him to hear her requests. For Mrs. M., her husband's witnessed expression of understanding and support was a source of significant help and a positive aid in putting her concerns into perspective.

The clinician's assessment of a couple's problems, functioning, and goals, and his or her level of expertise and available time, will determine the management plan. The clinician may, for example, wish to reassure the couple that their experience is a normal one, to provide them with needed information, to facilitate their interaction by making specific suggestions, to engage in short-term counselling, or to refer the couple to an appropriate specialist. These strategies parallel the interventions discussed in the chapter on working with families.

Validation and Normalization

Given the nature of our general education and socialization patterns, and the prevalence of unrealistic expectations about marriage, many couples do not realize that successful marriage can involve much hard work and compromise. The clinician often has an important role to play in helping couples to understand that some degree of marital strain is "normal" and that the realities of marriage may differ significantly from initial expectations.

If we return to the case of Mr. P., who was dissatisfied with his wife because she did not make him as happy as she "should," the physician was able to help Mr. P. to explore the basis of his expectations and to demystify some of his original myths about marriage. In part he accomplished this by encouraging Mr. P. to talk about his childhood perceptions of his parents' "happy" marriage; in part, by asking Mr. P. to read several chapters in *The Mirages of Marriage*,[16] a book which normalizes a number of common marital stresses.

The physician or nurse can also assure the couple that other couples in similar circumstances may be experiencing similar difficulties, and thereby help the couple to put their problems into a more informed perspective. For example, if a couple who are in their mid-50s come to the physician because they are questioning themselves and their marriage, the clinician can observe that at least part of this questioning is "normative" during this stage of their lives, and he or she can help the couple to differentiate between their concerns about themselves as individuals and as partners. As a result, the couple may gain the feeling that they are not "different," and that what they are experiencing "makes sense." Imparting the feeling to the couple that they are understood, and that their problems are shared is helpful in itself because the validation of their feelings can be a powerful new experience. The danger in "normalizing" too readily is the possibility of overlooking the uniqueness of each individual and providing hasty reassurances. Accordingly, the clinician should be cautious about choosing this mode of intervention.

When the physician considers normalization or validation to be inappropriate, he or she may opt for another intervention strategy.

Support

The clinician may choose to provide the couple with "support" during a difficult time, such as the loss of a job; the onset of a serious, chronic illness, or marital separation. Listening empathically to the couple's problems and concerns and helping them mobilize their own resources can be of significant help in stressful times.

If we return to Mr. R., the 48-year-old high school teacher who called his physician asking for help in telling his wife that he wanted a divorce, the physician invited Mr. R. to come in to discuss the problem. Although Mr. R. was not told what to do, he was given help in exploring the issues, in re-evaluating his decision, and in considering the consequences of embarking on such a course. Once Mr. R. had spoken with his wife, the physician was able to meet with them as a couple, on a number of occasions—not to "save the marriage," but to help to keep the divorcing process more "human". By providing the couple with a forum for discussion and support during the crisis period, the physician was able to help them to deal with some of the anger and sadness that they were feeling about their dissolving marriage. He was also able to explain to them some of the "tasks" involved in the process of separation. In this way he was able to combine support with the provision of information.

Some of the more instrumental tasks in separating include telling the family, telling friends, and making decisions regarding finances, shared belongings, etc. If children are involved, explaining the separation to the children and making decisions regarding custody and visitation rights are of paramount importance. Some of the more "emotional" tasks that people often face in separating include the need to "understand" what happened, the need to deal with the inherent sadness and anger, rejection and guilt, and disappointment in having "failed" at making the marriage succeed, and doubts about the decision, and the need to "start over again" and "refuel" a demoralized sense of self.

Mr. and Mrs. R. had thought about a number of the "instrumental" tasks which the physician had discussed with them. They had considerable difficulty in adjusting to the emotional demands of the separation. It was in talking about these feelings with the physician, and in reading *Marital Separation* by Robert Weiss[26] that they began to discover some sense of relief.

Mr. and Mrs. S., patients of Dr. C., had become increasingly depressed over the last 6 months, following the marriage of their 24-year-old daughter to a young man of whom they did not approve. Both parents were upset by their daughter's choice of husband and yet were unable to share these feelings with each other. For years they had entered a pattern of "protecting" each other from hurtful feelings, and it was difficult to break this habit. Following four conjoint interviews with Dr. C., in which they had the opportunity to express these feelings to each other and to question why they were unhappy about their daughter's choice, they were able to deal with the situation more effectively. Their symptoms of depression also decreased.

Education and Anticipatory Guidance

Anticipatory guidance refers to the preventive work of the family practitioner, and is particularly important before marriage, at each life cycle stage, and during the management of acute and chronic illness. In each situation the clinician can, on the basis of personal knowledge of the partners, assess whether the couple is able to meet its developmental tasks and can, if necessary, help the couple to prepare for the challenges ahead.

Occasionally, clinicians question the feasibility and utility of anticipatory guidance. For example, with respect to premarital counselling, it is questionable whether we know enough to predict "successful" marriages or whether a couple that has decided to get married is open to advice from any physician or nurse. The clinician may also wonder whether giving advice will harm an ongoing relationship of trust and respect. Although these questions cannot be easily answered, it is important for the physician to help the couple become aware of the relevant issues and concerns. The physician or nurse, by skillfully posing a number of questions to his or her patients during their premarital exam, can, for example, help them to reflect on their own "readiness" as well as the tasks which face them in getting married.[7] Similar issues arise at different moments in the life cycle.

Facilitation of Interaction and Specific Suggestions

At times, the physician or nurse can help the couple to become aware of their interactional difficulties by pointing out their "communication hazards" (blaming, talking indirectly about a problem, not taking responsibility for one's own feelings), and by suggesting alternative ways of communicating with each other. During an office visit, the nurse can encourage the couple to talk openly and directly to each other, to avoid blaming or wallowing in the past, and to not "second-guess" the partner. If the clinician sees that the couple is able to pick up on these suggestions, he or she may decide to see the couple for a number of sessions. If not, the clinician may discuss referral with them.

The physician or nurse may also help couples to improve their ability to problem-solve and negotiate. Although the clinician cannot solve the couple's problems, he or she can help the partners improve their "process" of communication.

> Mrs. N., a 24-year-old mother of two preschool children, came to see her physician, Dr. L., because of increasing feelings of fatigue. During the routine inquiry, Mrs. N. easily talked about the fact that she was feeling very tense and anxious in recent months. She felt that much of her stress was due to the fact that she and her husband, a 26-year-old laborer, were living in the country together with Mr. N.'s mother, who had been deserted by her husband 3 years before their marriage.
>
> Mrs. N. was currently feeling very isolated in the country. She was far from her own family and she had few friends. She felt that her mother-in-law was constantly criticizing her about the way in which she was raising her children ("I did it differently when I was your age."); and she felt that she did not have any time "alone" with her husband.
>
> When Dr. L. suggested that Mr. N. join Mrs. N. for her next appointment, she quickly agreed. In contrast to Mrs. N., Mr. N. was very quiet during the interview and reluctant to talk about his "wife's troubles." Nevertheless, he did express a willingness to do whatever he could to help his wife. He did not feel that he had any problems.
>
> As a result of Dr. L.'s careful, but nonthreatening questioning, Mr. N. began to question whether he, too, had a role to play in his wife's fatigue and anxiety. In talking about their move to the country, he realized that in many ways it had been his decision to live in a house adjacent to his mother's. His wife, on the other hand, realized that she had never openly told her husband that she didn't want to move to the country. She had grown up in a home fraught with tension between her parents, and she was determined to avoid problems with her husband "at any cost." In a way, she felt that the slightest disagreement might lead to threats of separation. Mr. N., on the other hand, had felt responsible for his mother for many years. His father, who had had a drinking problem, had physically abused his mother on a number of occasions, and Mr. N. had always felt that he had to protect her. For him, not living with his mother was equated with abandoning her, much in the way that his father had done.
>
> At the end of the interview, Mr. and Mrs. N. had begun to redefine their problem. Two weeks later, when they returned for a follow-up

appointment, they discussed a number of possible solutions to "their" problem. They chose the one with which they were most comfortable: they put their house up for sale!

The clinician may also decide to test out certain "specific suggestions" with couples. For example, during the regular prenatal visit of an expectant couple, the physician finds out that the woman is worried about her husband's future involvement in child rearing. She is concerned that he will be at work "as usual," and that she will be "stuck" in the house. The clinician has several options before him. He or she can allow the couple to express their worries and concerns; can trace the roots of their concerns to events in their past; or can suggest that both become involved in prenatal classes. At times, the latter suggestion may be the most helpful strategy for decreasing the woman's worries and concerns for she will see that her husband is "involved." However, if the couple is unable or unwilling to follow through with this suggestion, or if the clinician sees that the woman's worries are increasing, he or she can suggest further counselling to the couple.

> Jean Luc O., a 26-year-old unemployed construction worker returned to his physician on a number of occasions with "incapacitating" backaches for which no physical cause was found. Because he was becoming increasingly frustrated that the physician was not prescribing physical therapy or making further investigations, he decided to bring his girlfriend with him on the next visit, to "convince the doctor to do something."
> Jean Luc was sharing an apartment with his girlfriend, Suzanne L., a 24-year-old school teacher. They had been living together for the past year.
> During the interview, Suzanne talked earnestly about the problem. She was troubled by her boyfriend's pain and frustrated by the effect it was having on their social and personal lives. They had not gone out with friends for months and they rarely left the apartment. Although Suzanne questioned whether she would be able to stay in this relationship, she and Jean Luc rarely talked about what was happening to them as a couple. Rather, it appeared as if the focus of their relationship was on his "back aches."
> Shortly before the end of the interview, Suzanne, who had done most of the talking, asked what she could do to help Jean Luc. She said that she massaged his back whenever the pain seemed unbearable, and she was wondering whether she should continue to do so.
> Concerned about the couple's pattern of communication, and the role of Jean Luc's physical problems in their couple system, the physician suggested that they return for a number of sessions, to continue talking about their relationship and to explore alternative ways to communicate their feelings. Suzanne thought this was an excellent idea. Jean Luc said that he wasn't interested. He wanted "physiotherapy, not psychotherapy."
> The physician suggested that they not make a "hasty" decision, in any case, and that in the meantime, Suzanne continue to massage Jean Luc,

with one minor modification. Rather than massaging him when he was in pain, she was to massage him with a number of body lotions and oils when he was "pain free."

One month later, Suzanne phoned to thank the physician for his time. Although she did not understand why, Jean Luc's back problem had improved significantly.

Couples may also complain that they do not spend enough leisure time together; one of the partners may complain that they no longer go out together, or that too much time is spent with the children. Suggesting that the couple take one night for themselves may help the couple to break the vicious cycle of "not enough time."

Not all problems can be solved in the physician's office. Sometimes, however, discussing one's problems on neutral grounds can be helpful in itself. The couple can gain a new perspective on their problems, and possible solutions may become more evident.

Short-Term Counselling

Some physicians or nurses may wish to become involved in short-term counselling for particular couple problems. This decision will be based on their skill and expertise in counselling, their own interests and available time, the existence of appropriate community resources, and the nature of the couple's problems. Relatively circumscribed problems of recent onset are generally more amenable to short-term counselling, as are problems that can be dealt with in the present and do not require a thorough understanding of the past.

Patient characteristics also play a part in the clinician's decision. Motivation and insight on the part of the couple is key, as is the patient's belief that counselling can be helpful.[2] Moreover, if the clinician sees that the couple is able to use the office experience to their advantage and follow through on some of the specific suggestions made, this may be considered a positive indication for couple counselling. However, if it becomes evident that the couple is unable to agree on which problems need to be worked on, this will be a contraindication for short-term counselling.

If the physician or nurse does decide to follow through on short-term counselling, a number of principles should be kept in mind.

1. The clinician should establish trust and rapport with both partners. This may have been built up in previous encounters with the couple, or may be part of the current process.

2. The clinician, together with the couple, should establish clear-cut, specified goals for therapy. For example, the goal of a "happier" marriage cannot be worked on or achieved. What does a "happier" marriage mean? What would have to change for a couple to feel more satisfied? More specific

goals such as "spending more time together" or an "enhanced sexual life" need to be specified before therapy can begin.

Following the identification and clarification of the couple's problems, priorities should be determined, and one target for change should be chosen. Often, the stage of identifying goals and negotiating priorities is a helpful and "change-producing" process in itself.

3. The clinician and the couple should make a "contract" regarding the structure of counselling. This contract should include the frequency of visits, the length of each session, and the total number of sessions before re-evaluating change. Moreover, regular visits (that is, weekly or bi-weekly) should be scheduled if the clinician would like to observe change. Monthly visits become "check-ups" rather than "change-oriented" sessions.

4. The clinician should help the couple work towards change by focusing on the mutual exploration of problems, a discussion of possible solutions, and action-oriented interventions. The assignment of homework tasks, which enable the couple to work on change outside the clinician's office, should also be considered.

An awareness of "quid pro quo" principles and effective problem-solving strategies can be helpful to the clinician. "Quid pro quo" techniques[16,23] refer to a behavioral exchange model that is useful in working with mildly or moderately distressed couples. In this process, couples define the behaviors that they would like to see increased or changed in their partners and they make an agreement to "exchange" one new behavior for another. Although this strategy may appear simplistic at first glance, research has indicated that such training in communication and negotiation can help certain couples resolve their differences and increase their marital satisfaction.[15,23] Similar results have also been found in studies that have attempted to teach problem-solving strategies to couples.[12]

Given that couples often lack effective problem-solving strategies, the clinician can actually guide couples in becoming more adept in this process. The stages of effective problem-solving include the following:

1. identification of the problem;
2. communication of the problem and determining of priorities;
3. development of alternative action plans: "brain-storming";
4. deciding regarding suitable action;
5. action;
6. monitoring the action; and
7. evaluation of the success of the action

By going through a model such as this, the physician or nurse can help couples work through various problems without giving them advice or attempted solutions.

5. A method for evaluating change should be incorporated, as should a system for follow-up and maintenance of couple growth.

Referral

In order for the clinician to refer appropriately, he or she must be aware of the available forms of marital therapy, as well as their potential effectiveness.

Marriage counselling or therapy refers to the systematic application of techniques or interventions that are intended to modify the maladaptive or maladjustive relationships of married couples.[13] Generally, the major focus of change is the marital relationship.

The major forms of marital counselling include the following:

1. Individual counselling, whereby only one spouse is treated for the purpose of resolving marital difficulties;
2. concurrent marital counselling, whereby both spouses are treated in separate, individual interview sessions for the purpose of resolving marital difficulties; and
3. conjoint marital counselling, whereby both spouses are treated together in the same interview session.[8]

These above modalities can all occur in a group format (multiple individuals or multiple couples), and may vary according to the theoretical orientation of the therapist (that is, psychoanalytic, behavioral).

Conjoint counselling is the most widely used format for treating marital and sexual problems.[8,13] Although the relevant research is not conclusive, it does suggest that conjoint therapy is the most beneficial and effective strategy for resolving couple problems. Individual therapy, which is the least effective, has a significantly higher reported frequency of deterioration.[4,13]

At present, the expected improvement rate for couples involved in marital therapy is 66%.[13] Such an improvement rate is relatively encouraging, as interestingly, the spontaneous remission rate for marital problems is approximately 17%.[13] Changes that are expected to occur as a result of marital counselling include increased satisfaction towards the marriage, modifications in communication patterns, reduced hostility and conflict, and an improved self-image.[4]

Physicians and nurses can fulfill a number of tasks in referring patients to therapy. First, they can help the couple to "reframe" the problem. Often, when couples are in conflict, they tend to identify one or the other as the focus of the problem. The clinician can help the partners refocus on the relationship rather than on each other. Secondly, the physician can prepare the couple for therapy. By exploring the couple's problems and strengths, the clinician can set the stage for later couple therapy. He or she can also increase the couple's motivation for change by demonstrating his or her own confidence in the consultant and in the therapeutic process. Given that motivation is a key ingredient to therapeutic success, the clinician's initial work with the couple can be very helpful and productive. The clinician can also help the couple choose the right therapeutic modality; "consumers" of therapy are often not aware of what would be most helpful to them. The physician or nurse can guide couples appropriately, and then provide for follow-up and an evaluation of change. The process of referral is an essential aspect of the clinician's interventions with couple problems and one that should not be underestimated.

REFERENCES

1. Ables BS: *Therapy for Couples*. San Francisco, Jossey-Bass, 1977.

2. Anstett R, Hipskind M: Selecting patients for brief office counseling. *J Fam Prac* 13:195–199, 1981.

3. Bane MJ: *Here to Stay*. New York, Basic Books, 1976.

4. Beck DF: Research Findings on the outcomes of marital counseling, in Olson DH (ed): *Treating Relationships*. Lake Mills, Iowa: Graphic Publishing, 1976.

5. Bischoff LJ: *Adult Psychology*, ed 2. New York, Harper & Row, 1976.

6. Bissonnette R, Tapp J: Premarital marital counseling, in Taylor RB (ed): *Family Medicine: Principles and Practice*. New York, Springer-Verlag, 1973.

7. Burchinal LG: Trends and Prospects for Young Marriages in the United States. *J Marr Fam* 27:251, 1965.

8. Cookerly JR: Evaluating different approaches to marriage counseling, in Olson DH (ed): *Treating Relationships*. Lake Mills, Iowa, Graphic Publishing, 1976.

9. Crosby J: *Illusion and Disillusion: The Self in Love and Marriage*. Belmont, California, Wedsworth, 1976.

10. Duvall EM: *Marriage and Family Development*. Philadelphia, J.B. Lippincott, 1977.

11. Ellis A, Harper R: *A Guide to Successful Marriage*. California, Wilshire Book Company, 1974.

12. Epstein N, Bishop DS, Levin S: The McMaster model of family functioning. *Journal of Marriage and Family Counseling* 19–31, 1979.

13. Gurman AS, Kniskern DP: Research in marital and family therapy, in Garfield SL, Bergin AE (eds): *Handbook of Psychotherapy and Behavior Change*, ed 2. New York, John Wiley, 1976.

14. Haley J: Marriage therapy. *Archives of General Psychiatry* 8:213–234, 1963.

15. Jacobson NS: Problem solving and contingency contracting in the treatment of marital discord. *J Consult Clin Psychol* 45:92, 1977.

16. Lederer WJ, Jackson DD: *The Mirages of Marriage*. New York, W.W. Norton, 1968.

17. Medalie JH: Pre- and Early Marital Stage, in Medalie JH (ed): *Family Medicine: Principles and Applications*. Baltimore, Williams & Wilkins, 1978.

18. Okun BF, Rappaport LJ: *Working with Families: An Introduction to Family Therapy.* North Scituate, Massachusetts, Duxbury Press, 1980.

19. Satir V: *Conjoint Family Therapy.* California, Science and Behavior Books, 1967.

20. Satir V: *Peoplemaking.* California, Science and Behavior Books, 1972.

21. Smilkstein G: The family in trouble: How to tell. *J Fam Prac* 2:19–24, 1975.

22. Stahmann RF, Hiebert WJ (eds): *Klemer's Counseling Marital and Sexual Problems: A Clinical Handbook,* ed 2. Baltimore, Williams & Wilkins, 1977.

23. Stuart RB: An operant interpersonal program for couples, in: Olson DH (ed): *Treating Relationships.* Lake Mills, Iowa, Graphic Publishing, 1976.

24. Stuart RB, Stuart F: Marital Precounseling Inventory. Champaign, Illinois, Research Press, 1973.

25. Troll LE: *Early and Middle Adulthood.* Monterey, California, Brooks/Cole, 1975.

26. Weiss RS: *Marital Separation.* New York, Basic Books, 1975.

Chapter 28
Working with Couples:
Sexual Problems

Yvonne Steinert

Couples often present with sexual problems, which may, or may not, be related to other marital difficulties. According to Masters and Johnson (1970), approximately 50% of married couples have sexual problems. Although these problems may be the cause of marital discord, they more frequently represent expressions of underlying dynamics in the couple's relationship. The interplay between sexual problems and marital problems is not clear. Some couples who have sexual problems do not have any marital problems; some couples who have marital problems do not have any sexual problems. In all cases, however, sexual problems should be viewed within the larger context of the couple system.

As patients are often reluctant to discuss their sexual concerns with health professionals, these problems may present as physical complaints, or may only be hinted at during a visit for an apparently unrelated problem. It behooves the physician or nurse to ask specific questions about sexuality and to help patients to discuss their concerns in this area.

Often, careful questioning and the provision of information about sexuality and sexual response patterns may decrease anxiety or improve sexual functioning. At other times, more in-depth counseling may be required. If the clinician is unable to provide this service because of a lack of knowledge or skill, time, or comfort, he or she can refer the couple to an available resource. However, if the latter is unavailable, as in many rural areas, the clinician can facilitate the couple's communication about the problem and can provide them with limited information or specific suggestions.

COMMON SEXUAL PROBLEMS

The commonest sexual problems seen in office practice include premature ejaculation and impotence in the male; anorgasmia, dyspareunia, and vaginismus in the female; and a lack of sexual desire or interest in both partners.

Masters and Johnson define premature ejaculation as the "inability to

476

control the ejaculatory process for a sufficient length of time during intervaginal containment to satisfy the partner during at least 50% of coital intercourse."[11] Most individuals with the problem of premature ejaculation ejaculate just before or immediately upon entering the vagina. If the female is not able to be sexually satisfied for other reasons such as anorgasmia, dissatisfaction with the marriage, this definition does not apply.

Premature ejaculation is the commonest male sexual dysfunction. It is highly prevalent, and occurs in diverse patient populations; it is often unrelated to psychopathology or marital problems. Moreover, it is a normal phenomenon in certain situations such as the first contact during courting, during the first few months of marriage, during the first few contacts after separation, or during a convalescent period after an acute illness.[13] Anxiety can, however, increase the likelihood or severity of this problem, as can sexual difficulties in the partner. Orgasmic difficulties in the female may be associated with premature ejaculation or impotence in the male.

Impotence refers to the inability of the male to achieve an erection sufficient for intromission and maintenance of sexual intercourse.[11] In primary impotence, the male has never been able to achieve an erection; in secondary impotence, the male has been able to have an erection satisfactory for sexual intercourse in the past, but now no longer does, in at least 25% of his encounters. Secondary impotence is the second most commonly reported male sexual problem. The occasional failure that most men experience because of tiredness or distraction is not to be confused with secondary impotence.[3]

The interplay between physiologic and psychological factors in the etiology of impotence is critical. Impotence due primarily to psychological factors accounts for a high percentage of all cases (50% to 90%). Organic causes of impotence include certain systemic illnesses (diabetes), diseases of the nervous system (multiple sclerosis), and certain medications (antihypertensives).*

The problem of definition and classification becomes more complex in the female sexual dysfunctions. For example, the term "frigidity" has generally been used to refer to all forms of inhibition of female sexual response—from a total lack of responsiveness to orgastic inhibition. It is not a helpful concept. As Kaplan[8] has said, the need for a distinction between general sexual dysfunction and orgastic inhibition must be made. That is, one must distinguish between a woman who does not respond to sexual stimulation at all and one who is responsive, but not orgasmic.

---

*Please consult the following references for a good description of the effects of illness and medication on sexuality: Kaplan HS: *The New Sex Therapy.* New York: Brunner/Mazel, 1974. Kaplan HS: *Disorders of Sexual Desire,* II. New York, Brunner/Mazel, 1979. Drugs that Cause Sexual Dysfunction *Med Lett* 23:108, 1981.

General sexual dysfunction refers to the inhibition of the general arousal aspect of the sexual response; it involves a lack of erotic feelings subjectively, and physiologically, there is no vasocongestive response (no lubrication or expanding of the vagina). Primary orgasmic dysfunction refers to the situation in which a woman has never experienced an orgasm; the definition of secondary orgasmic dysfunction is more problematic. Most authors refer to the woman who cannot achieve orgasm during coitus, but who is able to have orgasm through masturbation or the husband's stimulation of the woman, as presenting with secondary orgasmic dysfunction. However, whether this is an actual "dysfunction" can be seriously questioned.

Recent research evidence has supported the finding that women are generally more frequently orgasmic with manual or oral stimulation than with coitus,[7] and it can therefore be questioned whether orgasm with alternative forms of stimulation is a dysfunction, or rather, a variant of sexual response.[8] Perhaps, the concept of "situational anorgasmia" would be more helpful.

Vaginismus refers to the involuntary spasm of the muscles surrounding the vaginal entrance which prevents penetration. Patients with vaginismus are usually phobic about coitus and vaginal penetration. Although vaginismus may be associated with general sexual dysfunction or orgastic inhibition, this is not always so. Many females are sexually responsive, and the phobic response may be due to other factors.

Dyspareunia refers to painful intercourse. This is a common complaint and is generally difficult for physicians to manage.[3] Both psychological and physiologic factors play a role in its etiology; failure to lubricate, infections, anatomic defects, or lacerations in the ligaments that support the uterus may all be causes of dyspareunia. A physical examination is obviously essential and may give additional clues to the problem; lack of pelvic and sphincter relaxation may correlate with sexual anxiety.

Low sexual desire is an increasing frequently presenting complaint. It is generally related to other marital problems, negative attitudes towards sexuality, or "intrapsychic" problems such as depression. How the couple sees the "function" of sexuality in their relationship may also determine the presence or absence of this concern.*

CAUSES OF SEXUAL DIFFICULTIES

Sexual problems may stem from a number of causes. Early experiences (sexual trauma, a strict religious upbringing, parental influences), a lack of

---

*For a more complete description of the common sexual dysfunctions please see: Masters WH, Johnson VE: *Human Sexual Inadequacy.* Boston, Little, Brown and Company, 1970. Kaplan HS. *The New Sex Therapy.* New York, Brunner/Mazel, 1974. Kaplan HS. *Disorders of Sexual Desire, II.* New York, Brunner/Mazel, 1979.

sexual knowledge or skill, poor communication, and interpersonal conflict seem to be the major causes of sexual dysfunction. Physical factors (illness, medications, aging) and psychological variables such as depression, guilt, or low self-esteem may also play an important etiologic role, as may a person's beliefs and cognitions about sexuality. Although factors in the individual's past may have initially caused the presenting problem, factors in the present usually maintain it. That is, physical, psychological and relationship variables interact in such a way as to sustain the dysfunctional sexual interaction.[6]

Anxiety is a key component common to most sexual problems. Masters and Johnson[11] have coined the terms "performance" and "spectator" anxiety. The former refers to anxiety about how one actually "performs" during sexual intercourse; the latter refers to the cognitive pattern in which people observe their responses, and thereby are unable to fully participate during love-making. Both anxieties have been frequently observed in couples with sexual problems, and should be dealt with in therapy.

In working with couples who present with sexual problems, it is important to note that problems that seemingly originate in one spouse may well be triggered by certain responses in the other. For example, in one couple with long-standing impotence in the male, felt by both spouses to be a deep-seated problem needing individual psychotherapy, it became apparent that the wife's complex relationship with men was behind a disinterest in sex that she only later acknowledged. In this case, had the man been seen alone, his wife's problems would have probably remained underground and his own erectile difficulties probably unchanged. As couples are interacting systems, it is best to assume that both partners play a part. Most sex therapists will not treat individuals without their partners.

THE CLINICIAN'S ROLE: ASSESSMENT AND INTERVENTION

The physician or nurse has a key role to play in the assessment and prevention of sexual problems. Studies have shown a direct correlation between the physician's behavior and the identification of sexual problems in patients. If clinicians do not take a sexual history, they identify sexual problems less than 10% of the time; if clinicians ask questions about sexual functioning, they identify problems 50% to 100% of the time.[15] The importance of asking questions about sexual functioning thus becomes self-evident.

There are two levels of history-taking that are important for the family physician or nurse. The first level of questioning occurs during the routine inquiry. It is at this point that the clinician attempts to inquire whether the patient has any concerns or problems around sexuality. The goal, here, is not to take a full sexual history, but rather, to give patients an opportunity to discuss their sexual functioning and to "open the door" to further discussions around sexuality. The clinician's own comfort in asking questions about sexuality and in discussing this topic with patients is essential.*

The second level of questioning involves a sexual history once a problem has been identified. It is at this point that clinicians aim to get a better idea of what the problem is so that they can best help their patients. Further help may include information from the physician or nurse, facilitation or specific suggestions aimed at improving the couple's sexual functioning, or referral. The goals of assessment, at this level are to provide a description or diagnosis of the problem, to clarify the cause, and to indicate appropriate treatment approaches.

Once a problem has been expressed, a sexual history should include the following:

1. *A good description of the problem.* This should include a history of the problem (for example, onset and course of the problem), a description of the circumstances under which it improves or gets worse, the partner's reaction to the problem, and the couple's own understanding of what the problem might be (that is, the patient's concept of the cause and maintenance of the problem). Couples' attempts at dealing with the problem should also be reviewed.

   In getting a description of the couple's sexual problems it is wise to avoid labels. For example, if a woman presents with a nonorgasmic response, it is important to distinguish whether she is actually not able to have an orgasm, or whether her sexual encounters are such that she is not able to become orgasmic. Similarly, when men present with the problem of premature ejaculation, it is important to question whether their partners are anorgasmic.

   Mrs. O., a 29-year-old married mother of two school-age children, came to see her physician, Dr. P., following a radio program on the treatment of sexual problems. Despite some initial hesitation, she wanted to know if he knew of a therapist who could help her become more "sexually satisfied." She had heard that certain treatment programs can help women become "orgasmic."

   Dr. P., told Mrs. O. that he did work with a number of sex therapists, but that he first wanted to get a more detailed description of the problem. In asking a number of relevant questions, it soon became apparent that Mrs. O.'s lovemaking with her husband, a 35-year-old

---

*Please consult the following references for a more elaborate discussion on techniques of sexual interviewing: Green R. Taking a sexual history, in Green R (ed): *Human Sexuality: A Health Practitioner's Text.* Baltimore: Williams & Wilkins, 1976. Hiebert WJ. Talking with clients about sexual problems, in Stahmann RF, Hiebert WJ (eds): *Klemer's Counseling in Marital and Sexual Problems: A Clinician's Handbook,* ed 2. Baltimore, Williams & Wilkins, 1977. Wiens A, Brazman R. A rationale and method for the sexual history in family practice. *J Fam Pract* 5:213, 1977.

career diplomat, was generally hurried. Both she and her husband were uncomfortable with lovemaking because they feared that their children might wake up or need them while they were making love. Foreplay was also very brief. Although Mr. O. had never enjoyed foreplay as much as intercourse, foreplay had decreased significantly in the last year. Mrs. O. had been orgasmic with manual stimulation in the past year, but she had not been "sexually satisfied" in this time period. She had never been orgasmic with intercourse.

At the end of the first interview, Dr. P. told Mrs. O. that he was not sure that "therapy" was indicated, for she and her husband might be able to improve their sexuality with his help. He also questioned whether she was "anorgasmic." He suggested that she return for a follow-up interview with her husband. Mrs. O. agreed willingly.

2. *Information on the couple's sexual repertoire and current love-making behavior.* Often, clinicians and patients feel that this is "private" information. A detailed description of the couple's sexual behavior is, however, required if the problem is to be clearly delineated. This information should include a description of "who does what to whom when," the frequency of various sexual behaviors (foreplay, manual and oral stimulation, masturbation, and coitus), the usual time and place of sexual encounters, and the amount of pleasure that both partners derive from their sexual interaction. The couple's ability to communicate around these issues is an additional area worthy of inquiry.

3. *Information on the couple's present relationship.* This should include a thorough assessment of the couple's marital relationship (as described in the previous chapter) as well as an evaluation of the interplay between their sexual and marital functioning, for a couple's sexual functioning cannot be viewed in isolation from other aspects of the couple system. Questions concerning individual problems and anxieties should also be included in this discussion.

Mr. and Mrs. W., a European couple in their mid-40s, came to see their physician, Dr. S., for "help" with a sexual problem. Mr. W., a university professor, and Mrs. W., a senior administrator in a university hospital, had been married for 15 years. They did not have any children. Mr. and Mrs. W. were concerned by their recent lack of sexual desire. Although they reported that they had enjoyed a "good sex life" for many years, they felt that their sexual "appetites" had diminished in recent years. They were unable to pinpoint what might have changed, but they did feel that they were more upset about the problem recently. Upon further questioning, they revealed that they had decided to seek help now because they "still had a number of good years left." Mrs. W. had celebrated her 45th birthday 2 weeks before this interview.

Although Mr. and Mrs. W. claimed that their couple life "was good, except for sex," their physician had the distinct impression that other marital problems were evident. It seemed that Mrs. W. was quite angry at Mr. W. for his recent travels to a number of professional conferences across the continent, and she wanted him to be "less involved" in his work. Mr. W., on the other hand, seemed to feel threatened by his wife's administrative position and by her "success" at work. He wanted her to be "more of a wife."

At the end of the interview, Dr. S. shared these impressions with the couple, and suggested that their lack of sexual desire was related to these issues. Moreover, he recommended couple therapy to them, rather than a therapy that would focus merely on the enhancement of their sexuality. Mr. and Mrs. W. did not accept this recommendation; they wanted a "sexual enrichment" program. Dr. S. asked them to think about his recomendation first, and if they still disagreed, he would refer them to an appropriate therapist. Two months later, Mrs. W. called to ask for a marital counsellor: she felt that she could no longer cope with her husband's absences, and perhaps she should "try" Dr. S's recommendation.

4. *A complete medical history.* Despite the finding that approximately 90% of sexual problems are related to psychological rather than physiologic variables, the role of physical or biological factors in sexual dysfunctions must always be carefully evaluated.

5. *A history of the couple's previous sexual experiences and relationships.* Inquiries about the individual's premarital—or pre-current relationship—experiences should include the following questions: When and how did you first learn about sexuality? When did you first masturbate? Was masturbation pleasurable or "sinful"? When did you first have intercourse? Was it pleasurable or painful? Did you have orgasms in the past? If so, under what conditions?

The person's sexual history should also include his or her ideas, cognitions, and fantasies about sexuality. Couples with sexual problems often adhere to self-defeating or erroneous beliefs around sex. These may include the belief that both partners must achieve an orgasm during every sexual encounter, that the male's sense of masculinity is dependent on his ability to give his partner an orgasm, that sex during menstruation is harmful, that masturbation is "wrong," or that orgasm with manual or oral stimulation is "incomplete." Such cognitions must be fully explored.

Taking a sexual history such as this can be therapeutic for patients in itself. By asking questions around sexuality, the clinician give the patient "permission" to feel sexual and to be concerned about his or her sexuality; he or she is also able to provide information to the couple. For example, if a middle-aged male is worried because he no longer has erections as quickly as he used to, his nurse may talk to him about the effects of aging on sexuality and reassure him appropriately. Without this information, the patient's fears may increase and he may, eventually, become impotent.

Similarly, a young, recently married couple may express concern because they do not have "simultaneous" orgasms. Again, information and clarification about the human sexual response can prevent the development of a more significant problem. Informing the couple that women are usually slower to reach orgasm than men, and that concerns about performance cause men to ejaculate more quickly and women to respond more slowly, may alleviate anxiety and improve sexual functioning.

To return to the earlier example of Mrs. O.: Dr. P.'s impression that Mr. and Mrs. O. could profit from a brief intervention was confirmed in the couple interview. Both Mr. and Mrs. O. seemed to be very motivated in improving their sexual relationship and they did not seem to have any other significant couple problems. Dr. P. therefore reiterated his earlier impression that he did not think Mrs. O. was "anorgasmic" and asked her whether she was aware that most women achieve orgasm more easily with manual stimulation. As neither she nor Mr. O. were aware of this, he suggested that they both read the *Hite Report*.[7]

Dr. P. then discussed the couple's concern and worry about the children waking up in the middle of the night and he helped them to discuss possible solutions to this problem. These included putting a lock on their door; going out to a hotel, once a week, for the next few weeks, to try to "break" the cycle of anxiety and concern; and "sneaking" home in the middle of the day.

Mr. and Mrs. O. wanted to try the second and third suggestions. However, as it was important to attempt only one new strategy at a time, it was decided that the couple try suggestion 2 in the coming week.

Dr. P. also recommended that the couple not attempt intercourse in the coming week. Instead, he prescribed Sensate Focus I and II, non-genital and genital mutual pleasuring (see next section). Mr. and Mrs. O. readily agreed with this suggestion and they planned to return for a follow-up appointment.

Two weeks later the couple returned saying that they had gone to a small hotel outside of town. They had enjoyed this experience tremendously, and they wanted to go again.

One month later Mrs. O. was no longer concerned about her lack of sexual "responsiveness." She had had an orgasm on two occasions—with manual stimulation—and both she and her husband were confident that their sex life would continue to improve. The cycle of "problem-anxiety-problem" had been broken.

In judging the appropriateness of treatment for a sexual dysfunction, the clinician should determine the existence of a sexual problem, the absence of any major marital, psychiatric, or physical problems, stable couple relations, and a commitment or motivation to engage in a sexual treatment program.[12] He or she should also remember that one partner should not be treated alone, for even if one partner does not complain of a sexual problem as such, he or she influences and is affected by it. Thus, "reframing" before referral can again be helpful.

THE TREATMENT OF SEXUAL PROBLEMS

Although the physician or nurse may not be the one who will eventually "treat" the couple's sexual problem, it is important for him or her to be aware of the major treatment approaches in this area. At present, the major components of sex therapy include:

1. Education and information-giving;
2. Skill training in communication and sexual techniques; and
3. Anxiety reduction and attitude change.

Masters and Johnson's treatment of sexual problems has been the most influential treatment strategy used to date. Short-term in nature, it is directed at symptom removal and not at the more conventional, psychodynamic goals of insight and resolution of unconscious conflicts. Although numerous adaptations of Masters and Johnson's basic treatment components have been made,[6,10] their approach still forms the central core of most treatment interventions. The three major components of the Masters and Johnson approach involve educative counseling, facilitation of open verbal and nonverbal communication, and a graded series of sexual tasks. The tasks are used to enable the couple to relax, to focus on incoming erotic stimuli, and to open channels of communication.* All therapy takes place within the context of the couple.

Although Masters and Johnson have developed a number of specific strategies for particular sexual problems (for example, premature ejaculation), their basic treatment "package" includes an emphasis on communication, the prohibition of intercourse, and the use of sensate focus. The prohibition of intercourse is helpful in alleviating a "pressure to perform" that most couples with sexual problems experience. Sensate focus is a process by which the partners learn to give and receive pleasure by touching and caressing each other's body. The couple is instructed to pick a time when and a place where they can relax freely, and where they can learn the pleasure of

---

*For a detailed description of Masters and Johnson's technique, please see: Masters WH, Johnson VE: *Human Sexual Inadequacy*. Boston, Little, Brown and Company, 1970. Readers interested in the treatment of sexual problems should also consult: Kaplan HS: *The New Sex Therapy*. New York, Brunner/Mazel, 1974.

communicating their likes and dislikes to each other, both verbally and nonverbally. Each partner is to spend time "pleasuring" the other. At the beginning, genital touching is not allowed. Gradually, the genital areas are included, and finally, intercourse is encouraged. An interesting aspect of this technique is that it teaches each partner to assume responsibility for his or her own sexuality instead of expecting the other to "mind read" or sense what they want or enjoy.[9] It is also beneficial in the reduction of anxiety, and in the relearning of "new skills."

Since sexual communication is the most intimate, nonverbal form of couple communication, training in this area may also become a highly potent form of facilitating other aspects of couple interaction. The actual steps of sensate focus include nonerotic physical contact, nongenital stroking and exploration of the body, breast and genital stroking, masturbation to orgasm, and, finally, intercourse.

Some of the more specific techniques for sexual problems include the "squeeze" technique for premature ejaculation, the use of masturbation in the treatment of primary orgasmic dysfunction in women, and the use of vaginal dilators in the treatment of vaginismus. The "squeeze" technique is designed to teach ejaculatory control by increasing the male's awareness of the feelings that immediately precede ejaculation. With the squeeze technique, the woman holds the penis between her thumb and the first two fingers of the same hand, and she squeezes fairly hard for three or four seconds just before ejaculation. The resulting pressure causes the male to lose his urge to ejaculate. Following the "squeeze," the stimulation begins again. Thus, the male learns to tolerate a considerable amount of stimulation before orgasm. This technique is integrated with intercourse after the couple has learned to apply it during sensate focus.

In masturbation training,[2,5,10] the woman is taught to become more comfortable with her body and her genitals, to examine and to explore her genitalia, and to stimulate herself to orgasm. Following the attainment of orgasm on her own (through masturbation or with a vibrator), she is to teach her partner what kind of stimulation she finds pleasurable. The use of erotic materials and fantasy may also be incorporated into her sexual repertoire. The most difficult problem to overcome with this technique is the woman's own attitudes toward masturbation; often, these attitudes become the initial focus of intervention.

The use of graduated dilators or fingers in the treatment of vaginismus enables the woman to learn to tolerate penetration. While this procedure is easy and direct, therapeutic issues in the couple's interaction often remain. Given that the sexual pattern may have previously focused on the woman's pain and anxiety, and the man's frustration, anger, and sometimes guilt,[6] taking away the pain does not guarantee a removal of the surrounding sexual interaction.

Regarding treatment effectiveness, the following information may be helpful to clinicians. Treatment of premature ejaculation offers the most dramatic and stable results. The most frequently used technique is the "squeeze" or "stop start" technique. Rates of success fall between 95% to 100%.[6] Response to this treatment is also little affected by the marital relationship or intrapsychic conflicts. Impotence is more difficult to treat. Moreover, primary impotence is less amenable to treatment than is secondary impotence. The 60% cure rate reported by Masters and Johnson[10] for primary impotence is the best cure rate reported to date. For secondary impotence, despite the problems of definition, Masters and Johnson report a success rate of 75%, whereas other averages fall between 60% to 80%.[6]

For women presenting with the problem of primary anorgasmia, 85% to 100% of the women treated are able to successfully have orgasm under some conditions[10]; there is greater success with orgasm to coitus for women with primary orgasmic dysfunction than for women who present with "secondary" orgasmic problems.[14] Although secondary orgasmic dysfunction should be considered a variant of sexual response rather than a "dysfunction" as such, the present treatment effectiveness rates for orgasm with coitus fall between 60% to 75%.[6,10] This is due to the fact that secondary orgasmic dysfunction is most often related to other marital problems.

Vaginismus compares with premature ejaculation in terms of its responsiveness to treatment. Success rates of 90% to 95% are common, using some variation of a physical dilation program.[4] Statistics on treatment effectiveness for "low sex drive" are not yet available.* However, since low sex drive is usually related to other marital problems, treatment effectiveness clearly depends on the success of marital counseling.

Annon[1] has described the PLISSIT model for the management of sexual problems: P refers to permission giving; LI refers to limited information; SS refers to specific suggestions; and IT refers to intensive therapy. This model is helpful in conceptualizing the involvement of physicians or nurses in the management of sexual problems. Many clinicians feel sufficiently comfortable in this area in order to give "permission" and "limited information" to their patients; "specific suggestions" or "intensive therapy" may depend more on the couple's presenting problem as well as the clinician's own interest and expertise in this area.

REFERENCES

1. Annon J: *The Behavioral Treatment of Sexual Problems, I.* Hawaii, Kapiolani Health Services, 1974.

---

*With regard to these statistics, it is worthwhile to note that the field of sex therapy is only 10 years old and that research in this area is still in its infancy.

2. Barbach G: *For Yourself—The Fulfillment of Female Sexuality*. New York, Doubleday & Company, 1975.

3. Belliveau F, Richter L: *Understanding Human Sexual Inadequacy*. New York, Bantam Books, 1970.

4. Fuchs K, Hoch Z, Paldi E: Hypo-desensitization Therapy of Vaginismus. *Int J Clin Exp Hyp* 21:144, 1973.

5. Heiman J, LoPiccolo J, LoPiccolo L: *Becoming Orgasmic: A Sexual Growth Program for Women*. Englewood Cliffs, New Jersey, Prentice Hall, 1976.

6. Heiman JR, LoPiccolo J, LoPiccolo L. The treatment of sexual dysfunction, in Gurman AS, Kniskern DP (eds): *Handbook of Family Therapy*. New York, Brunner/Mazel, 1981.

7. Hite S. *The Hite Report*. New York, Dell, 1976.

8. Kaplan H. *The New Sex Therapy*. New York, Brunner/Mazel, 1974.

9. Okun BF, Rappaport LJ: *Working with Families: An Introduction to Family Therapy*. North Scituate, Massachusetts, Duxbury Press, 1980.

10. LoPiccolo J, Lobitz WC: The role of masturbation in the treatment of orgasmic dysfunction. *Arch Sex Behav* 2:163, 1972.

11. Masters WH, Johnson VE: *Human Sexual Inadequacy*. Boston, Little Brown and Company, 1970.

12. Maurice WL, Stuart F, Szasz G: Sex therapy: Considerations in the selection of patients. *Can Med Assoc J* 115:317, 1976.

13. Medalie JH: *Family Medicine: Principles and Application*. Baltimore, Williams & Wilkins, 1978.

14. McGovern KB, McMullen RS, LoPiccolo J. Secondary orgasmic dysfunction: I. Analysis and strategies for treatment. In: LoPiccolo J, LoPiccolo L (eds): *Handbook of Sex Therapy*. New York, Plenum Press, 1978.

15. Pauly, TB: Human sexuality in medical education and practice. *J Psychiatry* (Australia/New Zealand) 5:206, 1971.

Chapter 29

Single-Parent and Reconstituted (or Blended) Families

Yves Talbot

The nuclear family as a structure now represents only 20% of Canadian families. Other family forms are increasing in frequency because of the rising divorce rate. The most prevalent is the single-parent family and the reconstituted or blended family. Understanding the differences in family structure and functioning of these families will enable professionals to better assist their patients to anticipate the different stresses related to the new family formation and support them through their adaptation.

SINGLE-PARENT FAMILIES

The single-parent family results from the death of a spouse, or from separation or divorce. This second category is becoming responsible for a larger proportion of single-parent families. Another group, yet very small, is that of people who decide to have children as a single adult.

In 1976, there were 300,000 single-parent families in Canada, representing approximately 13% of Canadian families. In 85% the single-parent was female, but the number of single fathers is steadily increasing. In these families are 631,360 children, of whom 25% are under 6 years old. In Canada, the average number of children per single-parent family is the same as two-parent families (2.1% to 2.3%).

The single-parent family represents a particular challenge for the family physician and nurse. The family organization with one parent, the role played by children, the lack of resources in the family and community often makes for particularly stressful adaptation in times of crisis such as illness. This chapter will outline some of the challenges in order to help the family practitioner develop an informed approach to the single-parent family. PRACTICE is used here as the structure to outline the effect on family functioning of single parenthood.

Presenting Problems. Often the parent presents to the clinician with signs of fatigue and tiredness, back pain or headaches, and organic illness caused by or aggravated by stress. Frequently, however, there may be a direct plea for help with problems in child rearing, and in emotional or financial distress or breakdown. If single parenthood results from a divorce there may still be tension between the ex-spouses and problems around parenting. A behavioral or physical problem in a scapegoated or stressed child may be the ticket of admission.

It is important for family physicians and nurses to realize that many of the difficulties encountered by single-parent families result from very real situations. The one adult filling the role of two increases the amount of energy required to cope on a day-to-day basis. Financial preoccupations add to the burden of parenting. Often the death of a spouse, usually the husband, or separation with maternal child custody results in a considerable loss of income. For example, only 12.7% of Canadian families with two parents are below the poverty line, whereas single-parent families represent 53% of the families below the poverty line.

Sudden loss of income is a major result of the change in breadwinner or the lack of employment of the parent. Of single men, 89% are fully employed, compared with only 45% of single women. This is often a result of a more traditional upbringing, of definite discrimination, of employers' attitudes toward single women with children, and lower pay scales. It is very important for the family practitioner to realize these facts; when turning to physician or nurse, the single parent may seem helpless, inadequate, or whiney. The male physician particularly may not be cognizant of real discriminatory practices and society's prejudices. The clinician should realize that the space for alternative care of children is often a fifth of what it should be in order to meet the needs only of families with single-parents (in Canada in 1976 there were 55,181 spaces for child care to meet the needs of 300,062 children of one-parent families). Other arrangements are often not possible. There may be neither an extended family near nor a reliable neighbor, and private babysitters and housekeeping agencies are impossible services to purchase for a low income, single-parent family.

The summer becomes a much more stressful period as the children who were in school now are at home, and this may be reflected in an increased demand for health services. Summer camps are again resources that are not as available because of their cost. For the younger child at school, the 2 to 3 hours before the mother comes home may be covered by a less than reliable person, such as a 14-year-old neighbor whose rates are affordable. More commonly the child fends for himself as best he can, the house key on a string around his neck. Guilt is a constant companion for such a mother. One divorced nurse had particular problems with her three children when she worked an evening shift (3:30 to 11:00 p.m.). The oldest, a rebellious teenager who needed her mother even more than her younger siblings, left notes around the house feeding the guilt: "We did ＿＿＿＿＿＿ because you WEREN'T HOME."

Illness in either child or mother can be a disaster. Income often decreases if the mother has to stay home and her job may be on the line if it happens frequently. Since children under 10 years old are often sick this is a constant worry. The lack of flexibility by many employers makes it very difficult for such women to take good care of their children or of their own health. For single fathers, staying at home to look after a sick child is tolerated even less and promotion may go to another male not too preoccupied with home duties.

For single-parent families, a larger proportion of income is spent on housing. Only 31% of Canadian single-parent families own a house, compared with 75% of two-parent families. There is no capital for down-payment, no money for mortgage, and yet there is much more difficulty in getting credit. Although housing often means renting an apartment, city landlords are often unwilling to tolerate children and look for adult-only occupancy. People in low income brackets are often forced to share living space; therefore, it is not unusual for family practitioners to be dealing with two single-parent women who have decided to share facilities. The housing situation is often so unstable that it requires frequent moves on the part of the single-parent family or at least more frequent moves than those of two-parent families.

Roles. In single-parent families roles may be reallocated. It is very important to be aware that an older sibling will often step into the position of the missing parent. As long as such a role is clearly defined and negotiated and the demands are not unreasonable for the developmental level of that child it can be a very functional way of getting by. Children may become companions and a replacement of the absent spouse that may make it awkward to make parenting demands on them and to enforce discipline. An older "parentified" child may resent the burden and, in later life, try to recapture their missing childhood or adolescence and avoid having children themselves. Mothers themselves have to fulfill both parental roles in the family.

In families in which the father was physically absent because of work or travel or an extramarital affair, the family was already functioning as a single-parent unit. Therefore, after separation the role reallocation may not be as much a problem as the drastic loss of income. The single-parent has to provide many things on their own: nutrition, limit setting and appropriate expectations of performance, fun and recreation, proper medical and dental care, education and role modelling, and emotional relationships. These represent a tremendous output of energy for somebody who also has to bring in the money for the household. These requirements are often handled with random bursts of energy, making the efforts less effective and the children more insecure.

Affect and Communication. This area of family functioning is of particular importance. The single-parent family overwhelmed with immediate practical problems, household chores, and financial planning may not have the time necessary to attend to the feelings of every family member. Often the question is "What does the single mother do with her feelings?". Does she share them with the children, and if so how can she do it in a way that is not also overburdening? If a widower is too close to an older daughter, or a divorcee in need of a son's time and affection, oedipal fantasies may be difficult for the adolescent to cope with. In the parent, an unconscious fear of incest may result in distancing or hostility as protection. In one family a mother alternated between open needy affection and outpouring of her problems to one of her sons and overcontrolling maternal behavior that provoked him into outbursts of rage. Confused and plagued at night by dreams of incest, he grew up with great difficulty; in relationships with women he oscillated between intense intimacy followed by panic and distancing.

Often a lack of other adults as resources or support may produce a build-up of different emotions, left over from past events or from the current situations, which are not easily shared. The primary care provider often plays the role of a confident and advisor in a family who has lost the second adult. Children also may withhold some of their feelings, being afraid to over burden an already fully employed parent. This is of particular relevance to the immediate period after a family separation but may later constitute a more chronic state given the lack of family resources. Resourceful children may confide in a friend, school teacher, or neighbor to ventilate feelings and problem solve outside the immediate household. If not, the clinician can be a temporary refuge but should encourage development of other resources as well as facilitating communication within the family.

On the positive side, however, many single parents experience enormous relief after separation or divorce, and are free for the first time in their adult lives to be themselves. One woman, who had married young to a dominant, inexpressive, wealthy male, changed her personality dramatically after divorce. Previously timid, mouse-like, and sexually frigid, she became expressive emotionally and sexually, and for the first time developed her own interests and career and eventually remarried. Her five children flowered along with her. Remarriage is an option for the young, chosen by many, but has its own challenges when there are children (see reconstituted families). Divorce counselling, if it occurred, may help the person to recognize reasons for failure of the first marriage (often a repeat of a childhood trauma or of the parents' marital pattern) and may help avoid a second similar failure.

For children as well there are positive aspects of divorce. The silent hostility of emotional divorce, or the constant turmoil and divided loyalty when parents are embattled but in the same house, probably do much more damage than divorce. If fighting continues through the children, the clinician should recommend divorce counselling to truly divorce the parents.

Time in the Life Cycle. A parent may find himself alone at any time in the cycle of individual and family development. Earlier in this century, death was the main cause of single-parent families. At present, divorce is the major cause, and there is a larger proportion of young single parents and families in the expansion phase of their development. For families with preschool-age children or school-age pre-adolescents there are several important tasks, as mentioned in the chapter on the life cycle, which have to be met. For example, the parent still has to learn to deal with outside systems (school) and provide the children with the necessary support for their own growth. If the end trauma of death or divorce occurs later in the life cycle, arrested development may result if the parent cannot cope alone so that separation and individuation of adolescents cannot occur. The clinician can gently nudge such a parent into developing his or her own resources and letting go of the child.

Illness. As mentioned earlier, illness can represent a major problem for working single-parents because of lack of other resources, low income, and the fact that they may have been cut-off from their previous community (separation often results in a move), and sometimes from their own family of origin. Illness may finally deplete resources in an already drained family. As has been pointed out,[19] repeated crises close together can cause the healthiest family to fall apart. Illness in the parent may be very frightening for the children, even more so if the missing parent is dead rather than divorced. In one family, recently bereaved, the two daughters in their early 20s had to care for their anorectic, depressed mother. Because the mother had a history of suicidal threats the daughters panicked when she retired to bed to mourn her husband. It was too reminiscent both of the mother's past and of the daughters' experience of their thin bed-ridden father dying of cancer. The family physician's role was to normalize mourning in this situation and help the daughters recognize their mother was not their responsibility. The physician's help in turn relabelled the mother as being able to cope, and soon after she was able to go out and get a job.

Coping. Coping will depend on the personality and past coping style of the single parent and also on the role of the parent now absent. For example, a divorcee incapable of earning her own living or of financial planning was given a generous settlement as well as financial advice by her ex-husband. While this situation was maintained she coped very well as she was quite competent in all other areas and had only depended on him for his money. When the parent who has now left the family was wholly responsible for one essential area, the role adjustment can be enormous. In these days of run-away wives, a man who devoted himself entirely to business may suddenly find himself having to be a parent for the first time in his life. His coping strategy will be determined by his self-image and past role models, the reaction of the children and of the extended family, the attitude of his work environment and peers, and the availability of other resources.

Environment. The quality of single parenthood is affected by the systems of which the family is a part. The attitude of some communities is so negative and rejecting that divorce in the first place may be long delayed, and once it occurs, the partners may both leave the community. Children are obviously affected through the attitude of teachers and school friends. For some ages of children (particularly ages 6 to 11), both divorce and death of a parent are so frightening to other children that the child is taunted, rejected or isolated by his peers.[10] Older children are more likely to be understanding so that ventilation of feelings to peers can take place. If divorce is common, or during periods when loss of a parent is common (post war), children with such experience may form a very effective support group for one another. Similarly for the parent the community may allow or promote self-help groups for single parents or for the widowed.

Cultural attitudes vary greatly and when negative can be destructive and promote secrecy, guilt, and isolation. Even the widow fares poorly in some societies and is seen as more of a threat to the married woman than is the divorcee. She will suddenly find invitations to couples' parties waning, as support and sympathy visible after the death begin to decrease. In some cultures it is the custom that she immediately remarry—usually to a male relative of her husband. Such customs, although protective and expected, may add to the adjustments necessary at such a time.

Religious groups are extremely helpful to the widowed with a faith, much less so to the divorced, in whom guilt is often an added burden. Economic resources have been discussed as has the attitude of the work environment. Educational resources may be deficient, and the single woman particularly may need to go back to school to qualify for a job. One resourceful if unscrupulous lady in Montreal threw her often unemployed husband out, applied for welfare payments, and then went back to school to retrain for 2 years. Most widowed or divorced women find themselves stuck with unchallenging jobs and no time to re-educate. Medical resources may be underused by the proud, the independent, or those afraid of what the doctor might find; or overused by the lonely, distraught, or helpless looking for a St. George to rescue them. Responding as St. George may be not only burdensome to the care-giver but in the long run not helpful as promoting dependency and limiting use of other resources. Fantasies of marriage to a male health professional may further complicate the relationship.

The Clinician's Role

Anticipatory guidance before the death of a parent (see Chapter 21) or before the separation or divorce can usually enhance decision-making and coping and may sometimes avert catastrophe. Referral for divorce counselling can be a major contribution avoiding the pain of a court battle over money and children and facilitating understanding of what went wrong. If the clinician perceives triangulation or scapegoating of children he or she should insist on couple counselling. This may be necessary even after the official divorce.

The family physician or nurse may be the first turned to in the grief and turmoil of the immediate circumstances, and he or she is in an ideal position as caregiver for the whole family. Facilitation of communication between parents and between parent and child, and of expression of repressed emotions can be enormously helpful. Normalization of the single-parent's distress, clarification of roles, emotions and problems in the children, and specific suggestions (use of support groups and community agencies) will enable the family to continue functioning. It is important to help the family organize itself and become competent in using outside resources; this is the role of coach rather than problem-solver. Since the clinician's essential role is health promotion and management of illness, interventions will usually be around these issues.

Two clinical examples illustrate the importance of the principles of working *with* families described in Section IV.

Example 1

John, a 13-year-old asthmatic, has presented more frequently to the emergency room in the last 6 months with severe dyspnea. Mrs. X., John's mother, has been a single parent for a few years since the death of her husband. Because of lack of money, she had shared an apartment with a female friend whose husband had left her a few years ago. This woman, Mrs. Y., had no children. She would often accompany Mrs. X. to the hospital when John required medical treatment. It was rarely the same physician who saw Mrs. X. in the emergency room and none would include Mrs. Y. in discussion and evaluation since she was perceived simply as a helpful neighbor.

After Mrs. X. joined a family practice unit, the family physician, when confronted with another asthmatic attack, decided to see Mrs. X. and Mrs. Y. together with John. During the interview, he noticed the very important role that Mrs. Y. took in decision-making around health care issues in the family. He was also struck by the intense bond between the two women. On finding out more information about their current living arrangement, the family practitioner discovered that Mrs. Y. was planning to rejoin her husband who had taken up a job a few hundred miles away from Montreal. It was then apparent that the two "parents" were dealing with impending separation in an important relationship, and that much of the tension had been transmitted to John. The decision had been made 6 months ago when the asthmatic attacks had begun to increase. The family physician then acted as facilitator and supported both women in the expression of their feelings.

It was interesting to note that, after this interview, John stopped having severe asthmatic attacks and, since the women have been separated, Mrs. X.

has been able to continue her care at the family medicine unit with her son. It is important for the family practitioner to be aware of this common dual family structure and not to exclude the other adults from the understanding of a current medical problem. Focusing on the child's asthma had prevented both family and physicians from understanding some of the current stressful life events that this family organization was undergoing.

Example 2

Mrs. J., a single parent, presented to her family physician with a request for orthopedic shoes for her 3 and ½ year old son. A year and a half previously, Mrs. J.'s husband had left home and never returned. Since she could not afford independent living she had moved to her mother's house, which allowed her to seek employment and to use her mother as a babysitter for her son. The use of extended family and this type of structure or reorganization is not unusual in single-parent families.

In defining the problem it was important for the family physician to find out who was defining the problem as John's feet. To his query, Mrs. J. replied that it was her mother who was concerned by the fact that his toes were pointing inwards and that her grandson therefore required some special heels. In such a situation it is important to meet all the players in the piece. The physician set up an appointment with the grandmother, Mrs. J. and her son. During the interview he found out that Mrs. J.'s mother was very concerned that, unless something was done for her grandson, he might develop club feet like her own son. At that point it was essential for the physician to be able to reassure the grandmother in person that her grandson did not have club feet and that he would probably do very well. This was all done in a very respectful manner, with the clinician recognizing the importance of the grandmother as a parent in the functioning of this single-parent family. Unless there is major discord between grandmother and mother, the use of a grandparent as a parent in a single-parent family can surely be a very adaptive way of dealing with the situation. Rather than excluding or reprimanding the grandmother, the family practitioner must work with the current family arrangement to increase the efficacy of his intervention. A more aggressive or antagonistic attitude towards the grandmother might have resulted in doctor-shopping or in iatrogenic conflict between mother and grandmother.

RECONSTITUTED (OR BLENDED) FAMILIES

The reconstituted family, often called the blended or step-family, is defined as a family in which at least one of the partners is acting as a step-parent. This definition includes families with or without custody of children as well as unmarried parents living in long-term couple relationships.

At the turn of the century, reconstituted families were mainly the result of remarriage after the death of a spouse (hence the expression step-families from the Old English prefix "steop," meaning bereaved or orphaned[12]). More recently, divorce has given rise to an enlarging proportion of reconstituted families: in 1979 there were approximately 59,000 divorces in Canada and of these, close to 15,000 occurred in Quebec.[20] This growth in the divorce rate, combined with a progressive decrease in age at divorce has resulted in the involvement of more and more children.[13,17] In 1975, remarriage accounted for 18.8% of marriages in Alberta, 23.6% in British Columbia, and 17.1% in Ontario.[18] Currently, at least one marriage in five has one previously married spouse, and one child in ten under age 18 (a total of 760,000) lives in a second-marriage family.[3] In the United States, the 1977 statistics estimated that 13% of families were reconstituted and 15% were single parent.[21] Because of the number of common-law relationships, not included in the census data, these statistics are clearly a gross underestimate of the actual number of reconstituted families. This omission has been rectified, however, and the 1981 census will provide a more accurate assessment of the number of such families.

Most of the popular literature about parenting and parent effectiveness is currently directed towards the natural family. Fairy tale literature abounds in myths about bad step-mothers who are never as good as natural mothers. Most cultural norms are also aimed at the natural family.[21] Children can be worried about knowing which set of parents they are supposed to invite to their graduation, how they should call this new man their mother is living with, and how they are going to introduce him to their friends. When filling out forms, the new step-parent may not know whether to write his or her name under "father" or "mother" or leave it all to the natural parent. All these subtle but powerful messages often put the step parent in a relatively isolated position.

The family clinician is often in the ideal position of having seen the progression of a family from the separation caused by divorce or the death of one of the spouses, through the single parent phase to the reconstituted family state following remarriage or common-law arrangements.

Research

Despite the paucity of research data on reconstituted families, Visher and Visher summarize such results as are available in the following terms.[21]

1. There appears to be a positive correlation between socioeconomic status and step-family success.[1,2,9] The higher the socioeconomic bracket, the more positive step-family interaction and functional characteristics were found.

2. Studies of adults indicate that persons growing up in step-father families do not differ according to measurements of social functioning from persons growing up in nuclear families.[25]

3. Step-mother/step-child relationships are more tentative and difficult than step-father/step-child relationships.[4]

4. Step-sibling relationships are relatively good, especially when there is a half-sibling to join the two groups together.[4]

5. Step-families experience more psychological stress than do intact families.[15]

6. Step-mothers have difficulties with the negative step-mother image.[21]

Visher concludes that research on step-families is plagued by methodological flaws and that there is a need for more logical studies to assess the tensions, the strivings, the failings, and the joys and successes of step-families. Research on the impact of divorce, single parent status, and death of one spouse is also very relevant to research on step families, because these past experiences are part of the adaptation that men and women carry with them to their new family experiences.

During periods of stress, patients tend to consult their physician for various ailments.[5,14] It is therefore important for the family doctor dealing with reconstituted families to understand the various aspects of family structure and their influence on the functioning of the reconstituted family. Such understanding will enable the clinician to help a new family in formation to anticipate and prevent the potential pitfalls associated with their new endeavor. It will also enable the physician to put the clinical problem (psychosomatic illnesses, behavioral problems, depression, etc.) in its proper perspective since it could be the result of, or be influenced by, the stresses of step-family formation.

Reconstituted Family Structure

In a nuclear family, the structure is a spouse subsystem, a parent subsystem, and a sibling subsystem.[16] Each of these subsystems is limited by a boundary indicating that groups of persons are members of a family system distinct from other families or in-laws in their community. The structure of the step-family is often very ambiguous. There is often disagreement as to who belongs to which family and whether it includes the children of this one versus the other one or both. The reconstituted family is clearly not a classic nuclear family and is almost always a much more complex structure. It can include up to eight sets of grandparents, four sets of parents, an unlimited number of step-siblings, and at least two households. The step-parents have no legal relation to the step-children, so they have functional responsibility but no legal power. Messinger[15] describes such families as having "permeable boundaries" that are different from the clear boundaries found in the nuclear family. Permeable boundaries may increase the susceptibility to conflict with the previous marriage relationship.

Visher and Visher[21] have summarized the potential problem areas resulting from the structural arrangements of the reconstituted family as follows:

1. The presence of a biological parent outside the reconstituted family and of a same sex adult within the household commonly give rise to power struggles in which the children are caught as the victims in between the two households. Such power struggles tend to increase when one of the two ex-spouses remarries. Room has to be made for a new set of values or perceptions on child rearing, for example.

2. Most children hold membership in two households, which gives rise to conflicts between the visitors and the members of the family. Lack of clear role definition and conflicts of loyalty are usually noted.

3. The role of the step-parent is ill defined. When ex-spouses are involved, their roles are not clearly defined in relation to outside institutions like health services, schools, etc.

4. The fact that reconstituted families come together from at least two previous historical backgrounds accentuates the need for tolerance of differences.

5. Step-relationships are new and untested, not given as they are in intact families.

6. The children in step-families have at least one extra set of grandparents. The grandparents' acceptance of step-children and of the new spouse is very important. Coalitions can be formed that undermine the child-rearing efforts of the blended family.

7. The final important characteristic concerns financial arrangements. If conflicts over money or alimony existed before the new marriage, they can easily be intensified. New marriages frequently upset a delicate balance, and alimony is well recognized as a fighting ground for couples who separate.

These structural characteristics represent potential pitfalls in the formation of reconstituted families. One cannot consider the step-family as a nuclear family; flexibility and good communication are major factors in the harmonious functioning of such families.

Functioning of the Reconstituted Family

The main function of the family is to integrate internal and external resources to foster the biopsychosocial growth of each of its members. Lewis and colleagues in the book *No Single Thread*[11] stress the importance of couple cohesiveness as a main characteristic of healthy families. For the reconstituted family this is even more important, since it will have to adapt immediately to a large number of events. The new partners have to think of recoupling, parenting, dealing with ex-spouses when present, the new neighborhood of one partner (most frequently the husband's), the attitudes of in-laws to the new marriage, the "puzzled neighbors" phase when children and parents have different names, and the imbalance of power and responsibility between custodian and the visitor. Not only do couples who remarry have to learn about the interactional style each has acquired from his or her family of origin, but also the carry-over from previous marital arrangements of at least one of the two members. Even within the family, the spouse who does not have children may feel excluded in some areas by the bonds already established between the partner and his or her children.

The relationship with the ex-spouse can generate a certain amount of stress on the new family in formation: a lack of clarity as to what should be discussed with the ex-spouse, as well as when and where, may have a variety of effects on the reconstituted family. Spouses recovering from a divorce may, for instance, react more sensitively to their new spouses' behavior.

Parenting presents some unusual challenges in reconstituted families. Since the number of involved parents can be as many as four, coordination and consistency of disciplining and of vocational expectations require a considerable expenditure of time and effort.

Parent-Child Relationship

Formation of a reconstituted family necessitates a whole process of negotiation, including an appraisal of the value of previous family arrangements in relation to those that the new family will attempt to create. When two households merge, previous functions, such as who takes care of the dog and who puts out the garbage, have to be renegotiated. Each group of children spends much time keeping track of "who is who's favorite?" The new parent cannot expect instant bonding from the children. He or she has to allow the children needed "space" to relate with their biological parents.

Studies on divorce[6,7,8,22,23,24] have shown that a good relationship with both sets of parents after divorce correlates with a much better outcome for the children. For some children, the remarriage represents the end of a reconciliation dream; the new family may appear tenuous and the risks of establishing a relationship with the new parent will be under constant test. Children are often the main link between the ex-spouse and the new family. They must not become the message carriers; parenting discussions must occur between the adults rather than through the children. This unduly powerful position is often uncomfortable for children and is not conducive to their optimal development, particularly because children often feel a conflict of loyalty between the two sets of parents even without this added burden. Duberman's research indicates that step-mothers and step-daughters have more difficulties than step-fathers and step-sons and that the most difficult relationship is between step-mothers and adolescent step-daughters.[4]

Sibling Relationships

When two families merge, the age order of children may be changed so that a younger or older child could suddenly become the middle child. Rooms may have to be reallocated, and a difference in status between the resident and the visiting children may become apparent. Chores and tasks may have to be renegotiated. When adolescents are involved, sexuality is more of an issue. Adolescents put together in the same household may be attracted to each other, or may be made uncomfortable at times by the increased sexual activity of the newlywed parents.

There are, then, a number of difficult areas in adaptation emphasizing the great need for flexibility and effective communication in the formation of a reconstituted family. The family physician or nurse practitioner has a very important function in assisting the reconstituted family. He or she is often the one constant figure who has followed a family through its disintegration, its single parent phase, and its reconstitution. In working with a reconstituted family, the clinician must be aware, not only of his or her own values and attitudes towards divorce and remarriage, but also of his or her previous alliance with one of the ex-spouses. These attitudes may color the clinician's judgment and may interfere with his or her ability to be helpful to the new family.

Many communities do not provide adequate support for step-families. The family doctor may then become a front-line provider to whom the family will turn for help. His or her role is that of providing anticipatory guidance to the family in formation, counselling or facilitation to help the family solve current transitional problems, or referral to mental health workers when the family's lack of adaptive capacity prevents it from making necessary and appropriate changes.

Anticipatory Guidance

Reconstituted families are unusually willing, during the process of their formation, to discuss any question that is relevant to the success of their new union. The family clinician is in a privileged position that allows him or her to offer the new couple the opportunity to sit down and review any questions they may have on parenting, relationships with ex-spouses and grandparents, and reactions of children to new members of the family, etc. By reviewing the various aspects of the new family structure and the functional adaptations required, the family and the clinician can jointly anticipate and prevent some of the difficulties that commonly occur during the formation of the reconstituted family. The doctor or nurse should stress the importance of the roles to be played by each of the parental figures in bringing about a successful transition. In so doing, he or she will cover any areas pertinent to their life as a new couple or as new parents.

Couple

1. How much time have you scheduled for yourselves, as a couple? The parental figures in reconstituted families are suddenly confronted with a large number of responsibilities to children and to community; it is easy for them to be left without the couple time that is essential to their long-term bonding.

2. How have your previous experiences changed your perspectives on the marriage? This question may allow the couple to deal with some of the fears they may have about repeating previous patterns; mothers who have come through a single parent phase may have had to increase their activities during the process and may not wish to return to a more traditional role assignment.

Parenting

1. How are the children reacting to the new marriage? This question may provide the opportunity to discuss some of the fears the parents may have about the effect remarriage might have on their children. Children will react differently according to their own stage of development. For example, school-age children or preschoolers may resent the new marriage, since it terminates their fantasies of a reunion of the parents; an adolescent who may have enjoyed a more adult status during the single parent phase may resent becoming one of the children again. An attitude of not rushing or pushing and of providing ample time for the children to develop their relationship with the new parent is usually more conducive to a successful transition. By not making too many demands on the children for affection, the new parents will alleviate the loyalty problems some children may have about biological parents and the step-family.

2. How are you planning to work out the sharing of child-rearing responsibilities? This broad area covers everything from disciplining to flexibility in adapting to a difference of values and approaches to child-rearing. The biological parent may often assume disciplining responsibility at the beginning, followed by a progressive transfer to a shared responsibility with the step-parent as his or her relationship with the child becomes consolidated. Step-parents should, nevertheless, be aware of the playmate trap that may have developed during the courting phase of their relationship. The support of the biological spouse will help the step-parent to feel comfortable in establishing his or her role as a parent.

3. What plans have been made for the necessary contacts and relationships with an ex-spouse? This question allows the couple to examine

their attitudes, flexibility, and comfort in dealing with such things as visiting and financial arrangements with the other biological parent, which will help the step-parent to feel comfortable in establishing his or her role as a parent. The more courteous and flexible the visiting arrangements, the more the children will be able to benefit from contact with the different adults involved. The parenting relationship within and between the families must remain at the parental level, so that the children are not ensnared as message carriers between the families.

Facilitation

Although anticipatory guidance is preferable as a form of prevention, patients more commonly present themselves when a specific problem arises. When the family physician is aware that a patient is part of a family in transition, he or she should elicit data pertinent to the different stresses generated by the transition. Whether the clinician deals with the symptoms of one of the spouses or a behavioral problem with one of the children, seeing the couple will allow a better grasp and understanding of the problem.

We have found that telling each patient how much importance we attach to the family as a unit in our practice facilitates their acceptance of the benefits to be derived from participating in such meetings. Couples welcome these discussions when they realize that their concerns are not at all uncommon to families in their situation.

Referral

Finally, there are situations where the family system does not have the flexibility required to adapt to unavoidable changes. Biological parents and children may be so close as to exclude the new step-parents; children can be caught between the two families as message carriers when there is virtually no other channel of communication, and situations may develop where the family cannot adopt simple suggestions, or the problem is of such long duration (over 6 months) that the family doctor should enlist the help of a mental health worker. As in other types of families, we prefer to use consultants with a family orientation. Even if the consultant may need to spend more time with different members of the family, his or her competence with the overall family system will be more efficient in the long run. Ex-spouses may need to be seen together to clarify various issues of visiting and child-rearing. Occasionally both families may need to be seen together to point out to the children that they need not be involved with adult matters. The physician's main contribution in such situations is his or her ability to clarify the problem for the family and to negotiate such interventions as may be necessary. If the physician is to play as constructive a role as possible, he or she must transfer the trust the family will have developed in him to the consultant.

The family clinician should be aware of other resources in the community; support groups for couples of reconstituted families are one of these resources often available through community agencies like the YMCA or social service agencies. The clinician can also provide a list of relevant books or other helpful literature for step families. The book by Visher and Visher is an excellent reference work for both professionals and step-families.[21]

REFERENCES

1. Bernard J: *Remarried: A Study of Marriage.* New York, Russel and Russel, 1971.

2. Bowerman CE, Irish DP: Some relationships of stepchildren to their parents. *Marr Fam Living* 24:113, 1962.

3. Carson S: Don't expect to be instant pals with stepchild. *Montreal Gazette* Dec 20, 1980, p. 69.

4. Duberman L: Step-kin relationships. *J Marr Fam* 35:283, 1973.

5. Gallin R: Life difficulties, coping and the use of medical services. *Cult Med Psychiatry* 4:249, 1980.

6. Hetherington EM, Cox M, Cox R: Divorced fathers. *Fam Coordinator* Oct:417, 1976.

7. Hetherington EM, Cox M, Cox R: The aftermath of divorce, in Stevens JH Jr, Matthews M (eds): *Mother-Child, Father-Child Relations.* Washington, D.C., NAEYC, 1978.

8. Hetherington EM: Family interaction and the social, emotional and cognitive development of children after divorce, in Brazelton TB, Vaughan VC (eds): *The Family: Setting Priorities.* New York, Science and Medicine Publishing Co., 1979, pp. 71-87.

9. Langner T, Michael ST: *Life Stresses and Mental Health.* New York, Free Press, 1963.

10. Le Shan E: *Learning to Say Goodbye When a Patient Dies.* New York, Avon Books, 1976.

11. Lewis J, Beavers WR, Gosset JT, et al: *No Single Thread: Psychological Health in Family Systems.* New York, Brunner Mazel, 1976.

12. *Living Webster Encyclopedic Dictionary of English Language.* Chicago, The English Language Institute of America, 1971, p. 957.

13. Maddox B: *The Half Parent.* New York, Evans, 1975.

14. Mechanic D: Response factors in illness: The study of illness behavior, in Jaco ED (ed): *Patients, Physician and Illness.* New York, Free Press, 1972, pp. 118-130.

15. Messinger L: Remarriage between divorced people with children from previous marriages: A proposal for preparation for remarriage. *J Marr Fam Counselling* 2:193, 1976.

16. Minuchin S: *Families and Family Therapy.* Massachusetts, Harvard University Press, 1975.

17. National Council of Welfare: *One in a World of Twos*. Ottawa, Government of Canada, 1976.

18. Roy L: Les remarriages, de plus en plus nombreux au Québec *Cahier québecois de demographie* 8:30, 1979.

19. Smilkstein G: Cycle of family function: A conceptual model for family medicine. *J Fam Pract* 11:223, 1980.

20. Statistics Canada: *Divorce and Marriage Rate for 1979*. Ottawa, Government of Canada, 1980.

21. Visher EB, Visher JS: *Step-Families: A Guide to Working with Stepparents and Stepchildren*. New York, Brunner Mazel, 1979.

22. Wallerstein JS, Kelly JB: The effect of parental divorce: Experience of preschool children. *J Am Acad Child Psychiatry* 14:600, 1974.

23. Wallerstein JS, Kelly JB: The effect of parental divorce: Experience of the child in early latency. *Am J Orthopsychiatry* 46:20, 1976.

24. Wallerstein JS, Kelly JB: The effect of parental divorce: The adolescent experience, in Koupernik C, Anthony J (eds): *Child in the Family, III*. New York, John Wiley, 1974, pp. 479-505.

25. Wilson KL, Zurcher LA, McAdams DC, et al: Stepfathers and stepchildren: An explanatory analysis from two national surveys. *J Marriage Fam* 37:526, 1975.

Chapter 30

Working with the Elderly and their Families

Dawn E. McDonald
Janet Christie-Seely

No community can call itself civilized if it treats its older generation with a lack of consideration. But consideration requires understanding, and everyone needs to know more about the process of aging and the difficulties it may bring. Ultimately, the quality of life of elderly people, especially the very old and frail, rest on the attitudes and perceptions of those younger than themselves.[19]

This quotation from *Growing Older*, published by the British government, underlines the need to understand aging. The social responsibility of a civilized nation for its elderly citizens is made operational in the day-to-day interaction between these elderly, their families, and a broad spectrum of care givers.

The "old old," those over 75 years of age, are the most frail and disabled, and often those in greatest need of support services. It is projected that this group will show the largest proportional increase in the next few years. At the same time, Kane[9] suggests that the number of siblings and children available as caretakers will decrease.

While health care professionals provide care for those elderly persons who come in contact with the health care system it is important to realize that a relatively small proportion (5% to 8%) of the elderly are in institutions.[15] Despite the prevelant perception that families do not care for their aged members, recent studies[9,18,20] have shown that many frail or sick elderly are cared for by a spouse, a child, or a sibling. Often these caretakers are assisted by helpers paid privately or via government programs.

ATTITUDES TOWARD THE ELDERLY AND THE THEORETICAL FRAMEWORK

Beliefs about old age determine the provisions made by the community for the elderly and the responses of both families and health care professionals to the care of the aged.[1] These beliefs are based on the prevailing values of the culture in question.

The belief system about provision of care toward the elderly is formed out of the clinician's experience in his or her own family, contacts with the elderly themselves, the clinician's stage in the life cycle, knowledge base, and conceptual framework. Physicians, nurses, psychologists, and social workers tend to emphasize different areas in work with the elderly and are guided by different theories, both of health care in general and the process of aging. Since teamwork of professionals involved with the elderly is essential, differences in beliefs about aging and goals for the elderly must be clarified and negotiated.

Myths and beliefs about the elderly are insidious and pervasive; it is therefore necessary that the practitioner be knowledgeable and be prepared to substitute well researched facts for these incorrect ideas. These myths and attitudes can be gathered under the general rubric of "ageism." Ageism is a very subtle prejudice whose effects are seen in decisions at many levels that affect policies, individual treatment, rehabilitation, and placement. For example, an administrator in a long-term care facility voices the conviction that the major goal in providing care for the elderly is to "keep them comfortable." This institution provides excellent physical care and nutritious food. There is no occupational therapy, little mental stimulation, or reality orientation. Staff are given a full orientation to custodial care but there is no continuing education. Anything more than washing, feeding, and moving from bed to chair is seen as a "frill."

There are certain physiologic and psychological changes that are found in varying degrees in individuals as they age. It is important to distinguish those changes that are considered part of normal aging and those which are seen as pathologic. Families often need help to recognize these often subtle differences as well. At the same time the realization that some physical changes occur should not be seen as a rationale for ignoring a new physical event or behavioral manifestation. "You're just getting older" is a potentially dangerous and defeatist oversimplification. Each change must be carefully evaluated when it occurs and in the total environment in which it occurs. For those insufficiently versed in the normal changes (most of us), Table 30.1 outlines some of these and suggests alterations to be made in professional practice and family life to accommodate them.[5,8,13]

Theories of aging, whether intuitive or formally labelled, necessarily affect the approach taken in providing service for the elderly. "Disengagement theory" suggests that there is a gradual mutual withdrawal from contact between the aging person and society and a giving up of roles. There is less willingness on the part of the older person to conform to the norms of society.[2] Belief in this theory of aging might lead the practitioner to accept some

Table 30.1 **Some Normal Changes in Aging and Professional and Family Accommodations to Meet Them**

Normal Changes	Professional and Family Accommodations
Alteration in the brain's cellular chemical composition and activity patterns leading to —memory loss —some degree of depression —altered sleep patterns	Nonjudgmental acceptance of decreased function Transmission of respect and awareness of "personhood" of the elder in spite of changes Determination of "best times" for interviews, teaching sessions, family visits, etc.
Decreased reaction time particularly in complex tasks	Scheduling longer periods for medical interviews or for shopping trips, visits (for example, 45 minutes) Teaching material in "chunks" with planned reinforcement Evaluation/performance tests not linked to time Evaluate environment for safety
Decreased response to pain sensation and temperature changes	Careful monitoring of any activity Alertness to temperature of environment and its safety
Diminished synthesis and secretion of some digestive enzymes, changes in sense of taste	Monitoring of quality and quantity of food and fluid intake
Slowed motility of the digestive tract and absorption	Evaluation of elimination Teaching of dietary aids to elimination for example, use of bran, fruits, and adequate fluid intake
Altered response to chemical changes, (slowed recovery to glucose overload, slowed liver metabolization)	Alertness to responses to drugs—family should also understand these —interactions —idiosyncratic responses Clinician awareness of differences in "normal" ranges in laboratory values and physiological measures
Changes in senses, altered/decreased —vision —hearing —balance	Use of more than one medium when communicating/teaching Willingness and ability to switch from visual to auditory media
Loss of teeth	Routine use of checklists, fact sheets, and presentation of these to patients so they may take the information away with them

Table 30.1 Some Normal Changes in Aging and Professional and Family
Accommodations to Meet Them (continued)

Normal Changes	*Professional and Family Accommodations*
	Routine checks to see if aids used, (glasses, hearing aids, false teeth) are clean, being maintained, and are in working order before information giving, teaching sessions and activities of daily living
	Selective use of items/activities that aid "orienting" functions in private homes, clinics and institutions
	—large print clocks, calendars, signs and name tags
	—high-contrast colors in furniture, rugs
	—maintenance of established routines
	—periodic repetition of vital information (date, time, names)
	—discussion of daily events, weather sports
Alterations in circulatory, musculoskeletal, and respiratory tracts leading to easier fatiguability	Monitor during any activity for fatigue Intersperse short activity periods with rest periods or "quiet" activities
Role changes due to —retirement —progression in individual and family developmental stages	As well as physical and mental status a full clinical assessment must include consideration of —capabilities in activities of daily living —support systems —family dynamics
Progressive multiple losses —friends and family through death —individual health, physical, and mental capabilities —living arrangements, (for example, move from family home to an apartment)	—recreation/diversion —usual patterns of social activity —living arrangements —coping/problem solving ability —availability and willingness to use community resources
Alteration in independence-dependence relationship	—financial status
Change in financial status	—individuals' or couples' plans and expectations re aging

degree of idiosyncratic behavior and gradual loosening of ties with family as usual behavior. This withdrawal from contact would not be seen as the norm if the practitioner espoused "activity theory," which "suggests that life satisfaction in older age occurs when the individual is involved in social interaction."[2] This practitioner would look for evidence of continuing ties and be prepared to initiate intervention(s) if social interaction began to wane. The practitioner who accepts "exchange theory" would examine the reward-cost balance of the elder's interaction with his environment and seek to foster greater usefulness and mutual satisfaction in social contacts, if interactions appeared to be decreasing. For example, babysitting can be suggested by a competent grandparent in exchange for transport and a good meal.

Systems theory as in other areas of health care provides a new orientation to the elderly. Expectations and family myths may be important determinants of health and relationships. "We all live to a ripe old age" suggests a satisfaction with this stage of the life cycle, and may be a self-fulling prophecy. A promise by one mother never to live with her children in old age resulted in a 95-year-old lady, completing the newspaper crossword before breakfast and teaching a grandson German. She died within a year after deafness and blindness necessitated care by an elderly family retainer in her own home. All her children followed the same pattern. "Good genes" are usually evoked in such families. In other families the elderly are expected to be dependent. The role reversal feared by the above family is encouraged either out of gratitude for parental caring ("She changed my diapers once, why should I complain about changing hers.") or as a means of turning the tables on a not-so-loved parent.

Baby talk to the elderly, taking over all decision-making, and control may thinly disguise hostility to a previously autocratic or unloving parent or anger at the burden they currently represent. Sometimes a gentle comment by the clinician about the possibility of such anger can give permission for its expression in a less destructive manner. Problem solving and improved communication are often prevented when such feelings remain repressed. Confrontation with the elderly about the past is rarely productive, but expression of negative feelings to the clinician may allow more positive feelings and positive memories to surface. Guilt can be decreased by normalizing statements (see Chapter 14) such as "I'd be fed up too if I was so tied to the house/had to keep changing the sheets/had my discipline of the children undermined."

Family myths and secrets play their role in the elderly. The myth that "Mum is weak and frail and must not be disturbed" can become more virulent in another form: "If you (at age 35) leave home she will have another heart attack and die." The strong woman in bed who rules the household may be impairing her own health further by lack of activity, and may be depriving herself of the real respect owed to her as someone who is tough and who is well able to organize those around her. Relabelling the woman as such may help her get out of bed and may help her children encourage her independence and eventually their own. Needless to say such families often resist change, but an awareness of their family pattern may contribute to prevention of such patterns in the next generation.

Family secrets can play a destructive role and are often more easily dealt with while those who perpetuated them are still living.

A father of three adolescents began to have marital problems after the death of his grandmother. Until the age of 16 he had been told by the two women who raised him that they were friends of his parents who had been killed in a car accident when he was a baby. Then when he was 16 years old, he accidentally discovered his birth certificate and found out that his two caretakers were in fact his mother and grandmother. They had hidden their true identities from him to protect him from the stigma of illegitimacy. He had met his father, a married man with a family, on three occasions but had not known who he was.

Thoroughly shocked by this revelation he had kept it a secret from his three children who were told the car accident story. He believed it was his mother's wish that the secret remain. He was encouraged by the clinician to discuss this with her. The following week in a family interview held for other reasons he announced that he had been mistaken about the car accident story. He told his three sons the truth with his mother's delighted permission. The oldest (19 years old) was "shocked" but not upset by it, the 16-year-old, who identified with his father, and the 13-year-old were "not at all surprised." As usual secrets are often conveyed at a nonverbal level. Revelation of this secret markedly improved the relationship with the grandmother 6 months before her death and contact increased. Her son's overly close relationship with his three sons to avoid his father's uninvolved role could now be discussed. The mother's role as "odd-woman out" could now be understood and corrected by all four males.

Triangulation of an elderly person can replace triangulation of children, particularly when the couple has a need to stabilize their relationship by detouring conflict through a third person and the children are of an age to leave home. This may be responsible for considerable distress and symptom formation in the old person.

The N. family took an elderly uncle into their home after the departure of their youngest child. The old man had always lived alone and was very difficult to live with. His annoying behavior (sloppy eating, forgetfulness, and poor personal habits) became a source of grievance and a topic of conversation for the couple, which served to bring the couple closer together. At the same time, however, it reduced the uncle's already low self-esteem and made it more difficult for him to relate to others. A decision was made to send him to live in a boarding home. His difficult behavior there resulted in his returning to live with the couple. Although tension had risen between the couple during the absence of the uncle, their relationship improved after his return.

In a situation such as this, where change would involve a major restructuring of the system, the ethics of interventions must be considered. The well-being of the uncle and of the couple must also be taken into consideration. Problems of adjusting to the empty nest and improving couple communication obviously must be dealt with. Resolving these problems will depend on their motivation for change. A comment that they seemed to get along better when the uncle was present might prompt a request for help and referral for family therapy. Community resources (see Chapter 8) might be able to provide a better environment for the uncle.

Systems theory provides the conceptual tools to assess the elderly in their family or social context. It presents simplistic solutions that do not take into account the total picture. It also provides a framework in which empathy with all parts of the system is facilitated, thereby reducing conflict of interests. So often professionals dichotomize between the elderly on the one hand and the family on the other and side with one against the other. This is particularly true of abuse of the elderly, a problem similar to child abuse and wife abuse in that it is complex, contributed to by all family members concerned and often undetected and unreported. A high index of suspicion and complete family assessment are mandatory.

The cornerstone of any intervention is assessment, or diagnosis: What is going on? How is this problem being aggravated or perpetuated by the family system, the community, or the health care system? Intervention can then be planned from a position of knowledge and detrimental effects kept to a minimum. Negotiation and communication play a major part in such management.

FAMILY CARE-GIVERS

When an elderly person requires assistance of any kind that need is often felt first in the family or support system. Much of the need is fulfilled by the family, and professionals are called in when the situation is beyond the support system's capabilities. As mentioned earlier, there is ample evidence that families continue to visit and aid their older relatives. Even though families tend to live in separate homes they often live close to each other and maintain contact[12,17] or communicate regularly by letter and telephone.

Usually family means those persons linked legally or by blood relationship. However, for an elderly person who has no descendants, whose close family has died or who is isolated for some reason from family, friends, neighbors, members of interest groups or professionals may become "family." The key requirement is a willingness to establish and maintain the affectional tie and provide aid in times of need.

Elders and their families must inevitably confront some or all of a number of issues which may require professional intervention. These include the following:

1. growth and development conflicts;
2. change in roles and relationships;
3. caretaker "burn out"; and
4. decisions regarding institutionalization.

Whether they are spouses, siblings, or children the caretakers often become as needy as the patient.[3] Health care professionals must be aware of these issues and be prepared to deal with them when necessary. Failure to do so may result in a proliferation of patients or earlier institutionalization of the initially designated patient, or both. The manner in which help is given and the type of support provided may make the difference between a family being able to continue caring for their aged member and having to institutionalize that elderly person.

Conflict of Developmental Tasks

If care-givers are children then conflict can occur between two sets of developmental tasks. If care-givers are spouses or siblings, the conflict may lie more in the realms of distribution of resources to meet the same set of developmental tasks for the carer and cared for. The problems encountered by middle-aged children and aging spouses as primary care-givers, are discussed later in this chapter, in the section on "Time in the Life Cycle."

Care-taker Burn-out

When shouldering the burden for an elderly parent or spouse, the care-taker is highly susceptible to overextension leading to exhaustion and inability to continue caring. The alerting event for the professional can be demands for precipitous institutionalization/hospitalization of the elder or health breakdown in the care-giver.

The role description of the female care-giving spouse reported in Fengler and Goodrich[6] is evocative of the tenuous balance in which many care-givers live. While the care-giving wife is being described, many aspects apply equally to care-giving children, siblings, or husband:

> She is not trained for her job, a priori. She may have little choice about doing the job. She belongs to no union or guild, works no fixed maximum of hours. She lacks formal compensation, job advancement, and even the possibility of being fired. She has no job mobility. In her work situation, she bears a heavy emotional load, but has no colleagues or supervisor or education to help her handle this. Her own life and its needs compete constantly with her work requirements. She may be limited in her performance by her own ailments.

Kane[9] outlines four variables important to a stable patient-caretaker situation:

1. the patient's level of disability and dependence;
2. the caretaker's own health and functional mobility;

3. the presence or absence of other assistants; and
4. the caretaker's other roles and responsibilities.

Each of these factors interacts with the others. There is a point in every patient-caretaker relationship, which is individually set, at which the caretaker becomes overloaded and breakdown is inevitable.

Conflict of duties is a major problem. Families often assign the role of caretaker to the member perceived as having the fewest other responsibilities. However, it may be the person closest to the patient or the family member who has always "shouldered the burden." In the case of the spouse it is a social expectation, particularly, that the wife cares for the husband. A family meeting, to discuss caretaking and division of responsibility, is often highly useful in confronting any abdicating members as well as pointing out to the caretaker the possibility of delegation. Care-givers may lack knowledge of sources of help to support their caregiving activities. It is not unusual to find care-givers totally unaware of resources readily available that could have prolonged their ability and willingness to care and perhaps prevented burnout.

Decision Making Regarding Hospitalization or Institutionalization

Institutionalization is often precipitated by caretaker burnout. Other reasons for institutionalization are the addition of one more factor such as incontinence to the caregiver load or additional health problems for the care-giver. A study by Sanford[18] estimated that 12% of geriatric admissions were made because relatives could no longer cope. Ninety-two percent of family members could identify which problem would have to be alleviated for them to have the elderly patient back home. The problem most frequently reported as causing the most difficulty was sleep disturbances. Others were incontinence, inability to be mobile or perform activities of daily living (A.D.L.), falls, behavioral problems, inability to communicate, and wandering away.

In spite of the burden of care and the length of time it has been carried, families and spouses often feel tremendous guilt at finally "placing" the patient. This guilt appears to be a combination of self-expectations and perception of societal expectations. The patient's response can do much to heighten or alleviate the care-giver's guilt.

The clinician can help the family or spouse include the patient in decision-making if possible, be aware of available alternatives, and work out a set of criteria for choosing an institution. Once the patient is institutionalized the clinician can help the family maintain contact, avoid unnecessary guilt, and avoid conflict with the new "foster family" of the institution.

FAMILY ASSESSMENT

The practitioner must be alert to family membership, interaction patterns, and developmental tasks. A systems orientation aids the practitioner as it provides direction for entry into the family system, assessment, interventions, and evaluation of those interventions.

Roles, Affect, and Communication

As in other areas of family function, the family with clear communication patterns, well-defined but permeable boundaries, and close affectional ties often deals effectively with the problems of an aged member. Entry to the family system is relatively easy and a supportive, noninvasive role is appropriate. When asked to, the practitioner provides information and anticipatory guidance, discusses alternatives, facilitates communication, and listens while planning an early withdrawal.

The B. family asked for an appointment with the nurse clinician in geriatrics. Mrs. B. wished to discuss the problems she saw arising with her 85-year-old mother, Mrs. D. Mrs. D. lived alone in the family home, an older house in a rundown neighborhood. Mrs. B. felt her mother could no longer live alone, her health was slowly deteriorating, she was becoming less functional in activities of daily living, and she had had two falls in the past 3 months. Fortunately Mrs. D. had only shaken herself up and sustained a few bruises.

The nurse clinician explored with the B. family what they felt the problem was and the basis for their identification of the problem. She asked what they felt would be a good solution and what alternatives they had considered. She also inquired if they had discussed the situation with Mrs. D.

It turned out that the B. family had given a great deal of thought to the problem and had considered leaving Mrs. D. where she was or taking her in with them, and had also explored a number of types of housing from senior citizens apartments to nursing homes. Their real needs were to work through feelings of guilt as they were unable to have Mrs. D. live with them and to be sure they had considered all resources. They also needed to plan a way of broaching the subject to Mrs. D.

The nurse clinician accepted their expressions of guilt and helped them realize that many of their feelings were shared by others in the same situation. She verified their information concerning living accommodations. An approach was planned that allowed the B. family to initiate the subject with Mrs. D., starting with their deep concern with her well-being. They would then ask her about her ideas regarding what would be best for her in the future.

It turned out that Mrs. D. was very worried about her future but was overwhelmed by the thought of planning a change. As the discussion developed it became clear that Mrs. D. did not want to live with the B. family as she felt this would be an imposition. Also, Mrs. D. had well-developed routines that supported her lifestyle and she did not want to change these patterns to accomodate to those of the B. family. She had a friend living in an apartment in a senior's complex that included a multi-level nursing home and was interested in such a solution for herself.

Three months later Mrs. D. moved in to an apartment in this complex. Her level of function improved. She enjoyed the socialization available and felt more secure.

In contrast, families may develop very rigid boundaries through which little information flows and professional entry is often difficult if allowed at all. In this case the professional may be able to help the family develop greater trust in outsiders, help problem solving within the family, or alternatively help the elder develop substitute supports in the broader social system. Some families are so disengaged or separated emotionally that there is little willingness to give assistance and the health profession becomes the family. The opposite end of the continuum is the family that is so enmeshed that there is little differentiation between family members and a problem with one member reverberates through the system, creating considerable stress. In this case the practitioner may take a more active role helping family members to define their roles, functions, and expectations more clearly. Facilitation of communication, education, and specific suggestions may all be necessary. A family may have developed problem-solving skills in the past but need assistance to see the application of these skills in a new situation. The elder's needs may be overly provided for, and help may be required to develop a greater degree of individuation and independence from a "smothering" or over-anxious family. Conversely, families may require help in dealing with an overly demanding parent.

Role reversal is the essential problem in many families. With incapacitated aged parents it is now the children whom the parents must depend on; the children must be dependable in their relationships with their parents.[9] The adult children may lack the maturity needed to stop looking for parental support and provide it instead. Faced with their own signs of the aging process they may deny their parents' aging and obvious mortality. They may react by withdrawing and decreasing visits and attention. If the parents did not, in the past, evoke affection in their children, such affection and caring will not be forthcoming now, particularly with the increase in irritability and selfishness that can occur in some elderly. Often, however, such behavior is a mask for fear—fear of death or loneliness or, more often, fear of loss of control and loss of independence. He or she may mask infirmities, such as deafness, and strenously resist any signs of role reversal.

Desperate attempts to maintain a role and meaning in life lead to bossiness, obstinancy, focusing on the past and past glories, all of which may further alienate family and friends. Helping the elderly to accept some dependency on others as a just return for a life of hard work, and to maintain meaningful activities and relationships can help them maintain health. There is considerable evidence that hopelessness and helplessness are associated with disease and death, and a sense of meaning with survival (see Chapter 9). A role in decision-making and a sense of some control over one's fate must be preserved for as long as possible. Some families do not understand the difference between support and interference and may be highly destructive if not abusive. These families often tax the professional's resources. At all times the practitioner must be prepared to refer families who require more in-depth intervention and treatment.

Time in the Life Cycle

Knowledge of the developmental stages of individuals and families helps the practitioner anticipate and plan for some obvious problems, as discussed in Chapter 5. Duvall[4] provides an outline of these tasks for both the individual and the family (see Tables 30.2 and 30.3). Duvall's tasks and stages are probably still valid for the elderly of today. However, as future generations age they may become less valid due to role changes presently occurring in North American society. The elderly person, developmentally, is in the final phases of life while her children are middle-aged. As people live longer it is becoming commoner to find both the older parent and the child or children in the final stages of life.[2]

Scrutiny of the developmental tasks suggest that conflicts may occur between the developmental stage demands of older parents and their children. Middle-aged children are often trying to cope with many changes that demand time and energy. Their own children are passing through adolescence and leaving home; a wife may now wish to pursue a long deferred career or develop a latent talent. Finances may be strained due to the demands of their children's education. The husband is peaking in his career and looking forward to or dreading retirement. Both are facing the inevitable evidence of their own advancing age. Just when they have the potential to relax, re-establish their relationship and look forward to a less demanding time, the needs of their own aging parent(s) may intervene. These aging parent(s) now have less energy to cope with bereavement, chronic health problems, and necessary changes in lifestyle or living arrangements. They may find it difficult to accept professional help or become excessively demanding of families or professionals.

Being aware of conflicts between the two generations' developmental tasks allows the professional to provide anticipatory guidance to both the elders and the "sandwich" generation:

Men and women pulled in three directions, trying to rear their children, live their own lives, and help their aging parents, all at the same time.[10]

Professionals can help the children deal with anger and guilt over some demands and develop strategies to meet them. Support may be needed in decision-making and implementation. Elders may need assistance in taking part in understanding and accepting decisions. Both elders and middle-aged children may need help to learn about and understand the normal demands of their own developmental stage and that of one another. Both individuals and the family system may need support to adapt to a new equilibrium.

Occasionally problems may be such that referral for family therapy may be required. It is also true that families in family therapy for other reasons may benefit from the addition of a grandparent in the sessions, particularly when the older person is closely involved with problems.[21] If grandparents are in the same household it is often essential they be part of the therapy.

Environmental Resources

Essential to the professional working with the elderly and their families is a comprehensive view of the services available in the community.[22] There are families who are only too willing to turn the care of their aging member over to the professionals. However, many families are ready to provide care to a degree that demands tremendous outlays of time and energy. It is important to realize that these families may only turn to the health care or social service system when they are in crisis due to a breakdown in their own strategies and resources. Availability of sources for assistance, support and respite care (1 to 2 weeks in an institution) may make the difference in the length of time a family is able to care for their older member.

The family often turns to the clinician who will be in a better position to help if fully cognizant of the availability of home care, Meals-on-Wheels, day centers, and temporary placement beds in care facilities, along with the eligibility criteria for the use of these services will be in a better position to help. The presence of a geriatric assessment unit or team in the community is an invaluable resource for the professional. The team can provide a pool of expertise to aid in perplexing diagnoses and treatment as well as provide support to family, patient, and practitioner, when difficult decisions must be made. Team members may be able to provide access to services to which the community practitioner cannot provide entry. If the individual is totally independent in self-care, and coping well with life events, the most appropriate action is to support this positive state as long as possible.

It is useful, while doing the complete assessment of the elderly individual to keep in mind a number of risk factors, several of which include the environment. While none of these alone is cause for concern, the accumula-

Table 30.2 Developmental Tasks in Ten Categories of Behavior

	Maturity (early to late active adulthood)	Aging (beyond full powers of adulthood through senility)
I Achieving an appropriate dependence-independence pattern	1. Learning to be interdependent—now leaning, now succoring others, as need arises 2. Assisting one's children to become gradually independent and autonomous beings	1. Accepting graciously and comfortably the help needed from others as powers fail and dependence becomes necessary
II Achieving an appropriate giving-receiving pattern of affection	1. Building and maintaining a strong and mutually satisfying marriage relationship 2. Establishing wholesome affectional bonds with one's children and grandchildren 3. Meeting wisely the new needs for affection of one's own aging parents 4. Cultivating meaningfully warm friendships with members of one's own generation	1. Facing loss of one's spouse, and finding some satisfactory sources of affection previously received from mate 2. Learning new affectional roles with own children, now mature adults 3. Establishing ongoing, satisfying affectional patterns with grandchildren and other members of the extended family 4. Finding and preserving mutually satisfying friendships outside the family circle
III Relating to changing social groups	1. Keeping in reasonable balance activities in the various social, service, political, and community groups and causes that make demands upon adults 2. Establishing and maintaining mutually satisfactory relationships with the in-law families of spouse and married children	1. Choosing and maintaining ongoing social activities and functions appropriate to health, energy, and interests
IV Developing a conscience	1. Coming to terms with the violations of moral codes in the larger as well as in the more intimate social scene, and developing some constructive philosophy and method of operation. 2. Helping children to adjust to the expectations of others and to conform to the moral demands of the culture	1. Maintaining a sense of moral integrity in the face of disappointments and disillusionments in life's hopes and dreams

Stage	Developmental Task	Specific Tasks
V	Learning one's psychosocio-biological sex role	1. Learning to be a competent husband or wife, and building a good marriage 2. Carrying a socially adequate role as citizen and worker in the community 3. Becoming a good parent and grandparent as children arrive and develop
VI	Accepting and adjusting to a changing body	1. Making a good sex adjustment within marriage 2. Establishing healthful routines of eating, resting, working, playing within the pressures of the adult world
VII	Managing a changing body and learning new motor patterns	1. Learning the new motor skills involved in housekeeping, gardening, sports, and other activities expected of adults in the community
VIII	Learning to understand and control the physical world	1. Gaining intelligent understanding of new horizons of medicine and science sufficient for personal well-being and social competence
IX	Developing an appropriate symbol system and conceptual abilities	1. Mastering technical symbol systems involved in income tax, social security, complex financial dealings, and other contexts familiar to Western man
X	Relating oneself to the cosmos	1. Formulating and implementing a rational philosophy of life on the basis of adult experience 2. Cultivating a satisfactory religious climate in the home as the spiritual soil for development of family members

Stage	Later-Life Tasks
V	1. Learning to live on a retirement income 2. Being a good companion to an aging spouse 3. Meeting bereavement of spouse adequately
VI	1. Making a good adjustment to failing powers as aging diminishes strengths and abilities
VII	1. Adapting interests and activities to reserves of vitality and energy of the aging body
VIII	1. Mastering new awareness and methods of dealing with physical surroundings as an individual with occasional or permanent disabilities
IX	1. Keeping mentally alert and effective as long as is possible through the later years
X	1. Preparing for eventual and inevitable cessation of life by building a set of beliefs that one can live and die with in peace

From Duvall EM: *Family Development*. Toronto, J.B. Lippincott, 1971.

Table 30.3 **Family Developmental Tasks**

Family Developmental Tasks in the Middle Years	*Developmental Tasks of Aging Families*
1. Maintaining a pleasant and comfortable home	1. Finding a satisfying home for the later years
2. Assuring security for the later years	2. Adjusting to retirement income
3. Carrying household responsibilities	3. Establishing comfortable household routines
4. Drawing closer together as a couple	4. Nurturing each other as husband and wife
5. Maintaining contact with grown children's families	5. Facing bereavement and widowhood
6. Keeping in touch with brothers' and sisters' families and with aging parents	6. Caring for elderly relatives
7. Participating in community life beyond the family	7. Maintaining contact with children and grandchildren
8. Reaffirming the values of life that have real meaning	8. Keeping an interest in people outside the family
	9. Finding meanings in life

From Duval EM: *Family Development.* Toronto, J.B. Lippincott, 1971.

tion of several should alert the clinician for the possibility of problems. Some of these risk factors are:

1. recent retirement;
2. recent bereavement;
3. solitary living;
4. very limited or no support system;
5. multiple pathology;
6. sensory deficits (for example, decreased hearing, vision, kinesthesia); and
7. changes in activities of daily living, especially when ADL become borderline or less than adequate for the environment in which the elder is living.

These risk factors do not necessarily indicate the need for immediate intervention. They are most useful as trigger points for closer observation and more data collection. Many people who have a spouse die go through a grieving process and then gradually re-establish their lives. However, a person who does not grieve or who has multiplied losses over a short period is highly at risk for somatic complaints, real physical illness, or death.[11,14] Some individuals have a life-long pattern of living alone and like it that way. But the person who has always lived with others may find even the prospect of living alone terrifying. Again, these data must all be evaluated in light of the existing situation and previous patterns.

The greatest health care challenge of the next 50 years will be improved care of the elderly.[7] Any professional can attest to the increasing number of elderly clients in daily practice. Statistics for most northern industrial nations show a steady rise in the number of those 65 years old and over in the population.[16] Projections indicate that this rise will continue into the next century. The age group of persons aged 65 to 74 years old will increase by 20% by the year 2000, the 75 to 84 group by 50%, the 85-year-old and older group by 80%. In 1982 there were 13,000 persons in the United States over 100 years old, compared with 3200 in 1970.[9]

In summary, professionals who give care to older clients have a complex, demanding role to play. The elderly client usually has multiple sources of difficulty ranging across physical, social, and psychological parameters. Families and social networks are vital to the elder and the elderly are a vital part of the family system; thus professionals must be prepared to work with them and the elder when providing care. Knowledge of aging in all areas is essential, as is awareness of community resources. A systems orientation to the family and the community will result in better assessment and management of the problems of older clients and their families.

REFERENCES

1. Bayne JRD: Placement of the elderly. *Can Fam Phys* 27:1589-1591, 1981.
2. Carnevali DL, Patrick M: *Nursing Management for the Elderly.* New York, J.B. Lippincott Co., 1979.
3. Davis AJ: Disability, home care and the care-taking role in family life. *J Adv Nursing* 5:475, 1980.
4. Duvall EM: *Family Development.* Toronto, J.B. Lippincott, 1971.
5. Eliopoulous C: Assessment and action in gerontological nursing. *Fam Comm Health* 1:81, 1978-9.
6. Feingler AP, Goodrich N: Wives of elderly disabled men: the hidden patients. *Gerontologist* 19:175, 1979.
7. Fuchs V: *Who shall live?* New York, Basic Books, 1974.
8. Herr JJ, Weakland JH: *Counselling Elders and Their Families.* New York, Spring Publishing, 1979.
9. Kane T: Family dimensions in the care of the elderly. Paper presented at the University of Michigan Conference, Ann Arbor, Michigan, June 18, 1982.
10. Kirschner C: The aging family in crisis: A problem in living. *Soc Casework* April, 209, 1979.
11. Kraus AS, Lilienfeld AM: Some epidemiological aspects of the high mortality rate in the young widowed group. *J Chron Dis* 10:207, 1959.

12. Kulys R, Tobin SS: Older people and their "responsible others." *Soc Work* 25: 138, 1980.

13. Laurence MK: Dealing with confusion in the elderly. *Can Fam Phys* 27:1565, 1968.

14. Lynch JJ: *The Broken Heart: The Medical Consequences of Loneliness.* New York, Basic Books, 1977.

15. Libow LS, Sherman FT: *The Core of Geriatric Medicine.* Toronto, Ontario, C.V. Mosby, 1981.

16. Marshall VW: *Aging in Canada.* Don Mills, Fitzhentry and Whiteside, 1980.

17. Miller JR: Family support of the elderly. *Fam Comm Health* 3:39, 1980-81.

18. Sanford JRA: Tolerance of debility in elderly dependents by supporters at home: Its significance for hospital practice. *Br Med J* 3:471, 1975.

19. Secretary of State: *Growing Older.* London, Queen's Printer, 1981.

20. Shanas E: The family as social support system in old age. *Gerontologist* 19:2169, 1979.

21. Spark GM: Grandparents and intergenerational family therapy. *Fam Process* 13(2):225-237, 1974.

22. Talsdorf CC: Social networks, support and coping: An exploratory study. *Fam Process* 15:407, 1976.

SECTION VI
THE FAMILY OF THE HEALTH PROFESSIONAL

Chapter 31
The Physician's Family

Janet Christie-Seely
Roxanna Fernandez
Gilles Paradis
Yves Talbot
Renée Turcotte

WHY MEDICINE?—FAMILY INFLUENCES
ON CAREER CHOICE

As was pointed out earlier, systems are so embedded in our everyday life that we become oblivious to their influence. We can more easily see patients as part of systems than look at the different systems that we are part of as health care workers, as fathers, mothers, sons, daughters. Nonetheless, it is not until we are capable and willing to look at ourselves and our own context that we can fully understand the complexity of interactions and the power of systems to mold behavior.

The choice of a career is scarcely ever haphazard. The interests of the peer group, the job opportunities in the community, and the role and position in one's own family all influence the decision. The weight each system has depends on its relative importance to the person. Hence, the influence of family is often a major one. One of the authors had thought that his decision to go into medicine was purely coincidental. It was not until he did his genogram that he was able to appreciate the extent to which his position and role within his family had influenced his career. Often the medical student has been in the role of family health care worker since adolescence—a role assigned to him because of his abilities, his position in the family, or even his name (John is like his cousin John, the M.D.).

Why *do* people enter medicine? Often physicians were motivated early by illness in their family; more often they are the family delegates. The force of the family system behind them propels them to perform or to achieve as a grandfather or father had achieved. Sometimes a parent wanted to go into medicine but was not able to for financial, academic, or family reasons; a son or daughter becomes a doctor instead, often unaware of this piece of parental history. Emotional deprivation in childhood sometimes plays a role. Unmet and denied dependency needs in the physician lead to the compensatory giving and caring for others. A lack of trust in getting his or her own needs met engendered in childhood makes feelings of dependence and recognition of need or vulnerability highly threatening. This is often part of the problem of the impaired physician.

THE IMPAIRED PHYSICIAN

"Doctor heal thyself" or "practice what you preach, doctor" are jokes made by many patients who are familiar with their physician and concerned enough to voice the obvious. Physicians as a group have largely stopped smoking but still drink to excess, often eat to excess or eat on the run, and certainly work longer hours than is good for their health or their families.[25,26] Alcoholism,[10] drug abuse,[10] suicide,[21,23] "burn-out,"[25] divorce,[6] marital and sexual problems[6] are all higher than in the rest of the population. Physician impairment has its causes within the individual who chooses medicine, within the profession, and within the culture.

The image of the dedicated Dr. Welby, the selfless, hard-working man who is devoted to his patients and available at all hours is perpetuated not only by the public but also by colleagues. A resident in a family medicine unit was criticized as not sufficiently dedicated because she was not usually around after 5:00 p.m., having gone home to look after her new baby. Hopefully the increasing number of women in medicine will enhance humane care for all physicians. Many female physicians must also cope with household and children; they must be "superwomen" if they are to continue the competitive struggle to keep up to date, publish, and maintain a practice (see later section on the female physician).

Blaming the profession avoids the essential problem: the emotional drive that propelled the individual into medicine, which is his or her undoing. Self-esteem becomes dependent on feedback from patients and colleagues, helping people becomes addictive, the ability to say "No" decreases, and demands on time and concern increase. Physicians are prestige oriented,[21,28] yet the prestige of doctors is decreasing, which increases the sense that more is demanded.

Often financial commitments escalate the need to see more patients. Our culture expects doctors to make money, and so do their families—but in many areas the salary is matched by hours double that of other workers. As the workload goes up, guilt about neglecting the family may increase the motive to compensate financially. A vicious cycle may develop with increasing business activities to escape from, escalating complaints from family, phone calls from patients, and too many committees or community organizations. Finally, inefficiency, irritability, insomnia, and early signs of incompetence ensue. Readily available drugs may be used to help sleep; social drinking becomes a regular use of alcohol to relax. These signs of early "burn-out" are described also in the next chapter on nurses. A conspiracy of silence[5] surrounds the problem. The conspirators include the physician himself or herself, the physician's family, community, professional colleagues, and nurses as well as hospital boards and administrators. They are all unable to reconcile deteriorating performance due to alcohol or drugs with an otherwise gifted professional who should know the dangers of substance abuse. There is enormous fear of labels such as "alcoholism" or "psychiatric illness." As Cohen[5] reports, "A Saskatchewan Medical Association Committee was formed in 1976 to penetrate the shroud of silence by identifying and rehabilitating impaired physicians. However, the committee's experience since that time has largely been frustrating because its function has been viewed as more punitive than therapeutic."

The Physician's Family

What is the role of the physician's family? While the family of origin sets the stage for personality, behavior, and career, the current family becomes the leading players. The wife (or husband) may have chosen a physician mate for the prestige or noble image or income, as well as for his or her personal characteristics. The more he works the higher the income; the more preoccupied with work, the nobler his image. It is very hard to complain to a man who can raise one eyebrow reprovingly and say he was only late for supper because he was saving Mrs. X.'s life.

Doctors' wives are particularly at risk for mental illness[8] and have a higher suicide rate than wives of any other group of professionals.[21] Vaillant[25] studied 268 male college students for 30 years; 47 became doctors. Compared to their nonmedical peers, half had bad marriages as against a third, and 36% resorted to drug abuse as against 20%. These ratings correlated with a high incidence of emotionally disadvantaged childhood backgrounds.

The children are also caught in the double bind: Daddy's work, or Mommy's work, is so important that they must understand if he or she has little time to play with them, or is called out in the middle of supper, or has to cancel the ballgame, fishing trip, or vacation they had planned together.

Family stress is aggravated by the medical member's tendency to avoid conflict and retreat to work when open discussion is needed. If both are conflict avoiders the marriage may become distant and lifeless or suddenly erupt without warning when one or the other becomes symptomatic.[8] Alcoholism or drug addiction, either spouse's having an affair, or physical illness may alter or further rigidify homeostasis. The physician partner may in fact encourage the sickness role of the partner by ignoring him or her until physical symptoms develop. It may be easier to deal with the spouse as patient rather than dealing with the emotional relationship. Conversely the partner may trigger violent anger if they dare to get sick and make the same demands as patients. Physicians proverbially make bad patients; their bedside manner with a spouse often leaves much to be desired.

Health Promotion

Not all physicians dig their graves early. Many are excellent at pacing themselves, lead contented lives with extraordinary job satisfaction, and maintain physical and mental health in sports and creative hobbies. Physicians often have a second career, farming, writing, painting, to name a few, which maintains a perspective on the "lay" world. Many have a social circle outside their colleagial relationships that prevents the phenomena of shop talk and the 18-hour-a-day focus on medicine.

Family mental health workshops are now being provided for physicians and their families. For example, the 1983 meeting of the Canadian College of Family Physicians offered such a workshop and counselling services (available anonymously).

Vincent[27] emphasizes the importance of recognizing the problem in colleagues and providing assistance. Suspicions of impairment may be aroused by the following:

1. a change in personality;
2. a loss of previous efficiency and reliability;
3. increase in sick days or accidents;
4. patients' complaints, especially noting a change in demeanor;
5. isolation, professional or social;
6. marital problems or divorce, or both;
7. problem children (related to #6);
8. frequent intoxication, particularly suggestive behavior in the absence of apparent alcohol use;
9. persistant overwork and fatigue, particularly with refusal to consider a vacation;
10. history of many moves from community to community or from group; and
11. legal problems.

If a quiet investigation through colleagues and hospital staff confirms suspicions the following may be done:

1. anonymously inform the nearest provincial or state organization which is there to help, not punish!;
2. speak to the wife (or husband): offer to be the doctor's advocate;
3. confront your colleague, preferably with someone else present. Usually the latter's response is relief, but it may be denial. The goal is to get him or her to admit the need for help and to offer practical and personal support for his or her rehabilitation.[27]

Doctors must often cope with very difficult and demanding patients, a major source of stress. Evans[7] provides a strategy for coping with these patients: 1) refuse the role of "doctor as God" and avoid the "Patient in Command" (or on the pedestal). Develop an "on the level" (egalitarian) relationship; 2) recognize and accept your negative feelings; 3) use those feelings to understand the patient's negative relationship with his environment; 4) look for the problem behind the complaint (read the rest of this book!); 5) involve the patient in his own care, share pessimism, allow adequate time and frequency of visits, use clear signals for termination of interviews, deal with one or two problems per visit, and avoid investigations and referrals; 6) don't book several such patients on the same day; and 7) know your limits of tolerance and share them without venting feelings of frustration and anger on the patient.

ILLNESS IN A COLLEAGUE OR FAMILY MEMBER

The Physician as Patient

An interesting and unfortunate aspect of the medical profession is its treatment of the sick physician. The peer system of physicians often seem to reject its dysfunctional members. Suffering from blindness, secondary to macular degeneration, Dr. DeWitt Stetten[22] "complained" of his opthalmologist's interests in restoring vision but lack of concern for blindness. The following case history exemplifies the problem:

> A 38-year-old orthopedist who had a very successful practice in a tertiary care hospital and who was highly regarded by staff, peers and students had a car accident when returning from vacation with his family. A daughter was killed instantly and both he and his wife suffered multiple and severe trauma. Ironically, they were brought to the emergency room of the hospital where he worked. Both underwent surgical procedures for multiple fractures, internal bleeding, etc. He was comatose for 2 months and remained in intensive care for weeks before being transferred to a regular hospital bed. His recovery was painful and long, and after 6 or 8 months he was transferred to a rehabilitation center and doubts were expressed about his ever practicing again.

When the author first heard of this event it was the talk of the hospital but gradually the topic disappeared. Even though he was hospitalized in his own hospital he was soon scarcely ever mentioned, and when he regained consciousness was rarely visited by peers or students.

The above case is an extreme example of what often happens in the health-care milieu. The experience of Dr. D. Rabin[18] who noticed that when his colleagues became aware that he suffered from amyotrophic lateral sclerosis they started avoiding and ignoring him, is particularly telling: "One day while crossing the little courtyard outside the emergency room, I fell. A longtime colleague was walking by. He turned, and our eyes met as I lay sprawled on the ground. He quickly averted his eyes, pretended not to see me and continued walking. He never broke his stride. I suppose he ignored the obvious need for help out of embarrassment and discomfort, for I know him to be a compassionate and caring physician." Dr. Rabin states further: "I state with total conviction that my colleagues never meant to hurt me. On the contrary, they grieved for me, yet were unable to express their grief."[18]

As a result of our medical training we are more apt to deal with the physical than the emotional aspects of diseases, particularly in chronic and progressive disease, although the greatest needs are in the field of emotional support. Medical students are given two messages: show empathy but do not become emotional or overinvolved (double bind?); for them it is easier to concentrate on the latter than the former. In addition, there is evidence that those who are "slightly introverted and neurotic" do well during their medical training but poorly later.[28] There may well be inappropriate selection for medical school; personality and family traits present before admission may relate to the doctor's attitude to illness[14] (particularly mental illness) and block his emotional response.

"To this fraternity of healers becoming ill is tantamount to treachery."[22] For clinicians who work daily with sick and dying patients and who have learned to block out their emotions, illness in someone as close as a colleague or a family member serves to remind us of our own vulnerability and mortality as well as our inability to cure or hold death indefinitely at bay.

The Sick Relative

The physician dealing with a sick family member may have his or her discomfort increased tenfold by feelings of inadequacy (missed diagnosis) and helplessness. When confronted with such stressful situations as illness in one's own family or oneself the emotional impact may be such that the first reaction of the physician is denial or anger. A common story is the physician experiencing sudden chest pain who insists on finishing his clinic before going to the emergency room. Sometimes a physician spouse or parent is overconcerned and overwhelmed with care of a symptomatic member. More frequently illness is underdiagnosed in physician's families.

An extreme example was of an anesthesist working in a tertiary care hospital. His two daughters (10 and 17 years old) were diagnosed by renal biopsy as having glomerulonephritis. The nephrologist advised his colleague that his daughter should be followed closely. Instead, the physician kept the diagnosis a secret for years. When the daughter started showing symptoms of renal failure, the physician and his wife (also a doctor) hid medical books so that their children could not find out what was happening. This lasted until the youngest daughter had to be brought in to the emergency room because of extreme weakness and anuria. When the father was shown his daughter's hemoglobin of 4 gm% he broke down in tears. She needed emergency hemodialysis. Shortly thereafter, the father brought the eldest girl to the nephrologist for follow-up.

Physicians reflect the larger culture and the stigma of disability or chronic disease. Recent articles on stigmatized health conditions (visible stigma such as burns,[15] dwarfism,[2] deafness,[4] and diabetes[13]) outline the coping mechanisms of persons affected. Ablon[1] and Goffman[11] point out that illness is seen as deviance. Many diagnoses (cancer, diabetes, mental illness) result in an identity that is "permanently spoiled,"[11] the degree of spoiling being proportional to the degree of stigma. (see Chapters 20 and 21). Since physicians have dedicated their lives to stamping out or preventing such anomolies they are likely to be those most upset by these conditions.

Finally, physicians, despite their apparent independence, are often highly dependent on their spouse. If the spouse gets sick, the anger can be enormous but is expressed by denial, distancing or "referral." If a sick parent (particularly of the opposite sex) was the trigger promoting the choice of medicine as a career, the old anger at the sick, unavailable, and uncaring parent may be directed at the spouse. Denial of dependency needs is also responsible for the difficulty the physician experiences with the patient role when he or she is sick.

The Female Physician

> Women are not sufficient for all the exigencies of medical practice either as regards their minds or their bodies. In particular, the impressionability and instability of their nervous systems are apt to land them in error and incompetency.
>
> All women are pregnant until proved otherwise. (The Lancet, 1883[20])

The first women physician, Elizabeth Blackwell, graduated in 1849, while Emily Stowe waited 20 years before entering the University of Toronto. Finally, she obtained her license in 1880.[9] In McGill University one woman disguised herself as a male in order to enter medical school and was only discovered after graduation.

In 1983, 100 years after the above quotation (taken from Lancet), it is interesting to speculate to what extent attitudes towards women in medicine and what they can achieve have changed. A century is over and women's role in medicine is not as easy as that of a male physician.[24] There is a higher rate of suicide and evidence of higher stress.[23]

The physician's wife is usually given undue responsibility for rearing children and managing the home. Her physician-husband often expects her to be a personable, cultured woman, equally at ease in the kitchen and in social gatherings, and who, by the decision of marriage, has accepted with equanimity the limitations and sacrifices inherent in her husband's career.

On the other hand, women physicians are often also wife-mothers of physicians. Traditionally they have been the caretakers, the healers, and the midwives and have doubled their responsibility with home and job. Their conflict can be enormous as they try to combine a demanding profession such as medicine with a family life.[12,16]

Increased sharing of responsibilities of household and parenting tasks is occurring in many younger families but the division of labor is still a major source of friction[3] and a very pressing issue in medical families. "Society" (including physicians' husbands and male physicians) receives the benefit from well-trained female physicians, but society has been slow to recognize women in medicine in their roles as mothers and keepers of a household. The necessity either of working full-time or part-time to avoid getting behind in medicine must be considered for women, with career interruptions only for birth.[12,16]

The lack of domestic help or day-care or the husband's unwillingness to work part-time forces women to drop out of medical training or practice. Suggestions such as creating more internships and residencies in which the mother could do 2 years part-time for one year gained would indicate acceptance of women in medicine.[17] This is no simple problem, however. In some family medicine programs half the residents are women and usually married, and three or four unexpected pregnancies can create havoc of rotations and resentment among those left behind to do the work. Half-time positions are expensive for the hospitals and complex to organize.

The literature on women in medicine mostly offers data on the number of female physicians working full-time, part-time, and the numbers in the different specialties.[12,17,19,24] There is little written on what happens in a female physician's family when she has children and when her husband is a physician, and how her attitudes and those of her husband and family influence her decision to make medicine a professional career and her choice of a specialty. It has been noted that medical husbands are more tolerant than other professionals towards married female doctors.[24] The most recent data are as follows: From September 1979 to July 1980, women held 23.1% of residency positions (8.3% of surgical positions) in the United States.[19] In December 1978, only 38.4% female physicians had board certification compared with 57% male physicians.

The proportion of female medical students has been rising since the late 1960's. Eva Ryten, research associate at the Association of Canadian Medical Colleges (ACMC), expects 45% of the graduating physicians to be women in 1990.[9] It is unclear how many of Canada's 43,192 active physicians, interns, residents, are women and which are working full or part-time. We do know that surgery is the specialty with the least female physicians and that more than one half go into either pediatrics, psychiatry, or family/general practice. Men most frequently specialize in surgery, internal medicine, and family/general practice. Ryten estimates about 15% of Canadian physicians are female; the proportion is increasing by 1% per year.[9] There is a very evident lack of female leaders in medicine, with some notable exceptions. In the hierarchy of academic medicine there are very few indeed among Deans and Chairmen.

In the past a quota for women in medical school was defended by the belief that a medical education was wasted on women who became housewives and mothers. This belief was not supported by follow-up studies of graduates, which showed that as many men left for law, politics or business and most women who did leave returned after a few years away.[12,17] The high incidence of alcoholism and addiction in male physicians is an additional "waste."

Opinions among women physicians differ (even among the authors of this book in which the women predominate!). Some feel there is little or no discrimination and that they are able to practice as freely as any male. One woman, however, tried to break into a group of male family physicians but was told by others they would never accept a woman as female attitudes to patients would be disturbing to them. She had to put up with constant jokes about women and about women physicians, apparently aimed at discouraging her attempt, and carefully maintained the image of meekness and acceptance holding in check her usual exuberance and independence.

Many female physicians feel that once in medical school (there seem to be attempts to discourage undergraduate premedical studies for women) there is no obstruction to nonacademic practice, but that leadership positions in the academic world go to men, even if they are less qualified than women in the area. For the woman with children trying to maintain a family priority, there is no doubt there is not only no help but disapproval and a subtle encouragement not to talk about her children and home or to let family interfere with work. The converse (medicine interfering with family life) is encouraged, as it is for the men, by long hours, evening meetings, etc.[16,24]

The hopeful side of this story is that it is now often said, by men as well as women, that the increasing numbers of women in medicine holds promise for needed change in medicine. Increased humanity to both patients and physicians is predicted to be the result.[9]

INTRODUCTION TO THE GENOGRAMS

We have found as a teaching faculty that our own families and those of our learners provide rich resources for understanding families and illness. Most physicians and nurses have memories of illness in themselves or relatives that may have significance for career choice. A session sharing such memoirs proved enlightening and illustrative of all the principles of families and health discussed in this book.

Anyone who has done their own genogram, particularly in the detailed manner suggested in Chapter 11 will attest to the resultant learning.

Awareness of triangulation, cut-offs and their significance, and repeated family patterns of illness and behavior heighten recognition of their importance in families. It also provides self-awareness of vulnerabilities and a humility that is essential in working in a democratic and therapeutic fashion with families. It is important to learn not to judge either one's own family, a student's, a colleague's, or a patient's. It is also important to be familiar with an experience we ask of our patients.

With some trepidation we have decided to practice what we preach and to do in print as we normally do when teaching students, residents, or fellow faculty at our own university or those we have visited. Hopefully, this will encourage the reader to take a look at his or her own family patterns and to help students of the family to do the same. We have found that in asking learners to reveal some of their own background it is necessary to start the process as role models.

It is important to make it clear that only information they feel quite comfortable in sharing with the group should be revealed, but also important to look beyond the simple names and dates. (A clear line must be drawn between comfortable self-revelation and mutual sharing, and requests for help or therapy. As in all work with groups, sensitivity and the setting of limits by a mature leader should ensure that no member dominates or is left out of the process). Visual display of genograms on large sheets of paper promotes openness and "normalizes" the process as it does with patients. A group size of seven to ten persons is optimal; a 5- or 10-minute limit per person prevents the verbose from giving their entire life history.

A most important by-product of the process is group cohesion. It is usually an enjoyable group experience that allows members to get to know and understand one another better. It is also a useful means of decreasing group tensions and scapegoating. For this reason it is essential that no members be left out of the process. For example, in faculty development workshops, it is important to have the department chairman present. It is also best to have a peer group rather than, say, a mixture of residents or nursing students and their teachers. A coach with an understanding of family patterns should be available, as in groups following Murray Bowen's lead in this area (we have not gone beyond a close look at current relationships to do work with the family of origin, as Bowen has with students of family therapy). We do stress as mentioned elsewhere in this book that knowledge of family dynamics and of one's own family usually produces two reactions in the learner: the first is the thought, "My family needs family therapy."; the second is the decision to go home and do it! Both should be discouraged.

The genograms depicted below are those of the physician authors of this work. They follow the pattern we usually suggest, indicating something about relationships and the role of the individual concerned, particularly in matters of illness in the family. We have answered the question, "What did you learn by doing your genogram?" In contrast to our practice when teaching, names have been omitted.

Physician Sample #1

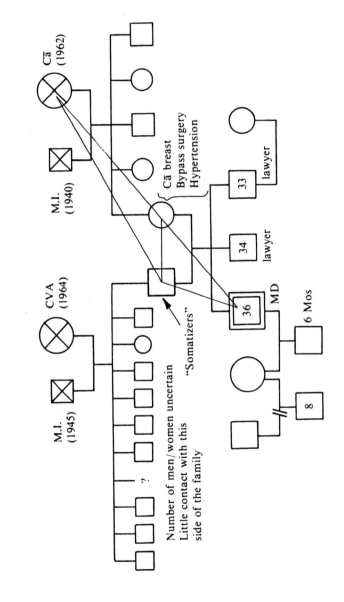

As a physician, having to do my own genogram turned out to be a stressful and revealing experience. This understanding occurred when, as a teacher, a colleague of mine looked at some of the information.

Position In The Family/Profession

Being the first of my family is not a surprising finding. As Toman points out (see Chapter 1), the eldest often becomes a doctor or nurse or some sort of helper and, as in my case, become role models for their siblings. This may isolate the physician member but it sets up the rule for an achievement orientation. I don't think that my brothers did too badly. I must have fulfilled my mission. (It is up to interpretation if that was a form of differentiation.)

I think that being the eldest in my family had a definite impact on my orientation in becoming a teacher and on always being so sensitive to the use of role modeling as a teaching method, often to the neglect of other methods.

The Dominance of Grandmother and Mother

It was pointed out to me that when I was teaching on the family I would often use examples pertaining to a powerful grandmother who needed to be joined for the sake of increasing compliance. This clearly relates to my experience; my grandfathers were not present and my grandmothers occupied a dominant place in my life. For example: I was diagnosed as a failure to thrive when I was 3 years old (I was a "spitter"). The doctors tried to reassure my mother that everything was all right and that I would get better, but my grandmother took it upon herself to cure me. She took me around a pilgrimage (not an unusual treatment for a French-Canadian family). We went through 3 sanctuaries and I was cured! Because of the unscientific way my grandmother proceeded, the next year we had to go back to all three churches, thanking the local saint, not knowing which one had done the job. My first orientation toward pediatrics could be interpreted as a way to rescue children from such treatment.

Triangulation, Loose Boundaries, and Lack of Conflict Resolution

Finally, I think my role as a go-between and a counsellor in my family has surely influenced my becoming a family therapist. When a person plays the role of the judge, he or she becomes acutely aware of nonverbal communication, especially in a family that avoids conflict. Mind and body reading is a skill. I probably learned more of this from my own family than in family therapy training. The training, and also marriage, simply made me aware of how well I had learned. In summary, the experience of doing one's own genogram is a powerful experience and demonstrates well the "invisible loyalty" (see Chapter 2) that one brings to his or her professional life.

Physician Sample #2

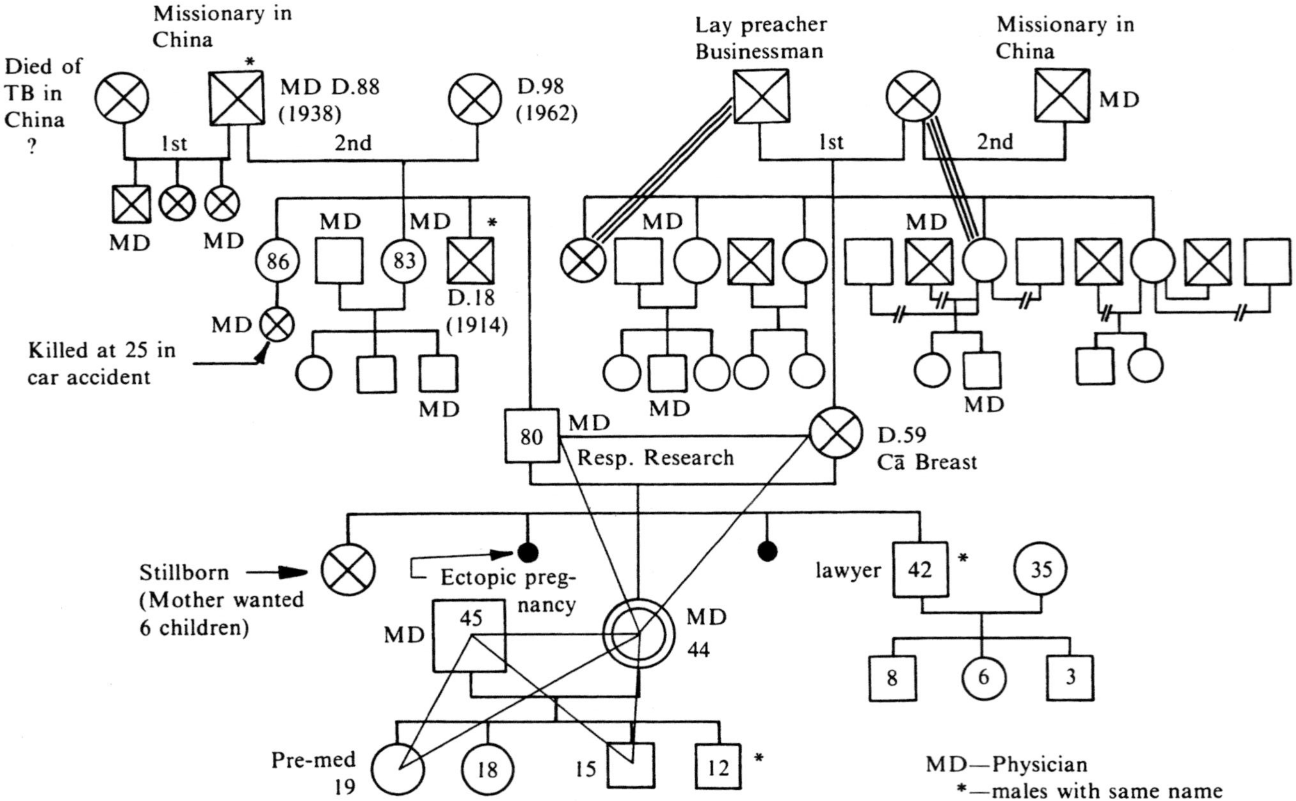

MD—Physician
*—males with same name

Medicine Is A Hereditary Disease

I am the 11th doctor in my genogram, and my daughter will be the 12th if she continues present plans. As the eldest, I was the family delegate. I realize that my missionary zeal in pioneering a family systems approach may be related to the fact that three of my grandparents were missionaries and my father was a pioneer in lung research. (I had to do 9 years of respiratory research—"a pure coincidence" I used to say—before I became individuated enough to leave the field.) The importance of family may also relate to my refugee status in the war, when from age 3 to 6 I stayed with a family in Montreal together with my brother of 1½ years because we were unable to return to my parents in England. Since training as a family therapist I have recognized the significance of that period; my husband looks extraordinarily like the man who was my foster father for those 3 years. I also learned early the coping style of looking after others under stress. I constantly worried about my brother, 1½ years younger, to avoid my own distress and because as the eldest I felt responsible.

Triangulation

My family was not without triangulation and I learned how difficult it is to "detriangle" and get out of the rescuer role. It took me 2 years to stop defending my eldest from my husband's occasional (displaced) anger. I also recognized the scapegoat and white knight in our two eldest children; I relabelled the latter as the "goody goody," and within 2 weeks their roles had reversed! Both are free of labels now.

Illness

My family had little illness but my mother developed breast cancer when I was 14 years old. I wasn't told until much later because she survived; it wasn't until both my brother and I left the nest, 15 years later, that I learned of the illness. This contributed to my interest in cancer and terminal care.

As a medical student (on orthopedic rotation!) I diagnosed myself as having congenital hip disease. I am sure four months in a plastic spica and six months on crutches taught me some understanding of chronic illness. It also illustrates the common problem of poor care for medical families, although there was less awareness of hip disease in that era.

Physician Sample #3

Family Roles and Professions

My career was decided early in my life. For as long as I can remember my mother kept telling me how tender I was and how I would make a good

Physician Sample #3

A   Alcoholism
S   Single
*   Chronic mental illness

doctor. She had dreamed that she would become a nurse when she was younger, and she took care of her dying father before getting married. I was therefore chosen to become a caretaker as she always had wanted to be.

Moreover, although I was adopted, I was always identified with her side of the family. My brother, also adopted, had dark hair and eyes like my father and I had light brown hair and blue-green eyes like my mother. She would say that I was very much like her: we had the same character, the same sensitivity, and we even shared the same susceptibility to illness (my bronchi were fragile, she would say).

Interestingly, my brother is a business man, which is the career identified with our father's side of the family, whereas I became a doctor, "to take care of my mother's side of the family," which was often identified as less healthy. My mother's family was enmeshed with a mother as a dominant figure. Two daughters developed chronic mental disease, three had alcoholic husbands, and the other two had to break from the family and move to another country to achieve their independence.

The fate of women in my father's family is particularly interesting. My paternal grandfather had a dominant mother and his wife was the dominant person in that couple. He was more withdrawn and he suffered from depression when younger. The two brothers in my grandfather's family of origin married and had children but two of their sisters became nuns and the other three never married. The two daughters of my grandfather would have the same fate; one would enter the convent while the other remained single. Moreover, the three sons all married women who would later in life develop some sort of "emotional illness" necessitating hospitalization.

Triangulation

My parents were very affected by not being able to have children of their own; consequently, my brother and I were overprotected. After adopting my brother my mother wanted a girl. Instead they chose me! My mother had bad feelings about having to take care of the family while my father was away. We were triangulated in this conflict and I remember siding with my mother in these arguments. I was the white knight in my family: never in trouble, always getting good marks at school, etc. This and the way roles were assigned in my family paved the way for my interest in family therapy and medicine.

Physician Sample #4

I come from a Roman Catholic, French-Canadian family of eight children. We lived on a farm in a rural area on an island near Quebec City. My father was an administrator as well as a farmer and my mother a teacher before she married. We were very close to our extended family, often visiting each other.

Physician Sample #4

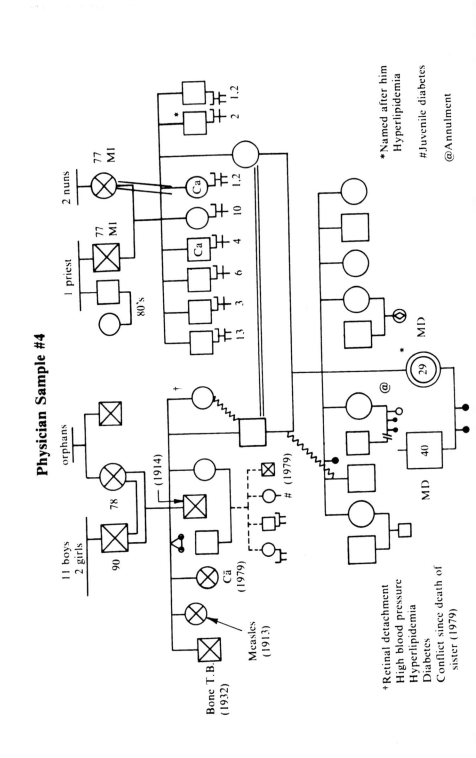

*Named after him
Hyperlipidemia

#Juvenile diabetes

@Annulment

2 nuns

1 priest

11 boys
2 girls

orphans

Bone T.B.
(1932)

Measles
(1913)

Cā
(1979)

(1914)

(1979)

MD

MD

+Retinal detachment
High blood pressure
Hyperlipidemia
Diabetes
Conflict since death of
sister (1979)

Position In The Family

I always thought I was the fourth child of the family, and although not really in the middle, I always felt that I was the one in the middle. When I did my genogram, I realized that in fact I really was in the middle, because my mother had had a miscarriage. I also realized that given the sequence of boy, girl, boy, girl, I should have been a boy. My name is also a male name, which made me hate it. I asked my parents why I was named like that while my other sisters had such beautiful feminine names. I was named after my god-father, who was single at that time, because my parents didn't know which name to choose. I always felt I was a "tom-boy"and hated that. I wanted to be feminine and gracious but couldn't stand the stupid games that girls were playing. Boys' games were so much more interesting! Recognizing my position in the family genogram helped me understand better why it was like that.

Career Choice

My father influenced me a great deal in my career choice. He was my model and I followed him when he worked on the farm (when my mother could not go). I was more serious than the others. I was staid, logical, and responsible (the "goody-goody") to please him and not make him angry. I still have difficulties standing up to angry male patients as well as to my husband. Anger feels like rejection.

My father used to talk about the value of being free, being one's own boss. This attitude influenced me as well as did his religious values. My father also said sometimes that he would have liked to be a physician. My older brother wanted to be a doctor but he had problems in high school. So, I decided to be a physician. I didn't realize how much I was competing with my older brother who was the black sheep of the family. I do not understand yet why I'm not actually more competitive with men. But my husband tells me that I am bossy!

An Illness Cluster in the Family

While doing my genogram, I was struck by the number of illnesses that occurred in the same period. My 19-year-old cousin committed suicide in 1978. My god-mother had cancer at that time and died in 1979; her sister, who was living with my god-mother, had retinal detachment a few times before her death soon after. In the same year my mother's sister had breast cancer, her husband developed hypertension; my mother also got sick and her brother died of myocardial infaction. That was the year I finished my residency program and started my practice. It was also the year I began to date my husband. My sister was separating from her husband, my other sister had conflicts with her husband for one year, and my younger brother started to date his current girlfriend. My parents are very religious people and all those events caused a lot of stress in my family.

About Death

I always questioned myself why some physicians have difficulty touching people when they are dead, while it seems so natural for me. I think I know the answer now. My grandmother died when I was around four. She was laid out in the living room at our house. I remember that I was alone in the room and trying to kiss her in her coffin when my grandfather called me saying, "Don't do that, come here." I felt guilty and sad, having the impression that I could not bid her goodbye. I remember also that a few times before her death I teased and disobeyed her. My grandfather gave me a slap on the behind, which made me feel more guilty and rejected for a while. Perhaps I felt responsible for my grandmother's death and in a way was trying to be forgiven by trying to kiss her in her coffin.

It has always been important to me to learn the story of my family. I listened for many hours to conversations of my aunts and uncles about our ancestors when I was a child. On both sides of my family, we know all the names of our ancestors, from the first one who arrived in Canada. Hence my interest in the family.

Physician Sample #5

Being asked to do my own genogram led to the analysis of my family in depth for the first time.

Role In The Family

I am the youngest of six children brought up in a Latin American country. The importance of family issues to me are obvious, for mine was a family with many secret problems under its financially secure, successful exterior. I remember looking up my birth certificate, which was necessary for my entering elementary school, and finding out that my parents were married 5 days before our birth (my brother and I were non-identical twins). This was the third time they married each other and the fourth marriage for my father, for he had married once before.

Between the 4th or 5th month of pregnancy, health problems began in my mother. She had gall stones and acute peritonitis; surprisingly, it was not until surgery that the medical staff knew she was pregnant. Neither she nor my father knew it. My twin brother died in infancy. In my mother's family and ancestors there have been twins in every generation. I learned to take care of people in my own family under stress. I used to be my mother's "pillar" and

Physician Sample #5

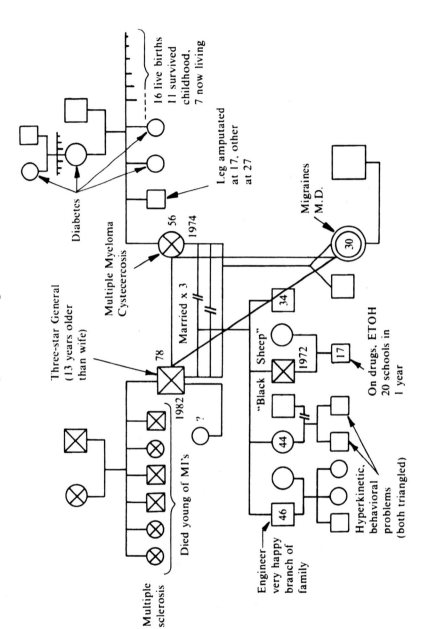

Diabetes

16 live births
11 survived
childhood,
7 now living

Leg amputated
at 17, other
at 27

Migraines
M.D.

Multiple Myeloma
Cystecercosis

Three-star General
(13 years older
than wife)

56
1974

30

Married x 3

34

"Black Sheep"

1972

17

On drugs, ETOH
20 schools in
1 year

78

1982

?

44

Died young of MI's

Multiple
sclerosis

Engineer —
very happy
branch of
family

46

Hyperkinetic,
behavioral
problems
(both triangled)

constantly worried about her problems and sickness and difficulties with my father and the rest of the family.

Triangulation

I was abused physically by both parents, but particularly by my father. I was triangled between my parents. My mother protected me too much, which aggravated my relationship with my father. I loved my mother very much, my father less so. The other four children were from my parents' first marriage, mine from their third, which my in-utero existence precipitated (perhaps that's why I felt the obligation to be the family therapist). My eldest brother was also abused by my father and similarly triangled. So was the second child, a girl who was also raped during adolescence. (I too was almost raped at age 5, but was rescued by my nanny. We lived in a rather violent environment in Latin America.) She grew up to be very bitter, she sought in material possessions the affection she had missed. The older ones suffered a great deal from the stormy on-off marriage relationship of my parents.

The third child, who looked very much like my father, was the "black sheep," always in conflict with both parents and his older brother and sister. His marriage was forced as his fiancée was pregnant. He did not complete high school and drank excessively. He was in three serious accidents; the third was the last: he was accidentally shot-down by one of his employees at the age of 32 and on my mother's birthday in 1972. My mother never recovered. Her illness increased dramatically and she died in 1974.

It was not until my mother's death that I could "detriangle" and get rid of the rescuer role, which upset not only my father, but also my brothers and sister. I was 19 years old.

Illness

Illness was present since my mother's pregnancy (see above). But the illness that most impressed me was in 1959. I was 5 years old when I heard that my mother had multiple myeloma. This term meant nothing to me until I heard the word "cancer." I realized that my mother was in danger and I couldn't do anything at all to stop it. Fortunately, she survived until 1967, when new treatments made a cancer diagnosis less negative. Later, between 1971 and 1974, she had cystecercosis, which became abruptly worse after my brother's accidental death. She died in 1974.

In addition, one paternal aunt had multiple sclerosis, there were several women with diabetes in my mother's family, and my uncle had a mysterious medical disease that resulted in the amputation of one leg at the age of 17 and of the other at the age of 27. My mother often told me medical stories about the family. No doubt, such a background of disease and constant visits to doctors influenced my decision to become a doctor.

REFERENCES

1. Ablon J: Stigmatized health conditions. *Soc Sci Med* 15B:5, 1981.

2. Ablon J: Dwarfism and social identity: Self-help group participation. *Soc Sci Med* 15B:25, 1981.

3. Bader E, Microys G, Sinclair C, et al: Do marriage preparation programs really work? A Canadian experiment. *J Mar Fam Ther* 6:171, 1980.

4. Becker G: Coping with stigma: Lifelong adaptation of deaf people. *Soc Sci Med* 15B:21, 1981.

5. Cohen S: The conspiracy of silence. *Can Fam Phys* 26:847, 1980.

6. Duffy JC, Litin EM: Psychiatric morbidity of physicians. *JAMA* 189:989, 1964.

7. Evans CE: Physician survival: Should the doctor come first? *Can Fam Phys* 26:856, 1980.

8. Evans JL: Psychiatric illness in the physician's wife. *Am J Psychiatry* 122:159, 1965.

9. Gray C: How will the new wave of women graduates change the medical profession. *Can Med Assoc J* 123:798, 1980.

10. Gilbert JA: Alcohol and drug addicted physicians: The scope of the problem. *Can Fam Phys* 26:851, 1980.

11. Goffman E: *Stigma.* Englewood Cliffs, New Jersey, Prentice Hall, 1963.

12. Heins M: Productivity of women physicians. *JAMA* 236:1961, 1976.

13. Hopper S: Diabetes as a stigmatized condition: The case of low-income clinic patients in the United States. *Soc Sci Med* 15B:11, 1981.

14. Hunter RCA: Prince RH, Schwartzman AE: Comments on emotional disturbances in a medical undergraduate population. *Can Med Assoc J* 85:989, 1961.

15. Knudson-Cooper MS: Adjustment to visible stigma: the case of the severely burned. *Soc Sci Med* 15B:31, 1981.

16. Nadelson C: The woman physician. *J Med Ed* 47:176, 1972.

17. Pool JG, Bunker JF: Women in medicine. *Hosp Pract* August:109, 1972.

18. Rabin D, Rabin PL, Rabin R: Compounding the ordeal of A.L.S. Isolation from my fellow physicians. *N Engl J Med* Aug 19:506, 1982.

19. Rinke C: The economic and academic status of women physicians. *JAMA* 245: 2305, 1981.

20. Roberts S: All women are pregnant until proven otherwise. *Lancet* July:89, 1978.

21. Safinofsky I: Suicide in doctors and wives of doctors. *Can Fam Phys* 26:837, 1980.

22. Stetten D Jr: Coping with blindness. *N Engl J Med* Aug 20:458, 1981.

23. Steppacher RC, Mauser JS: Suicide in male and female physicians. *JAMA* 228: 323, 1974.

24. Swerdlow AJ, McNeilly RH, Rue ER: Women doctors in training: Problems and progress. *Br Med J* 281:754, 1980.

25. Vaillant GE, Sobowale NC, McArthur C: Some psychologic vulnerabilities of physicians. *N Engl J Med* 187:372, 1972.

26. Vincent MO, Robinson EA, Latt L: Physicians as patients. *Can Med Assoc J* 100:403, 1969.
27. Vincent MO: The impaired physician and you. *Can Fam Phys* 26:861, 1980.
28. Walton HJ: Effect of the doctor's personality on his style of practice. *JR Coll Gen Pract* 16:113, 1968.

Chapter 32
The Nurse's Family

Celia Oseasohn
Jenny Craig

To be a nurse is to care about others. But a balance must be found between work, family, friends, and time for oneself. There is no set formula for this. People vary in the amount of time they need for themselves, which varies with the responsibilities they have to family and changes over time. But we all need some time for ourselves and we need to be able to assess our own needs or the result is increasing stress or burn-out and family dysfunction. A professional commitment may require more than the 8 hours we are paid for, but none of us can tolerate a 24-hour involvement in our work, nor can our families.

Symon MacMillan, a teenager whose mother is a nurse[3] complains that his "mother can never get away from the fact that she is first a nurse, second a mother." Even when they are driving somewhere, she must stop at every road accident and often ends up in the emergency room or in some strange house comforting the family. She is on the phone for hours talking to someone who is in need of her help and in the neighborhood she is the poor man's doctor, dispensing pills and potions.

Another concern of children growing up in such families is that the world seems to consist of nurses, doctors, and sick people. These people tend to "talk shop" with little attention to other happenings in the world around them. It can give a child a distorted view of the world.

Very little has been written about the nurse's family, in contrast to the large amount of literature on the physician's family. Perhaps this is partly because nursing was so long viewed as a temporary career ended by maternity clothes if not by wedding bells. With the changing role of women and the increasing interest in the relationship between health professionals, more research into the role of nurses both at work and at home will probably be forthcoming. The "doctor-nurse game"[6] is one in which nurses maintain the hierarchical authority and responsibility of the physician's role while conveying information and suggestions in such a way that decisions appear to be made by the physician. This game, which has been described with sympathy for both players by Stein,[6] may reflect the traditional role of women "power behind the throne" but is becoming increasingly difficult to maintain in the modern battle for power between the sexes. Since many nurses marry doctors (more in the past when interns had no time for a social life outside the hospital) this professional relationship is likely to be reflected or rebelled against at home. At present the types of marriage typical of nurses, and the incidence of divorce or family problems can only be a matter for anecdote or speculation.

BURN-OUT

Much has been written recently about the phenomenon of burn-out in professionals, especially those working with psychosocial problems. But behind each burnt-out professional there may be a family affected by and perhaps contributing to the burn-out. There is little written on the effects on the family system nor on the effects of family role assignment. The nurse is often unable to ask for help or caring when she is in need, but expects and is expected to be the giver and caretaker.

The work of a nurse is often emotionally taxing and stressful.[5] To work on an accident unit and see mutilated victims of motorvehicle accidents or some young person who has over-dosed on drugs is traumatic. It is also hard to work with the dying—whether they are young or old. It is recognized that those particularly at risk are those with poor family support who cannot ventilate at home the accumulated stress of the day. However, spouses and children constantly exposed to painful hospital stories will have their own problems.

In primary care settings, the nurse is faced with the problems of life and illness and social distress. It is easy to become depressed by the inability to help all who ask for it and to forget to replenish the self in order to continue giving.

"Burn-out" has come into common usage. It can be defined as stress gone out of control.[4] It can exist when learned ideas conflict with the real world of health care. It can start with the transition of student to staff nurse or with the curtailment of budget and reduction of staff, so that the nurse is unable to do what he or she would like to do or is unable to meet patients' legitimate requests. He or she may try to keep up with his or her ideals and take on more tasks and work overtime,[7] and run faster just to stay in place. At some point either a recognition of reality takes place, priorities are set, and tasks are re-evaluated and re-assigned, or the nurse succumbs to burn-out with feelings of failure and outrage against the school or institution that "failed to prepare her"[2] for the work world.

What are the symptoms of stress or burn out? They are chronic fatigue, disturbed sleep, feelings of inadequacy, an increase in somatic complaints and increasing bouts of sickness.[1] Many nurses easily recognize these symptoms in others but not in themselves. They also tend to "doctor" themselves in the mistaken belief that this crisis is unique, that it will soon pass: "One who is his own doctor, has a fool for a doctor." This practice may lead to addiction to drugs.

Making a commitment to oneself or, better still, a commitment to another may be helpful to stay on that diet or exercise program. A planned program of exercise—to jog, swim, or walk—is important for physical and mental well-being. Many nurses disclaim such a need, saying they get plenty of exercise at work. They do, but it is not the kind that reduces stress. A nurse's mental health can be questioned if he or she does not find time for personal care.

Do you tend to try to be all things—super nurse, wife, mother, student, and community worker? Have you any social supports? Is there someone with whom you can talk, share some of your concerns, bounce off some of your ideas, and who would help you? Nurses tend to overextend themselves at work and fail to nurture their relationships with family and friends. This often leads to increased anxiety. Some nurses encourage the sick role in a spouse or child because it is easy to respond to that role and is a comfortable role for them. Do you tend to get more involved with patients because they are more grateful or because they are easier to control than family?[8]

In today's society, the role of women is in a state of flux. They have broadened their scope and have assumed new roles but have not given up many of their traditional responsibilities. In addition, the nurse is expected to be professionally responsible to continue her education and keep up with the literature in her field. There is movement toward compulsary continued education to maintain licensure in both nursing and medicine. A graduate degree is increasingly expected for nurses working in a community setting, for administrators of nursing services, and for nurses who wish to teach in a school of nursing. We need to find better ways to deal with and balance our professional and personal lives.

Nurse Sample #1

After the Russian Revolution in 1917, the country was in turmoil. We lived in a small village in southern Russia near the Black Sea. At this time many private armies were running rampant through the countryside, looting and raping. During those unsettled times, the community leaders, Greek Orthodox and Jewish, frequently met and planned together to deal with these "armies." They bribed them with food and money to leave the village and surrounding countryside alone. As the chaos continued for years, food and money became scarce, and the community government gained control of the state and church. The landed gentry and church leaders, looking for a scapegoat, blamed the Jews for their plight. Anti-Semitism was never far below the surface. The local leaders aroused the peasants in the area, who

Nurse Sample #1

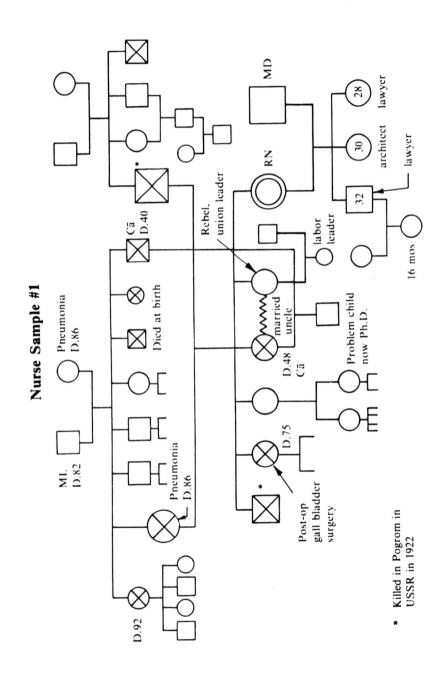

* Killed in Pogrom in
  USSR in 1922

called the Jewish men to a meeting, and murdered them all. My father, an elder of the village, and my brother were among them. A peasant boy revealed the massacre. I was aged 1 and ½ at the time.

When the news of the pogroms reached the United States our relatives there banded together to raise money and send my mother's brother to rescue the remnants of the family. The expedition took 1 whole year, there were many crises along the way. There were delays, there were illnesses; a border could not be crossed without bribes. There were arrests. The path often was circuitous, and promised passage on train and boat was often not available. I know of all this only through stories.

A full year later, when the family finally arrived at the United States, they moved into a small apartment in Brooklyn, New York. The three older girls and mother went to work to support the family and attended night school. The two younger girls went to day school: My sister, aged 12, went to junior high school; I started in kindergarten and so had the best opportunity to integrate into the "melting pot" that was New York City.

Motivations Behind a Nursing Career

The value of free education and the opportunities afforded in the United States were repeatedly stressed. We were obligated to take full advantage of these opportunities by studying, by learning, and by being useful human beings. The 1930s saw the birth of fascism in Germany, Adolph Hitler was at its helm with his doctrine of anti-Semitism. The concentration camps, the displacement of peoples all over Europe, the extermination of those not purely "Arian," all these events recalled the stories I had heard as a child of how the Jews were persecuted. I wanted to do something. All over Europe people were experiencing situations similar to those our family had suffered. My chance came with the development of the Cadet Nurse Corps in the United States. I joined and hoped to serve overseas after my graduation. The war ended in 1945 before I could go overseas.

Marriage

In 1948 I married a physician. We have no problem in discussing health issues. Each respects the other's area of expertise. What is interesting is to see how family, friends, and neighbors have dealt with us about health matters over the years. Some, the better schooled, tend to want everything to go to the doctor; others, less sophisticated, tend to ask me questions about their family's health. Early in our marriage, I was often the go-between for friends and neighbors to the doctor. But more and more they come to me with their problems, most likely the result of the changing view of nursing as nurses' education increases and their role expands.

Primary Care

After many years of hospital nursing, I became interested in primary care when we lived in Banglahdesh for 2 years. There was a great need to help families with health maintenance, to avoid infections, and to understand the need for immunization and how to care for a family member when he or she became ill. I realized that for a society to develop and to improve its standards of living you need people who are well and able to work.

When we returned from overseas I went to the Frontier Nursing Service in Kentucky to learn more about primary care. This service has for over 50 years devoted itself to meeting the health needs of the people in that part of Appalachia. They helped me to see the family as the primary unit in which health behaviors are learned and in which health habits are developed.

I found that skills, like history taking and physical examination, are not only useful in gathering data and identifying problems; they can be the basis for developing a trusting relationship so that family problems will be dealt with. Our aim has to be to help and allow families to develop and take responsibility for their health. I also saw first hand how health professionals can damage the family by moving in and taking over important functions when a member is incapacitated or ill.

Nurse Sample # 2

Illness

What a remarkably healthy family! I know of no chronic or disabling diseases. My mother is being treated for hypertension and so am I, although the onset of my condition was at age 33 and was attributed to the pill rather than to my mother.

The Role of Women

All the women except me have remained at home after having children. There have been no divorces or separations except mine. I can see why I was indoctrinated with the idea that my role as a woman was to get married and live happily ever after. Nursing and teaching were considered acceptable for women. Feminism is an emotionally laden issue because it is considered the cause of the decline of the family and the lowering of society's morals. None of the marriages were without problems but they all weathered their various storms. My parents have learned to live with what I see as constant discord; my father puts my mother down and she reacts by shouting.

Nurse Sample #2

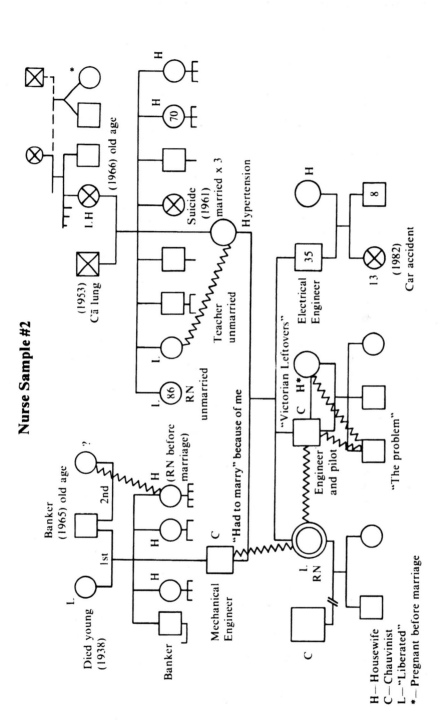

H — Housewife
C — Chauvinist
L — "Liberated"
* — Pregnant before marriage

Repeat Patterns

What did I learn by doing this? I recognized that the male chauvinism and unwed pregnancies might be interconnected, and that the former might be a defense against the latter. Fear of pregnancy might be the reason why careers were so discouraged. Sons were allowed liberty; daughters had to be docile and sweet. Surprisingly, both my grandmothers were "women's libbers" for their time. Such awareness then skipped a generation. My father is a chauvinist and my mother a martyr; my brother is a worse chauvinist. I married one such chauvinist, but then divorced him; I agree that "one marries one's childhood's worst nightmare," although I didn't recognize it at the time (see Chapter 1).

I also connected with this theme the family skeleton: twins, a man and a woman 60 years old, who surfaced after a death-bed confession. They were the illegitimate children of a great uncle's mother, who confessed her sin before dying. The great uncle was a vicar and I remember his mother as pious and a regular churchgoer. The family, always very cohesive and supportive of members in distress, took these two to its bosom, despite the scandal of illegitimacy.

It was not until the age of 34 that my brother shocked me with the information that my parents "had to" marry because my mother was pregnant with me. I was amazed that I had not guessed; it explained my parents' unsuitable marriage and some of my aunt's attitudes towards my mother.

REFERENCES

1. Freudenberger HJ: The staff burnout syndrome in alternative institutions. *Psychother Theor Res Pract* 12:73, 1975.

2. Kramer M: *Reality Shock.* St. Louis: C.V. Mosby, 1974.

3. MacMillan S: Living With mother. *Nurs Times* 76:1207, 1980.

4. Saunders C, Miller M: Stressed? Or burn out? *Can Nurse* 76:28, 1980.

5. Shubin S: Burnout: The Professional hazard you face in nursing. *Nursing '78,* 8:22, 1978.

6. Stein L: The doctor-nurse game. *Arch Gen Psychiatry* 16:699, 1967.

7. Storlie FJ: Burnout: The elaboration of a concept. *Am J Nursing* 79:2108, 1979.

8. Vachon LS: Care for the caregiver. *Can Nurse '76* 9:28, 1980.

ANNOTATED BIBLIOGRAPHY

Systems Theory

Bateson, G. *Steps To An Ecology of Mind.* New York: Ballantine Books, 1972. An anthropologist who studied schizophrenics and dolphins, Bateson was the father of family theory and applied cybernetics to communication and human systems. In this complex book he discusses levels of experience (logical types) and the interactional or circular nature of reality as opposed to the "billiard table model," or linear Newtonian model of cause and effect.

Bertalanffy, Ludwig von. *General Systems Theory.* New York: Braziller, 1968. Pioneering mind who analyzed the science of systems so that basic theory could apply not only to the natural and social sciences, but to the life sciences as well.

Brody, H. "A Systems View of Man: Implications for Medicine, Science and Ethics." *Perspectives in Biology & Medicine,* Autumn, 1975, pp. 71-91. Inspired by Laszlo's book, Brody as a medical student (now a family physician) pioneered the application of systems thinking to the various systems levels assessed by the clinician: cell, organ system, person, family, community, etc. This "hierarchy of systems" was then used by Engel.

Engel, George L. "The Need for a New Medical Model: A Challenge for Biomedicine. *Science* 196, no. 4286 (1977): 129-136. Provocative, frequently cited article, calling for a biopsychosocial model to manage disease.

Laszlo, Ervin. *The Systems View of the World.* New York: Braziller, 1972. An interdisciplinary thinker traces the systems view from its origins to the current understanding of nature and of man. Very helpful as an introduction to systems theory, suggesting that medicine is somewhat behind other sciences who have embraced a cybernetic model as more productive than the reductionist linear "scientific method" of the early twentieth century.

Shapiro, Johanna. "A Revisionist Theory for the Integration of Behavioral Science into Family Medicine Departments." *Journal of Family Practice* 10, no. 2 (1980): 275-282. Skillful, imaginative essay describing the cycle of infatuation followed by disillusionment frequently encountered when the family physician and the behavioral scientist collaborate. Sensible suggestions for relieving the problem.

Family Systems

Ackerman, Nathan W. *The Psychodynamics of Family Life.* New York: Basic Books, 1958. Older work by a major family theorist; important for its descriptive understanding of family relationships.

Barnhill, Laurence R. "Healthy Family Systems." In *The Family Coordinator* 28, no. 1 (January, 1979): 94–100. Defines eight basic dimensions of family mental health and pathology; well-integrated review of major family therapists; useful in understanding both the healthy and the dysfunctional family unit (see also Chapter 2).

Epstein, Nathan B., Bishop, Duane S., and Levin, Sol. "The McMaster Model of Family Functioning." *Journal of Marriage and Family Counselling* 4, no. 4 (October, 1978): 19–31. Utilizes a general systems theory approach in an effort to describe the structure, organization, and transactional patterns of the family unit. Six family functions are described: problem solving, communication, roles, affective responsiveness, affective involvement and behavior control. (see also Chapter 15).

Garique, Philippe. *La Vie Familiale des Canadiens Francais.* Montreal: Les Presses de l'Université de Montréal, 1962. Overview of French Canadian family life useful in understanding this cultural lifestyle.

Ishwaran, K. *The Canadian Family.* Toronto: Holt, Rinehart & Winston, 1970. Sociological survey of diverse Canadian family lifestyles; useful in understanding unique features of families observed in one's distinctive cultural heritage.

Lewis, Jerry M., Beavers, W. Robert, Gossett, John T., and Phillips, Virginia Austin. *No Single Thread: Psychological Health in Family Systems.* New York: Brunner/Mazel, 1976. Pioneering study, which enumerates the family system characteristics that contribute to family health and optimal functioning; contrasts with the many studies focusing only on family dysfunction.

Napier, A. Y. and Whitaker, C. A. *The Family Circle.* New York: Bantam Books, 1978. A delightful paperback describing a family's experience with family therapy. Sprinkled with chapters explaining systems theory and the reasons for the interventions made by the two family therapists. A window into family therapy, and a "hard to put down" introduction to systems, this book is highly recommended for residents, who rarely know as much about the function of family therapists as they do about surgeons and other consultants to whom they also refer patients.

Papp, P. "Family Sculpting in Preventive Work with 'Well Families'." *Family Process* 12, no. 2 (1973): 197–213. An excellent article for both patients and clinicians, introducing them to the concepts of healthy family functioning.

Westley, William A. and Epstein, Nathan B. *The Silent Majority.* San Francisco: Jossey-Bass, 1969. Important long-term psycho-social study, which investigates the relationship between student emotional health and the organization of their family of origin; one of the few studies of healthy families.

Family Systems and Disease Processes

Christie-Seely, J. "Life Stress and Illness: A Systems Approach." *Canadian Family Physician* 29 (1983): 533-540. Lists the stress-illness literature in a systems context; family distress may be expressed through illness.

——. "Preventive medicine and the family." *Canadian Family Physician* 27 (1981): 449-455. An approach to primary, secondary, and tertiary prevention of illness using a family system model and the concepts of high-risk families and high-risk stages of the life cycle.

——. "Teaching the Family System Concept in Family Medicine." *Journal of Family Practice* 13, no. 3 (1982). 391-401. Outlines the research linking family and illness that should be taught early in the training of family medicine residents, one of five strategies for teaching a family systems orientation.

Craven and Sharp. "The Effects of Illness on Family Functions." In *Nursing Forum* 11, no. 2 (1972): Clear demonstration of family dislocations in the face of serious illness.

Family Systems Medicine. A journal at the confluence of family therapy, systems theory, and modern medicine. Editor, Donald Block. First issue, Spring, 1983. Published by Brunner/Mazel. A milestone heralding a marriage between family therapists interested in medicine and family systems oriented physicians, which promises to fill the gap outlined above by Weakland.

Kaplan, Berton H. and Cassel, John C. *Family and Health: An Epidemiological Approach.* Chapel Hill, North Carolina: University of North Carolina Press, 1975. Rigorous scientific documentation of the interrelationships between family dynamics and the determinants of health and disease.

Madanes, C. "Marital Therapy When a Symptom Is Presented by a Spouse." *International Journal of Family Therapy* 2 (1980): 120-136. A description of the family system in which a symptom, physical or psychological, is used to balance the power in the relationships. The "weak" or "sick" one gains power through the symptom and through frustrating the efforts to help of the caretaker spouse (and of the doctor). The system is organized around the symptom and will resist attempts to treat it (see chapter 20).

Medalie, J. H. *Family Medicine, Principles, and Applications.* Baltimore: Williams Wilkins, 1978. An important basic text for family physicians, organized around the family life cycle, describing all the major aspects of illness in families. It classifies the clinical approaches to the family, which is the context of health if not always the unit of care.

Minuchin, S, Rosman, B. L., and Baker, L. *Psychosomatic Families, Anorexia Nervosa in Context.* Cambridge: Harvard University Press, 1978. One of the most important books for the family-oriented clinician, Minuchin describes his research on children with labile diabetes, severe asthma, and anorexia nervosa. Stress at the level of the family system is translated into decreased lung function, keto-acidosis or weight loss in these children, while family therapy improves these same meassures. Biochemical evidence for transfer of stress from one part of the system to another is shown by a study of families of labile diabetes.

————. "A Conceptual Model of Psychosomatic Illness in Children: Family Organization and Family Therapy." *Archives of General Psychiatry* 32 (1975): 1031-1038. One of the most useful articles for residents, this clearly outlines Minuchin's concept of psychosomatic families, the theory and sequence of therapy, and its results.

Pratt, Luis. *Family Structure and Effective Health Behavior: The Energized Family.* Boston: Houghton-Mifflin, 1975. Analysis of the interface between family dynamics and personal outcomes of good health. One of the best descriptions of the role of the family in its own health care.

Schmidt, David D. "The Family as the Unit of Medical Care." *Journal of Family Practice* 7, no. 2 (1978): 303-313. Superb review of the interrelationships between family dynamics and disease disturbances; review of the literature under four rubrics: (1) "The Family's Contribution to the 'Cause' of Disease"; (2) "The Family's Contribution to the 'Cure' of Disease"; (3) "The Family's Response to Serious or Chronic Disease"; and (4) "The Family's Desire and/or Need for Family-Oriented Care."

Talbot, Yves. "Anorexia Nervosa: A Lifestyle Disorder." *Canadian Family Physician* 29: 553-557. An outline of the family basis of this illness for the family physician. Therapy for the family system is clearly more effective than individual therapy; the referral skills necessary for the family physician include relabelling this illness as a family problem.

Weakland, J. H. "Family Somatics—A Neglected Edge." *Family Process* 16 (1977): 263-272. This article points to the area of focus of this book, illness in the family system, as one neglected by both family therapists and family medicine. Little direct research of an interactional nature has been applied to the vast arena of physical health.

Marital Therapy

Berman, Ellen M. and Lief, Harold I. "Marital Therapy from a Psychiatric Perspective: An Overview." In *American Journal of Psychiatry* 132, no. 6 (June, 1975): 583-592. Excellent survey of various methods of marital therapy; considers the power, intimacy, and marital boundary dimensions of marital psychodynamics and relates each one to the marital life cycle.

Lederer, William J. and Jackson, Don D. *The Mirages of Marriage*. New York: W. W. Norton, 1968. An incisive analysis of marriage in modern North America, delineating the major elements in a satisfying marriage.

Martin, Peter A. *A Marital Therapy Manual*. New York: Brunner/Mazel, 1976. One of the first basic texts in the field; analyses of four of the most commonly observed pathological marriage patterns with discussion of appropriate marital therapy techniques.

Paolino, Thomas J., Jr. and McCrady, Barbara S. *Marriage and Marital Therapy*. New York: Brunner/Mazel, 1978. Collection of essays edited by two marital therapists that seeks to evaluate the psychoanalytic, behavioral, and systems theory perspectives; the conceptual is melded with treatment approaches in each of these three schools of thought.

Sager, Clifford J. *Marriage Contracts and Couple Therapy*. New York: Brunner/Mazel, 1976. Good focus on the conscious and unconscious contracts couples negotiate in a marriage; therapeutic principles and techniques used in marital therapy discussed and illustrated with case histories.

Sexual Dysfunction Therapy

Chavelle, Anna H., Leversee, John H., and Smith, Charles Kent. "Sexual Problems in Family Practice." In *Medical Aspects of Human Sexuality* 8, no. 7 (July, 1974): 45–50. Roundtable discussion by three family medicine clinicians of commonly seen office problems concerning patient sexuality.

Kaplan, Helen Singer. *The New Sex Therapy*. New York: Brunner/Mazel, 1974. Authoritative and comprehensive approach that integrates the psychoanalytic and sex therapy techniques; basic principles and procedures to be used on an out-patient basis, usually by a solo therapist.

Katchadourian, Herant A. and Lunde, Donald T. *Fundamentals of Human Sexuality*. 2d ed. New York: Holt, Rinehart & Winston, 1978. Classic university text covering the biophysiological, psychosocial, literary, legal, and moral aspects of human sexual behavior; extremely useful for reference and the preparation of lectures on human sexuality.

Lief, Harold I. *Medical Aspects of Human Sexuality*. Baltimore: William & Wilkins, 1975. Superb text for office reference; uses question and answer approach to respond to most of the 'minor' sexual dysfunctions that the primary care practitioner will encounter.

Masters, William H. and Johnson, Virginia E. *Homosexuality in Perspective*. Boston: Little, Brown & Co., 1979. Definitive text describing the clinically tested programs for treating homosexual dysfunction and dissatisfaction.

————. *Human Sexual Inadequacy*. Boston: Little, Brown & Co., 1970. Classic text describing the range of sexual dysfunctions, both male and female, and their treatment plans; conjoint team approach.

————. *Human Sexual Response*. Boston: Little, Brown & Co., 1966. Classic text describing the biophysiological phases of human sexual response for both the male and female.

Trainer, Joseph B. "The Physician as a Marriage Counselor." In *The Family Coordinator* 22, no. 1 (January, 1973): 73–80. Overview of both marital and sexual problems the health practitioner may uncover in the office from a physician who has written frequently on the office management of various sexual problems.

AUTHOR CITATION INDEX

SUBJECT INDEX

Abdominal pain
  in childhood, 375, 376; and depression, 400
Abortion, 95, 100, 109, 183
Abuse, 411–420
  of child, 103, 389–391, 413–416; of elderly,
  418–419, 511; mortality rate in children, 412;
  risk factors of, 412, 416–417; and
  S.I.D.S., 359
Accidents, 286
  cases of, 294, 306; as cause of sudden death,
  355; in children, 412; hip fracture in elderly,
  319; and low social support, 146; and
  secondary and tertiary gain, 321; and stress,
  135, 138
Acculturation, 80, 81, 87, 93
  and traditional healers, 81
Activities of daily living (ADL), 513, 520
Adaptability, 16, 229
  exaggeration of or failure of leads to illness,
  9, 10, 18, 32–35, 152–155
Addiction. See Drugs
Adolescence, 220, 244, 245
  and death, 353, 362, 385; individual therapy
  for, 51; pregnancy in, 93, 103; responsibility
  versus autonomy, 48; stage 5 of life cycle,
  48–51
Advocacy, 343
  of impaired physician, 527; of patient by
  clinician, 103, 325; of patient by family,
  100; of sibling of sick child, 340
Affect, 212, 215, 217, 223, 224, 462
  in couple, 462. See also Practice
Agenda, patient's, 457. See also Ticket of
  admission
Aging, 505, 521
  developmental tasks of, 518, 519; normal
  changes of, 506, 508; stage 8 of life cycle,
  55–58; theories of, 506
Agoraphobia, 273–274, 398–399
Alcoholics Anonymous (and Alanon, Alateen,
  Alafam), 314, 436, 441
Alcoholism, 139, 422–445
  "acid test" of, 438; as adaptive response to
  system, 10; and adolescents, 50, 424; and
  community; 70, 71, 286, 436, 441; in health

professional, 525, 532; as label, 126; and
  tuberculosis, 141; values clarification in, 103
Alexithymia, 154
Alliances, 223. See also Coalition
  of clinician with family member, 455
Amputation, cases of, 300
Amyotrophic lateral sclerosis, case of, 528–529
Animal studies
  Harlow's monkeys, 41; peripheral animals,
  human parallels with, 51; social systems,
  154
Anorexia nervosa
  family therapy and, 161, 164, 330; as
  symptom of couple conflict, 35, 125, 147,
  376
Anticipatory guidance, 19, 238, 272, 273. See
  also Family life cycle; Hospitalization
  empty nest in enmeshed family, 410; in
  prenatal, neonatal period, 40, 384; and pre-
  retirement counselling, 53; with
  preschoolers, 385; reasons for awareness of
  family life cycle, 34
Anxiety, 398–400
  reduction in alcoholism, 460; and sexual
  performance, 479, 481; in terminally ill,
  354
APGAR. See Family APGAR
Arachnoiditis, case of, 228, 330, 331
Arthritis
  case examples, 126, 303; impact on family,
  21; ankylosing spondylitis, case of, 298;
  and stress, 134, 330, 368
Assessment. See also Family assessment
  of elderly, 514–517; prerequisite to intervention, 216, 466
Asthma
  cases of, 237, 244, 261, 338; and family
  therapy outcomes, 161, 163; in
  psychosomatic family, 125, 147, 375;
  reflecting life-cycle stress, 35, 368
Autonomy, 153, 220, 221. See also
  Individuation
  age-appropriate, 50, 386–388; in
  community, 63, 95; from in-laws, 37
Autopsy, 358, 359–360

571